Cardiopulmonary Point of Care Ultrasound

Hatem Soliman-Aboumarie ·
Marcelo Haertel Miglioranza ·
Luna Gargani · Giovanni Volpicelli
Editors

Cardiopulmonary Point of Care Ultrasound

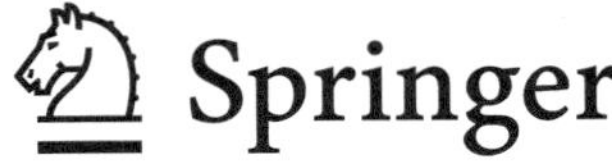
Springer

Editors
Hatem Soliman-Aboumarie
Department of Anaesthetics
and Critical Care
Royal Brompton and Harefield
Hospitals
London, UK

Luna Gargani
Department of Surgical
Medical and Molecular Pathology
and Critical Care Medicine
University of Pisa
Pisa, Italy

Marcelo Haertel Miglioranza
Federal University of Health
Sciences of Porto Alegre (UFCSPA)
Porto Alegre, Brazil

Giovanni Volpicelli
San Luigi Gonzaga University Hospital
Orbassano, Italy

ISBN 978-3-031-29474-7   ISBN 978-3-031-29472-3   (eBook)
https://doi.org/10.1007/978-3-031-29472-3

This Springer imprint is published by the registered company Springer Nature Switzerland AG
The registered company address is: Gewerbestrasse 11, 6330 Cham, Switzerland

Foreword by Jagat Narula

Unchanged patterns of bedside cardiovascular examination have continued to be practiced with inspection, palpation, percussion, and auscultation being the four pillars. The physical examination remains highly valued even though a robust evaluation of the accuracy and precision of physical examination has never been undertaken. The ingrained practice and convenience of physical examination have obviated the need for critical appraisal that evolving diagnostic technologies have to face. However, physicians currently less frequently use bedside examinations because of presumed limited returns and shorter available time for patient visits. Even when physical examination is attempted physicians do not fare well regardless of the level of training, and yet the rigorous teaching efforts do not improve proficiency. This leads to unnecessary downstream testing, which has not adequately alarmed the healthcare system because physical examination is *mistakenly* considered to be inexpensive.

The most promising technology that could improve the accuracy of diagnosis at the bedside is point-of-care ultrasound using small hand-held systems. When it was first introduced 200 years ago, the stethoscope (*stethos*, chest and *scope*, to see) was named so because it allowed the physicians to indirectly visualize the chest through auscultation, and now that the ultrasound indeed helps look in the chest, the stethoscope could be downgraded to a *stethosphone*, and a hand-held ultrasound device instead be designated as the true bearer of the stethoscope designation! Selective use of bedside ultrasound (or, *insonation*) can then be added as another pillar of physical examination. It should permit superior bedside decision-making and appropriate downstream testing. Consistent miniaturization of ultrasound into an independent transducer coupled with widely available mobile phones would allow the incorporation of technology into physical examination as a much-needed enhancer of the bedside examination.

The use of hand-held systems without carefully defining how best to use them has caused some anxiety even in believers. These devices have been meant to supplant physical examination, and are not to be considered the replacement for echocardiography imaging. The young students are tech-savvy, and we need to start training early in medical schools. There is a need for the development of curricula for medical school teaching wherein ultrasound-assisted anatomy and physiology teaching might take place in the first year, followed by differential assessment of pathology in subsequent years. Medical students should be able to develop algorithms for differential diagnosis for common clinical complaints by the time they complete their medical school training. During the residency and fellowship training imaging should become the second nature. Emergency room physicians, intensivists, and pulmonologists have been leading the coursework and the cardiologists are joining the motivation.

With this end in view, Hatem Soliman, Luna Gargani, Marcelo Haertel, and Giovanni Volpicelli have gathered the finest ultrasound exponents from Europe to put together an exquisitely illustrated compendium for the training of cardiology fellows and early career cardiology faculty. They meticulously divide the presentation into 5 parts devoted to basic principles, use of insonation in diagnosis, following up on the disease course, and use in guiding interventions. The final section addresses the outlook which deals with training and accreditation in cardiopulmonary ultrasound, safety and governance in cardiopulmonary ultrasound, and potential applications in the ensuing years. Being a staunch proponent of the use of insonation in a cardiovascular examination, I am overjoyed with a painstakingly crafted manuscript and do hope that you will enjoy reading it as much as I have.

Jagat Narula, M.D., Ph.D., MACC
Philip J. and Harriet L. Goodhart Chair of Medicine;
Chief, Division of Cardiology, Mount Sinai Morningside;
Professor of Medicine, Radiology and Global Health; Associate Dean
for Global Health, Icahn School of Medicine at Mount Sinai;
Director, Cardiovascular Imaging, Mount Sinai Health System;
Executive Editor, Journal of the
American College of Cardiology;
President-elect, World Heart Federation

Foreword by Rosa Sicari

In 2011, I prepared on behalf of EACVI, the first European document on hand-held devices. The first really portable machines were becoming available, and echocardiography was moving fast outside the conventional echo lab. At that time, there was a need for standardization but mostly for classification of what the technological development was giving us for everyday life in several clinical settings and scenarios. The echo-cardiological community had the strange feeling of losing control and power over this technology. More than ten years have passed, more documents have been written, and more definitions have been given ("focused echocardiography," "hand-held echocardiography," "hand-carried echocardiography," "point of care echocardiography," and "directed echocardiography " ASE guidelines), but the final result is widespread use of ultrasounds, in the hands of a wide variety of specialists. Terminology is more appropriate when the definition is related to the net result of the exam: complete versus limited (reduced number of images) versus focused (specific question). It is, then, a history of success because ultrasound did not seem to have provided all its potential, due to a certain conservatorism inside the cardiology community. Ultrasounds have always been a portable technique because machines move on wheels. Proximity to patients, technology that moves toward patients also outside hospitals, is one of the greatest achievements of our time, in medicine. This book is a practical and graphic representation of this evolution where the use of ultrasound is in the hands of a wide range of specialists in acute settings, in monitoring critical conditions, in assessing and guiding interventions. Imaging the heart but not only the heart: imaging of the lungs for combined assessment which is able to diagnose and risk stratify patients. The time-honoured complete echocardiogram to be replaced, in several conditions, by a fast and quick application that becomes a prosthesis of eyes and hands of the physician for the difficult patient. No matter how you call it, you know you need it.

Rosa Sicari, M.D., Ph.D.
CNR
Institute of Clinical Physiology
Rome, Italy

Foreword by André Y. Denault

Some 315,000 years ago, an upright-walking species appeared in Africa: *Homo sapiens*, a hunter-gatherer living in small groups. Then, about 12,000 years ago dawned the age of the agricultural revolution, during which more stable settlements led to larger populations. Much later came the industrial revolution, replacing hands with machines in manufacturing. Today, *Homo sapiens* lives within a digital revolution. *Homo sapiens* now has access to a tool that is revolutionizing medicine—the ultrasound.

My first contact with ultrasound was in 1989 as a second-year internal medicine resident at the Royal Victoria Hospital in Montreal. In the fall of that year, a code blue was called in the hemodynamic suite. When I arrived as part of the code team, I was surprised to hear the cardiologist in charge of the hemodynamic lab calling his echocardiographer colleague, Dr. Rahal, to help. Dr. Rahal arrived briskly, switched on this huge echocardiographic machine with a tiny snowy screen, took the ultrasound probe in his right hand and confidently directed it on the subxiphoid region. Within 15 seconds, he declared: "OK guys, continue cardiac massage, there's no tamponade". This was my very first contact with POCUS. I never forgot that moment which was the beginning of a passion for learning how to use this technology for patient care. Over the subsequent 30 years, I had the privilege to witness the development of this amazing technology, which has been called "the fifth pillar of physical examination". (1) In the echocardiographic lab in 1991, I initially learnt transthoracic echocardiography from outstanding cardiologists who opened and led the field to what would later become POCUS.

As clinicians, ultrasound provides us with the ability to rapidly diagnose life-threatening conditions affecting not only the heart but also the brain, chest, abdomen, vascular system, muscular skeletal system, and soft tissue. We are even exploring the role of high-frequency ultrasound in the diagnosis of septic inflammation models by looking at red blood cell aggregation. (2) There is literally no part of the body that cannot be screened and analyzed, either today or in the not-so-distant future, using ultrasound ranging from the lowest to the highest frequency and using M-mode, 2D imaging, Doppler, strain, and now 3D reconstruction, and all this without any radiation, at the bedside of our patients and with POCUS instruments miniaturized to fit in the pocket of all future doctors regardless of their specialties. The real challenge now lies in how we can teach POCUS.

This is precisely the goal of "Cardiopulmonary POCUS": to bring ultrasound to the bedside when dealing with patients with acute cardiopulmonary conditions. The book is divided into five sections and 30 chapters with more than 300 figures and 100 videos. Basic principles in the use of POCUS, POCUS diagnosis, POCUS monitoring, and its role in guiding interventions are presented in the first four sections, while the last section explores important issues such as training, safety, and what future lies ahead of POCUS. This is the most up-to-date POCUS textbook of the twenty-first century. The authors of the book are internationally known and recognized clinicians with unique expertise in the area of POCUS. They are basically the new ultrasound *Homo sapiens* of modern clinical medicine. The readers of "Cardiopulmonary POCUS" will remain grateful to the authors for sharing their unique knowledge and expertise. Those authors are among our leaders in the ultrasound revolution.

André Y. Denault, M.D., Ph.D., FRCPC, ABIM-CCM,
FASE, FCCS, Anesthésiologiste, Intensiviste;
Institut de Cardiologie de Montréal, Montréal (Québec), Canada;

Professeur Titulaire de Clinique;
Directeur du Progrmme de Fellowship en Échographie Ciblée;
Département d'Anesthésiologie;
Département de Pharmacologie;
Affilié au Département de Médecine
Département de Chirurgie, Division des Soins Intensifs
Institut de Cardiologie de Montréal, Montréal, Canada

References

1. Narula J., Chandrashekhar Y., Braunwald E. Time to Add a Fifth Pillar to Bedside Physical Examination: Inspection, Palpation, Percussion, Auscultation, and Insonation. JAMA cardiology. 2018;3(4):346–50.
2. Tripette J., Denault AY., Allard L., Chayer B., Perrault LP., Cloutier G. Ultrasound monitoring of RBC aggregation as a real-time marker of the inflammatory response in a cardiopulmonary bypass swine model. Crit Care Med. 2013;41(8):e171–8.

Preface

We believe this 'ultrasound stethoscope' is very useful for the differential diagnosis ... it allows quick screening of ill patients with doubtful physical symptoms and signs since visualization of intra-abdominal organs or processes is readily available. The instrument can therefore be considered as an 'extended palpation' ... Immediate and on-the-spot assessment of patients is now possible with this miniaturized, self-contained and battery powered ultrasound device ... It is expected that this miniaturized and automated instrument will have an important impact on the diagnostic use of ultrasound and the further development of ultrasonic equipment.

Dr. Jos Roelandt, Dutch Cardiologist and POCUS Pioneer, 1978 AD

In the year 1821 AD and in a teaching hospital in Paris, a French physician was able to use the stethoscope for the first time in history to listen to his patients' chests. Ever since, and despite the enormous technological innovations spanning over the last two centuries, physicians are somehow still relying on stethoscopes in the clinical evaluation of their patients. However, the landscape has shifted dramatically over the last 40 years with the technological advancement in point of care ultrasound and the increasing utilization of that powerful tool by various practitioners from a wide range of specialties.

The current revolution in point of care ultrasound powered by the technological advances and the miniaturization of ultrasound equipment enables clinicians to perform POCUS almost everywhere—in hospitals wards, battlefields, remote deserts, and even in space. In various medical specialties including cardiology, critical care, anesthesiology, emergency and even general internal medicine, an enormous interest of clinicians and wider members of the multidisciplinary team.

POCUS, however, has been deemed a basic focused assessment for many years. The widespread use of ultrasound and the development of international accreditation of echocardiography for non-cardiologists has led to more advanced utilization of POCUS at the bedside. Moreover, this was fostered by the ongoing technological breakthroughs in hand-held and mobile ultrasound machines which brings spectral and even tissue Doppler into hand-held ultrasound platforms.

Therefore, POCUS has become a standard bedside tool especially in the management of cardiopulmonary disorders and is now included as a training requirement by various international fellowship and residency programmes in Europe, Australia, the USA, and Canada.

Cardiopulmonary Point of Care Ultrasound is the first manual of its kind dedicated to both basic and advanced applications of POCUS in cardiopulmonary disorders.

The book brings together an international panel of world renowed experts and pioneers in cardiac and pulmonary ultrasound and aims to serve as a handy bedside practical guide to all POCUS learners. It also represents a powerful multidisplinary collaboration as the authors represent multispecialty collaboration (intensive care medicine, cardiology, emergency medicine, anaesthesia, thoracic surgery, radiology, respiratory medicine, as well as nursing and cardiac physiology). We hope the book will serve as a practical learning guide for the novices as well as a refresher for the experts.

The book is divided into five sections and a total of 30 chapters. Section I is dedicated to basic principles of POCUS, and Section II discusses the role of POCUS in the diagnosis of various cardiopulmonary disorders. Section III is dedicated to the role of POCUS in monitoring acute heart and lung disorders. Section VI briefly touches upon POCUS-guided cardiac and pulmonary interventions, and finally Section V discusses future perspectives as well as the vital aspect of safety and governance and the status of training and accreditation in cardiopulmonary POCUS.

The editors believe that the explosive development of POCUS is changing the way we practice medicine and improves the quality of care we deliver to our acutely ill patients. We also believe that POCUS is evolving into levels of practice and competence (from basic to intermediate to advanced) which should be supported by local, national, and international accreditations. Until advanced POCUS evolves into a solid body governed by established training and governance, Cardiac POCUS practitioners should keep in mind that it is not a substitute for an expert comprehensive Echocardiographic assessment.

<table>
<tr><td>London, UK</td><td>Hatem Soliman-Aboumarie</td></tr>
<tr><td>Pisa, Italy</td><td>Luna Gargani</td></tr>
<tr><td>Porto Alegre, Brazil</td><td>Marcelo Haertel Miglioranza</td></tr>
<tr><td>Orbassano, Italy</td><td>Giovanni Volpicelli</td></tr>
</table>

Acknowledgements

To my late beloved father Abdullah and my beloved mother Noor for their unconditional love and for teaching me that hardwork and genuine compassion while staying true to yourself can make the impossible possible.
To my wife Yara for being my backbone and main support. To my children Lilian and Adam for inspiring me everyday. Thanks for tolerating my absences and many sleepless nights while working on this book.
To all my mentors in Egypt and the UK, to all my colleagues and patients, I'm forever grateful, thank you for everything.
—Hatem Soliman-Aboumarie

To Eugenio and Rosa who taught me the beauty and the power of ultrasound.
To Ugo, Bernardo and Bianca who taught me the beauty of life.
—Luna Gargani

To my loving family.
To my wife, for her unwavering support, and my daughter Laura, the sunshine of my life. And to my baby boy who is on the way, I am so excited to welcome you into this world and watch you grow.
To all my teachers and all my patients, for the invaluable lessons.
—Marcelo Haertel Miglioranza

Dedicated to all my past, present and future patients.
—Giovanni Volpicelli

Contents

The Evolution of Point of Care Ultrasound   1
Vicki E. Noble
References   5

Physics of Ultrasound and Doppler   7
Marcus Peck, Jonny Wilkinson, and Ashley Miller
Introduction   8
Generation   8
Tissue-Ultrasound Interactions   9
    Reflection   10
    Reverberation   10
    Refraction   10
    Scattering   11
    Attenuation   11
Penetration Versus Resolution   11
Resolution   11
    Axial Resolution   12
    Lateral Resolution   12
    Elevational Resolution   12
    Temporal Resolution   13
Knobology   14
    Depth   14
    Width   14
    Zoom   14
    Gain   14
    Time Gain Compensation   14
    Focus   15
    Dynamic Range   15
    Tissue Harmonic Imaging (THI)   15
Doppler Ultrasound   15
    Generation   15
    Pulsed Wave Doppler   15
    Colour Doppler   16
    Power Doppler   16
    Continuous Wave Doppler   16
    Tissue Doppler Imaging   17
Conclusion   17

Image Optimization and Artifacts 19
Segun Olusanya and Adrian Wong
Introduction... 19
   What are Artefacts?..................................... 20
   Artefacts Related to 2D Imaging.......................... 20
   Reverberation Artefacts................................. 20
   Attenuation Artefacts................................... 21
   Side Lobe Artefacts.................................... 21
   Beam Width Artifacts................................... 23
   Refraction Artefacts.................................... 23
   Artefacts Related to Doppler Imaging...................... 24
   Miscellaneous Artefacts................................. 26
Conclusion 27
References.. 27

Fundamentals of Transthoracic Echocardiography 29
Marcus Peck, Ashley Miller, Jonny Wilkinson,
and Aleksandar N. Neskovic
Introduction... 29
   Machine Set-Up.. 30
   Probe Handling.. 30
   Cardiac Axis.. 31
   Windows... 32
Basic 2D Views 32
   Parasternal Long-Axis View.............................. 32
   Parasternal Short-Axis View.............................. 36
   Apical 4-Chamber and 5-Chamber Views................... 37
   Subcostal 4-Chamber View............................... 38
   Subcostal Short-Axis Views (Including Inferior
   Vena Cava View) 40
Additional Views 42
   Right Ventricular Inflow and Outflow Views 42
   Apical 2-Chamber and 3-Chamber Views................... 43
   Suprasternal View...................................... 44
Beyond 2D Imaging 45
   Colour Doppler.. 45
   Pulsed Wave Doppler................................... 46
   Continuous Wave Doppler 48
   Tissue Doppler 49
Conclusion 50

Fundamentals of Transesophageal Echocardiography 51
Fabio Guarracino and Marcelo Haertel Miglioranza
Introduction... 51
Indications and Patient Selection............................ 52
Patient Preparation 52
Probe Manipulation and Insertion 53
Goal-Directed TOE in Critical Care 53

Training and Technical Skills 59

Conclusion 60

References... 60

Fundamentals of Lung and Diaphragmatic Ultrasound 63

Giovanni Ferrari and Gianmaria Cammarota

Introduction... 64

Ultrasound Assessment of the Lungs 64

Patient Position 65

Transducer Selection (Fig. 3) 65

LUS in Lung Disease 69

Limitations of LUS... 71

Fundamentals of Diaphragmatic Ultrasound 71

   Technical Aspects and Measurements 72

   Clinical Applications of Diaphragmatic ultrasound 75

   Diaphragmatic Paralysis 76

   Chronic Obstructive Pulmonary Disease (COPD) 76

   Novel Coronavirus-19 Disease (COVID-19) 76

References... 77

POCUS in Diagnosis: Acute Heart Failure 79

Luna Gargani and Alberto Palazzuoli

Focus Cardiac Ultrasound (FoCUS) and Standard

Echocardiography 80

   Global Left Ventricular Systolic Function and Size............. 82

   Global Right Ventricular Systolic Function and Size........... 84

   Pericardial Effusion 84

   Intravascular Volume Assessment and Inferior Vena Cava 85

   Major Signs of Chronic Cardiac Disease..................... 85

   Gross Valvular Abnormalities 85

   Large Intracardiac Masses................................. 86

Echocardiography in AHF Beyond POCUS 86

   Hemodynamics 87

Lung Ultrasound.. 87

   Methodology.. 87

   Diagnostic Role of LUS in AHF........................... 88

   Prognostic Role of LUS in AHF........................... 88

   Limitations 89

Integrated Cardiopulmonary Ultrasound 90

References... 90

POCUS in Acute Myocardial Ischaemia 93

Anthony J. Barron and Hatem Soliman-Aboumarie

The Patient's Presentation.. 94

   Patient Findings—Typical and Atypical 94

   What to Do if Unsure 94

Evidence for Timely Intervention 95

The Ischaemic Cascade and Its Utility 95

How the Myocardium Differentially Responds to Ischaemia........ 96

Perfusion Abnormalities of the Left Ventricle   96
Left Ventricular Diastolic Abnormalities   97
Left Ventricular Systolic Abnormalities.   99
Other Motion Abnormalities Including LBBB. 103
Further Abnormalities 105
Prognosis. 106
Regionality and Benefit in Identifying Culprit Vessel Ischaemia. 106
Myocardial Infarction with Non-obstructed Coronary Arteries
(MINOCA) 107
Conclusions. 108
References. 109

POCUS in Diagnosis: Acute Pulmonary Embolism 111
Peiman Nazerian and Matteo Castelli
Introduction. 112
Lung Ultrasound (LUS) 112
Focused Cardiac Ultrasound (Focus). 113
Compression Ultrasound (CUS) 114
Multiorgan Point of Care Ultrasound 114
References. 116

Lung Ultrasound in Pneumonia Diagnosis 117
Francesco Corradi, Francesco Forfori, Giada Cucciolini,
and Danila Trunfio
Introduction. 118
Clinical Aspects of Pneumonia 118
How to Perform Lung Ultrasound. 121
Anatomopathological Modifications in Pneumonia 122
Sonographic Findings in Pneumonia. 123
Ultrasound in COVID-19 126
Usefulness of Lung Ultrasonography in Pneumonia 127
Limitations of Lung Ultrasonography in Pneumonia. 128
Conclusions. 130
References. 130

Pneumothorax 135
Giovanni Volpicelli
Introduction. 135
Imaging Process in Pneumothorax 136
Ultrasound Signs. 137
Lung Sliding 137
Importance of Additional Signs. 137
Parenchymal Signs 138
Lung Pulse 139
Lung Point 139
Combination of Signs 139
Ultrasound Technique 139
Ultrasound Probes 141
Clinical Conditions and Settings 142

Comparison with Chest Radiography and CT   142
Quantification and Monitoring.   143
Pitfalls and Complex Pneumothorax   143
   Double Lung Point   143
   Septated Pneumothorax   144
   Hydropneumothorax   144
   False Lung Sliding and False Lung Pulse   144
References.   144

POCUS in Monitoring: Cardiogenic Pulmonary Oedema   147
Pierpaolo Pellicori and Luna Gargani
Introduction.   148
What Should I Monitor?.   148
   The Heart: Structure, Function and Hemodynamics.   148
   The Lungs: B-Lines and Pleural Effusion   153
   Intravascular Fluids: Inferior Vena Cava   154
Future Perspectives   155
References.   155

POCUS in Monitoring: Non-cardiogenic Pulmonary Oedema   159
Erminio Santangelo, Silvia Mongodi, and Bélaid Bouhemad
Introduction.   160
Main LUS Findings   160
   B-Lines   160
   Pleural Effusion and Consolidations   161
Cardiogenic Pulmonary Oedema and Non-cardiogenic Pulmonary
Oedema: The Differences   162
   Mixed Pulmonary Edema   163
Non-cardiogenic Pulmonary Oedema and LUS Monitoring.   164
   Positive End Expiratory Pressure (PEEP) Setting   164
   Prone Positioning   166
Conclusion   166
References.   166

POCUS in COVID-19 Pneumonia   169
Hatem Soliman-Aboumarie, Luna Gargani, and Giovanni Volpicelli
Introduction.   170
The Revolution of POCUS in COVID-19.   170
LUS in COVID-19 Pneumonia   170
   LUS in the Diagnosis of COVID-19 Pneumonia.   170
   LUS in Monitoring COVID-19 Pneumonia.   173
Clinical Scenarios   173
Clinical—Ultrasound Integration for the Diagnosis of COVID-19
Pneumonia   174
Risk of Spreading Infection.   174
Future Perspectives   174
Conclusions.   175
References.   175

POCUS in Monitoring: Volume Responsiveness 177
Xavier Monnet and Jean-Louis Teboul
Introduction. 178
The Concept of Fluid Responsiveness. 178
Static Indices of Cardiac Preload. 180
Respiratory Variations in LV Outflow Tract Flow Velocity 180
    Phenomena Causing the Respiratory Variability
    of Stroke Volume 180
    Stroke Volume Surrogates Used to Measure Its Respiratory
    Variation 180
    Limitations of the LVOTVV 181
    In Summary. 183
Variability of the Diameter of the Venae Cavae 183
    Phenomena Causing Respiratory Variability in the Diameter
    of Venae Cavae. 183
    Reliability 183
    Limitations 183
    In Summary. 183
Mini Fluid Challenge 184
    In Summary. 184
Respiratory Occlusion Tests 184
    Principle 184
    End-Expiratory Occlusion Test 184
    Combination of End-Inspiratory and End-Expiratory
    Occlusions. 184
    Limitations 185
    In Summary. 186
Passive Leg Raising 186
    Principle 186
    Reliability 186
    Cardiac Output Measurement Techniques 186
    Limitations 187
    In Summary. 188
Conclusion 188
References. 188

Systemic Venous Congestion. 191
Korbin Haycock, Rory Spiegel, and Philippe Rola
Introduction. 191
The Hepatic Vein 193
The Portal Vein. 195
Intrarenal Venous Doppler 196
Conclusion 197
References. 197

**POCUS in Monitoring: LV Diastolic Function and Filling
Pressures**   201
Matteo Cameli, Maria Concetta Pastore,
and Marcelo Haertel Miglioranza
Introduction   202
Diastolic Function and LV Filling Pressures   202
    POCUS Parameters of Diastolic Function   202
    Pulsed-Wave Doppler (PWD)   203
    Tissue Doppler Imaging (TDI)   205
Classification of Diastolic Dysfunction   206
Additional Parameters   207
    Left Atrial Volume Index (LAVi)   209
    Tricuspid Regurgitant (TR) Jet   209
    Pulmonary Veins Velocity   209
    IVRT   210
    LA Strain   210
Clinical Applications of Diastolic Function by POCUS   210
Limitations   211
Conclusions   212
References   212

**POCUS in Monitoring: LV Systolic Function and Cardiac
Output**   215
Francisca Caetano and Hatem Soliman-Aboumarie
Introduction   216
Diagnosis of Cardiogenic Shock with Echocardiography   216
Tailored Management of Cardiogenic Shock
with Echocardiography   218
    Heart Rate   219
    Preload   219
    Afterload   219
    Myocardial Contractility   219
Segmentation of the Left Ventricle   224
Visual Assessment   224
Regional Abnormalities in the Absence of Coronary Artery
Disease   224
Conclusion   226
References   227

**POCUS in Monitoring: Right Ventricular Function
and Pulmonary Hypertension**   231
Arif Hussain, Rajkumar Rajendram, and Guido Tavazzi
Introduction   232
Assessment of the Right Ventricle   232
Anatomy   235
Physiology and Pathophysiology   235
Assessment of Right Ventricular Function   236
Measurement of Right Ventricular Size and Wall Thickness   236
Measurement of the Shape and Area of the Right Ventricle   237

Visual Assessment of Right Ventricular Contractile Function   239
Right Ventricular Fractional Area Change.   239
Tricuspid Annular Plane Systolic Excursion by M-Mode   239
Tissue Doppler S'   240
Right Ventricular Myocardial Performance Index   240
Right Ventricular Strain   241
3D Assessment of Right Ventricular Volumes and Ejection
Fraction.   241
Estimation of Tricuspid Regurgitation, Right Ventricular Systolic
Pressure and Pulmonary Artery Systolic Pressure   242
POCUS Assessment of Pulmonary Hypertension   243
M-Mode and Bidimensional Views.   244
Measurements of Pulmonary Artery Pressure   244
    Systolic Pulmonary Artery Pressure.   244
Pulmonary Flow   246
Conclusion   247
References.   248

Assessment of Valves at the Point-of-Care   251
Shelley Rahman Haley
Introduction.   252
Overview.   252
Recommended Reading.   271
References.   271

**POCUS in Monitoring: Echocardiography After Cardiac
Surgery**   273
Nicholas J. Lees and Ana I. Hurtado-Doce
Introduction.   274
Reasons for Performing Scans.   274
Acute Heart failure After Cardiac Surgery   275
    Focused Versus Comprehensive Echocardiography
    in Postoperative Patients   276
    Common Conditions in Postoperative Cardiac Surgical Patients
    Readily Evaluated by Echocardiography   276
    Left Ventricular Assessment and Dysfunction   277
Diastolic Dysfunction   278
    Cardiac Output Assessment.   280
    Right Ventricular Failure.   280
Methods of Assessment.   280
Pulmonary Hypertension   283
    Valvular Heart Disease   284
    Volume Status Assessment and Hypovolaemic Shock.   285
    Distributive Shock and Vasoplegic Syndrome.   285
    Cardiac Arrest.   286
References.   286

Echocardiography in Mechanical Circulatory Support 289
Susanna Price and Guido Tavazzi
Background 289
Cardiogenic Shock and Acute Mechanical Circulatory Support 290
Types of MCS 290
Key Information Required for Emergency Decision-Making 290
Exclusion of Contraindications 291
Cannulation and Institution of Support for VA-ECMO:
The Role of FoCUS 291
    Immediate Effects of VA-ECMO Seen on FoCUS 292
Troubleshooting and Complications 293
Assessment of Offloading and Weaning 295
Summary and Conclusions 296

Point of Care Ultrasound in Chest Trauma 299
Serena Rovida, Salman Naeem, and Andrew Kirckpatrick
Ultrasound for the Chest Wall 300
Ultrasound for the Pleura 300
Ultrasound for Lung Parenchyma 304
Ultrasound of the Heart 305
POCUS for Procedural Guidance in Chest Trauma 306
References 307

**POCUS in Monitoring: How Monitor Pulmonary Aeration/
Deaeration?** 309
Aileen Tan, Antonio Rubino, Sundeep Kaul,
and Hatem Soliman-Aboumarie
References 313

POCUS in Cardiac Arrest 315
Liana Shirley and Christopher Shirley
Introduction 316
Part I: What Information Can Point of Care Ultrasound (POCUS)
Give Us? 316
Tamponade 317
Pulmonary Embolism 317
Coronary Embolism 317
Hypovolaemia–Hypercontractile 'Kissing' Ventricle 319
Tension Pneumothorax 319
Part II: The 'Right Tool', Used in the 'Right Way' 320
The Window of Opportunity 321
Training: *Train, Train, & Train Again* 321
Planning and Preparation 322
Communication 323
Teamwork 324
Conclusion 326
References 326

POCUS in Pericardial Effusion and Cardiac Tamponade   327
Eftychia Galiatsou and Clara Hernandez Caballero
Introduction.   328
Anatomy and Physiology of the Pericardium   328
Image Acquisition and Interpretation.   330
Cardiac Tamponade.   332
Drainage   335
Pearls and Pitfalls   335
References.   340

POCUS-Guided Assessment and Drainage of Pleural Effusion . . .   343
Nora Mayer and Paras Dalal
Assessment of Pleural Effusion.   344
Drainage of Pleural Effusion   346
Preassessment and Requirements.   347
Conclusion   352
References.   352

Teaching and Accreditation in Cardiopulmonary POCUS.   355
Serena Rovida, Giampaolo Martinelli, and Nick Fletcher
Introduction.   356
The Educational Challenges   356
Key Education Concepts.   357
   Knowledge Base   357
   Technical Skills.   357
   Simulation   357
   Reporting.   358
   Mentoring/Supervision.   358
Development of Basic Cardiac Ultrasound Teaching Protocols.   358
Advanced Echocardiography.   359
Intermediate and Modular Accreditations   359
Lung Ultrasound Training and Accreditation.   359
Development of Lung Ultrasound Teaching Protocols   360
Intermediate and Modular Accreditations   360
Future Perspectives   361
References.   362

Safety and Governance in Cardiopulmonary Ultrasound.   363
Thor Edvardsen and Lars Gunnar Klaeboe
Introduction.   363
Availability, A Safety Concern?   364
Structure and Organization of POCUS   364
Reporting POCUS.   365
Conclusion   365
References.   365

Future Applications of Handheld POCUS.   367
Craig Fryman and Paul H. Mayo
Handheld Ultrasonography Devices.   367
Artificial Intelligence and POCUS.   369

Artificial Intelligence and Echocardiography 369
Artificial Intelligence and Lung Ultrasonography 370
Limitations of Combining AI and POCUS 371
Conclusion 371
References 371

Index 375

The Evolution of Point of Care Ultrasound

Vicki E. Noble

Future generations of doctors will find it hard to believe that, in 2013, many clinicians were still relying on the vague findings of a 200-year-old traditional physical examination and were compromising clinical efficacy when direct information was available from point-of-care echocardiography. History will undoubtedly show that point-of-care echocardiography was the beginning of a 'new glorious age' of the physical examination.

Dr. Jos Roelandt–Cardiologist & POCUS pioneer (1938–2014)

Abstract

To review the history of how point of care ultrasound evolved—both clinically and technologically—world wide. The early history of clinical applications will be reviewed and the early pioneers in this field will be highlighted.

Keywords

Point of care ultrasound · Clinical ultrasound · Ultrasound technology

One version of the point of care ultrasound origin story involves a clinician with a clinical dilemma. The protagonist in these stories is a physician—surgeon, intensivist, emergency physician—who is working at night or in an under-resourced environment and has a patient care question. Our protagonist struggles and thinks some more diagnostic information might be useful to help guide his or her decision making. Is there fluid in the abdomen? Is the heart working well? Are the lungs wet or dry? Our protagonist may "borrow" an ultrasound machine. The value of direct visualization of a patient's physiology is immediately apparent. Straight to the operating room. Diuresis. Added positive end-expiratory pressure. Lo and behold the patient improves. The clinician feels a sense of satisfaction and confidence in facilitating a clear intervention or treatment. The patient's care becomes more efficient if not more efficacious. This clinician feels empowered and becomes an evangelist for the technology. These stories are discussed at conferences all over the world and other clinicians think how they could use this technology. Not just in the ways described but "wouldn't it be nice" scenarios where visualizing any number of clinical conditions and physiology would add to their post-test confidence and

V. E. Noble (✉)
Department of Emergency Medicine, University Hospitals Cleveland Medical Center, Cleveland, USA
e-mail: vicki.noble@uhhospitals.org

Case Western Reserve Medical School, Cleveland, OH, USA

diagnostic and treatment abilities. Papers start to be published.

In these early days, however, technology had yet to catch up with these physician pioneers. Machines were heavy and hard to move. There was a lot of skill required in image acquisition including buttons and levers to adjust things like frame rate, minimizing artifacts and so barriers in spreading imaging skills to these non-traditional sonographers remained high. However, even as early as the 1970s the utility of portable sonographic technology was obvious to innovators like Dutch physician Dr. Jos Roelandt [1]. In 1978, Dr. Roelandt published what has to be one of the earliest descriptions of a portable ultrasound machine (Image 1). There were no clinical protocols and it was not entirely clear where this machine would find its place but the allure of visualizing anatomy and physiology was certainly revolutionary. Indeed, as Dr. Roelandt comments in his summary, "Immediate and on-the-spot assessment of patients is now possible with this miniaturized, self-contained and battery powered ultrasonic device" [1]. He goes on to outline many of the theoretical applications which have since become standard of care; needle guidance, obstetric assessments and evaluation of basic cardiac function.

And so we come to the second chapter of our point of care ultrasound origin story. The clinical potential the early physician pioneers saw required that engineers and others who create ultrasound technology saw the same opportunity—perhaps from a market driven "new user" capitalism—but also from an innovation sense of what ultrasound could do. The technology and its potential were too tantalizing to ignore. And indeed these engineers saw the potential of visualized physiology perhaps with less of the bias that physicians held regarding hierarchy of technology propriety. They began to think about how to mold the technology for a wider audience and how to influence the user experience. Over time a few core principles in the requirements for this new imaging modality evolved. The machine user interface needed to be more intuitive and simplified. Software to automate image optimization was useful. Durability for non-traditional use environments was necessary to make the machines more rugged and able to survive non-traditional use environments. Finally, the formed image needed to projected on a screen that was portable and clear.

The engineering part of the origin story is equally as important to the success of point of care ultrasound as the clinical. A company known at the time as ATL was tasked by the United States government with a military DARPA (U.S. Government Defense Advanced Research Projects Agency) grant in 1994 to

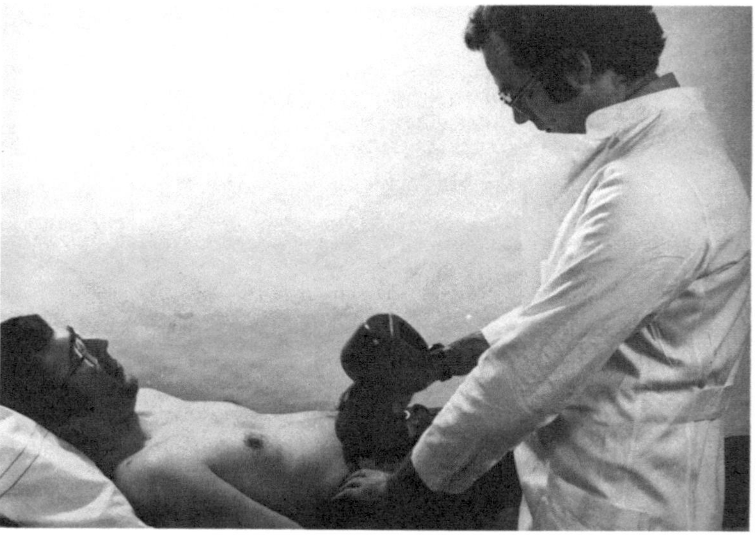

Image 1 Dr. Roelandt and his portable ultrasound machine

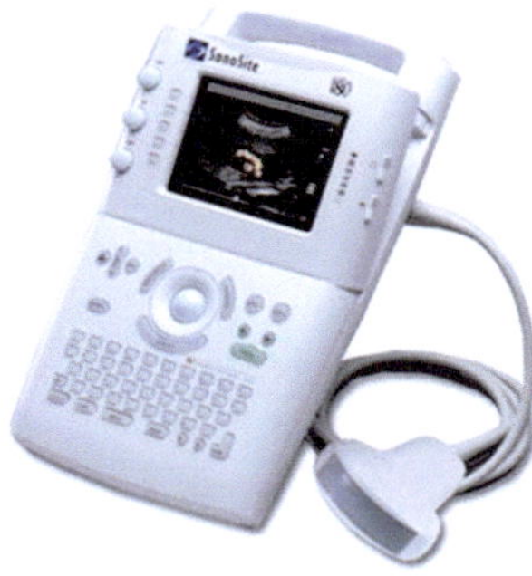

Image 2 The Sonosite 180 machine

develop diagnostic imaging that could be brought to far forward military outposts [2]. This technology had to have the core principles as mentioned above. It had to be portable, durable and user friendly so it didn't require lots of training and technical know-how to use. It was also useful if the imaging modality was non-ionizing. This grant led to a spin-off company and Sonosite Incorporated developed the first battery powered mobile diagnostic ultrasound unit in 1998; the Sonosite 180 (Image 2). Without this push the subsequent timeline of engineering that continued to enable this technology and its democratic spread would not have occurred (Fig. 1).

The retrospective look at the evolution of how this technology was harnessed is a case study in creativity, innovation, meticulous attention and tireless organization. It is also a fascinating look at human behavior. Does disruptive technology attract a certain kind of maverick mind or is it the maverick mind that seeks out disruptive technology? These two origin stories collided in the 1990s when the physician innovators and the engineering potential became aligned and the democratic potential of the newly engineered ultrasound went world-wide.

One of the first physicians who saw the clinical potential of point of care ultrasound was Dr. Erik Sloth. Dr. Sloth and his group in Aarhus Denmark developed one of the first point of care ultrasound training courses in 1989. The innovation of his training was that he saw the need to direct a clinicians evaluation of physiology in a protocoled way so that competency and an understanding of how to use the technology safely was ensured. His course was open to clinicians of all specialties from all over the world and their protocol was called FATE (Focused Assessment with Transthoracic Echocardiography) (Fig. 2) [3]. The FATE protocol was a simplified sonographic scanning protocol for the clinician to assess at the bedside a patient's basic cardiothoracic physiology and to identify immediate life-threats. The course involved didactic lectures as well as hands-on image acquisition training and set the standard for what was to come. It also set the standard in that the education in point of care ultrasound could not just be theoretical or how to interpret images but had to include practical training in how to use an ultrasound machine and acquire images. The power of the portable ultrasound machine was in the clinician's ability to both acquire and interpret.

The 1990s saw an explosion of publications that started to define the clinical conditions and scanning protocols where point of care ultrasound had a meaningful impact on patient care. Dr. Plummer and his group described a mortality difference in patients with penetrating trauma to

Fig. 1 Portable ultrasound machine engineering timeline

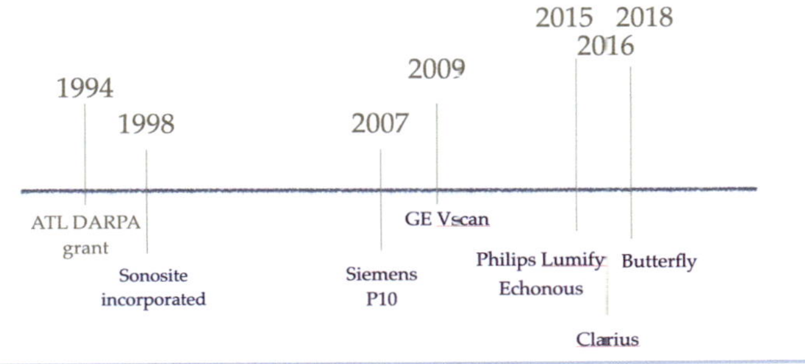

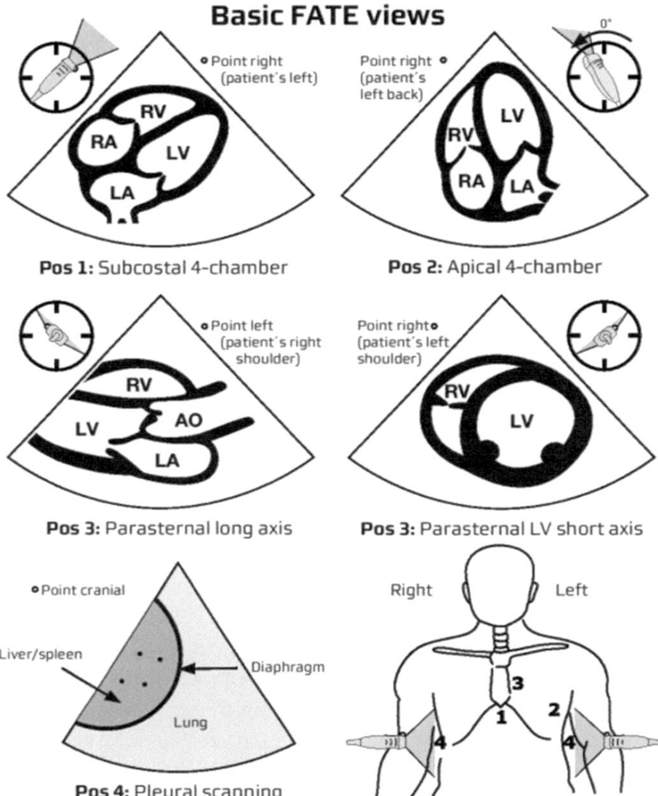

the chest when point of care ultrasound was used to identify pericardial injury at the time of presentation [4]. Dr. Rozycki codified the term FAST (Focused Assessment with Sonography in Trauma) and described how ultrasound could be used to localize the source of bleeding and prioritize patients who needed operative intervention [5]. Dr. Lichtenstein described novel techniques for assessing numerous pulmonary conditions—indeed when conventional wisdom had written off the thoracic cavity because of the "inability" of ultrasound to insonate air [6, 7]. Dr. Breitkreutz and his team saw the potential for ultrasound protocols to do more holistic assessments—in the spirit of the FATE exam—by describing a FEEL (Focused Echographic Evaluation in Life support) protocol for cardiac arrest and near-arrest patients [8].

The importance of these publications was that bedside diagnostic imaging was not just replicating traditional imaging algorithms. Nontraditional sonographers had been training in imaging techniques for decades but mostly to replicate traditional sonographic applications [9, 10]. The revolution in the 1990s was that the technology now made possible a host of holistic applications that looked beyond traditional protocols and tried to quantify a patients physiology, to understand pathologic conditions that required time-sensitive diagnostic abilities to empower the clinician to make clinical interventions based on this holistic assessment. The publication of the Rapid Ultrasound for Shock and Hypotension (RUSH) protocol in 2001 capitalized on this emphasis on symptom based ultrasound protocols. For a clinician trained in point of care ultrasound techniques the use of ultrasound to assess the cardiovascular system could help to categorize the etiology of hypotension and suggest treatment strategies. This has only grown to other users who developed a hepatic vascular interrogation for volume assessment (VExUS protocol) [11, 12].

The question remained how to organize this new kind of diagnostic imaging. Point of care imaging by a clinician required three levels of competency: image acquisition, image interpretation and image integration. National and International organizations rose to the challenge. The American College of Emergency Physicians (ACEP) published one of the first national guidelines for ultrasound training in a nontraditional imaging specialty in 2001 [13]. Their guidelines described not just scanning techniques and applications but began the discussion of what constituted competency in the three spheres of acquisition, interpretation and integration. The World Interactive Network Focused on Critical Ultrasound (WINFOCUS) organized in 2001 and brought the concept of "holistic" ultrasound to a global audience [14, 15].

Now the acceptance for this tool is widespread. It is being taught in medical schools which means that a generation of students is bringing this skill forward to all specialties [16]. Family medicine and pediatrics now incorporate ultrasound skills in their training [17, 18]. Surgery, obstetrics and gynecology, nephrology and even dermatology have found applications that relate to the care of their patients necessitate diagnostic imaging at the bedside [19, 20]. It would be hard to under-emphasize the importance of this skill world-wide and the impact it continues to deliver on how clinical care is practiced.

In many ways, the story of point of care ultrasound highlights the best of the collaboration between engineering and innovators. When technology is brought to bear with end-users guiding utilization, amazing progress can happen. Patients may not yet perceive how this collaboration impacts their access to care with respect to portable diagnostic imaging but clinicians have definitely understood that this diagnostic autonomy makes their practice more efficient and effective. The best is yet to come.

References

1. Roelandt J, Waldimiroff JW, Baars AM. Ultrasonic real time imaging with a hand-held scanner. II: initial clinical experience. Ultrasound Med Biol. 1978; 4:93–6.
2. http://www.fundinguniverse.ccm/company-histories/sonosite-inc-history/
3. Jensen MB, Sloth E, Larsen KM, Schmidt MB. Transthoracic echocardiography for cardiopulmonary monitoring in intensive care. Eur J Anaesthesiol. 2004;21(9):700–7.
4. Plummer D, Brunette D, Asinger R, Ruiz E (1992) Emergency department echocardiography improves outcome in penetrating cardiac injury. Ann Emerg Med 21(6):709–12
5. Rozycki GS, Ballard RB, Feliciano DV, Schmidt JA, Pennington SD (1998) Surgeon-performed ultrasound for the assessment of truncal injuries: lessons learned from 1540 patients. Ann Surg 2228(4):557–67
6. Lichtenstein DA, Menu Y. A bedside ultrasound sign ruling out pneumothorax in the critically ill. Lung sliding. Chest. 1995;108(5):1345–8.
7. Lichtenstein D, Mézière G, Biderman P, Gepner A, Barré O (1997) The comet-tail artifact. An ultrasound sign of alveolar-interstitial syndrome. Am J Respir Crit Care Med 156(5):1640–6
8. Breitkreutz R, Price S, Steiger HV, Seeger FH, Ilper H, Ackermann H, Rudolph M, Uddin S, Weigand MA, Müller E, Walcher F, Emergency Ultrasound Working Group of the Johann Wolfgang Goethe-University Hospital, Frankfurt am Main. Focused echocardiographic evaluation in life support and peri-resuscitation of emergency patients: a prospective trial. Resuscitation. 2010;81(11):1527–33; American College of Emergency Physicians. ACEP emergency ultrasound guidelines. Ann Emerg Med 2001;38(4):470–81.
9. Loch EG, Linhart P, Frank K. Prerequisites for offering ultrasound services in general practice. Ultraschall Med. 1982;3(2):47–9.
10. van Dongen L. Training the obstetrician in ultrasonography. Minimum requirements. S Afr Med J. 1981;60(9):355–6.
11. Rose JS, Bair AE, Mandavia D, et al. The UHP ultrasound protocol: a novel ultrasound approach to the empiric evaluation of the undifferentiated hypotensive patient. Am J Emerg Med. 2001;19:299–302.
12. Rola P, Miralles-Aguiar F, Argaiz E, Beaubien-Souligny W, Haycock K, Karimov T, Dinh VA,

Spiegel R. Clinical applications of the venous excess ultrasound (VExUS) score: conceptual review and case series. Ultrasound J. 2021;13(1):32.

13. American College of Emergency Physicians. ACEP emergency ultrasound guidelines—2001. Ann Emerg Med. 2001;38(4):470–81.

14. Price S, Via G, Sloth E, Guarracino F, Breitkreutz R, Catena E, Talmor D, World Interactive Network Focused on Critical UltraSound ECHO-ICU Group. Echocardiography practice, training and accreditation in the intensive care: document for the World Interactive Network Focused on Critical Ultrasound (WINFOCUS). Cardiovasc Ultrasound. 2008;6(49).

15. Neri L, Storti E, Lichtenstein D. Toward an ultrasound curriculum for critical care medicine. Crit Care Med. 2007;35(5 Suppl):S290-304.

16. Fox JC, Schlang JR, Maldonado G, Lotfipour S, Clayman RV. Proactive medicine: "The UCI 30", an ultrasound-based clinical initiative from the University of California, Irvine. Acad Med. 2014;89 (7):984–9.

17. Hall JW, Holman H, Bornemann P, Barreto T, et al. Point of care ultrasound in family medicine residency programs: a CERA study. Fam Med. 2015;47 (9):706–11.

18. Good RJ, Ohara KL, Ziniel SI, Osborn J, et al. Point of care ultrasound training in pediatric residency: a national needs assessment. Hosp Pediatr. 2021;11 (11):1246–52.

19. Niyyar VD, O'Neill WC. Point of care ultrasound in the practice of nephrology. Kidney Int. 2018;93 (5):1052–9.

20. Hadian Y, Link D, Dahle SE, Isseroff RR. Ultrasound as a diagnostic and interventional aid at point of care dermatology clinic: a case report. J Dermatol Treat. 2020;31(1):74–6.

Physics of Ultrasound and Doppler

Marcus Peck, Jonny Wilkinson,
and Ashley Miller

The science of today is the technology of tomorrow.

Edward Teller– Hungarian–American theoretical physicist (1908–2003)

Abstract

Physics explains everything that we see and do with ultrasound. Understanding physics and knowing how to utilise it to your advantage will make you a skilled operator. This chapter introduces how ultrasound is generated, transmitted and received by transducers to produce two-dimensional images. It explains how ultrasound beams behave inside the body in terms of reflection, refraction, reverberation and scattering, which produce attenuation and artefacts. And it discusses in depth the factors affecting the cornerstones of image acquisition—penetration and resolution. Everything within this chapter stays completely relevant to knobology and image optimisation. For more advanced POCUS operators, this chapter introduces the fundamental principles of Doppler ultrasound and how these explain the characteristics, strengths and weaknesses of all the various Doppler imaging modalities.

Keywords

Wavelength · Resolution · Artefacts · Doppler

Key Messages

- Understanding of ultrasound physics is crucial for performing POCUS
- It is important to familiarize yourself with the ultrasound machines in your department
- A good understanding of physics prepares POCUS practitioners to optimally use their equipment and consequently obtain high quality ultrasound images which is essential for optimal evaluation of patients.

M. Peck (✉)
Consultant in Anaesthesia and Intensive Care Medicine, Frimley Park Hospital, Surrey, UK
e-mail: marcus.peck@nhs.net

J. Wilkinson
Consultant in Intensive Care and Anaesthesia at Northampton General Hospital, Northampton, UK
e-mail: jonathan.wilkinson3@nhs.net

A. Miller
Consultant in Intensive Care Medicine and Anaesthesia, Shrewsbury and Telford Hospitals NHS Trust, Shrewsbury, UK

© The Author(s), under exclusive license to Springer Nature Switzerland AG 2023
H. Soliman-Aboumarie et al. (eds.), *Cardiopulmonary Point of Care Ultrasound*,
https://doi.org/10.1007/978-3-031-29472-3_2

Introduction

Everything inside and around us has the potential to receive and transmit mechanical energy in the form of pressure oscillations (compression and rarefaction) known as sound. In the audible frequency range (20 Hz–20 kHz) this energy vibrates our bony ossicles, triggering our auditory system, and we can hear it. Above this, we can't. Fortunately, however, 'ultrasound' continues to behave predictably, and we can utilise these properties to image body tissues.

The word physics strikes fear into some, passion in others. But knowing something about how ultrasound images are generated helps us to understand the 'knobology' of the machine and how to get the best out of it. This chapter will focus on exactly what you need to know to become an ultrasound master.

Generation

Ultrasound is generated and propagated as pressure waves with oscillating peaks and troughs, similar to those of a sine wave. And like sine waves, propagation velocity (c), frequency (F) and wavelength (λ) are related, according to the equation $c = F \times \lambda$. The importance of this is that as frequency increases, wavelength decreases.

In most transducer probes, ultrasound is produced by piezoelectric crystals, while in some this is done using newer silicone or microchip technology. These media vibrate at very high frequency when exposed to electrical current, and they can also do the reverse—absorb ultrasound and convert this into an electrical signal. In this way, the same probe can send and receive pulses of ultrasoundspaced periodically enough that one returns before the next is sent—and determine where the reflection occurred based on the time it takes to return. To do this, a transducer typically spends 1% of its time transmitting and 99% receiving.

Ultrasound pulses consist of bursts of ultrasound containing multiple wavelengths (Fig. 1). For resolution purposes, the shorter these pulses are the better, so behind the generation zone of any probe is damping material that absorbs ultrasound and reduces the 'ring-down' time (the time taken for the ultrasound-generating material to stop vibrating).

Transducer probes generally emit columnar ultrasound beams, which diverge in all directions

Fig. 1 A schematic diagram representing an ultrasound pulse

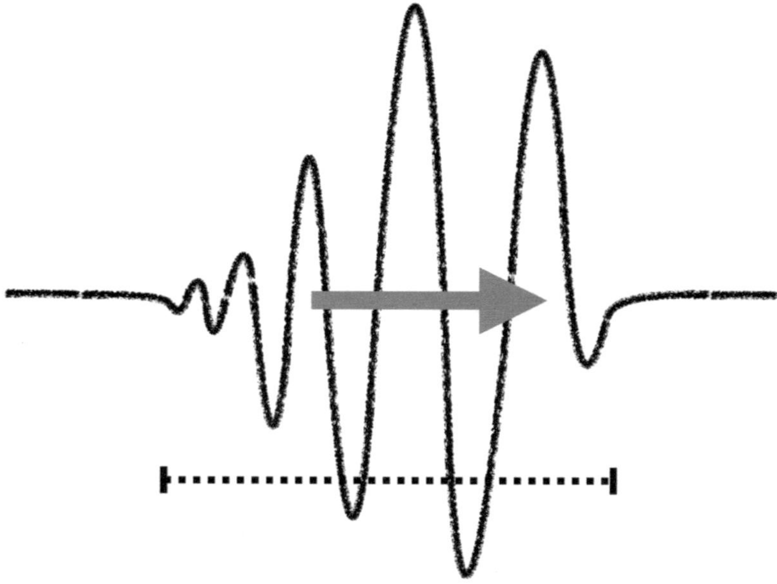

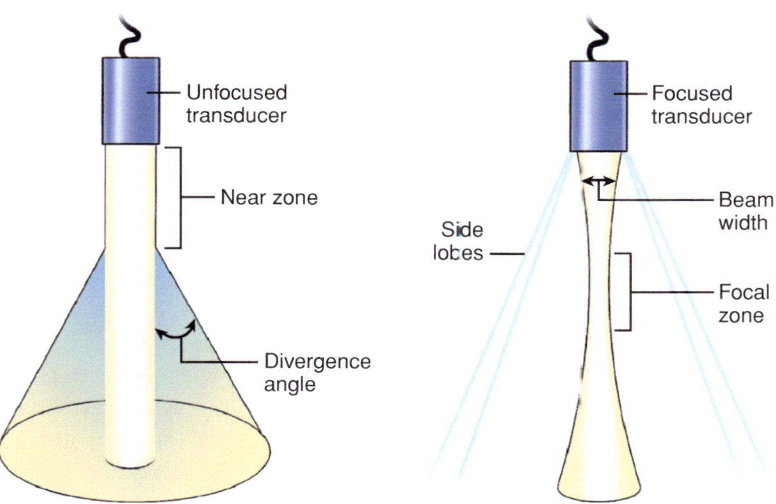

Fig. 2 Figure 1–6 from Textbook of Clinical Echocardiography, Fourth Edition, Saunders Elsevier

after a certain point, much like a flashlight does. Divergence makes it difficult to discriminate between two objects lying closely side by side in the far field, which may otherwise be seen as a single object. Lateral resolution is discussed later in this chapter. To minimise divergence and focus the beam in the middle of the field, piezoelectric crystals are arranged in a concave shape, or an acoustic lens is placed in front of them. See Fig. 2.

The degree of beam divergence is inversely related to the frequency and physical width of the transducer. This means that a high-frequency (2.5–12 MHz) linear array probe can afford to be narrow and emit a rectangular beam, while a low-frequency (1–7.5 MHz) curvilinear transducer 'abdominal' requires a wide aperture. The curvilinear probe emits a wide beam in the same radiation as its convex surface, which gives it good near-field resolution (high beam line density) while also being able to image deeper structures in a wide field of view. Of all the transducers, the low-frequency (2–7.5 MHz) phased array 'cardiac' probe has the narrowest aperture but can still emit a wide beam because its crystals can be fired differentially, allowing the wavefront of the beam to be 'steered'. This feature enables you to look through intercostal spaces and image structures that would have otherwise been obscured by rib shadows, while having a wide field of view.

All ultrasound transducers emit less-energetic side lobes that fan out at equal points on either side of the main lobe. See Fig. 2. In addition, phased array probes emit more powerful grating lobes spaced at a wider angle from the main lobe. All of these can be reflected by structures outside the field and return to the transducer, causing a horizontal, smear-like artefact, known as a side-lobe artefact (For more information on this and other ultrasound artefacts, see Chap. Image Optimization and Artifacts).

Tissue-Ultrasound Interactions

Not all transmitted ultrasound waves reach the far field, let alone back to the transducer to create an image. However, those that do get amplified and generate a signal that the machine can recognise and plot on the 2D sector, depending on where on the transducer they were detected and how long they took to return. This happens across the entire field up to 100 times a second, building a dynamic map of the structures within it. All returning signals derive primarily from reflection.

Reflection

The propagation velocity (c) of ultrasound travelling through soft tissues of the body is fairly constant at 1530 m/s. However, in stiff, high-density tissues c increases (bone 3000 m/s) and in elastic, low-density tissue c decreases (lung 700 m/s) by increasing and decreasing in wavelength, respectively.

The ratio between the acoustic pressure wave and the particle velocity it causes in the medium is known as '*acoustic impedance*'. Differences in acoustic impedance cause acoustic mismatch. And the more acoustic mismatch, the more energy is reflected back to the transducer to create an image. *This explains why hard, dense objects tend to reflect sound better than soft, light ones.*

'Specular reflectors' are flat-surfaced objects associated with high acoustic mismatch lying perpendicular to the transducer, such as the pericardium in a subcostal 4-chamber view. Like a mirror, these reflect transmitted signals extremely well and produce the clearest images. However, as the angle of intercept increases, the likelihood that the reflected beam will return to the transducer decreases. For instance, *in an apical 4-chamber view, the right ventricular free wall is often invisible due to its complete alignment with the ultrasound beam.*

Reverberation

Two strong reflectors lying parallel to each other with high acoustic impedance mismatch can reflect ultrasound signals back and forth. If this signal is received by the transducer, it forms repeat images behind the first, usually at multiples of the distance between the two reflectors. *Reverberation artefacts produce A lines and B lines in lung ultrasound.* See Fig. 3.

Refraction

Acoustic mismatch also causes refraction, which bends the ultrasound beam in the same way that optic lenses bend beams of light. When it occurs in the near-field, refraction can produce 'double-image' or 'ghosting' artefacts, whereby two identical images lie side by side in the far field.

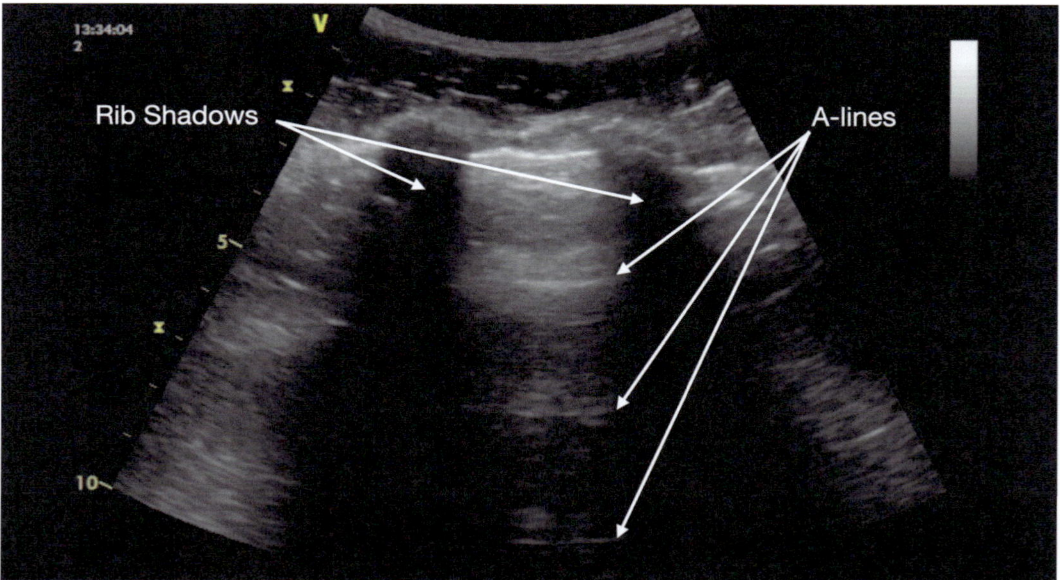

Fig. 3 A lung ultrasound image demonstrating: Rib shadows due to attenuation; A-lines due to reverberation artefacts

For more information on this and other ultrasound artefacts, see Chap. Image Optimization and Artifacts.

Scattering

Particles smaller than the wavelength of the ultrasound beam, such as circulating red blood cells, cause the transmitted signal to be scattered in all directions leading to less returns to the transducer. An analogy is the attenuation of light by heavy fog. The higher the ultrasound frequency, the shorter its wavelength and the more this phenomenon occurs.

Despite scattered signals returning to the transducer with 100–1000 times less energy than those of specular reflectors, these produce most of an ultrasound image. Scattering is utilised positively in two other ways: it is the basis of Doppler ultrasound (discussed later in this chapter) and 'speckle-tracking', which takes advantage of backscattering within the myocardium to create a reliable speckle pattern that can then be traced to provide detailed regional wall motion information. Speckle-tracking forms the basis of strain and strain rate assessment, an evolving tool used to assess atrial and ventricular function.

Attenuation

Attenuation describes the combination of reflection, refraction, scattering and absorption, and each tissue has an attenuation coefficient. The attenuation coefficient of air is about 1000 times that of soft tissue, which is why acoustic gel is required to see beyond it and into the body.

Attenuation, such as that caused by ribs, can be so extreme that it causes acoustic shadows in the far-field behind them, whereby no image (2D or Doppler) can be generated behind them. See Fig. 3.

Penetration Versus Resolution

Optimal imaging depth is limited to about 200 wavelengths, which means that to clearly image deep structures (20–30 cm below the skin) you need a high-wavelength, low-frequency (1–2 MHz) transducer, such as that found in the curvilinear probe.

The lower the transducer frequency, the longer ultrasound wavelength it produces and the better its penetration into the tissues, but the poorer its resolution. Conversely, the higher the transducer frequency, the shorter ultrasound wavelength it produces and the better its resolution, but the poorer its penetration. *All ultrasound imaging involves a trade-off between these two ideals.*

The biggest decision is which transducer probe to use. Beyond this, some machines have pre-sets that promote penetration or resolution by altering the transducer frequency, power and tissue harmonic imaging (THI, described later); others have manual frequency controls—lowest for penetration and highest for resolution.

In the sine wave analogy, the amplitude of each wave represents acoustic pressure or energy, which is measured against a reference value and presented in decibels (dB). Decibel is a logarithmic scale, so a 6 dB rise indicates a doubling in energy and quadrupling in intensity (or loudness). Just as in the audible range—when the louder you shout, the more likely you are to hear an echo—so it is in ultrasound. Energy per unit time represents power, and power per unit area represents intensity (=power^2).

Resolution

Spatial resolution has three elements—axial, lateral and elevational—and describes how well you can differentiate two points lying side by side. Temporal resolution describes how these points are seen to move over time.

Axial Resolution

Axial resolution is determined by the ability to differentiate two points lying vertically (one above the other) in the sector. If reflected ultrasound pulses overlap, these points will blur together. See Fig. 4. The term pulse length describes the length of each transmitted pulse (and equals the number of cycles multiplied by their wavelength). Bandwidth describes the range of frequencies within each pulse—being wider indicates that it includes smaller wavelengths. So, axial resolution is improved by using a higher transducer frequency, with shorter pulse length and wider bandwidth.

Lateral Resolution

Lateral resolution is determined by the ability to differentiate two points lying horizontally (side by side) in the sector. While the above factors are all important, scan line density is paramount, so beam focusing is key. Lateral resolution is optimal at the focal zone and deteriorates in the far-field as the beam diverges, particularly when using a curvilinear probe. See Fig. 5. Using the highest frequency transducer with the widest aperture will help, as will using the focus function if the transducer has one.

Elevational Resolution

Elevational resolution is determined by the ability to differentiate two points lying next to each other within the slice of ultrasound. The thicker the beam, the more likely it will pick up signals from objects outside the desired slice. This is minimised, somewhat counter-intuitively, by using a transducer with a thicker face and an acoustic lens to focus the beam. Despite these properties, however, a low-frequency curvilinear probe may still produce a beam thickness of over 2 cm in the far field. See Fig. 5.

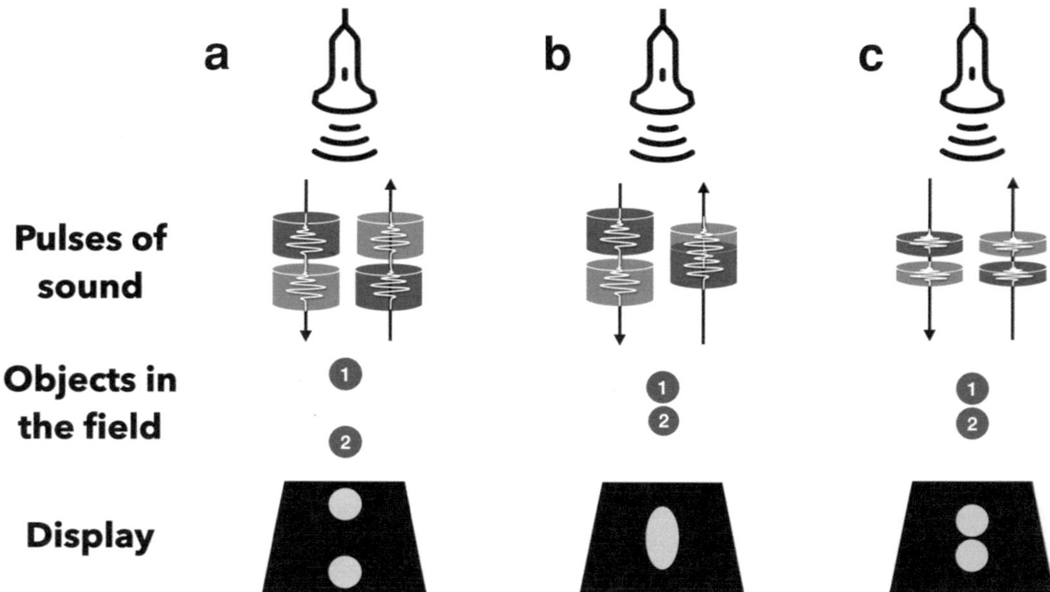

Fig. 4 A schematic diagram demonstrating axial resolution: **a** objects 1 and 2 are far enough apart that the reflected pulses do not overlap and they are displayed as separate objects; **b** objects 1 and 2 are so close together that the returning pulses of sound overlap, meaning the ultrasound machine cannot distinguish them; **c** the pulse duration has been shortened by increasing the frequency (shortening the pulse length) so that the reflected pulses do not overlap and the two objects, despite being close together, can now be distinguished

Fig. 5 Example of how rows of the same sized reflective spheres at increasing depths would look due to the diverging beam. This is an example of lateral resolution becoming compromised. Shallow depth and an appropriately positioned focus point will limit these effects

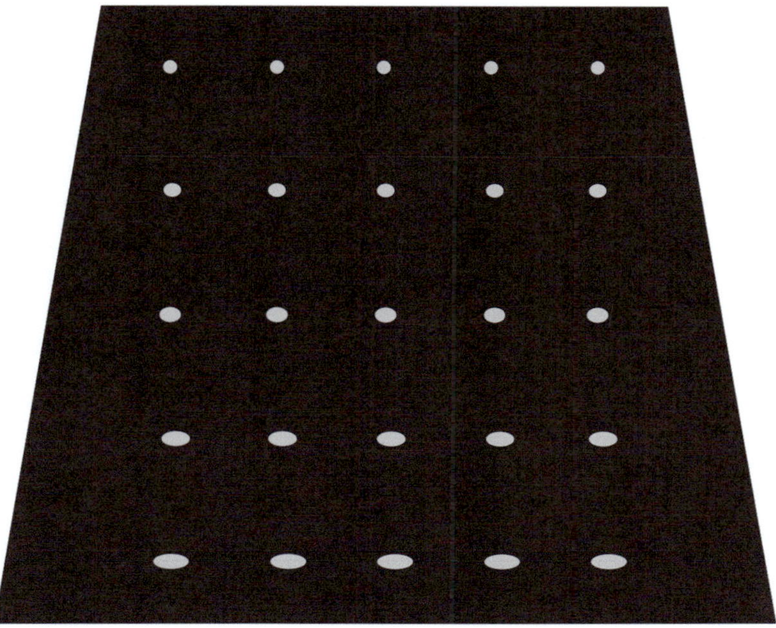

Temporal Resolution

Temporal resolution is determined by how well the image can detect and display movement. This is important for cardiac structures that move quickly, such as valve leaflets. A transducer sends pulses down a set number of beam lines within each field. Each one must send and receive before the next one is triggered, and signals from all beam lines must be received to create a single frame. To create a moving image, this process must be repeated many times per second (Fig. 6).

Frame rate describes the number of images displayed per second. Echocardiography needs a frame rate of about 30 frames per second (FPS). Frame rates below 20 FPS cause the image to appear jerky and may miss important frames. Higher frame rates allow you to slow playback down and observe movement in more detail. For comparison, movies play at 24 FPS, television at 30 FPS and GoPro cameras at 60 FPS.

Fig. 6 Figure 1–10 from Textbook of Clinical Echocardiography, Fourth Edition, Saunders Elsevier

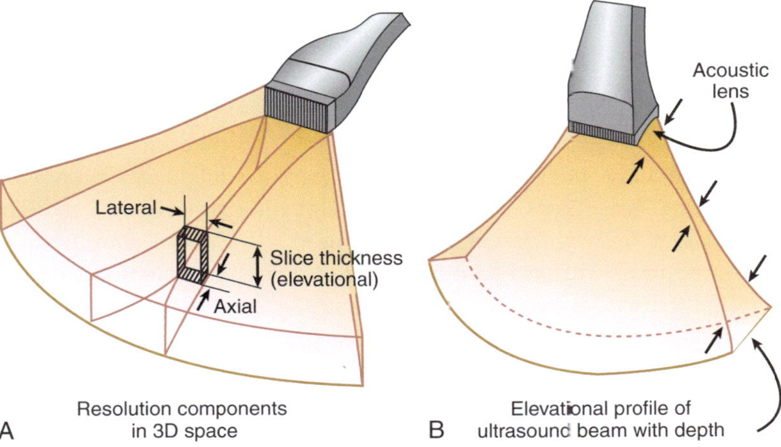

Because M mode has only one beam line, it has the highest frame rate of all modalities at over 1000 FPS.

The number of pulses delivered and received per second is known as the pulse repetition frequency (PRF). The deeper the field, the longer it takes for ultrasound to travel out and back, so the lower the PRF. By this mechanism, frame rate is compromised by increasing sector depth. However, frame rate is compromised far more by increasing field width because more beam lines are required to image a wider area. It is possible to manually reduce beam line density to accommodate for this, but at the expense of lateral resolution.

Knobology

So far, we have covered the physical principles of how ultrasound is produced and how to choose and set-up the right transducer. Now we need to understand how the buttons work.

Depth

By filling the whole sector with the object of interest and placing any measurement targets in the middle, you will optimise lateral resolution (at the focal zone) and frame rate. In comprehensive echo, for instance, after an apical 4-chamber view has been recorded, practitioners reduce sector depth, losing the atria, to further evaluate left ventricular wall motion.

Width

A phased-array transducer has beam-steering technology that allows you to narrow and tilt the angle of the sector left or right without moving the probe. Curvilinear transducers can also do this, but linear ones usually can't. Reducing sector width significantly increases the frame rate.

Zoom

There are two types of zoom—read and write—that enable you to magnify part of an image sector. Read zoom quickly magnifies the object lying in the middle of the screen using post-processing and no change in frame rate. Write zoom involves an extra step whereby the user places a box on the sector to predetermine the area to be enlarged. Once activated, write zoom stops evaluating outside this area, which increases PRF, reduces the number of beam lines and increases the frame rate.

Gain

Not all subjects are easy to scan, and poor ultrasound images usually need amplification to become diagnostic. Conversely, images that are too bright can also be suboptimal because the tissues lack definition. The gain control allows you to modify amplification of the received signal of the whole sector, making it brighter or darker, until you have reached the optimal image.

Some machines have a modifiable auto-gain button, which can be helpful. However, to get the best out of this function, it is worth setting it up with a machine engineer.

Time Gain Compensation

Loss of signal by attenuation is expected, so ultrasound machines accommodate for this by automatically amplifying received signals progressively down the sector. Despite this, the far-field can sometimes appear too dark (e.g. very deep images) or because of this it can appear too bright (e.g. posterior acoustic enhancement of the pericardium). Fortunately, separate to the gain control, some machines have a near- and far-field gain control, while others have between five and eight independent sliding gain controls, known as time-gain compensation (TGC), that allow you to optimise gain differentially at corresponding depths to make the whole sector look uniformly bright.

Focus

Beam focus is essential for optimal lateral resolution. In some linear and curvilinear probes, focus is fixed optimally in the centre of the sector; in others (and all phased array transducers), you can set the focus at any depth. For optimal lateral resolution, you should set the focal zone just deep to the object of interest.

Dynamic Range

The grey-scale of the displayed image can be adjusted using 'dynamic range' (opposite to 'compression', which is analogous to the contrast setting on a television). Turning dynamic range down amplifies the difference between light and dark; turning dynamic range up adds shades of grey and makes the image appear more homogenous.

Tissue Harmonic Imaging (THI)

When ultrasound penetrates body tissues it generates harmonic frequencies that peak between 4 and 8 cm depth. Harmonics behave differently to the fundamental frequency, which is subject to attenuation and artefact generation (near-field and others). So, by preferentially receiving harmonic frequencies the signal-to-noise ratio can be improved, but at the expense of poorer axial resolution. For instance, *endocardial border definition is significantly improved by THI, but valves may appear thicker than they should.*

Doppler Ultrasound

Generation

When ultrasound hits motionless objects less than its wavelength in size, the signal is scattered in all directions with no change in wavelength. When these objects have motion, the scattered wavelengths change depending on the direction they are travelling in: shorter in front of the object; longer behind. Shorter wavelength increases the frequency, and vice versa, and this frequency shift can be detected and converted to velocity according to the Doppler equation.

Spectral Doppler modes—Pulsed Wave (PW) and Continuous Wave (CW) Dopplerutilise this phenomenon to measure blood flow, which has a much higher velocity than tissues. Like 2D, spectral Doppler modes have power, gain and dynamic range controls. Unlike 2D, spectral Doppler uses a high-pass filter to reduce interference from wall motion.

Angle of intercept significantly affects velocity measurement. An ultrasound beam that is fully aligned with blood flow will create a maximal Doppler shift and register its true peak velocity; a beam perpendicular to blood flow will create zero Doppler shift. Any angle of intercept causes progressive underestimation of true velocity, so you should aim to minimise this by careful probe manipulation. Angle-correct technology, found on some machines, can accommodate for known angles of intercept using the cosine function.

Pulsed Wave Doppler

PW Doppler measures blood velocity at a certain point, set manually by placing the 'sampling volume' (a small gate lying on the sampling line) at the area of interest. Once a transducer transmits a pulse, the distance to the sampling volume determines the travel time ('waiting time') and the size of the sampling volume determines the receiving time. The complex information received by the transducer is processed by the machine and displayed as a spectral waveform (velocity over time) with movement towards the probe conventionally above the baseline and movement away below it. The intensity of the received signal (at all velocities) is displayed on the grey scale, with highest being white and lowest black.

In laminar flow, most measured velocities will be close to the peak, so a PW trace typically has a characteristically dark inner and bright outer envelope (e.g.: PW Doppler of LVOT flow). In turbulent flow, there will be a wider range of velocities and the PW trace will appear more filled in (e.g.: PW Doppler at the aortic valve). Contrast this with CW Doppler, which is always completely filled in as there are multiple velocities along the sampling line.

Due to the listening time involved, there is a limit to the velocity that PW can be measured. Much like moving helicopter rotors can erroneously appear stationary (or even move backwards) when recorded (sampled) by video, PW can't determine the direction of travel if the sampling frequency is too low. The maximum Doppler shift that can be reliably detected is known as the *Nyquist Limit*; when this is exceeded the associated error is known as *aliasing*.

Aliasing occurs when the Doppler shift exceeds half the PRF, so it becomes more likely as you increase the sector width and depth. In PW Doppler, aliasing velocities are translated to the opposite site of the spectral waveform baseline.

A high-pass wall-filter is used to reduce the likelihood of noise from slow-moving tissues. This can be seen on a PW trace as a signal-free space either side of the baseline.

Further discussion about clinical applications and artefacts associated with PW Doppler can be found in Chaps. Image Optimization and Artifacts and Fundamentals of Transthoracic Echocardiography.

Colour Doppler

Colour Doppler is based on PW Doppler technology, so it has the same strengths and weaknesses. But instead of deploying a sampling volume within the sector, in colour Doppler you deploy a box. And because the same send-receive sampling process is repeated on every sampling line within this box, the wider and deeper you make it the lower the aliasing velocity and frame rate will be. The scale, usually displayed next to the image, sets the aliasing velocity and frame rate. A low frame rate in colour Doppler has the same effects on playback as it does in 2D imaging.

Blood flow within the box is mapped over the moving 2D image in red or blue, depending on whether it is towards or away from the transducer, respectively. Full saturation of either colour reflects the velocity at the Nyquist limit; shades of either colour represent lower velocities. Aliasing in colour Doppler is represented by an area with a mosaic of the opposite colour (or green if the variance setting is activated).

Power Doppler

While colour Doppler detects the frequency shift caused by the moving red blood cells, power Doppler detects their density. The greater number of red blood cells there are moving inside a vessel or chamber, the higher the amplitude of the scattered signal. Because power Doppler does not indicate direction of travel, it is not limited by angle of intercept or aliasing. In fact, it can readily delineate vessels running at right angles to the beam of ultrasound. Power Doppler is more sensitive than colour Doppler, so it can image smaller, low-flow vessels. And it is particularly good at identifying vessel boundaries while targeting them for spectral Doppler.

Power Doppler maps vessels over a moving 2D image and represents higher amplitudes by a colour change from red to yellow.

Continuous Wave Doppler

As the name suggests, CW Doppler is a form of spectral Doppler that emits pulses continuously. It uses two crystals simultaneously to do this—one transmitting; another receiving—and instead of a sampling volume or box, a CW Doppler sector displays only a sampling line. While CW Doppler imaging is active, the 2D image usually freezes.

There is no limit to the blood velocity that CW can measure, but it can't determine where on the sampling line this originated from.

Otherwise, PW and CW Doppler share similar waveform conventions and angle of intercept limitations.

Because CW Doppler registers all velocities simultaneously, the spectral trace is always completely filled in. Contrast this with PW Doppler, which has an enveloped trace.

Tissue Doppler Imaging

Relative to blood flow, ventricular walls are brighter specular reflectors and move slowly. To exclude noise from blood flow and interrogate only wall motion, Tissue Doppler Imaging (TDI) uses PW Doppler technology with no wall filter, reduced gain, and a low-pass filter.

Like PW Doppler, a TDI trace has a distinct envelope and accurate TDI data depends on a minimal angle of intercept.

Conclusion

Knowing how ultrasound is generated, transmitted, attenuated, reflected, received, displayed and optimised will enable you to get the best out of it. Physics underpins every button on the machine and every image that it generates. This chapter has covered the foundations of knobology and introduced the principles of Doppler, which will be built on in further chapters. We hope that you found it useful and we wish you all the best for your point of care ultrasound careers.

Image Optimization and Artifacts

Segun Olusanya and Adrian Wong

I at length resolved to throw the fluid immediately into the circulation. In this, having no precedent to direct me, I proceeded with much caution.

Courtesy of Thomas Latta (Lancet (1832a) Leading article. 2: 731–5)

Abstract

Ultimately, the key to making the correct diagnosis and hence management with ultrasound is a high-quality image. Hence it is imperative that the user is able to optimize the image obtained whilst taking into account the physical properties (alongside the limitations) of the ultrasound wave. Artifacts give the appearance of objects appearing on the image which are not present in the actual object being scanned. In this chapter, we cover the most comment artifacts encountered and how they can be minimized.

Keywords

Artifacts · Reverberation · Attenuation · Aliasing

Key Messages

- **Ultrasound artifacts** are commonly encountered, and understanding and familiarity are necessary to avoid interpretation errors and false diagnoses
- Some artefacts are avoidable and arise due to improper scanning technique, others are inevitable and are generated by the physical limitations of the modality
- They should not be confused with transducer artefacts which are due to hardware failure
- The ability to recognize and resolve potentially correctable artifacts is crucial for image quality improvement and optimal patient care.

Introduction

A working understanding of the physics of ultrasound beam formation is essential to the acquisition of optimal ultrasound images. The previous chapter has reviewed this in great detail; here we will discuss situations whereby the image obtained does not exactly reflect what is actually present—the science (and art) of ultrasound artifacts.

S. Olusanya (✉)
Consultant in Intensive Care Medicine, St. Bartholomew's Hospital, London, London, UK
e-mail: segs@doctors.org.uk

A. Wong
Consultant in Intensive Care Medicine, King's College Hospital NHS Foundation Trust, London, London, UK

What are Artefacts?

As defined by Kremkau and Taylor [1], these are "display phenomena that do not represent, properly, the structures to be imaged". They occur because the ultrasound machine makes several idealised assumptions about the sound waves it transmits and receives:

- The ultrasound beam travels in a narrow straight line without deviation;
- Ultrasound is reflected back along the same narrow straight line on which it travelled;
- The speed of ultrasound is 1540 m/s regardless of the medium;
- Attenuation is uniform regardless of the medium;
- All echoes arise as a result of the most recent transmitted pulse.

In reality, ultrasound within tissues does not conform to these rules. There are three sets of these artifacts to deal with; those generated during the use of 2D/B-mode imaging; colour Doppler artefacts; and 3D/4D imaging artefacts. We will also consider techniques to optimise imaging through reduction of these artifacts.

Artefacts Related to 2D Imaging

The main artifacts to consider here are:

- More distant than the object:
  - Reverberation artifacts (moves parallel to the object). These include "comet tail" and "ring down" artifacts.
  - Refraction artifacts (moves opposite to the object). These include Ghosting and Mirror image artifacts.
- Same distance as the object:
  - Side lobe artifacts.
  - Beam width/slice thickness artifacts.
- Attenuation artifacts : posterior acoustic enhancement, posterior acoustic shadowing and edge shadowing.

Reverberation Artefacts

Reverberation artifacts arise from multiple reflections of the ultrasound beam before returning to the transducer. Since the processor assumes all returning signals to be directly generated by objects in the ultrasound path, it represents each of these returning signals as discrete objects along the path of the beam. This results in nonspecific lines, bright areas, or duplicate structures appearing elsewhere on screen, at a greater depth than that of the original object.

Reverberations may be generated by the ultrasound transducer itself or other strong reflectors in the path of the ultrasound beam such as the pericardium. Doppler flow display can also generate reverberation artifacts.

Whilst these artifacts can sometimes be used to our advantage, for example the A and B line artifacts in Lung Ultrasound (LUS), they can also be problematic; a reverberation artifact is commonly seen in the descending aorta during TOE examination, which can be confused for a dissection flap.

Where there is a suspicion, the following criteria can help to confirm that the image is artifactual in nature [2];

- Indistinct boundaries;
- Non-plausible anatomy;
- Extension across normal surrounding structures;
- Disappearance with changes in sector depth setting, imaging planes and transducer position;
- Absence of independent motion, but rather demonstrates movement which parallels that of the reverberation source (where identifiable), and
- Absence of influence on blood flow as assessed by color Doppler, showing flow crossing the artifact without turbulence or changes in direction or velocity. Foreign materials, most often catheters and prosthetic valves, typically contain metal, plastic, and/or pyrolytic carbon that strongly reverberate the ultrasound beam.

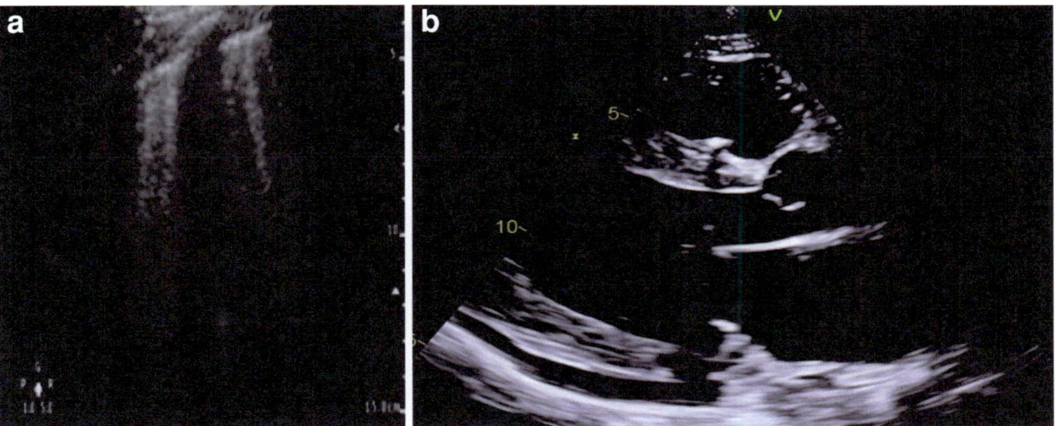

Fig. 1 **a** Reverberation artefactin this case B lines on lung ultrasound. **b** Reverberation artefact from a pacing wire in the right ventricle

A "*comet tail*" artifact is a specific reverberation artifact where multiple echoes appear close together to generate a continuous bright line. This can be seen occasionally with needles when performing ultrasound-guided procedures and is commonly seen as the B line artifact in LUS.

A "*ring down*" artifact is a comet-tail like artifact that occurs in the presence of trapped gas bubbles. There is some debate in the literature as to whether it is a true reverberation artifact or attributable to a slightly different mechanism [3].

Near field clutter is a less common artifact that results in false signals within the near field particularly on echocardiography. The mechanism is poorly defined but has been attributed to reverberation by some authorities [4].

Figure 1 shows some examples of reverberation artifacts.

Attenuation Artefacts

This is a group of artifacts related to altered attenuation of the ultrasound beam along its path.

If the ultrasound beam hits an object or medium which significantly attenuates it, the result will be reduced signal intensity behind the structure—*posterior acoustic shadowing*. The reverse occurs if it hits an object or medium that has lower attenuation properties than the

surrounding tissues—the structures deeper to the tissues become "bright"; this is *posterior acoustic enhancement*. While these changes are strictly artifactual, they are often useful as diagnostic clues:

- Fluid-filled structures can be recognised by the associated posterior acoustic enhancement
- The presence of Gallbladder stones, renal stones and bony structures (such as ribs) can often be confirmed by their strong posterior acoustic shadowing. The latter is particularly useful in LUS; the signature "Merlin's space" described by Daniel Lichtenstein can be recognised by being bounced by 2 ribs, with a lung window in between [5].

Figure 2 demonstrates examples of attenuation artifacts.

Side Lobe Artefacts

These fascinating artifacts arise from the mistaken assumption that the ultrasound beam is straight and uniformly narrow. All waves (including microwaves) display a "main beam", but also multiple smaller and less powerful adjacent "side beams". Under normal conditions, these side beams (or "*side lobes*" when referring to

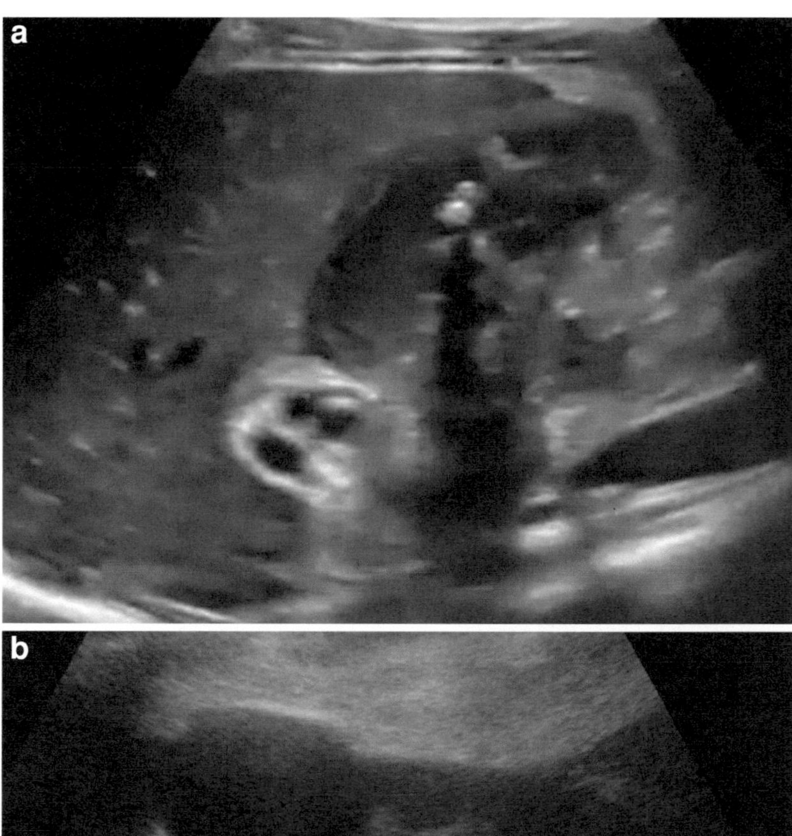

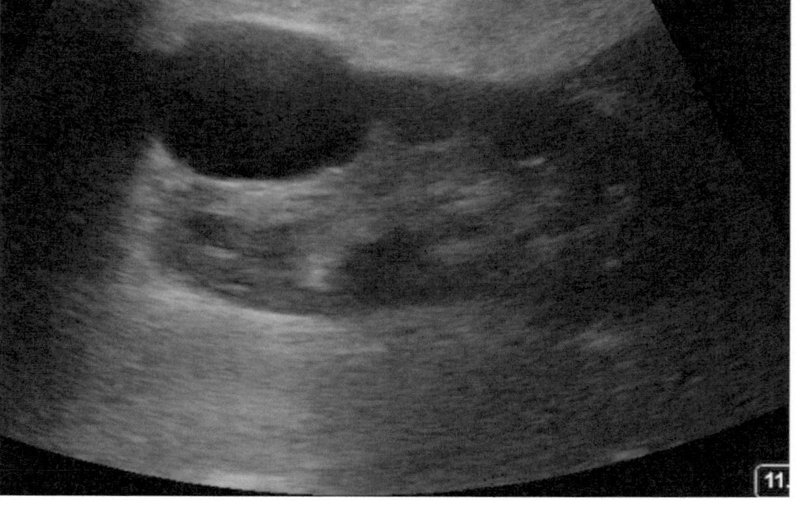

Fig. 2 **a** Posterior acoustic shadowing from gallstones in GB with sludge. **b** Posterior acoustic enhancement from a renal cyst

ultrasound) are too weak to yield significant echoes. However, a strong reflector next to a side lobe may generate sufficiently detectable backscattered signal. Since the processor presumes all reflected signals originate from the central beam/path, side lobe artifacts will appear projected over the primary central ultrasound beam. Their classic appearance is of an arc-shaped image, over a strong reflector, which fades as the reflector is moved away. Side lobes can be minimised by changing the transducer angle and the use of harmonic imaging.

Figure 3 demonstrates examples of side lobe artifacts.

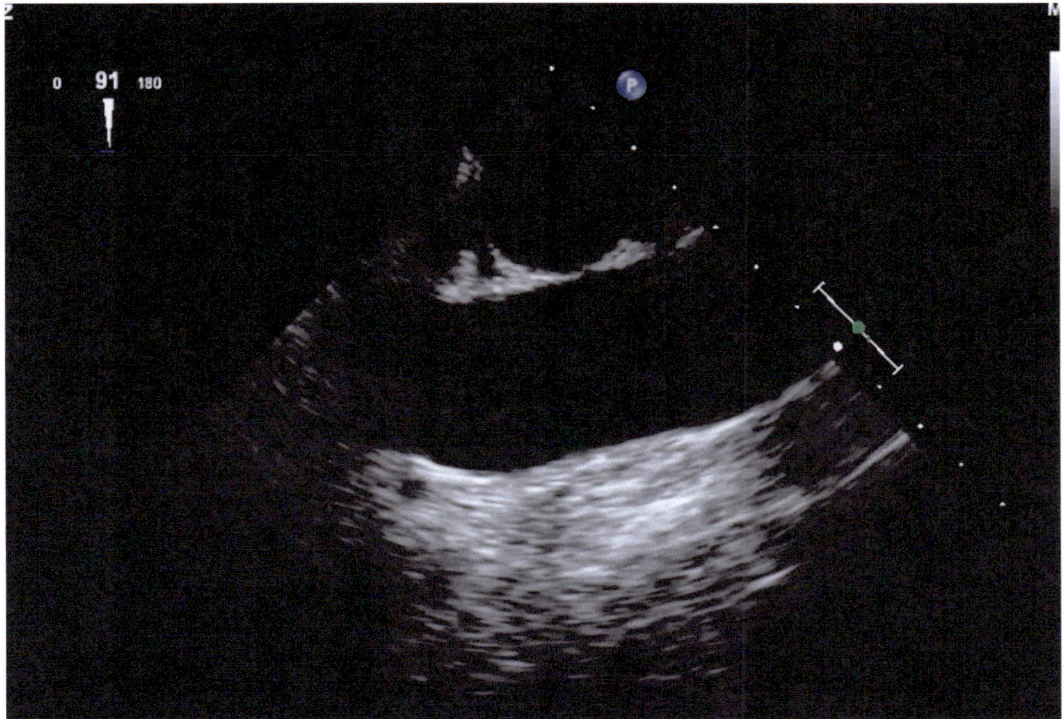

Fig. 3 Side lobe artefact—a thin line seen in the lumen of the aorta on this TOE can easily be mistaken for a dissection flap

Beam Width Artifacts

Whilst not an artifact per se, divergence of the ultrasound beam can distort the appearance of cardiac structures in the far field—a phenomenon often referred to as "beam width" effect. This can be reduced by the use of "matrix" transducers.

Figure 4 demonstrates an example of a beam width artifact.

Refraction Artefacts

These artifacts are generated whenever the ultrasound beam encounters a significant change in acoustic impedance as it travels through different media or tissues. This results in a refracted beam with an amplitude proportional to the difference in velocities of the ultrasound beam between the two media. Any backscatter from this refracted beam is presumed to have travelled in a straight line between the transducer and the point of backscatter; this generates a variety of false images including enlargement and contraction of structures.

The most common refraction artifacts include:

- *Ghosting/double-image artefacts*: this—occurs when the refracted beam is close to the original beam, producing an "after image" of the original structure.
- *Mirror image*: This occurs when duplicate structures are observed on either side of a strongly reflective interface. This is classically seen in transthoracic echocardiography (where the pericardium can result in a mirror image of cardiac structures seen on the parasternal long axis view) and in LUS (a perfect mirror image of the liver can be visualised above the diaphragm).

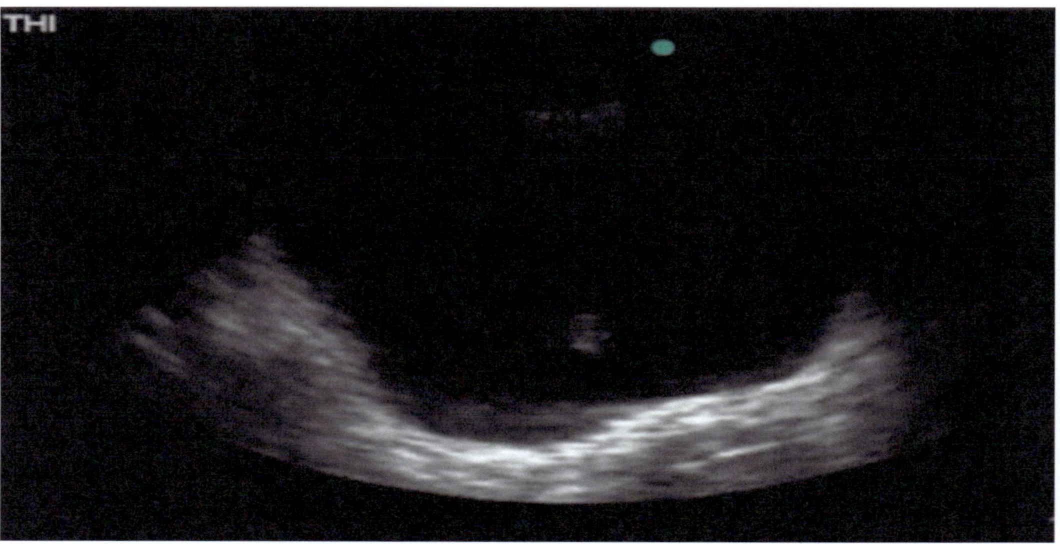

Fig. 4 Beam width artefactgiving the appearance of "sludge" in an empty bladder

Artefacts Related to Doppler Imaging

There are two main artifacts to consider that are related to Doppler imaging:

- Aliasing
- Range ambiguity.

Aliasing: is a specific feature of pulsed wave (and by extension, colour) Doppler. As described in the previous chapter, these modalities transmit ultrasound in intermittent short bursts, which allows for the precise determination of direction of travel and velocity within a specific region of interest. With the transducer having to alternate rapidly between receiving and transmitting ultrasound, Doppler imaging is associated with a number of limitations:

- The delay between the transmission and the receipt of the signal is depth-dependent. This means that the rate of burst transmission (known as the Pulse Repetition Frequency, or PRF) is also affected by depth.
- There will be frequencies that exceed the transducer's detection capability. This limit of detection—the Nyquist limit—is exactly half of the PRF. Frequencies above the Nyquist limit will be

displayed as travelling in the opposite direction of true travel. An analogous phenomenon occurs in daily life, when spinning objects (such as car wheels or helicopter rotor blades) initially seem to be travelling in one direction, until they exceed a certain speed, beyond which they appear to be rotating 'backwards'.

The apparent "backwards" movement of the Doppler signal is displayed on a pulsed wave tracing as a "wrap around" signal (the signal extending above the top of the screen and reappearing on the bottom), while in colour Doppler it is seen as a change in signal colour. This is called 'aliasing', and is demonstrated in Fig. 5.

Aliasing is an important artifact to manage because it can result in inaccurate measurements. A stepwise approach to managing aliasing is as follows:

- Shifting the baseline to accommodate the "wrap around" signal;
- Changing the Doppler velocity scale;
- Reducing the frequency;
- Reduce the depth;
- Switch to "High PRF" imaging, if your machine has that capability;
- Use continuous wave Doppler.

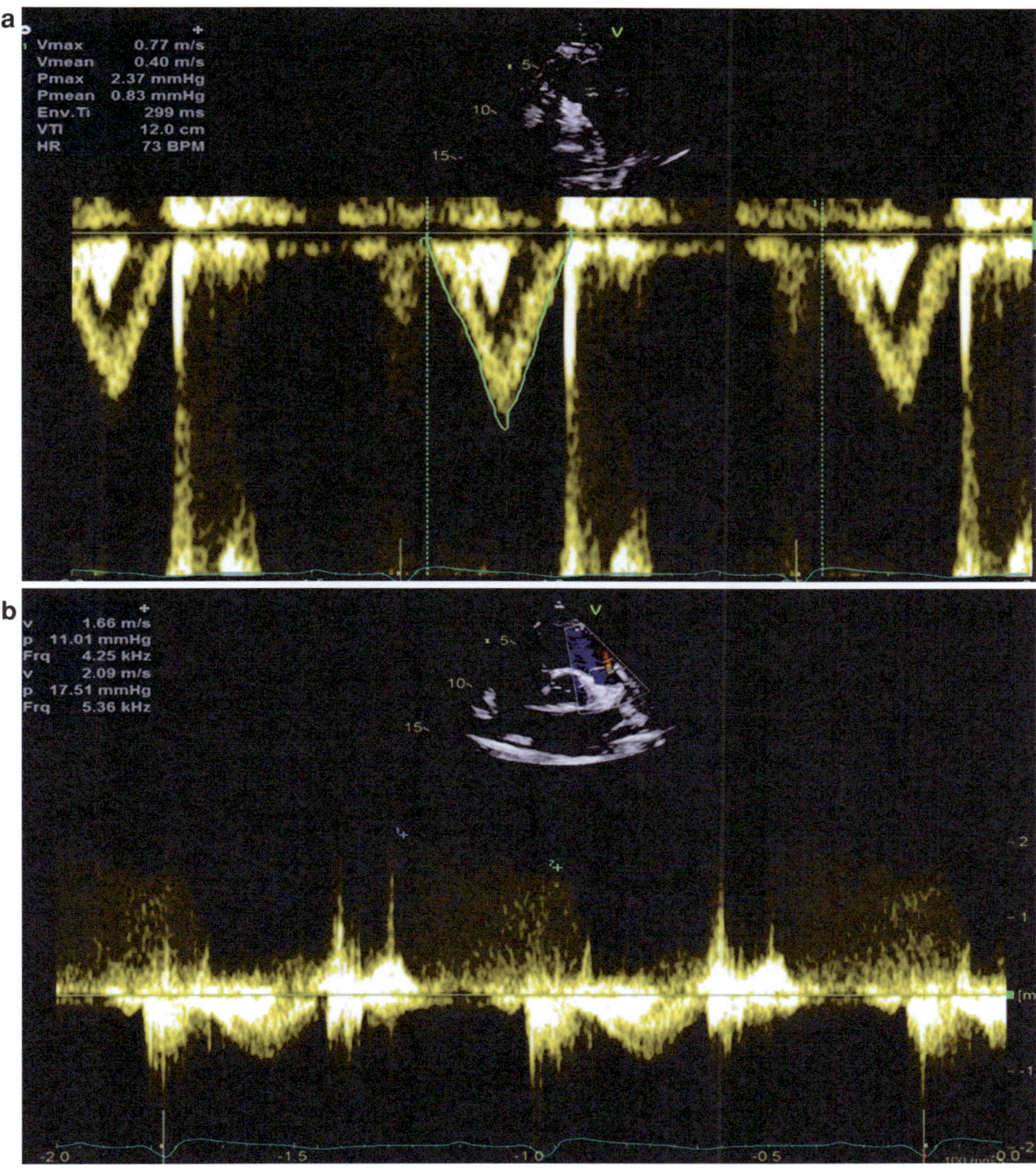

Fig. 5 **a** Aliasing (1)—this PR signal can be seen "wrapping round". **b** Aliasing (2)—same PR signal as above, using CW and having the scale and baseline adjusted

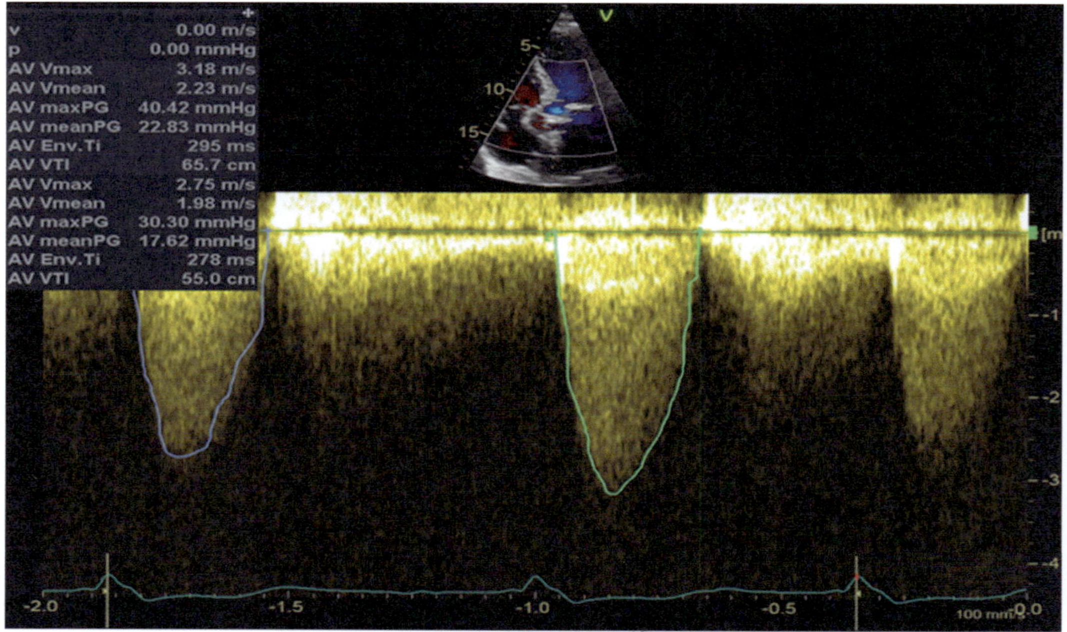

Fig. 6 Range ambiguity—this patient has a degree of aortic stenosis from an artificial aortic valve, and also a sigmoid septum. This CW doppler trace cannot resolve whether the raised gradient detected here is from the valve or the subvalvular component

Range Ambiguity: The latter two modalities, which allow for higher velocities to be recorded, also result in a secondary artifact of their own. Both high PRF and continuous wave doppler rely on the transducer spending more time "listening", resulting in a range of velocities being displayed as opposed to single velocities from a specific region. Consequently, individual velocities cannot be resolved; the peak velocity seen could have occurred at any point along the ultrasound beam path. This is called 'range ambiguity' and can present a problem. For instance, when trying to resolve the location of LVOT obstruction on continuous wave Doppler, a cursor placed along the path of the LVOT could be detecting a high velocity from anywhere along this path—including the mid cavity, sub aortic root, and aortic valve.

Figure 6 shows an example of range ambiguity.

Miscellaneous Artefacts

Electrocautery produces a characteristic, fan-shaped interference pattern artifact precluding proper 2D and colour Doppler imaging. It is unique and easily identified because it appears only during electrocautery use. This is most relevant during intraoperative TOE.

The presence of a second Doppler source (such as an oesophageal Doppler probe) results

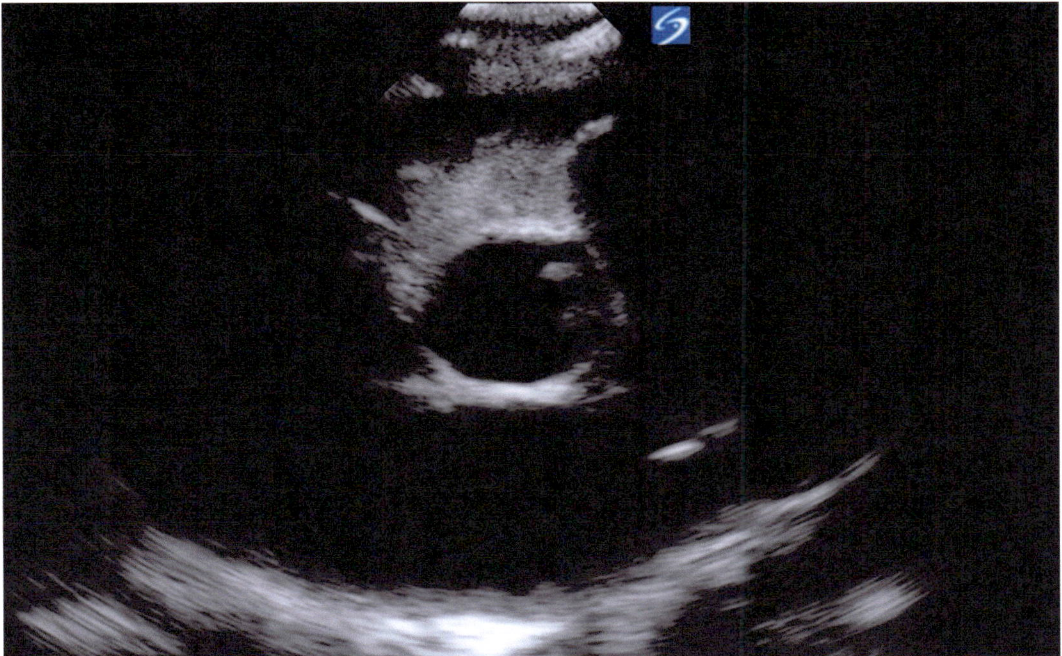

Fig. 7 "Ghosting" artefact—two aortic roots are seen in this short axis view

in a characteristic artifact which reduces in intensity as the two transducers are moved further apart.

Conclusion

A clear understanding of ultrasound artifacts is essential for optimal image acquisition and image interpretation when performing point of care ultrasound. We hope that the reader is now better equipped to deal with any potential "false news" they may encounter during their diagnostic and procedural journey with point of care ultrasound.

References

1. Kremkau FW, Taylor KJ. Artifacts in ultrasound imaging. J Ultrasound Med. 1986;5:227–37.
2. Vignon P, Spencer KT, Rambaud G, et al. Differential transesophageal echocardiographic diagnosis between linear artifacts and intraluminal flap of aortic dissection or disruption. Chest. 2001;119:1778–90.
3. Avruch L, Cooperberg PL. The ring-down artifact. J Ultrasound Med. 1985;4:21–3.
4. Schmailzl KJG, Ormerod O. Ultrasound in cardiology. Oxford: Blackwell Science; 1994.
5. Lichtenstein D. Novel approaches to ultrasonography of the lung and pleural space: where are we now? Breathe (Sheff). 2017;13(2):100–11.

Fundamentals of Transthoracic Echocardiography

Marcus Peck, Ashley Miller,
Jonny Wilkinson,
and Aleksandar N. Neskovic

Any fool can know. The point is to understand.
Albert Einstein–German–born theoretical physicist (1879–1955)

Abstract

Bedside transthoracic echocardiography is among the most important point of care imaging tools. It enables the assessment of cardiac anatomy, physiology as well as represents an extension of bedside cardiac examination.

Keywords

POCUS · FoCUS · Spectral Doppler

M. Peck (✉)
Consultant in Anaesthesia and Intensive Care Medicine, Frimley Park Hospital, Surrey, UK
e-mail: marcus.peck@nhs.net

A. Miller
Consultant in Intensive Care Medicine and Anaesthesia, Shrewsbury and Telford Hospitals NHS Trust, Shrewsbury, UK

J. Wilkinson
Consultant in Intensive Care Medicine and Anaesthesia, Northampton General Hospital, Northampton, UK

A. N. Neskovic
Clinical Hospital Center Zemun, Faculty of Medicine, University of Belgrade, Belgrade, Serbia

Key Messages

- TTE is an important imaging tool for the bedside diagnosis and assessment of cardiac disorders
- Learning and mastering TTE views acquisition is a crucial step in learning cardiac ultrasound. Any further echocardiographic calculations should be based on optimal acquisition of TTE windows
- TTE findings should be interpreted in the context of patient's physiology and clinical status especially in acute and critical care medicine
- Understanding limitations of TTE will enable clinicians to interpret results and avoid misdiagnosis

Introduction

The heart is a remarkable organ that can perfuse the body through a wide range of loading conditions in both health and disease. However, it can fail in different ways. And unless you know how, it is very difficult to treat the patient it belongs to.

Some diagnoses are notoriously difficult to detect clinically because their physical signs are unreliable in critical illness, while others require specialist input or transferring the patient—with time, resource and safety implications. When performed at the bedside, transthoracic echocardiography (TTE) allows us to look inside the chest—in ways we could previously have only dreamt about—and make the right diagnosis, at the right time, and in the right place.

The scope of TTE lies on a continuum from basic two-dimensional (2D) visual assessment (known as "focused echocardiography", "focused cardiac ultrasound" or simply "FoCUS") to a full advanced study using a minimum dataset (known as "comprehensive echocardiography"). Thus, the principal difference between the two is in the amount of information that can be obtained. The more complex TTE becomes, the more information it can deliver, but more training and experience are required to perform it accurately. These issues, as they relate to FoCUS, are explored further in the position and guideline documents of the European Association of Cardiovascular Imaging (EACVI).

This chapter will explain how to perform a TTE examination and introduce how Doppler can potentially add value—and pitfalls—to the haemodynamic assessment of critically ill patients.

Machine Set-Up

Radiology and cardiology developed diagnostic ultrasound independently and chose to display the screen marker on opposite sides of the sector: radiology on the left, cardiology on the right. Machines will set this automatically when you confirm which probe you plan to use. But this can be a source of confusion for people extending their skillset and moving from one convention to another.

To perform POCUS, it is important to connect ECG leads, as this improves the accuracy of waveform analysis, timing of cardiac cycles and sharing your clips (playback is better).

Images recorded in bright clinical environments often look fine at the time but tend to be too bright ("over-gained") when reviewed later. Therefore, if possible, try to optimize the gain accordingly.

Probe Handling

The phased array probe is designed for echocardiography. With a small footprint and broad range of ultrasound frequencies, it can image between the ribs and visualise both superficial and deep structures well. It should generally be held like a pen, although there are exceptions to this (the subcostal window and a left-handed apical window).

Which hand to hold the probe in is determined by personal preference; there are advantages and disadvantages to each. The important thing is to get as comfortable as possible since good ergonomics leads to good image acquisition. Resting the heel of your hand on the patient's chest wall helps stabilise the probe/image and is usually more comfortable for both the operator and the patient.

The pressure required to get good images varies and the "ALARA" (as low as reasonably achievable) principle applies. Firm pressure is sometimes needed—as is pressing down on the adjacent rib (to open up the window)—but these manoeuvres may be uncomfortable for the patient.

Because the heart is relatively deep inside the chest, small movements of the probe cause large changes to the image—as the beam moves through it. Therefore, while learning, it is important to make these movements slowly and deliberately, one at a time, so you can undo them if the image gets worse.

Since the head and tail of the probe move in opposite directions, when communicating, it is important to be clear about which one you are describing. To avoid any confusion, in this chapter we will always refer to movements of the beam.

Various terms are used to describe probe kinematics, but all relate to three elemental movements—sliding, tilting and rotating. Sliding means moving the beam to a different point on the chest wall. This can be in any direction, so this must be stated. Some use the word "sweep" specifically to describe sliding from long side to long side of the probe. Tilting can also be done in any direction, but in TTE these tend to be in two perpendicular planes: "fanning" (or "angling") means tilting the beam from long side to long side of the probe; "rocking" means tilting the beam from short side to short side of the probe. Rotating means turning the beam clockwise or anticlockwise on the footprint of the probe. See Fig. 1.

Fanning causes the image to change in shape, as the beam cuts through different structures, and allows you to look at different levels of the object (e.g. the different parasternal short-axis views). Rocking causes the same image to swing sideways in the field, as the beam cuts into structures either side of it, and allows you to centre an object in the middle of the screen (e.g. the left ventricle in the parasternal short axis).

Cardiac Axis

The heart lies obliquely within the chest, with its base behind the upper sternum in the midline and its apex somewhere near the 5/6th intercostal space in the mid-clavicular line. However, the apex can vary remarkably between patients—from the left sternal edge in some to the axilla in others—so expect varying degrees of probe rotation to find its true axis. See Fig. 2.

'Long axis' describes a chamber along its full length (a normal left ventricle is bullet-shaped). 'Short axis' describes a chamber across its full width (a normal left ventricle is circular). Each is perpendicular to the other, so rotating the probe 90° will move between them. Visualising a chamber 'off axis' means that it will not appear as it should, and its shape and dimensions may not be true.

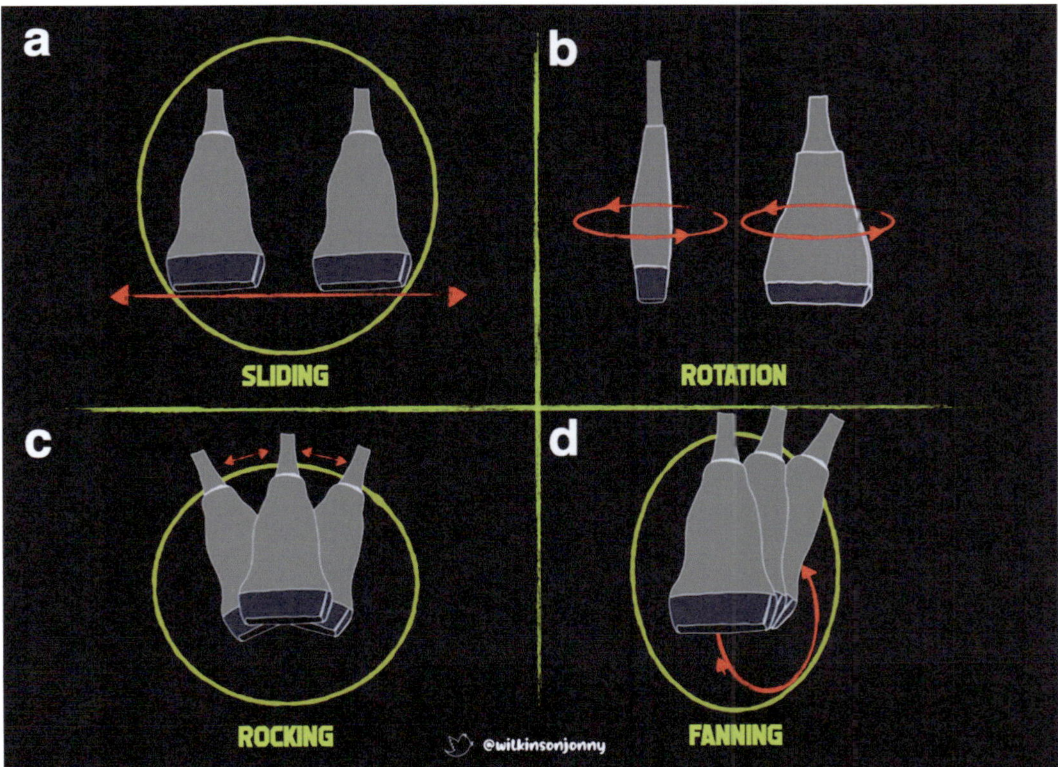

Fig. 1 Schematic demonstrating probe kinematics: **a** sliding; **b** rotation; **c** rocking; **d** fanning

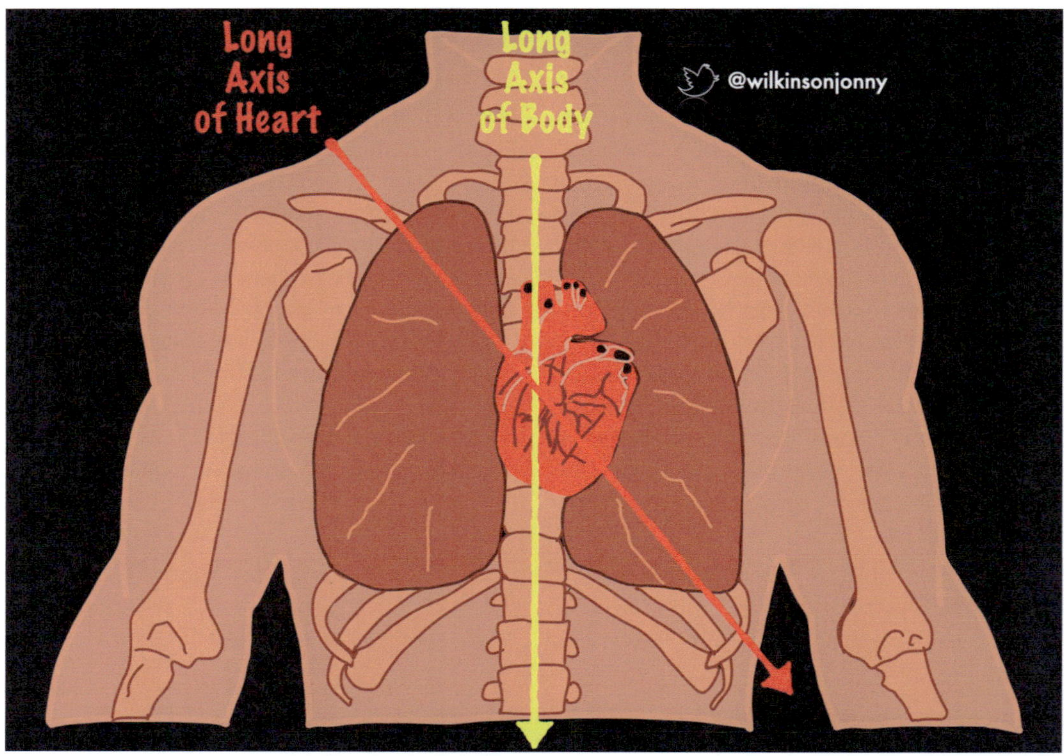

Fig. 2 Schematic demonstrating how the cardiac axis relates to the axis of the body

Windows

The heart is mostly surrounded by lungs, so it is a wonder it can be seen at all. Fortunately, there are three windows on the chest wall where this is minimal—these are known as the parasternal, apical and subcostal windows. See Fig. 3.

The left parasternal window is found at the left sternal edge between the 2nd and 5th intercostal spaces. The apical window is found around the 5th/6th intercostal space in the mid-clavicular line. However, it can be more inferior or lateral depending on the patient's body habitus or pathology. The subcostal window is found between the epigastrium and right upper quadrant of the abdomen.

Within each window, multiple views of the heart can be achieved by careful manipulation of the probe and beam.

Basic 2D Views

Parasternal Long-Axis View

Sonoanatomy

The left parasternal long-axis (PLAX) view is one of the most reliable views in TTE, which is why basal dimensions are measured from it in comprehensive echo. It visualises most major left-sided structures, the right ventricular outflow tract (RVOT), pericardium, aortic root and descending aorta. See Fig. 4.

There are three PLAX views—high (a), mid (b) and low (c). See Fig. 5. The high view images the aortic root on the right of the field and the base of the heart on the left. The mid view (the ideal view) images the base and mid sections of the heart with the left ventricular (LV) cavity

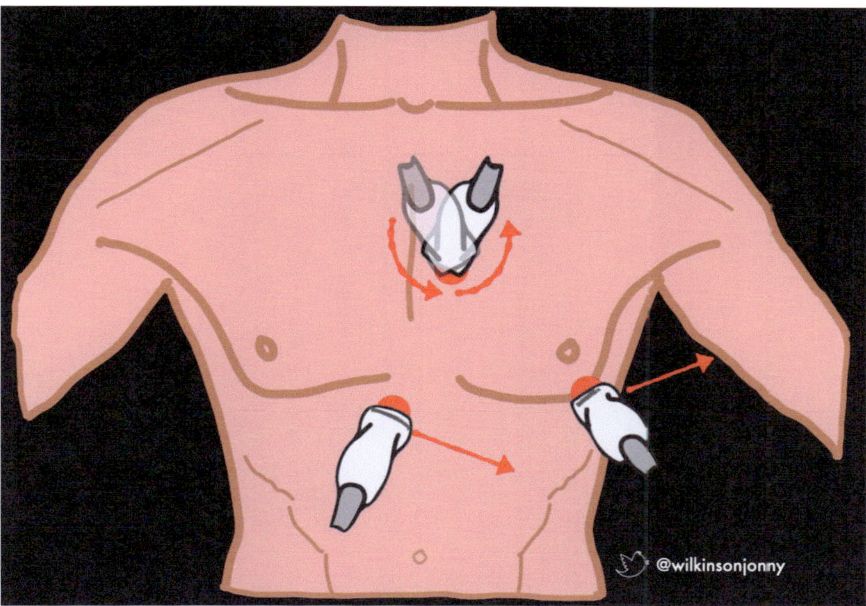

Fig. 3 Schematic demonstrating the three main echocardiographic windows—parasternal, apical and subcostal

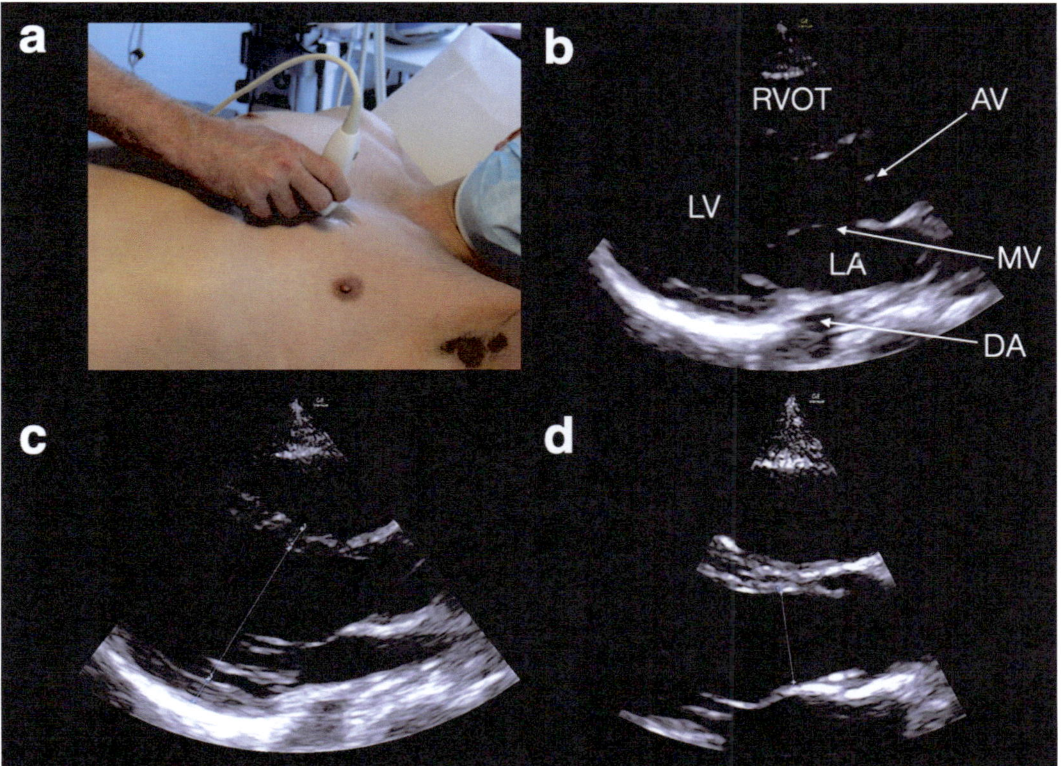

Fig. 4 The left parasternal long-axis view: **a** photo of probe position; **b** the ideal (mid) PLAX view; **c** image with line demonstrating the correct position for measuring LV basal dimensions; **d** image with line demonstrating the correct position for measuring LVOT diameter [LA, left atrium; LV, left ventricle; RVOT, right ventricular outflow tract; AV, aortic valve; MV, mitral valve; DA, descending aorta]

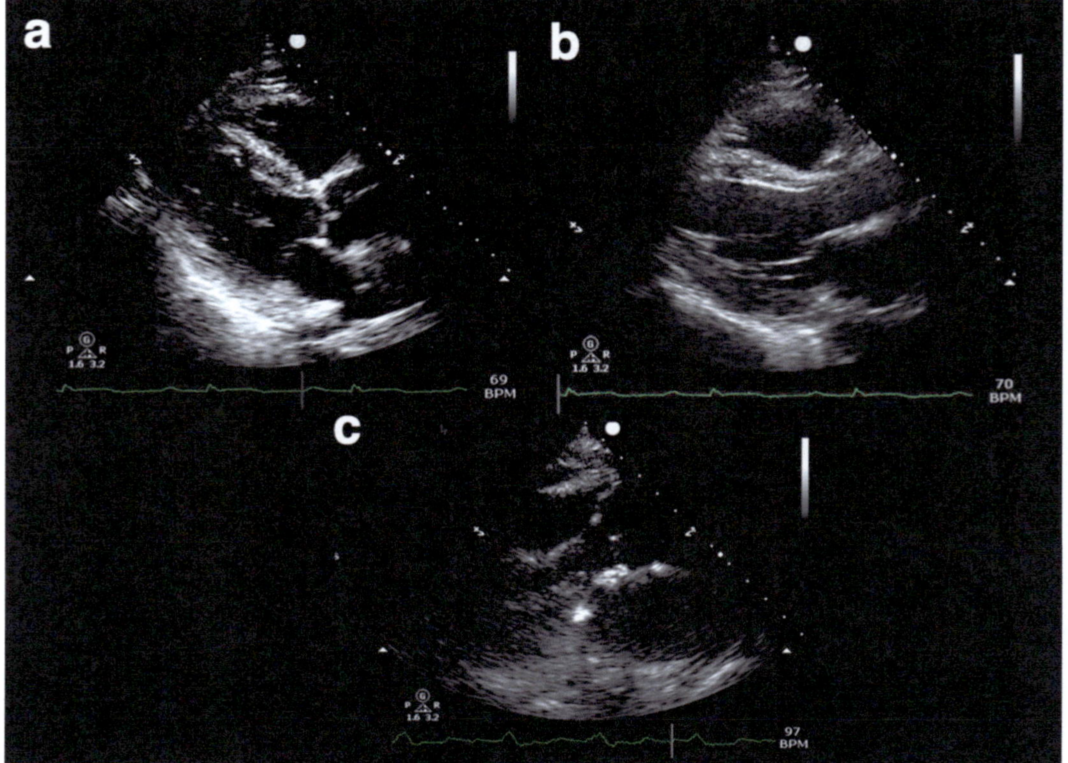

Fig. 5 The 3 left parasternal long-axis views [all images from the same patient]: **a** the low PLAX view (the easiest to find in critically ill patients—with the LVOT lower than the LV chamber); **b** the mid PLAX view (the ideal view for measurements—with the LVOT at the same level as the LV cavity; **c** high PLAX (with the LVOT higher than the LV cavity; note how the aortic root here appears larger than the others) [images courtesy of Professor Sharon Kay]

lying horizontally at the same level at the aortic valve. The low view (the most commonly found PLAX view in critically ill patients) visualises the left ventricle lying at an angle across the image. Seeing what looks like an apex in PLAX means that your beam is either malrotated or in a rib-space too low, or lateral towards the apex, and any measurements you take may be inaccurate.

Acquisition

1. Turn the patient as near as possible to the left lateral position
2. Hold the probe perpendicular to the skin at the left sternal edge with the probe marker pointing towards the patient's right shoulder
3. Slide it up and down using broad movements until you see something recognisable as PLAX (ideally the mid view)
4. Set the depth so you can visualise the descending thoracic aorta at the bottom of the field (deeper only briefly to look for a left pleural effusion)
5. Fan the probe slowly one way, then the other, until you have the aortic and mitral valves sharply in view at the same time. The LV cavity will now be at its widest
6. Rock the beam until the LV cavity lies as horizontally as possible, with the mitral valve leaflet tips centred in the image
7. Rotate the beam slowly one way, then the other, until the LV cavity opens out and any 'apex' disappears completely off the left side

of the screen. You have now identified the left ventricle in its long-axis

8. Adjust the gain to make the chambers as black as possible, while keeping the structures clearly defined
9. Record your clip [PLAX]
10. Finally, make a mental note of the direction the ultrasound beam is pointing—somewhere laterally along this line you will find the apex and the apical window.

Interrogation

Important LV basal dimensions in diastole include: interventricular septal wall thickness, LV internal dimension and inferolateral (also known as posterior) wall thickness. The only basal dimension usually measured in systole is LV internal dimension. These measurements form the basis for diagnosing LV dilatation and calculating fractional shortening (a surrogate of LV ejection fraction).

Measuring basal dimensions:

1. Connect an ECG if possible
2. Obtain an optimal PLAX (mid view if possible)
3. Freeze it at end-diastole (just before the QRS complex or the frame before mitral valve closes)
4. Place a 2D measurement caliper across the basal LV cavity, perpendicular to its long-axis, at the level of the open mitral valve leaflet tips
5. Measure basal dimensions
6. Scroll forward to mid-systole (mid QRS complex or a frame with fully open aortic valve leaflets)
7. Measure basal dimension.

One of the most difficult measurements to perform accurately is the left ventricular outflow tract (LVOT) diameter. Any error made doing so will be squared in the stroke volume calculation. So, take great care when measuring this or avoid it altogether and use LVOT velocity-time integral (VTI) alone as a surrogate of stroke volume.

Measuring LVOT Diameter:

1. Obtain an optimal PLAX view
2. Zoom in on the LVOT
3. Freeze the image in mid-systole
4. Place a caliper across the LVOT (inner edge to inner edge), perpendicular to its long-axis, as close as possible to the aortic annulus
5. Measure LVOT diameter.

Interpretation

The PLAX view provides lots of information, including:

- Chamber size (right ventricular [RV] outflow tract, base of the left ventricle, left atrial [LA] diameter)
- LV wall thickness
- LV basal systolic function ('Fractional Shortening')
- Identifying (and distinguishing between) pericardial and left pleural collections according to their relationship with the descending thoracic aorta
- LVOT diameter
- LVOT pathology (e.g. systolic anterior motion of the mitral valve [SAM])
- Aortic root pathology.

Pitfalls

The low PLAX view often images the papillary muscles and primary cords, which can overestimate fractional shortening (and LV function). To measure basal LV dimensions accurately, whenever possible, use the mid PLAX view.

Despite the high PLAX view imaging the aortic root well, when the beam is rocked towards the left ventricle, the aortic root can appear falsely dilated (see Fig. 5). To measure aortic dimensions, whenever possible use the mid PLAX view (or the high PLAX view with the beam rocked towards the aorta).

Parasternal Short-Axis View

Sonoanatomy

The parasternal short-axis (PSAX) view is another stable view that images all major left-sided structures, both ventricles and the pericardium. See Fig. 6.

There are four PSAX views, depending on how the beam is fanned—the aortic (most superior), mitral, mid-papillary and apical levels (most inferior). The aortic level images the aortic valve leaflets, interatrial septum, tricuspid valve (TV), right ventricle (RV), pulmonary valve, main pulmonary artery and bifurcation. The mitral level images both ventricular cavities and both anterior and posterior mitral valve leaflets (resembling a 'fish mouth') with cords. The mid-papillary level images both ventricular cavities and papillary muscles (anterolateral and posteromedial) as they embed into the LV wall. The apical level images only the LV apex.

Acquisition

1. Optimising your PLAX view first is essential so that you subsequently get an optimal PSAX view
2. Whatever left-sided structure is in the middle of the screen in PLAX will be the level you visualise when you rotate, so rock the beam gently to optimise this
3. Rotate the beam 90° clockwise, taking care not to do any other movement; though counter-intuitive, watching the probe, not the screen, usually helps
4. Rock the beam to place the LV cavity in the middle of the screen

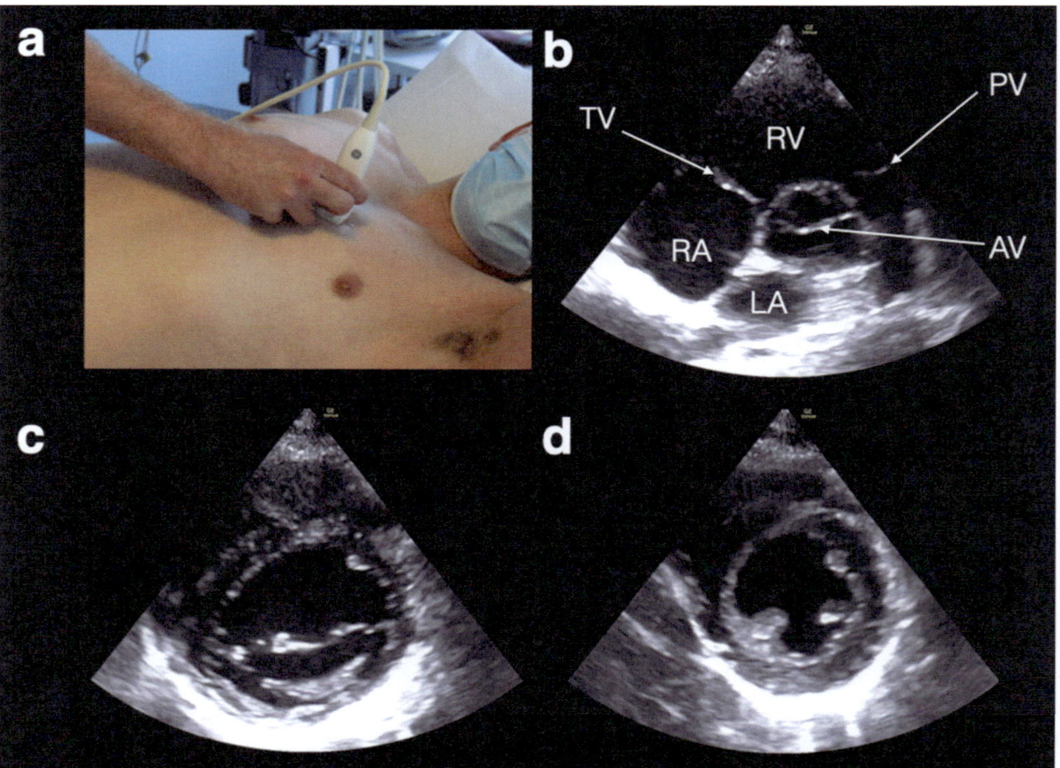

Fig. 6 The left parasternal short-axis view: **a** probe positioning; **b** the PSAX-AV view; **c** the PSAX-MV view; **d** the PSAX-MP view [AV, aortic valve; MV, mitral valve; MP, mid-papillary; LA, left atrium; RA, right atrium; LV, TV, tricuspid valve; RV, right ventricle; PV, pulmonary valve]

5. Fan slowly up and down to image the desired level
6. Record your clips
7. Finally, if you located the LV apex, make a mental note of where—as this is where you should find the apical window.

Interpretation

The PSAX view provides lots of useful information, including:

- Relative chamber size (both ventricles)
- Global and regional LV wall motion abnormalities
- Ventricular interdependence (a D-shaped interventricular septum)
- Atrial interdependence (fixed bowing of the interatrial septum)
- Gross aortic and mitral valve disease.

Pitfalls

In an off-axis or low PSAX view, the left ventricle will be oval-shaped and may give a false impression that the septum is D-shaped. Additionally, an off-axis cut of the myocardial walls may falsely suggest hypo- or hyperkinetic regional wall motion. Take care to rotate no more or less than 90° from the mid-PLAX view.

Apical 4-Chamber and 5-Chamber Views

Sonoanatomy

The apical 4-chamber (A4C) is the go-to view for comparing left and right-sided structures. It images the entire long-axis of both ventricles, including their apices, and the mitral and tricuspid valves. See Fig. 7.

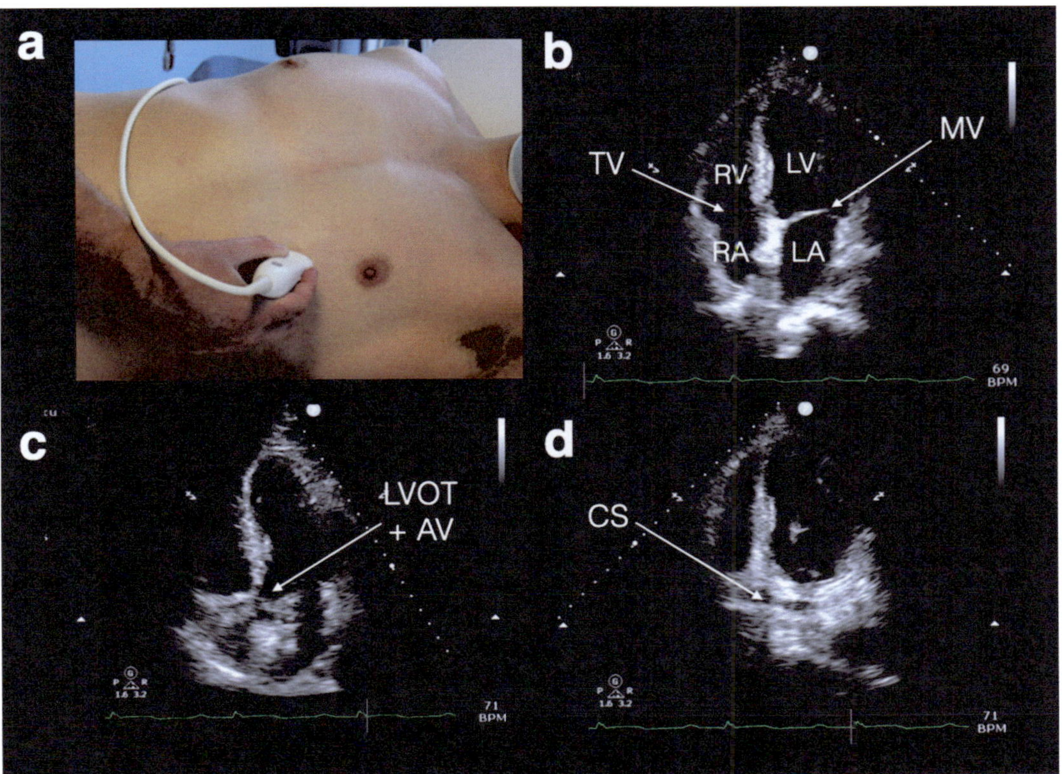

Fig. 7 The apical 4-chamber and 5-chamber views: **a** probe positioning; **b** the ideal A4C view; **c** the ideal A5C view; **d** the coronary sinus view [LV, left ventricle; MV, mitral valve LA, left atrium. RA, right atrium; TV, tricuspid valve RV, right ventricle; LVOT, left ventricular outflow tract; AV, aortic valve; CS, coronary sinus]

The apical 5-chamber (A5C) includes the LVOT.

Acquisition

1. Turn the patient as near as possible to the left lateral position (if possible)
2. Slide the probe to where you have identified the apex should be. Alternatively, start with the 5th/6th intercostal space, mid-clavicular line
3. Rotate the probe marker pointing towards the left, in line with the rib space
4. Fan the beam slightly upwards until you see a recognisable A4C
5. Slide down to the lowest rib-space that this can be seen
6. Adjust the depth so that both atria are in full view
7. Slide the beam out along the rib space until the LV apex is located in the middle of the near field
8. Rock the beam until the interventricular septum lies vertically in the middle of the screen
9. Fan the beam to open up both atria, including the pulmonary veins in the far field if possible (visible coronary sinus = too low; visible LVOT = too high)
10. Check if the LV apex is motionless and if it is the thinnest of all visible LV walls: if so, you are spot-on the true apex; if not, you may be foreshortening the ventricles. See Fig. 8.
11. Adjust the gain to make the chambers as black as possible, while keeping the structures clearly defined
12. Record your clip [A4C]
13. Fan upward to include the LVOT to obtain the A5C view
14. Record your clip [A5C].

Interpretation

The A4C and A5C views provide a huge amount of information, including:

- Relative chamber size (both ventricles)
- Global and regional wall motion (both ventricles)
- Atrial interdependence (fixed bowing of the interatrial septum)
- Gross mitral and tricuspid valve disease
- LVOT pathology (e.g. SAM) [A5C]
- Gross aortic valve disease [A5C]
- Doppler interrogation of stroke volume [A5C].

Pitfalls

In a foreshortened A4C (usually caused by imaging through a rib-space too high) all chambers appear short and round, and similar in shape and size. This is a common reason that right ventricular size is overestimated. Additionally, important apical wall motion abnormalities/pathologies (e.g. thrombus) can be missed and global LV systolic function can be overestimated. To avoid foreshortening, image the heart as low as possible and check that you are directly on the apex (see above).

Subcostal 4-Chamber View

Sonoanatomy

The subcostal 4-chamber (S4C) view is a useful view, particularly in a mechanically ventilated patient, when hyperinflated lungs can make other views difficult. It is the first-choice view during cardiac arrest since it can be integrated into cardiopulmonary resuscitation without interfering with chest compressions.

Acquisition

1. Turn the patient supine and, if possible, ask them to bend their knees and breathe in deeply; these manoeuvres bring the heart into view
2. Hold the probe with your hand over the top— like a flashlight (overhand grip), not a pen (as you have for other views)
3. Place it one probe width to the right of the xiphisternum and slide up to the costal margin with the probe orientation marker facing towards the patient's left; this avoids bony interference, minimises patient discomfort, and improves the image by using the liver as an acoustic window

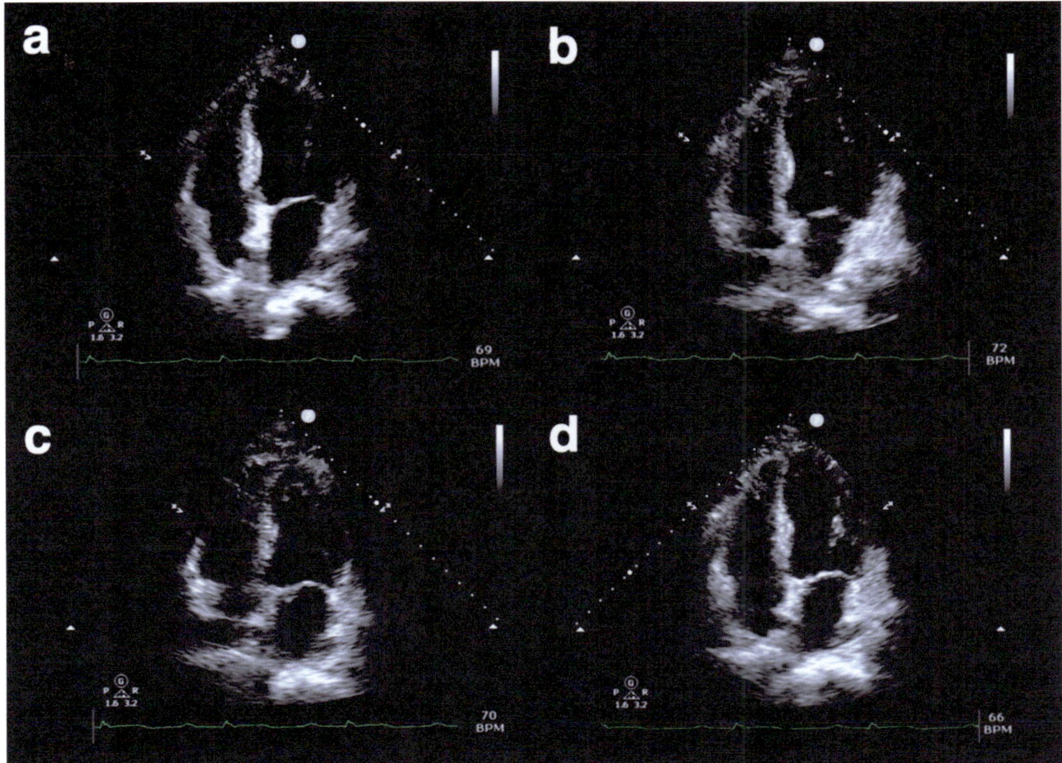

Fig. 8 Foreshortening in A4C [all images from the same patient]: **a** the ideal A4C view (the RV apex inserts short of the LV apex, the LV apex is the thinnest of all LV segments, the atria are fully opened up, and the right lower pulmonary vein (RLPV) is clearly seen in line with the IAS); **b** a foreshortened A4C view caused by sliding the beam to a rib space too high (the commonest error in ICU patients; the atria are too short, you can't see the RLPV, and intercostal ligaments obscure the RV free wall, making the right ventricle appear enlarged); **c** a foreshortened A4C view caused by fanning the beam too anteriorly (the RV 'apex' appears at the same level as the LV apex, making the right ventricle appear enlarged); **d** a foreshortened A4C caused by rocking the beam too medially (the RV 'apex' appears at the same level as the LV apex, making the right ventricle appear enlarged) [images courtesy of Professor Sharon Kay]

4. Rock the probe towards the patient's left shoulder and fan anteriorly until you see a recognisable S4C
5. Fine-tune these movements to open up the ventricles as much as possible, avoiding the LVOT if you can
6. Rotate the beam to visualise as much right ventricle as possible
7. Adjust the gain to make the chambers as black as possible, while keeping the structures clearly defined
8. Record your clip [S4C].

Interpretation

The S4C views provide a huge amount of information, including: see Fig. 9

- The pericardium (especially to guide pericardiocentesis)
- RV free wall thickness
- Interatrial septum

Pitfalls

S4C is not as reliable as A4C when it comes to assessing chamber size—small movements can

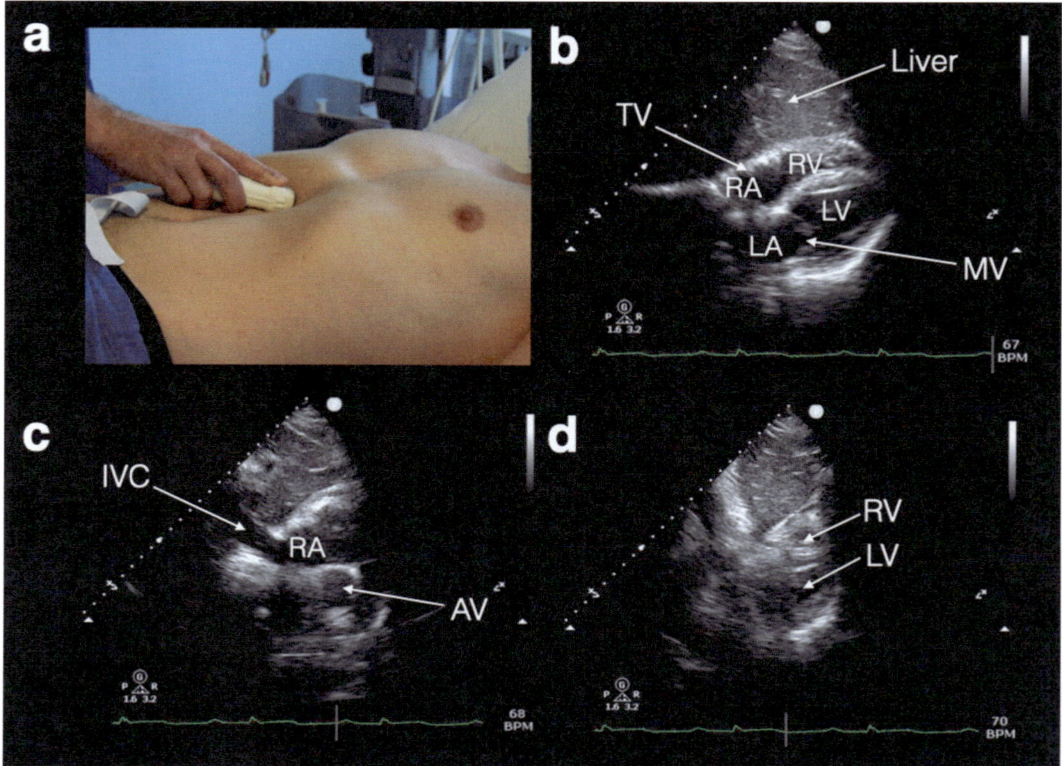

Fig. 9 The subcostal 4-chamber view: **a** probe positioning; **b** the ideal S4C view; **c** the IVC view; **d** the SSAX-MP view [LV, left ventricle; MV, mitral valve LA, left atrium; RA, right atrium; TV, tricuspid valve RV, right ventricle; IVC, inferior vena cava; images courtesy of Professor Sharon Kay]

make the right ventricle appear large or small—so exercise caution when observing RV dilatation. This is a reason why chamber sizes are not measured in this view.

S4C is often a difficult view to obtain, particularly when parasternal and apical view are easy, due to anatomical relationships within the chest. Using the liver as an acoustic window and pressing firmly both really help.

Subcostal Short-Axis Views (Including Inferior Vena Cava View)

Sonoanatomy

The subcostal short-axis (SSAX) views image the heart in the same way that PSAX views do. They share similar anatomical features, but SSAX images appear smaller and rotated in an anti-clockwise fashion.

Acquisition

1. Optimise your S4C view
2. Rock the beam so that the right atrium is located in the middle of the screen
3. Tilt the beam downwards slightly until the right atrium becomes the inferior vena cava in short-axis, keeping this in the middle of the screen; you will see the liver edge brightly enhance in the far field at this point
4. Rotate the beam anti-clockwise (up to 90°) until you visualise the long-axis of the inferior vena cava, running horizontally, and the superior hepatic vein joining it, running vertically in the near field

5. Adjust the gain to make the chambers as black as possible, while keeping the structures clearly defined
6. Record your clip [inferior vena caval (IVC) view]
7. If you wish to measure IVC diameter, do so within 1 cm of the superior hepatic vein
8. Fan the beam downwards to replicate all PSAX views
9. Record your clips [PSAX views].

Interpretation

The SSAX views provide useful information, including:

- Similar to that from PSAX views
- IVC size and variability

Pitfalls

When trying to find the inferior vena cava in long-axis, you can easily mistake the right hepatic vein for it and grossly underestimate IVC dimensions. See Fig. 10.

If assessing IVC variability in long-axis using M-mode, it is important to visualise the bright endothelial signal throughout. Otherwise, you might be imaging the vessel as it is being moved out of plane by spontaneous or mechanical ventilation.

Compared to PSAX views, SSAX views are smaller, which makes them harder to interpret, and their segments are rotated so take care not to misinterpret the territories of any regional wall motion abnormalities.

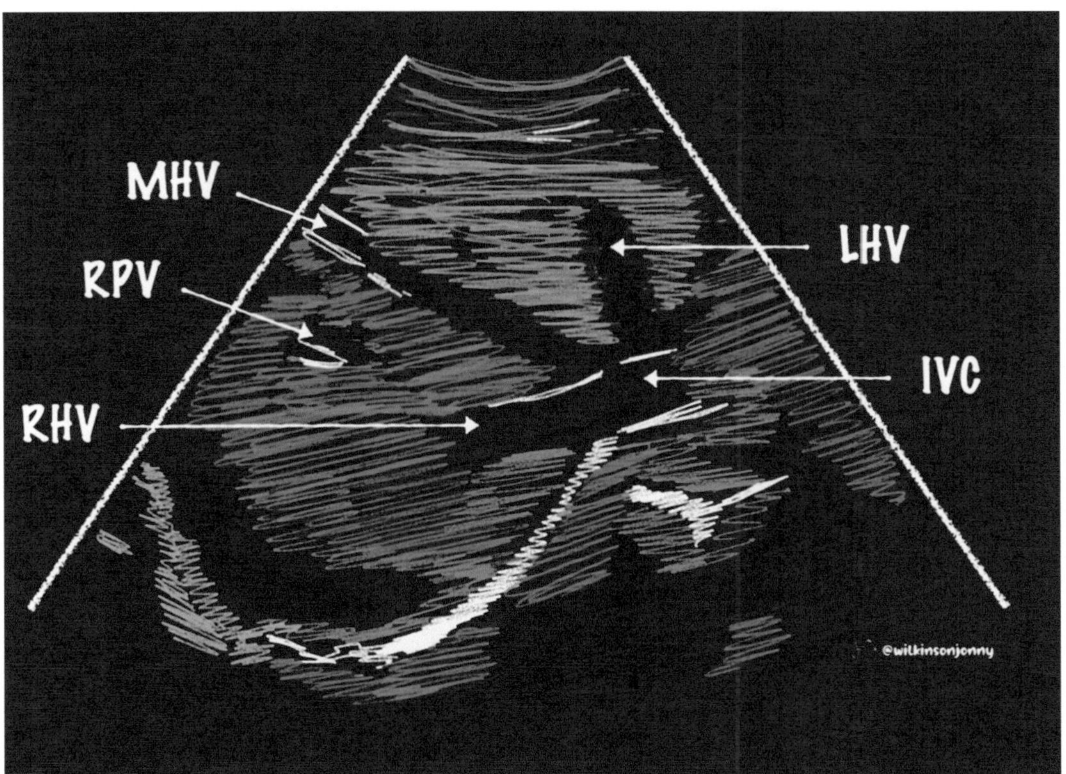

Fig. 10 A schematic demonstrating the close relationships between the inferior vena cava and hepatic veins; note how easy it might be to mistake the right hepatic vein for the IVC [RHV, right hepatic vein; RPV, right portal vein (anterior branch); MHV, middle hepatic vein; LHV, left hepatic vein; IVC, inferior vena cava]

Additional Views

Right Ventricular Inflow and Outflow Views

Sonoanatomy

The right ventricular inflow (RVI) and outflow (RVO) views are extremely close to PLAX—sometimes only 10° of fanning away—but image completely different structures. RVI visualises the inferior vena cava, coronary sinus, tricuspid valve and right ventricle. RVO visualises the RVOT, pulmonary valve, main pulmonary artery and occasionally the left and right pulmonary arteries. See Fig. 11.

Acquisition

1. Optimise your PLAX view
2. Fan the beam down towards the right hip until you see a recognisable RVI
3. Record your clip [RVI]
4. Fan the beam upwards, past PLAX until you see a recognisable RVO
5. Record your clip [RVO].

Interpretation

The RVI and RVO views provide useful information, including:

- Gross tricuspid valve pathology [RVI]

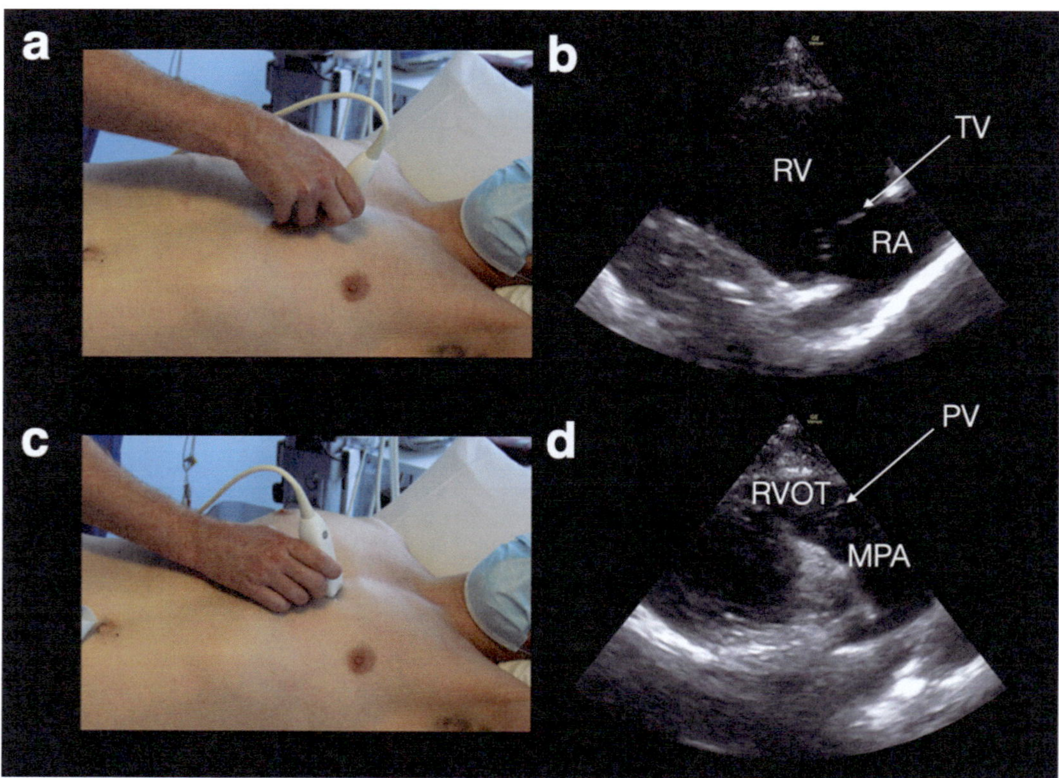

Fig. 11 The right ventricular inflow and outflow views: **a** probe positioning for RVI; **b** the ideal RVI view; **c** probe positioning for RVO; **d** the ideal RVO view [RV, right ventricle; TV, tricuspid valve; RA, right atrium; RVOT, right ventricular outflow tract; PV, pulmonary valve; MPA, main pulmonary artery]

- Colour and pulsed wave (PW) Doppler interrogation of the tricuspid valve [RVI]
- Gross pulmonary valve pathology [RVO].

Pitfalls

The degree of downward fanning will determine whether the inferior RV wall or the septum is in view. This alters which valve leaflets are seen.

Apical 2-Chamber and 3-Chamber Views

Sonoanatomy

All apical views contain the mitral valve, LA and LV cavities. The A4C view visualises the inferoseptal ('septal'), apex and lateral LV wall. Rotating the beam anticlockwise (probe orientation marker towards patient's head) produces the apical 2-chamber (A2C), which visualises the anterior and inferior LV walls without visualisation of the right ventricle. Further anti-clockwise rotation (orientation marker towards patient's right shoulder) produces the apical 3-chamber (A3C) (long-axis) view, which visualises the anterior septum and inferolateral ('posterior') LV wall in a similar way to PLAX. See Fig. 12.

Acquisition

1. Optimise your A4C view
2. Rotate the beam approximately 50° anticlockwise
3. Press down and out onto the lower rib; this opens up the space and makes the image clearer
4. Adjust the gain to make the chambers as black as possible, while keeping the structures clearly defined
5. Record your clip [A2C]

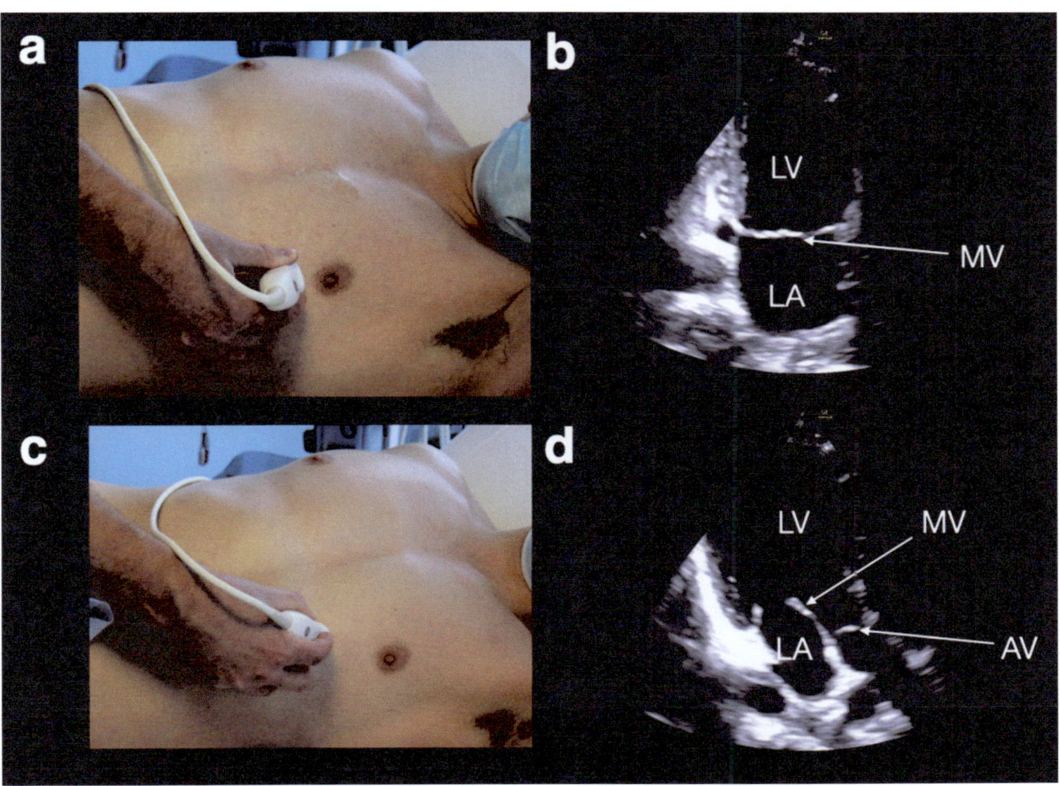

Fig. 12 The apical 2-chamber and 3-chamber views: **a** probe positioning for A2C; **b** the ideal A2C view; **c** probe positioning for A3C; **d** the ideal A3C view [LV, left ventricle; MV, mitral valve, LA, left atrium; AV, aortic valve]

6. Rotate a further 80° (130° from A4C)
7. Record your clip [A3C].

Interpretation

The A2C and A3C views provide useful information, including:

- Global and regional LV wall motion abnormalities
- Gross mitral valve disease
- LV ejection fraction [A4C and A2C]
- LVOT pathology [A3C]
- Doppler interrogation of stroke volume [A3C].

Pitfalls

The A2C is a difficult view to obtain in critically ill patients, partly because the apical view is difficult and partly because the imaging plane is oblique to the rib-space.

Suprasternal View

Sonoanatomy

The suprasternal (SS) view looks at the aortic arch and its branches—including the brachiocephalic ('innominate'), left common carotid, and left subclavian arteries—and the descending aorta. It also visualises the right pulmonary artery in short-axis beneath the arch. See Fig. 13.

Acquisition

1. Extend the patient's neck, if possible, in the supine position
2. Place the probe in the suprasternal notch with the marker towards the patient's left ear
3. Tilt the beam slightly inferiorly until you see a recognisable SS view

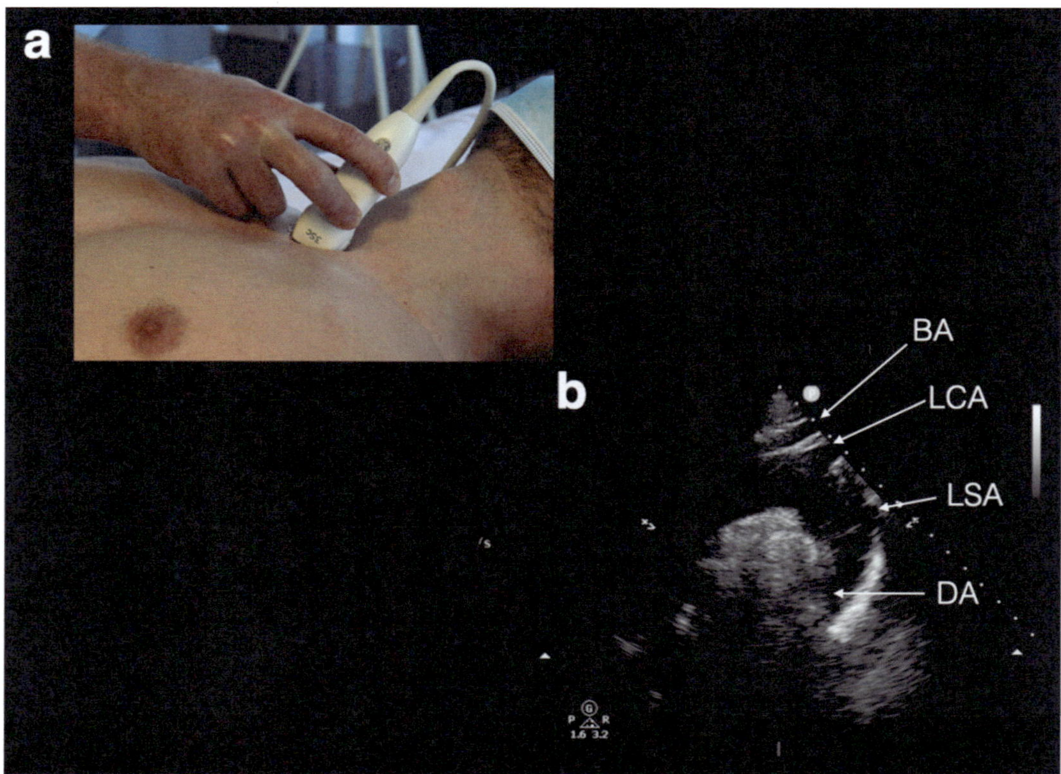

Fig. 13 The suprasternal view: **a** probe positioning; **b** the ideal SS view (note that the LSA is just out of view in this field) [BA, brachiocephalic ('innominate') artery; LCA, left common carotid artery; LSA, left subclavian artery DA, descending aorta; image courtesy of Professor Sharon Kay]

4. If this proves difficult, turn on colour Doppler as this can help you identify structures more easily

5. Record your clip [SS].

Interpretation

The SS view provides useful information, including:

- Aortic arch pathology.

Pitfalls

Patients' necks are sometimes difficult to access with a phased array probe; tracheostomies make this impossible.

Endotracheal tubes can distort anatomy.

SS imaging can be unpleasant in the awake patient.

Beyond 2D Imaging

Colour Doppler

This uses pulse wave technology to determine the velocity of blood, as it travels through chambers and vessels, and maps this in either red or blue over the 2D image according to its magnitude and direction. Like PW Doppler, colour Doppler has a limit above which it cannot determine velocity—known as the Nyquist limit—and it displays regions of blood flowing above this velocity as mosaics of the opposite colour (or green if the variance setting is activated). This is known as "aliasing". See Fig. 14.

Regurgitant jets usually cause aliasing primarily by generating high-velocity blood flow.

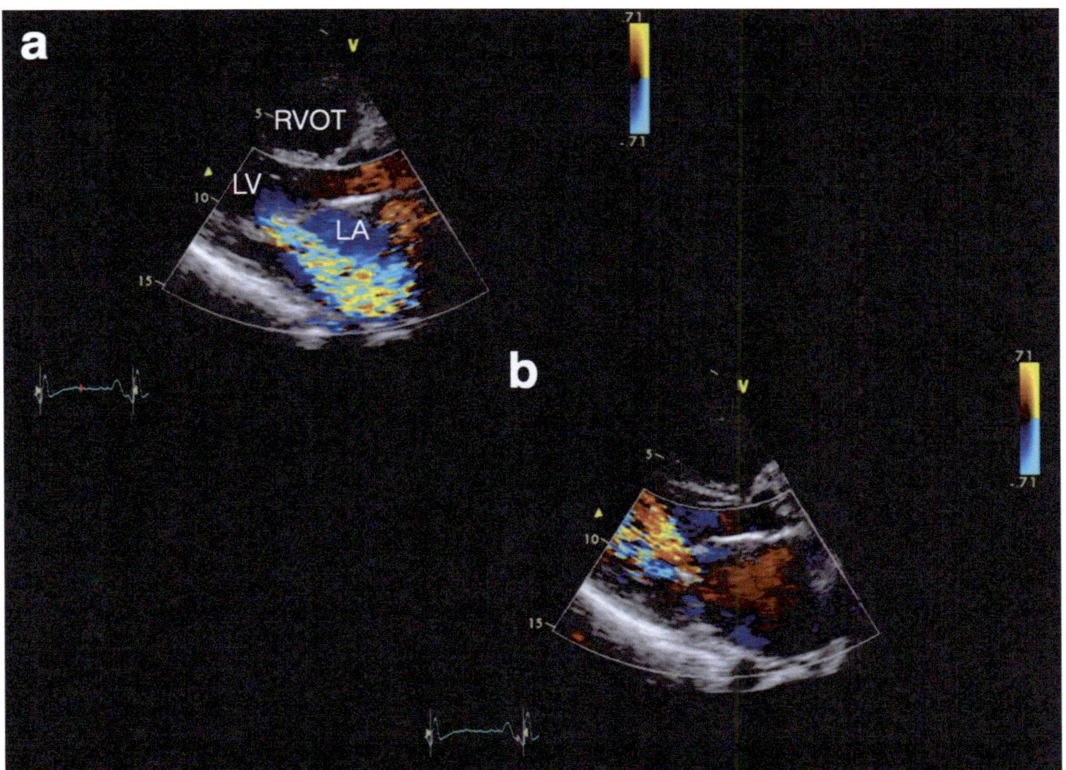

Fig. 14 Parasternal long-axis views with colour Doppler [images from the same patient with rheumatic heart disease] demonstrating: **a** high velocity flow in the left atrium during systole caused by mitral regurgitation; **b** turbulent flow in the left ventricle during diastole caused by mitral stenosis [LV, left ventricle; LA, left atrium; RVOT, right ventricular outflow tract]

They are particularly easy to see when directed into low-pressure chambers such as the atria, where their wave fronts cause preexisting red blood cells to swirl in different directions, contributing to the mosaic appearance. Generally speaking, how much area of the receiving chamber is taken up by aliasing determines the degree of regurgitation. However, there are caveats to this (see pitfalls below). Stenotic valves can cause similar mosaic patterns in downstream chambers, due to a combination of high velocity and turbulent flow.

Targets for colour Doppler interrogation include both sides of all valves, and each one should be imaged in more than one view. For instance, the tricuspid valve can be seen in PSAX, RVI, A4C, S4C and SSAX views.

Acquisition

1. Turn on colour Doppler
2. Set the area of the box over the chamber of interest and make it as narrow and shallow as possible to maximise frame-rate (temporal resolution) and Nyquist limit
3. Turn up the colour Doppler gain until everything inside the box becomes speckled with colour (due to random background noise), then turn it down until this just disappears; this avoids underestimation of flow signals
4. Set the baseline to zero
5. Set the scale to 50–60 cm/s to avoid under and overestimation of flow signals
6. Record your clip.

Interpretation

Colour Doppler provides useful information, including:

- Valvular regurgitation
- Valvular stenosis
- Shunts, communications
- Vessels that are difficult to see with 2D (e.g. SS view).

Pitfalls

Because colour Doppler is based on PW Doppler, when flow is perpendicular to the angle of intercept, the observed flow signal will be zero. However, zero signal does not mean that there is zero flow.

Setting the scale too high will underestimate the flow signal; setting it too low will overestimate it.

Regurgitation can hug the wall of a chamber —known as the Coanda effect—and may cause it to be visually underestimated.

Colour Doppler may underestimate valvular regurgitation when loading conditions change suddenly—such as the apparent reduction in mitral regurgitation (on lowering of blood pressure) after induction of anaesthesia.

Pulsed Wave Doppler

PW Doppler enables you to measure the velocity of blood flowing wherever you place the sampling volume. This is displayed on the screen as a continuous parabolic velocity-time trace, above and/or below the baseline depending on whether flow is towards and/or away from the probe. Because intracardiac blood flow tends to be laminar and the sampling volume is small, PW traces usually have a bright outer envelope and characteristically dark interior. See Fig. 15a.

PW Doppler has the same limitations of colour Doppler. It can only measure velocities up to the Nyquist limit, and anything above this will be displayed as an overlapping trace on the opposite side of the baseline. Adjusting the baseline towards this aliasing trace will cut/paste it back to the appropriate direction—but only up to point, after which it will recur.

Non-parallel imaging will underestimate velocity, so you should minimise the angle of intercept wherever possible. However, up to 20° either side is generally considered acceptable for measurement as this underestimates velocity by only 6%.

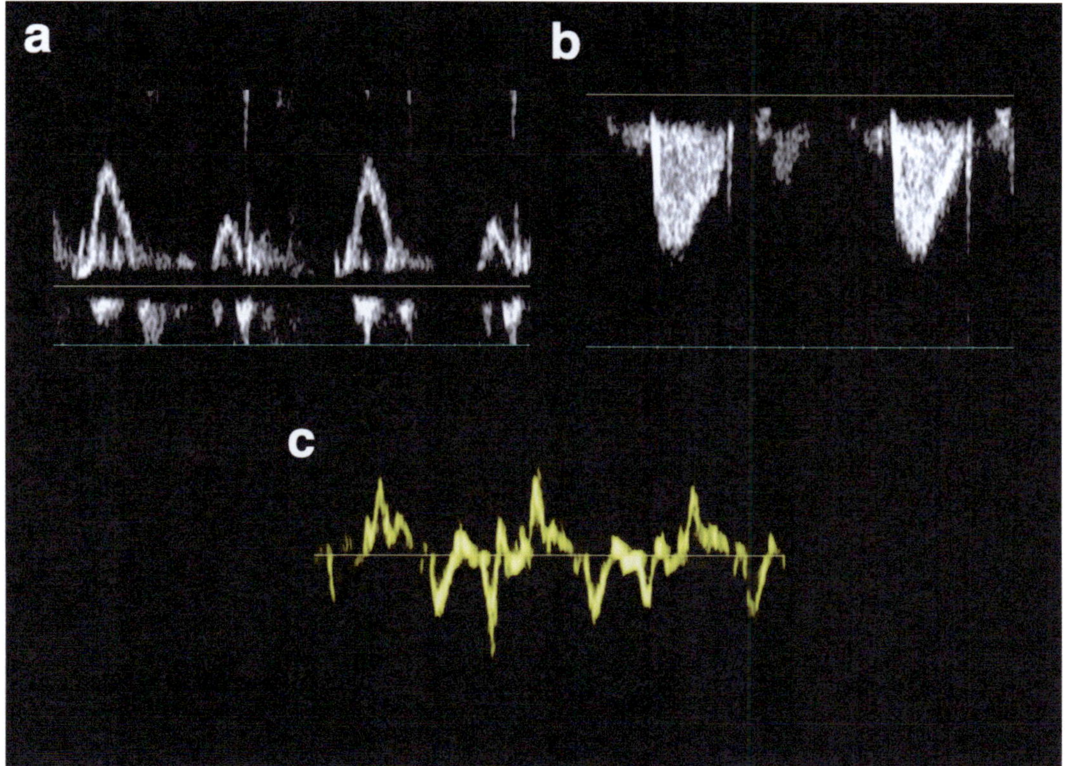

Fig. 15 Characteristic spectral doppler traces of: **a** PW Doppler (mitral inflow); **b** CW Doppler (aortic outflow); **c** tissue Doppler imaging (at the lateral MV annulus)

Acquisition

1. Turn on PW Doppler
2. Set the sampling volume at 3 mm
3. Place the sampling volume over the area of interest
4. Click PW again to activate the PW trace (the speaker will produce a moderately-pitched noise)
5. Adjust the baseline to maximise the trace of interest on the screen (i.e. entirely negative trace for LV outflow in A5C) and minimise any aliasing
6. Adjust the scale to maximise the height of the trace
7. Adjust the sweep speed to display three to five cardiac cycles
8. Freeze the image and track back to the most representative three cycles (five in the presence of atrial fibrillation)
9. Measure peak velocity and/or trace their perimeter using the velocity time integral (VTI) function
10. Record your clip.

Interrogation

Targets for PW Doppler interrogation include the LVOT [A5C; A3C] and mitral inflow [A4C]. Sampling volume placement is important for each of these: the same distance from the aortic valve that LVOT was measured, and between the open mitral leaflets, respectively.

Interpretation

PW Doppler provides useful information, including:

- LVOT VTI
- Mitral inflow: Early passive LV filling and active atrial contraction ('E and A waves').

Pitfalls

Placing the PW sampling volume within the aortic valve in the LVOT can cause overestimation of LVOT VTI due to eddy currents that are generated by flow acceleration at this point.

High velocities are uninterpretable with PW; continuous wave (CW) Doppler is required for this. For instance, peak tricuspid regurgitation velocity typically requires CW Doppler in the A4C or RVI views.

In arrhythmias, measurements may be increased or decreased depending on the duration of the previous cardiac cycle. This can be minimised by averaging measurements or using a single beat where the two preceding RR intervals have similar timings.

Continuous Wave Doppler

Like PW, continuous wave (CW) Doppler will underestimate velocity with non-parallel imaging, so it is very important to minimise the angle of intercept, particularly for high-velocity targets. Non-standard windows may be required to achieve this. See Fig. 15b.

Unlike PW, CW Doppler has no limitation to the velocities it can measure. However, it cannot determine where along the sampling line the peak velocity was generated. And because it measures all velocities simultaneously, a CW velocity-time trace is characteristically filled-in.

Acquisition

1. Turn on CW Doppler
2. Place the sampling line over the area of interest
3. Click CW again to activate the spectral trace (the speaker will produce a high-pitched noise)
4. Adjust the baseline to maximise the trace of interest on the screen
5. Adjust the scale to maximise the height of the trace
6. Adjust the sweep speed to display three to five cardiac cycles
7. Freeze the image and track back to the most representative three cycles (five in the presence of atrial fibrillation)
8. Measure peak velocity and/or trace their perimeter using the VTI function
9. Record your clip.

Interrogation

An important target for CW Doppler is the tricuspid valve. A small amount of regurgitation is common in the general population, and CW can be used to measure tricuspid regurgitation peak velocity (TR Vmax). TR Vmax >2.8 cm/s is an indicator of raised ventricular pressures, so if TR is seen with colour Doppler in PSAX, RVI, A4C, S4C and SSAX, further measurement techniques are necessary.

CW Doppler traces can also be used to calculate valve gradients, according to the simplified Bernoulli equation (peak gradient from peak velocity; mean gradient from VTI).

The only caveat to this is ruling in aortic stenosis using 'Dimensionless Index' (DI). In aortic stenosis, trans-aortic CW Doppler produces two simultaneous traces overlaid on one another—one tall (from the aortic valve); one short (from the LVOT). DI = LVOT/valve peak velocity ratio, and a value of <0.25 indicates severe aortic stenosis. DI avoids most of the major pitfalls associated with measuring gradients: effects of blood flow, LV impairment, sex and body size (and to some extent even angle of intercept) are all minimised by this technique.

Interpretation

CW Doppler provides useful information, including:

- Tricuspid regurgitation peak velocity (TR Vmax)
- Dimensionless index across the aortic valve

Pitfalls

A complete CW waveform should be parabolic. If it is truncated, you may not have included the whole target in the CW sampling line. And you should make very slow and small movements to see if this improves. Otherwise, peak velocity will be underestimated.

CW can't determine where along the sampling line the peak velocity came from. Therefore, it is possible to mistake one jet for another and make erroneous conclusions. For example, medially-directed eccentric mitral regurgitation can be easily mistaken for aortic outflow with CW Doppler in an A4C view.

In arrhythmias, measurements may be increased or decreased by the duration of the previous cardiac cycle. This can be minimised by averaging measurements or using a single beat where the two preceding RR intervals have similar timings.

Tissue Doppler

Tissue Doppler Imaging (TDI) uses PW Doppler with a low-pass filter to exclude high velocity targets, such as blood and valves, and image tissue movement inside the sampling volume. Velocity data is then mapped over the 2D image in red or blue, depending on direction and magnitude of tissue movement. See Fig. 15c.

TDI data is used in the assessment of systolic and diastolic ventricular function.

Acquisition

1. Turn on TDI
2. Place the sampling volume over the area of interest (usually the medial and lateral tricuspid or mitral valve annulus)
3. Click TDI again to activate the TDI trace (the speaker will produce a low-pitched noise)
4. Adjust the baseline to maximise the trace of interest on the screen
5. Adjust the scale to maximise the height of the trace
6. Adjust the sweep speed to display three to five cardiac cycles
7. Freeze the image and track back to the most representative three cycles (five in the presence of atrial fibrillation)
8. Measure desired velocities
9. Record your clip.

Interrogation

TDI is particularly useful for assessing systolic and diastolic performance of the bases of the ventricles. Placement and alignment of the TDI sampling volume is crucial for accuracy. Measurements of the left ventricle are usually taken at both the medial and lateral mitral valve annuli, then averaged.

Interpretation

TDI provides useful information, including:

- LV basal wall peak early diastolic velocity (e′)
- LV basal wall peak systolic velocity (LV S′)
- RV basal wall peak systolic velocity (RV S′).

Pitfalls

Care must be taken to measure the correct part of the TDI trace, which should have a crisp white edge. Resonance can cause a fuzzy 'beard' that should be avoided. The inner black-white envelope usually follows the same shape as the true outer white-black envelope, so tracking the former can help you avoid overestimating the latter.

Basal ventricular regional wall motion abnormalities will underestimate TDI values at that point.

Conclusion

TTE provides unparalleled insight into the structure and function of the heart. Coupled with other aspects of POCUS, it enables a considerably thorough assessment of the patient's pathophysiology and haemodynamics. TTE encompasses a broad range of skills, some of which require more experience than others. So, when progressing your skillset beyond the basics it is important to be supported by good supervision. In this chapter, we have outlined the core skills involved in POCUS and introduced some more advanced modalities to explain their fundamentals. These will be built upon in subsequent chapters to give you all the tools you need to assess critically ill patients using cardiopulmonary POCUS.

Fundamentals of Transesophageal Echocardiography

Fabio Guarracino and Marcelo Haertel Miglioranza

Learning is the only thing the mind never exhausts, never fears and never regrets.
Leonardo da Vinci. Italian Polymath (1452–1519 AD).

Abstract

Transesophageal echocardiography (TOE) is becoming more frequent imaging tool for the emergency evaluation of unstable patients at the point of care. TOE has clear advantages, providing additional diagnostic information for embolic sources, endocarditis, aortic dissection, intracardiac shunt, loculated pericardial effusion, and superior vena cava assessment. This chapter outlines the process and sequence of image acquisition involved in TOE. Further assessments will be discussed in subsequent chapters which will give you all the tools you need to assess critically ill patients with TOE POCUS.

F. Guarracino
Department of Anesthesia and Critical Care Medicine, Cardiothoracic and Vascular Anesthesia and Intensive Care at Azienda Ospedaliero Universitaria in Pisa, Pisa, Italy

M. Haertel Miglioranza (✉)
Echocardiography Lab—EcoHaertel/Mãe de Deus Hospital, Porto Alegre, Brasil
e-mail: marcelohaertel@gmail.com

Federal University of Health Sciences of Porto Alegre, Porto Alegre, Brasil

Keywords

TOE · TEE · Transoesophageal echocardiography · POCUS

Key Messages

- Transesophageal echocardiography (TOE) is becoming more frequent imaging tool for the emergency evaluation of unstable patients at the point of care
- TOE has clear advantages over TTE, providing additional diagnostic information for embolic sources, endocarditis, aortic dissection, intracardiac shunt, loculated pericardial effusion, and superior vena cava assessment
- Safety of performing TOE is crucial to minimise risk of complications.

Introduction

Even though transthoracic echocardiography (TTE) is well established as the principal methodology in critical care assessment, transesophageal echocardiography (TOE) is becoming more frequent for the emergent evaluation of

Table 1 List of absolute and relative contraindications to TOE

Absolute contraindications	Relative contraindications
– Perforated viscus – Esophageal stricture – Esophageal tumor – Esophageal perforation, laceration – Esophageal diverticulum – Active upper GI bleed	– History of radiation to neck and mediastinum – History of GI surgery – Recent upper GI bleed – Barrett's esophagus – History of dysphagia – Restriction of neck mobility (severe cervical arthritis, atlantoaxial joint disease) – Symptomatic hiatal hernia – Esophageal varices – Coagulopathy, thrombocytopenia – Active esophagitis – Active peptic ulcer disease

unstable patients. TOE has clear advantages, providing additional diagnostic information for embolic sources, endocarditis, aortic dissection, intracardiac shunt, loculated pericardial effusion, and superior vena cava assessment. A better therapeutic decision-making process for hemodynamic instability and hypoxemia management is also provided [1]. In addition, a significant parcel of critical care patients has suboptimal image quality TTE studies. Around 45% of the patients with ventilatory support have lung hyperinflation and inadequate TTE images. Obesity, edema, subcutaneous emphysema, inability to position the patient, and the presence of wounds and chest devices are the other common factors related to the TTE's low performance. The proximity of the esophagus to the heart and great vessels possibility an excellent ultrasonic window bypassing most of the TTE images limitations. Thus, a goal-directed TOE has been proposed as an advanced-level skill in critical care ultrasound.

Indications and Patient Selection

The main indications include evaluating cardiac and aortic structure and function in situations where the results of TTE are nondiagnostic, and the TOE findings may potentially alter management [2, 3]. Usually, these situations include compromised TTE image quality; hemodynamic instability and hypoxemia in critically ill patients; evaluation of prosthetic heart valves and paravalvular abscess; masses and embolic sources

evaluation; and the detailed evaluation of the structures that are typically in the far-field, such as the aorta and the left atria appendage [1, 3].

Despite being a minimally invasive and safe procedure, some potential rare complications could occur. The most frequent are esophageal abrasion, perforation, bleeding, dysphagia, and laryngospasm [4–6]. Thus, the procedure's safety should be carefully evaluated on a case-by-case basis in the face of relative contraindications (Table 1) to determine if the benefits exceed the potential risks. The TOE should be contraindicated when the overall procedure risk exceeds the potential diagnostic benefit (Table 1).

Patient Preparation

The TOE examination is usually performed with the patient under conscious sedation or anesthesia. Thus, general measures are required to secure airway protection and patient stability (e.g., cardiac and oxygen saturation monitoring, noninvasive blood pressure, supplemental oxygen, intravenous access). A fasting period of six hours is desired, mainly for non-intubated patients. During the procedure, the patients should be placed in a left lateral decubitus position, with the head of the bed elevated 30° to prevent aspiration. Local anesthesia of the oropharynx and appropriate doses of intravenous narcotic and/or sedative agents are recommended. Patients intubated on mechanical ventilatory support require less airway preparation. In these cases, the intravenous sedation should be augmented, if necessary, to provide unconscious during the examination.

Probe Manipulation and Insertion

The TOE probe is inserted orally into the esophagus in the same manner in which an orogastric tube is placed, keeping the face of the transducer positioned anteriorly. With the probe at the esophageal inlet, the patient is asked to swallow while the operator advances the probe. A jaw lift maneuver could help the insertion, and the advancement should carefully continue unless resistance is met. The probe is kept in a neutral position during any advancement or withdrawal. In mechanically ventilated patients, a standard intubating laryngoscope could be used to insert the TOE probe into the esophagus under direct vision. Alternatively, the TOE probe may be inserted "blindly". This process may be facilitated by neck flexion, jaw thrust, and ensuring a midline insertion while avoiding rotation of the probe. If resistance is met at any point during intubation or the performance of the study, force should never be applied to advance the endoscope. It should be noted that the inflated cuff of the orotracheal tube could compress the esophagus, making it difficult to pass the probe. For cardiac imaging, the probe introduction ranges from the upper esophagus (visualization of great vessels), mid and lower esophagus (visualization of the left atrium and main heart structures) to the stomach (left and right ventricle). Before passing the probe, a bite block should be placed to protect the shaft from teeth or gums.

After insertion of the TOE probe into the esophagus, several composed movements are used to alter its position and orientation, generating different two-dimensional image cut-planes (Table 2). Thus, each echocardiographic view results from a specific position and orientation of the ultrasound beam achieved through maneuvers concerning the heart. Therefore, understanding the imaging plane orientation is essential for visualizing and interpreting the cardiac structures.

Goal-Directed TOE in Critical Care

The American Society of Echocardiography (ASE) chas described 28 standard TOE views of the heart (Fig. 1) for a comprehensive examination, which could have some alternative or additional particular views [4]. Although, this thorough evaluation is not always feasible in the critical care scenario. Usually, the physician should balance between a fastidiously complete and a focused examination to address a specific diagnostic question.

Whether focused or comprehensive TOE examination, it should evaluate all pertinent heart structures (valve and chambers) and myocardium segments in at least two orthogonal planes. There is no "correct" systematic and sequential approach to the exam. A commonly accepted method is based on progressive esophageal advancement of the probe to evaluate cardiac anatomy and function, followed by progressive withdrawal for the aorta evaluation.

– Mid Esophageal ascending aortic short-axis view (Fig. 1, image 8)

From the initial position, after introduction into the esophagus, the probe is slightly advanced approximately 30 cm until the proximal aorta is seen. The probe angle is then rotated, usually between 0° and 45°, until a true short axis is seen. The main pulmonary artery bifurcating is seen, and the right pulmonary artery will lie posterior and perpendicular to the proximal aorta. This view helps identify pulmonary artery catheter placement and visualize thromboembolism in the pulmonary artery.

– Mid Esophageal right pulmonary vein view (Fig. 1, image 9)

From the previous view, the probe is turned to the right to display the right pulmonary vein entering into the left atrium. Minimal changes in depth and angle may be needed to optimize this view. Usually, the superior vena cava is often seen in the short axis.

Table 2 Maneuvers during the transesophageal echocardiographic probe manipulation

Maneuvers	Description
Advancement/withdrawal	Changing the transducer distance from the month, possibly the position in the upper, middle, and lower esophagus or intragastric (distances noted on the endoscope shaft). The degree of insertion can be determined by the depth markings imprinted on the shaft
Flexion	Performed by rotation of the control knobs on the shaft of the endoscope. The large knob movement results in anteflexion of the probe face or retroflection of the probe face. The small knob movement results in right and left flexion of the probe face
Turn	Twisting the probe shaft in a counterclockwise (left side of the patient) or clockwise motion (right side of the patient)
Rotation	Correspond to the changing of the plane of orientation of the crystal within the endoscope. The angle indicator represents the exact orientation of the transducer on the screen with values between 0○ and 180○

– Mid Esophageal ascending aortic long-axis view (Fig. 1, image 7)

After turning back, the probe to the left, the ascending aortic short-axis view is reacquired. The probe angle should be rotated to visualize the proximal aorta in the long axis. The right pulmonary artery is seen in cross-section.

– Mid Esophageal aortic valve short-axis view (Fig. 1, image 10)

The imaging plane is rotated back to 30-45°. Then the probe is advanced approximately to 35 cm to visualize the aortic valve (AV) in short-axis, positioned in the center of the screen. To achieve a "true" short axis of the AV, a clear

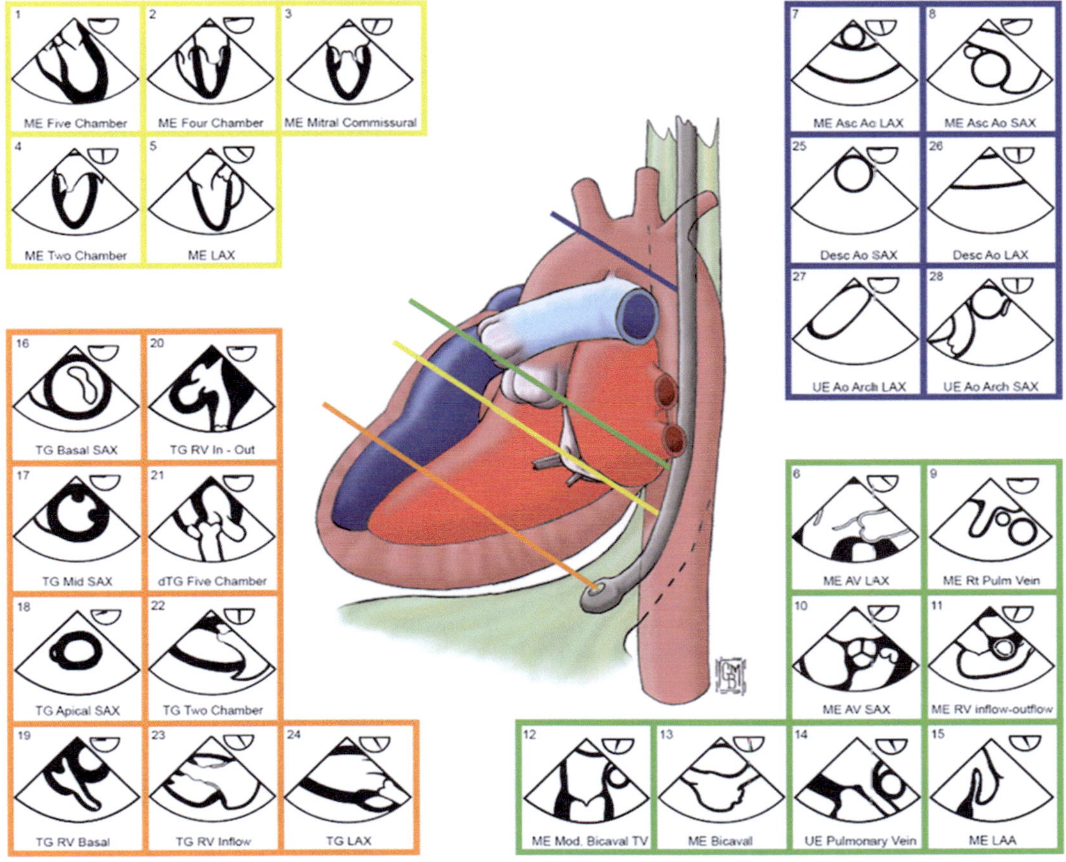

Fig. 1 Comprehensive transesophageal echocardiographic views (this schematic figure is from the book–Perioperative Transesophageal Echocardiography in Cardiac Surgery Procedures–Springer)

view of all three aortic valve leaflets and commissures with a coaptation point should be seen.

– Mid Esophageal Right Ventricular Inflow–Outflow (Fig. 1, image 11)

After completing the ME short-axis view of the aortic valve, three views will be obtained at the aortic valve level in the longitudinal plane. For the first view, start at the ME aortic valve short-axis and change the rotation angle of the imaging to approximately 60° to 90° without moving the probe. We will visualize the tricuspid valve, right ventricular outflow tract (RVOT), and proximal pulmonary artery for this acquisition. This view may help confirm the location of a pulmonary artery catheter. In addition, an echo-dense linear

image corresponding to the pulmonary artery catheter will be seen in the proximal pulmonary artery if it is in the correct position.

– Mid Esophageal Modified Bicaval Tricuspid Valve View (Fig. 1, image 12)

Turning the probe to the right, a ME-modified bicaval tricuspid valve view is obtained. Noneccentric tricuspid regurgitation jets are usually adequately interrogated in this view.

– Mid Esophageal Aortic Valve Long-Axis View (Fig. 1, image 6)

The ME aortic valve long-axis view is obtained by slightly turning the probe toward the patient's left and rotating the imaging angle to approximately 110° to 130°. This projection should display the left ventricular outflow tract (LVOT), AV, and proximal ascending aorta. Additional structures to observe are the mitral valve, the sinus of Valsalva, the sinotubular junction, and sometimes the coronary artery ostium (slight probe twist). The primary objective is to evaluate aortic valve function and dimensions of the LVOT, aortic annulus, and sinotubular junction. In addition, the proximal ascending aorta wall should be inspected for integrity. An important limitation of this view is the impossibility of visualizing the distal ascending aorta.

– Mid Esophageal Bicaval View (Fig. 1, image 13)

By turning the probe clockwise to the patient's right and slightly reducing the image angle by 5–15°, the ME bicaval view is then obtained. The key structures in this view are the left and right atria, inferior and superior vena cavae, interatrial septum, and right atrial appendage. In addition, a minor adjustment to probe depth and multiplane angle will often bring the tricuspid valve or coronary sinus into view. The primary diagnostic goals of this view are to examine for atrial chamber enlargements and the presence of a patent foramen ovale or an atrial septal defect and to detect intra-atrial air. In addition, the integrity of the intra-atrial septum should be evaluated by color Doppler or bubble contrast.

This view may be helpful in the assessment of catheters' positions, superior vena cava thrombus, and assessment of volume responsiveness.

– Mid (Upper) Esophageal Right and Left Pulmonary Vein View (Fig. 1, image 14)

The acquisition of pulmonary vein views is tough to be obtained in all patients. Each patient has slightly different images angles, and the lower pulmonary veins are in the extreme near field and perpendicular to the ultrasound beam. To visualize the right veins, the probe should be turned rightward from the ME bicaval view, and sometimes a slightly withdraw, or angle correction is needed. The right upper vein will be seen entering into the left atrium from the approximate 4 o'clock position, heading posteriorly toward the apex of the imaging sector. The probe should be turned leftward (counterclockwise) from the ME bicaval view to visualize the left-sided veins.

– Mid Esophageal Five-Chamber and Four-Chamber Views (Fig. 1, image 1 and 2)

The imaging angle is turned to 0°, and the TOE probe is advanced to the mitral valve level. Depending on the patient, either the four-chamber or five-chamber view will be seen. The five-chamber view is obtained, moving the probe slightly cranially from the four-chamber view. In the five-chamber view, portions of the LVOT and AV will be seen, and the tricuspid valve is often obscured or not seen in its entirety. General chamber morphology and sizes can be interpreted in this view, but the four-chamber view is more consistently obtained. The probe and slightly advancing or rotating the imaging plane to 5° to 10° should produce the ME four-chamber view by retroflection. It is essential to notice that the true left ventricular apex is not visualized at these acquisitions. The probe should be twisted right for a more dedicated right chambers view.

The ME four-chamber view is one of the most diagnostically valuable views in TOE. The fundamental structures to observe are the left atrium, left ventricle, right atrium, right ventricle, the mitral and tricuspid valves, and the inferoseptal and anterolateral walls of the myocardium. The diagnostic goals of this view include evaluation of chamber size and function, valvular function (both mitral and tricuspid), and regional motion of the septal and lateral walls of the left ventricle.

– Mid Esophageal Mitral Commissural View (Fig. 1, image 3)

Rotating the ultrasound beam to approximately 60°, the mitral valve will be displayed in a characteristic P1-A2-P3 appearance. In this view, both the posteromedial and anterolateral papillary muscles will be visible, with chords seen going to the anterior and posterior leaflets. This view is fundamental to the localization of structural mitral valve pathology.

– Mid Esophageal Two-Chamber View (Fig. 1, image 4)

The ME two-chamber view will be obtained by rotating the imaging angle to approximately 60° to 90°. This view is identified by the appearance of the left atrial appendage and the absence of right-sided heart structures. It allows visualization of the anterior and inferior walls of the left ventricle. Occasionally, the left ventricle is foreshortened, and the true apex is not seen. When the true apex is visualized, ventricular thrombus or hypokinesis at the apex is often best appreciated in this view. The primary goals of this view are to evaluate left ventricular function (especially the apex) and anterior and inferior regional wall motion. It can also be used to look for a thrombus of the left atrial appendage.

– Mid Esophageal Left Atrial Appendage View (Fig. 1, image 15)

From the ME two-chamber view, a slight probe manipulation is done to focus and maximize the left atrial appendage (LAA) opening and apex.

– Mid Esophageal Left Pulmonary Vein View.

From either the two-chamber or LAA view, withdraw the probe slightly to visualize better the left upper pulmonary vein entering the left atrium. Again, minimal manipulation of the probe is needed to open up the course of the upper vein.

– Mid Esophageal Long-Axis View (Fig. 1, image 5)

After evaluation of the left-sided pulmonary veins, the probe is further rotated to approximately 120° or until the LVOT is seen. Small amounts of rotation and flexion will allow for maximizing the diameter of the outflow tract. This view is similar to the ME aortic valve long-axis. However, most left ventricular cavities, mitral valve (inflow), and LVOT are seen. This view allows for the identification of mitral valve prolapse, the systolic anterior motion of the mitral valve, and localization of the A2 and P2 scallops of the mitral valve. In addition, assessment of regional wall motion and global function of the anteroseptal and inferolateral walls of the ventricle is possible in this view.

– Transgastric Basal, Midpapillary and Apical Short-Axis Views (Fig. 1, image 16, 17, and 18).

The probe is advanced, entering into the stomachs, and then withdrawn and anteflexed to obtain the TG basal short-axis view of the left ventricle. The probe is then advanced, anteflexed, and withdrawn until contact with the stomach wall. The ultrasound beam should be rotated back to 0°. The "fish mouth" view indicates a basal view. Anterior leaflet chords are seen on the left and posterior chords on the right. All six basal left ventricular wall segments are seen in this view.

The TG midpapillary short-axis view is obtained by advancing the probe. The fundamental structures to visualize are the left ventricular walls and cavity in addition to the posteromedial and anterolateral papillary muscles. A true short-axis cross-section of the left ventricle is confirmed when the two papillary muscles are approximately equal in size. If chordae tendineae are visible, the probe is too high and should be advanced. If no papillary muscle is visible, the probe is often too low and should be withdrawn. The primary diagnostic goals of this view are assessment of left ventricular systolic function, left ventricular volume, and regional wall motion. All six midpapillary left ventricular wall segments are seen in this view.

The probe is then slightly advanced and anteflexed (if necessary) to visualize the apical left ventricular cavity in a short axis for the apical TG view.

– Transgastric Two-Chamber View (Fig. 1, image 22)

The probe should be positioned to the midpapillary short-axis view, and the imaging angle should be rotated to approximately 90°. This provides an image of the left ventricle and the mitral valve. The primary diagnostic goal of this view is the analysis of regional wall motion. In addition, this is the preferred view for evaluating the support structures of the mitral valve because they lie perpendicular to the ultrasound beam.

– Transgastric Long-Axis View (Fig. 1, image 24)

The probe is rotated to approximately 120°, and the LVOT and aortic valve should come into view at 4 o'clock. This view is especially helpful in the spectral Doppler interrogation of the aortic valve and LVOT, essential for hemodynamic evaluation.

– Transgastric Right Ventricular Inflow View (Fig. 1, image 23)

The probe angle is rotated back to 90° and then turned right until the right ventricular inflow view is seen. This view helps evaluate right ventricular wall thickening and tricuspid valve pathology.

– Deep Transgastric Five-Chamber View (Fig. 1, image 21)

With the probe rotated back to 0°, advanced toward the left ventricular apex, then maximally anteflexed and slightly withdrawn, the deep transgastric view is achieved. This view allows spectral Doppler interrogation of the LVOT and aortic valves. Probe rotation may be necessary to optimize the Doppler interrogation.

– Transgastric Right Ventricular Basal View (Fig. 1, image 19)

From the deep transgrastric five-chamber view, the probe is anteflexed, withdrawn slightly, and turned rightward to obtain the right ventricular basal view. Minor manipulations will be required to optimize this view. All three leaflets of the tricuspid valve should be seen with the septal leaflet on the right, the posterior leaflet in the near field, and the anterior leaflet in the far-field. The RVOT and pulmonic valve are seen progressing toward the image far field.

– Transgastric Right Ventricular Inflow–Outflow View (Fig. 1, image 20)

The probe is then rightward flexed to obtain the right ventricular inflow–outflow view.

This view allows general inspection of the right ventricle's tricuspid inflow and pulmonic outflow.

– Descending Aorta Short-Axis View (Fig. 1, image 25)

After completion of the evaluation of the ventricles, the probe is rotated to 0°, and the shaft is turned to the patient's left and slightly withdrawn until a transverse view of the descending aorta is obtained (the descending aorta short-axis view). Some maneuvers are necessary to optimize aortic imaging. First, the image depth is reduced to enlarge the displayed aortic image. Second, the time gain compensation in the near field may have to be increased because it is often set at low levels during the cardiac examination. Finally, the frequency of the transducer can be increased to enhance resolution. The aorta is then examined along its course as the probe is slowly withdrawn. When the aorta begins to appear elongated, the probe has reached the level of the aortic arch.

– Upper Esophageal Aortic Arch Long-Axis View (Fig. 1, image 27)

At the level of the arch, the probe is turned rightward to visualize the distal ascending aorta and arch on the long axis. This view is often helpful in evaluating the distal ascending aorta for the presence of parietal abnormalities.

– Upper Esophageal Aortic Arch Short-Axis View (Fig. 1, image 28)

The imaging angle is then turned to 90° to obtain the upper esophageal aortic arch short-axis view. A slight left and right turn of the probe shaft will allow you to interrogate the arch for calcification, enlargement, and foreign bodies. You may see the origins of the great vessels at approximately 3 o'clock in the short axis of the aortic arch. The innominate vein and the origin of the left subclavian artery are visualized in this view. The pulmonary artery lies parallel to the imaging beam affording excellent Doppler interrogation.

– Descending Aorta Long-Axis View (Fig. 1, image 26).

After completion of the aortic arch views, the probe is slowly advanced to obtain the longitudinal view of the descending aorta (the descending aorta long-axis view). During the probe is advancement, slight left and right turns will permit better interrogation of the aortic walls.

In the critical care environment, we recommend starting the examination focusing on the clinical question in the context of patient's instability. In this case, an abbreviated or focused study plays a crucial clinical role is appropriated. The physician should be facile with a comprehensive exam but dynamically abbreviate the exam and add accessory views according to clinical picture and TTE or TOE findings. The aim should do the minimum number of views that provide the information in the shortest time.

Training and Technical Skills

The competency for training and certification in TOE differs among countries and medical societies [4, 6–10]. There are several guidelines addressing the prerequisites for learning and practice. In general, TOE is seen as an advanced echocardiographic procedure that must be performed just by experienced and certified physicians. To achieve the TOE level competence a cardiology-based training, a primary prerequisite is first to domain the knowledge of the TTE (Table 3). A minimal number of 75 to 150 TOE exams performed under supervision is recommended for complete training according to different medical societies. However, for the anesthesiology-based training, the competence of TTE is not required.

Table 3 Cognitive and technical skills required for competence in transesophageal echocardiography

Cognitive skills	Technical skills
• Basic knowledge for echocardiography and TTE	• Proficiency in using conscious sedation safely and effectively
• Knowledge of the appropriate indications, contraindications, and risks of TOE	• Proficiency in performing a complete transthoracic echocardiographic examination, using all echocardiographic modalities relevant to the case
• Understanding of the differential diagnostic considerations in each clinical case	• Proficiency in safely passing the TOE transducer into the esophagus and stomach and in adjusting probe position to obtain the necessary tomographic images and Doppler data
• Knowledge of infection control measures and electrical safety issues related to the use of TOE	• Proficiency in operating the ultrasonographic instrument correctly, including all controls affecting the quality of the displayed data
• Understanding of conscious sedation, including the actions, side effects, and risks of sedative drugs, and cardiorespiratory monitoring	• Proficiency in recognizing abnormalities of cardiac structure and function as detected from the transesophageal and transgastric windows, distinguishing normal from abnormal findings, and recognizing artifacts

(continued)

Table 3 (continued)

Cognitive skills	Technical skills
• Knowledge of normal cardiovascular anatomy, as visualized tomographically by TOE	• Proficiency in performing qualitative and quantitative analyses of the echocardiographic data
• Knowledge of alterations in cardiovascular anatomy that result from acquired and congenital heart diseases and of their appearance on TOE	• Proficiency in producing a cogently written report of echocardiographic findings and their clinical implications
• Understanding component techniques for transthoracic echocardiography and TOE, including when to use these methods to investigate specific clinical questions	
• Ability to distinguish adequate from inadequate echocardiographic data and distinguish an acceptable from an inadequate TOE examination	
• Knowledge of other cardiovascular diagnostic methods for correlation with TOE findings	
• Ability to communicate examination results to the patient, other health care professionals, and medical records	

Adapted from Quinones et al. [10]

Conclusion

Goal-directed (focused) TOE examination is an advanced diagnostic method in critically ill patients, providing additional information mainly for hemodynamic instability and hypoxemia management. This semi-invasive approach is indicated in situations when the TTE is suboptimal or nondiagnostic, enabling a better visualization of far-field structures. Goal-directed TOE encompasses a broad range of advanced-level skills, including the knowledge domain of the TTE. Therefore, supervision training is fundamental during the learning process. This chapter outlines the process and sequence of image acquisition involved in TOE. Further assessments will be discussed in subsequent chapters which will give you all the tools you need to assess critically ill patients with TOE POCUS.

References

1. Heidenreich PA, Stainback RF, Redberg RF, Schiller NB, Cohen NH, Foster E. Transesophageal echocardiography predicts mortality in critically III patients with unexplained hypotension. J Am Coll Cardiol. 1995;26(1):152–8. https://doi.org/10.1016/0735-1097(95)00129-N.
2. Peterson GE, Brickner ME, Reimold SC. Transesophageal echocardiography. Circulation. 2003;107(19):2398–402. https://doi.org/10.1161/01.CIR.0000071540.97144.89.
3. ACCF/ASE/AHA/ASNC/HFSA/HRS/SCAI/SCCM/SCCT/SCMR 2011 Appropriate Use Criteria for Echocardiography. J Am Soc Echocardiogr. 2011;24(3):229–267. https://doi.org/10.1016/j.echo.2010.12.008.
4. Hahn RT, Abraham T, Adams MS, et al. Guidelines for performing a comprehensive transesophageal echocardiographic examination: recommendations from the american society of echocardiography and the society of cardiovascular anesthesiologists. J Am Soc Echocardiogr. 2013;26(9):921–64. https://doi.org/10.1016/j.echo.2013.07.009.
5. Shanewise JS, Cheung AT, Aronson S, et al. ASE/SCA guidelines for performing a comprehensive intraoperative multiplane transesophageal echocardiography examination: recommendations of the american society of echocardiography council for intraoperative echocardiography and the society of cardiovasc. Anesth Analg. 1999;89(4):870. https://doi.org/10.1097/00000539-199910000-00010.
6. cFlachskampf FA, Badano L, Daniel WG, et al. Recommendations for transoesophageal echocardiography: update 2010. Eur J Echocardiogr. 2010;11(7):557–76. https://doi.org/10.1093/ejechocard/jeq057.
7. Beller GA, Bonow RO, Fuster V. ACCF 2008 recommendations for training in adult cardiovascular medicine core cardiology training (COCATS 3) (Revision of the 2002 COCATS Training Statement).

J Am Coll Cardiol. 2008;51(3):335–8. https://doi.org/10.1016/j.jacc.2007.11.008.

8. Cahalan MK, Stewart W, Pearlman A, et al. American society of echocardiography and society of cardiovascular anesthesiologists task force guidelines for training in perioperative echocardiography. J Am Soc Echocardiogr. 2002;15(6):647–52. https://doi.org/10.1067/mje.2002.123956.

9. Béïque F, Ali M, Hynes M, et al. Canadian guidelines for training in adult perioperative transesophageal echocardiography. Can J Cardiol. 2006;22(12):1015–27. https://doi.org/10.1016/S0828-282X(06)70317-8.

10. Quiñones MA, Douglas PS, Foster E, et al. ACC/AHA clinical competence statement on echocardiography a report of the American College of Cardiology/American Heart Association/American College of Physicians-American Society of Internal Medicine Task Force on Clinical Competence. J Am Coll Cardiol. 2003 Feb 19;41(4):687–708. https://doi.org/10.1016/s0735-1097(02)02885-1

Fundamentals of Lung and Diaphragmatic Ultrasound

Giovanni Ferrari and Gianmaria Cammarota

The danger of a non-invasive exam lies not in its performance but in its interpretation

Anonymous

Abstract

Lung ultrasound (LUS) is a tool of indisputable usefulness for diagnosis and monitoring of various lung diseases. Basic principles of LUS and lung artifacts will be described in this chapter, in order to learn how to perform a scan of the thorax and how to recognize and differentiate a normal from a pathological lung. This chapter also describes the evaluation of the diaphragm with ultrasound (DUS), highlighting the techniques to assess movement and thickening of the diaphragm. DUS is useful in several situations from assessing diaphragm dysfunction in the critically ill patients or as an index for weaning from mechanical ventilation.

Keywords

POCUS · Ultrasound · Diaphragm and lung

Key Messages:

- LUS is a safe, rapid and repeatable imaging tool that can evaluate a variety of lung parenchymal and pleural disorders
- LUS is superior to CXR in evaluating pleural effusion, consolidation, pulmonary congestion and pneumothorax
- Diaphragmatic ultrasound can be used effectively in evaluating difficulty weaning from mechanical ventilation due to diaphragmatic weakness.
- Integration of LUS with Echocardiography is crucial in evaluating cardiopulmonary disorders in critical care and emergency settings.

Supplementary Information The online version contains supplementary material available at https://doi.org/10.1007/978-3-031-29472-3_6.

G. Ferrari (✉)
Pneumologia e Unità di Terapia Semi-Intensiva Pneumologica, AO Mauriziano, L.go Turati 62, 10128 Torino, Italy
e-mail: giovanniferrarister@gmail.com

G. Cammarota
Department of Medicine and Surgery, Università degli Studi di Perugia, Service of Anesthesiology and Intensive Care Unit 2, Azienda Ospedaliera di Perugia, S. Andrea delle Fratte, 06156 Perugia, Italy

Introduction

Lung ultrasound (LUS) is a relatively simple and useful technique, requires a few minutes to be performed, especially in the critically ill patients and is an important tool for diagnosis and monitoring. LUS allows differential diagnosis in dyspnoeic patients differentiating conditions that despite having similar clinical presentation, they require different treatments. Moreover, LUS doesn't expose patients to ionizing radiation, can be easily performed at the bedside avoiding mobilization of unstable patients. LUS is an accurate tool for diagnosis, has a similar accuracy to Chest Computed Tomography (CT) for the diagnosis of pneumonia, has a higher accuracy than chest X-Ray for diagnosing pneumonia and pneumothorax, has a high sensitivity for the detection of pleural effusion and, finally, is a tool of indisputable value for procedural guidance (Table 1). Furthermore, LUS can be performed repeatedly at the bedside as a part of clinical assessment and follow up of patients [1].

All these advantages explain the widespread use of LUS in daily clinical practice.

Ultrasound Assessment of the Lungs

LUS can be performed in the two-dimensional mode (2D mode) or in motion mode (M mode) imaging. The former allows to visualize a two-dimensional image, while the latter allows to visualize a moving image over time along a single scan line.

When the transducer is placed on the chest, over intercostal spaces, US waves penetrate through the skin, muscles, soft tissues, reaching the visceral pleura and the ribs. At the level of the ribs, almost all echoes are reflected: the ribs appear as a hyperechoic structure and underneath is a dark anechoic shadow (video 1).

At the level of tissue/pleural interface there is always a high acoustic impedance and more than 80% of the US waves are reflected like a mirror, generating a hyperechoic, horizontal image that represents the pleural interface. The sliding of the two pleural layers, parietal and visceral, appears as a dynamic movement, synchronous with respiration (video 1). The lung sliding is an important indicator of ventilation in the evaluated thoracic area. Below this hyperechoic line, other artifact generated can be observed. Since US beam is reflected several times from the pleural interface, this to and fro phenomenon makes a misleading interpretation by the US software that the pleural interface is deeper. This reverberation artifact produced by the rebound of the ultrasound wave between the pleural interface and the transducer, generates artifacts, the so called 'A lines', appearing as horizontal lines, separated each by a distance that corresponds to the distance from the transducer and the pleura (video 2).

When alveolar air is reduced and fluids or inflammatory material is increased, the mirror effects disappear. This phenomenon happens because the acoustic impedance of tissues and alveoli flooded with fluids are close to one other and US wave can spread easily, generating a real image [1].

Table 1 .

Advantages of lung ultrasonography
Rapid evaluation
Useful for differential diagnosis (dyspnoea, chest pain, pulmonary oedema, pleural effusion)
Guide/assistance in invasive procedures (thoracentesis, chest drainage, lung biopsy, central venous catheters)
Assess diaphragmatic dysfunction
Evaluation of pleural pathology
Monitoring lung pathologies (evaluation of reaeration/dearetation (recruitment/derecruitment) during mechanical ventilation, proning, following recruitment manoeuvres etc.)

Table 2 A line is a static artifact parallel to the pleural interface. It is observed in the normal lung. In presence of a pneumothorax, A lines are visualized, but no sliding is observed. B line is a dynamic artifact, it begins at the pleural interface and spreads towards the edge of the screen. B lines are a pathological sign observed when there is a moderate loss of aeration. Tissue like appearance of the lung (as occurs in pneumonia or in atelectasis) is no longer an artifact but a real image of the lung whit total loss of aeration. When fluid accumulates in the pleural space, ultrasonography can rapidly help to identify liquid and estimate the amount of pleural fluid

Clinical condition	Artifact	Artifact
Normal lung	Air	A lines, sliding
Pneumothorax	Air	A lines, no sliding
Interstitial syndrome	Mild to moderate loss of areation	B lines
Pneumonia	Total loss of areation	Tissue like appearance (consolidation)
Pleural effusion	Fluid between the two pleural layers	Anechoic space; echoes in the fluid suggestive of exudative or complex effusion

An intermediate condition occurs when fluids are increased in the interlobular septa and alveolar air is slightly decreased, the altered balance between air and fluid in the interlobular septa and the consequent thickening creates a reverberation of the US beam creating vertical artifacts, the so called 'B lines (video 3). Appearance of the lung in different clinical conditions is summarized in Table 2. B lines are defined as vertical—laser like—artifacts, synchronous with respiratory movements, arising from the pleural interface, extending to the bottom of the screen never fading down, erasing A lines. Many factors (included US machine settings) may influence B lines visualization: tissue harmonic imaging, transducer type and frequency, focus setting, gain and frame rate [2].

In 2D mode, in the normally aerated lung, placing the transducer in vertically shows the characteristic "bat sign" with two rib shadows at the edge of the screen and the pleural interface in between at the center with the sliding of the two pleural layers (video 1). In M-mode, the pleural sliding will be depicted as 'sea-shore sign' or 'waves on a sandy beach' because the motion in the normally aerated lung creates artifacts that return to the US machine creating a speckled appearance (the *seashore* sign) Fig. 1. In pneumothorax, 2D mode will demonstrate loss of sliding (video 4) and in M-mode there will be no movement detected below the pleura, creating a linear appearance 'barcode or *stratosphere* sign' (Fig. 2).

Patient Position

The patient is generally evaluated in the supine or semi-recumbent position. Scanning position depends also on the pathology that is suspected: supine position and scanning of anterior chest wall is requested for assessing pneumothorax, while a comprehensive scan of anterior, lateral and posterior areas of the thorax will be necessary in suspected lung parenchymal disease. To explore dorsal regions, lateral decubitus is a good alternative to sitting position if the patient can't assume the latter position.

Transducer Selection (Fig. 3)

Ultrasound machines are generally equipped with the following transducers:

- Linear transducer: high frequency (2–15 MHz), poor penetration and high resolution; useful for pleural line and diaphragm visualization.

Fig. 1 Seashore sign: the parallel lines over the pleural interface correspond to the thoracic wall, while the "sandy" pattern below the pleural interface represents the dynamic artifact of lung parenchyma

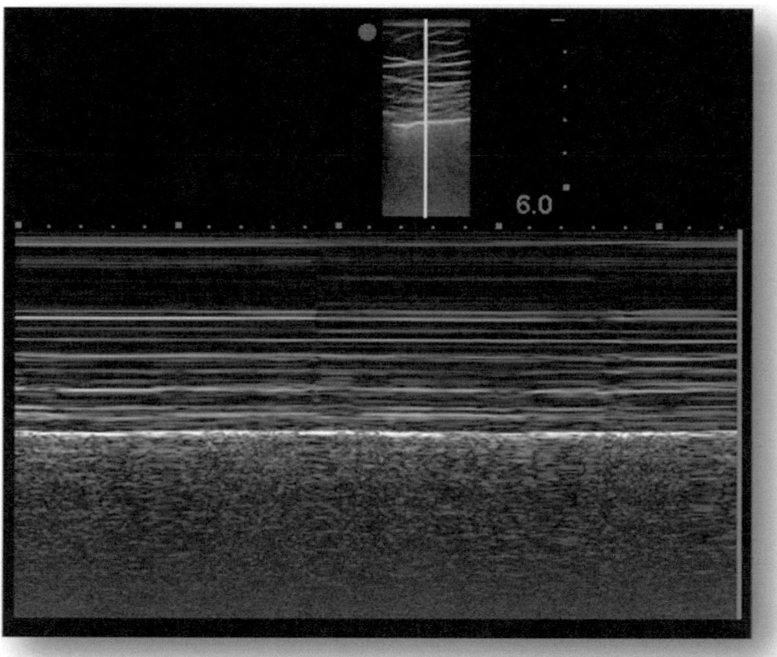

Fig. 2 Stratosphere sign: in the presence of a pneumothorax (lung sliding absent), the seashore sign is replaced with uniform horizontal lines named the stratosphere sign or bar-code sign

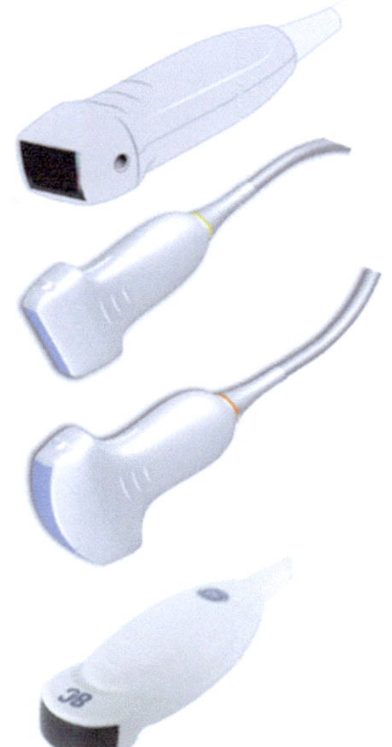

Fig. 3 Different ultrasound transducers used to perform lung ultrasound: the phased array, the linear, the curvilinear and the microconvex transducer

- Curvilinear transducer: low frequency (2–10 MHz), acceptable resolution, good penetration; suitable for parenchymal assessment
- Phased array: low frequency (2–7.5 MHz), good penetration. suitable for parenchymal assessment
- Microconvex transducer: (2–22 MHz), acceptable resolution and good penetration. Suitable for pleural as well as parenchymal assessment.

Each transducer has pros and con, but ideally each one can be used whichever is available. An important issue is to set up the US machine to achieve a good image: choose lung preset if available, set the focus point at the level of interest, adjust frequency according to the anatomical site of interest (high frequency for pleural interface/diaphragm—low frequency for effusion/parenchyma), optimize depth should be set to 10 cm when scanning the parenchyma; exclude tissue harmonic imaging, optimize gain and time gain compensation (TGC).

How and where to perform a scan:

The US probe should be placed in the intercostal spaces in each of the 6 areas of the two hemithoraces. These areas are anterior, lateral and posterior and are identified as follows (Fig. 4a–c):

(a) Anterior area is limited by parasternal line and anterior axillary line;

(b) Lateral area is located between anterior and posterior axillary lines;

(c) Posterior area is located between posterior axillary line and paravertebral line. Part of the posterior area is difficult to assess due to the presence of the scapula.

Each area is also divided into superior and inferior zones with an imaginary line passing through the fourth intercostal space.

An approach suggested is to place the transducer in a longitudinal (vertical) position over an intercostal space, so that at the centre of the screen there will be a hyperechoic artifact (i.e. the pleural line) and at the two edges of the

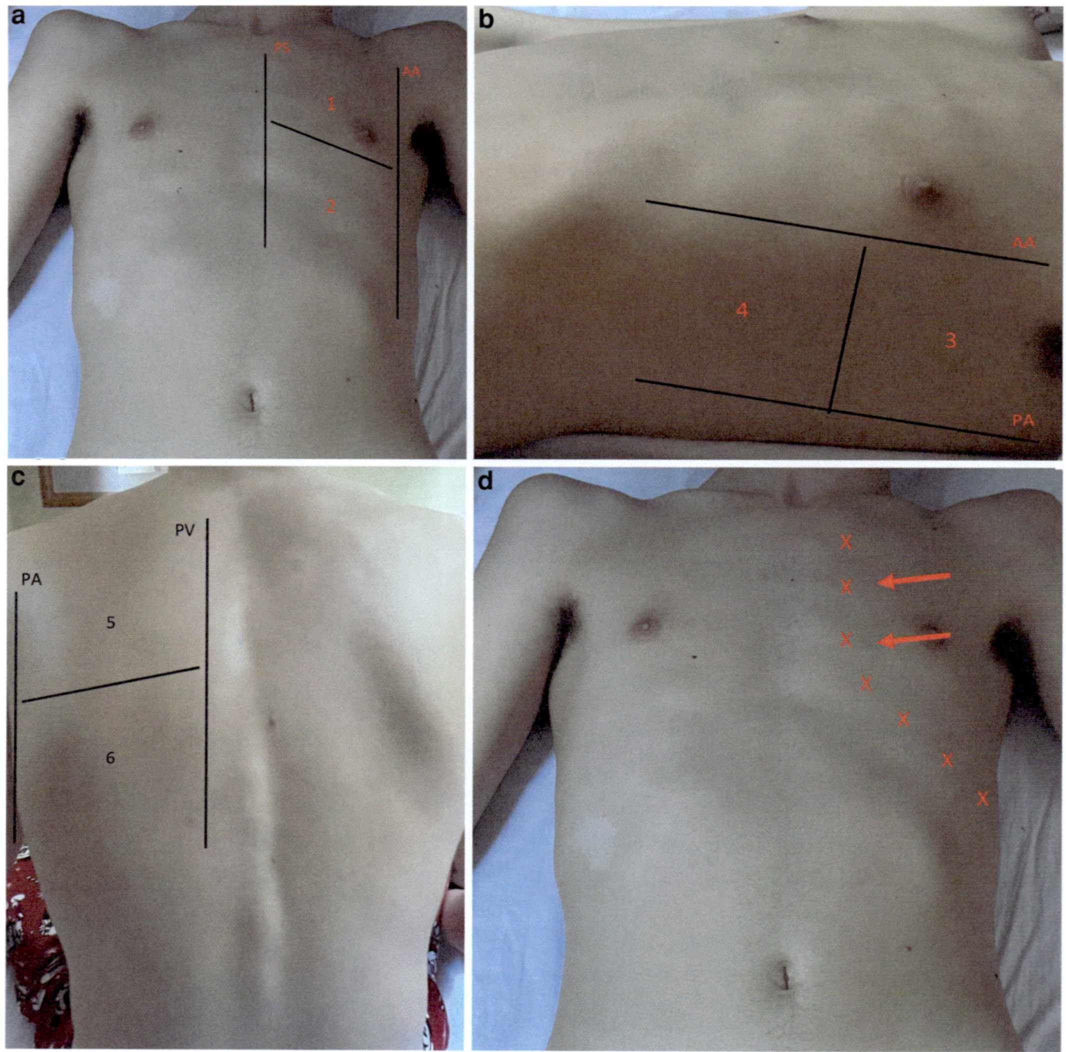

Fig. 4 a, b Scanning technique of the anterolateral zones of the chest. PS: para-sternal line; AA: anterior axillary line; PA: poster axillary line. 1: upper anterior zone; 2: lower anterior zone; 3: upper lateral zone; 4: inferior lateral zone. c Scanning technique of the posterior zones of the chest. PA: poster axillary line; PV: para-vertebral line. 5: upper posterior zone; 6 inferior posterior zone

screen, the two hyperechoic edges of the ribs with posterior hypoechoic shadows, depicting the so called "bat sign" (Fig. 5, video 1). Later the probe should be rotated counter-clockwise and placed in an oblique position in alignment with the intercostal space which allows a more extensive visualization of pleural surface [3].

Once the pleural line is identified, three US signs should be evaluated:

– Sliding: lung sliding is a horizontal movement of the pleural line, synchronous with the respiratory cycle that indicates the movement of the visceral pleura over the parietal pleura (video 1). In presence of a pneumothorax, air separates the two pleural layers, the sliding disappears (video 1a).

– A lines: associated with lung sliding, they are horizontal reverberation artefacts of the

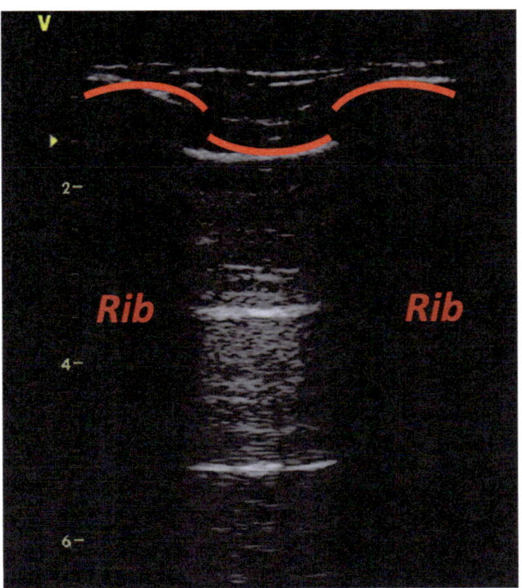

Fig. 5 The bat-sign: at the edge of the screen, the ribs resemble the wings of the bat, while in the center of the screen the pleural line seems the body of the bat. A correct visualization of this sign is observed with the probe in the longitudinal scan. The bat sign is always observed, except in subcutaneous emphysema

pleural line. Due to the difference to acoustic impedance, A lines result from US reflection between two interfaces with a high reflection coefficient (air and tissue) and are visualized below the pleural line at multiples of the distance of the probe and the pleural interface (videos 2a and b).

– B lines: they are vertical (laser-like) artifacts, originating from the pleural interface, hyperechoic, synchronous with respiratory movement, extending to the bottom of the screen, erasing A lines. You can see up to two individual B lines in one scanning zone in the normal lung especially in dependant zones. They originate at the interlobular septa and are created by the reflection of the US beam in areas where there is an increase in extravascular lung water (videos 3a, 3b and 3c) [3].

Another sign than should be assessed is the lung pulse, the rhythmic, vertical movement of the pleura, synchronous with cardiac beats, meaning that the two pleural layers attached, ruling out pneumothorax (video 5).

Other structures that should be identified are the liver, the kidneys and the diaphragm, that appears as a hyperechoic surface if evaluated with the curvilinear probe or as a three-layered structure if a linear probe is used.

A complete evaluation should assess ideally all the zones of the thorax. Several approaches are described in the literature, however there has been no consensus on which protocol to choose. As previously observed, the thorax is divided into zones (6 zones for each lung).

– Another simple approach consists of a 3 point examination of each hemi-thorax (BLUE Protocol). This approach can be used in the intensive care unit.
– Another approach uses an 8 zones scanning protocol (4 for each side) assessing anterior and lateral areas. This approach suggested for the interstitial syndrome, however, it doesn't include the evaluation of the posterior areas.

Briefly, we can conclude that different approaches are available and the scanning protocol can be chosen according to the clinical context (ICU/HDU, cardiology ward, emergency room etc.) and the evaluated pathology.

LUS in Lung Disease

The normal lung is generally characterized by the presence of lung sliding, A lines, absence of pleural effusion, very few B lines in the dependent areas: up to two B lines in a single intercostal space (often in the elderly, seldom in younger patients).

In the following paragraph, a brief summary of LUS in different lung diseases will be discussed:

– **Pneumothorax**: when air accumulates in the pleural space, the movement of the two pleural layers will not be seen (i.e.: loss of pleural sliding) (videos 1a and 4). A lines will be seen, but there will be no sliding, because the presence of intrapleural air prevents the transmission of movements to parietal pleura. In M-mode, the stratosphere pattern is present (Fig. 2). If no sliding is observed, but B lines are present, pneumothorax can be ruled out, because B lines originates at the level of the pleural line in the interlobular septa. A specific sign of pneumothorax is the presence of the lung-point, The transition zone between an area of lung sliding and an area with no lung sliding (videos 6 and 6a). M mode is helpful in assessing the absence of sliding with the appearance of a linear artifact (the *stratosphere* sign).

How to examine the chest in search of POCUS signs of pneumothorax (Fig. 4d)?

- The presence of normal lung sliding rules out a pneumothorax at the site of probe application.
- The absence of lung sliding suggest the presence of a pneumothorax and the presence of a lung point is diagnostic of a pneumothorax.
- Use a high frequency probe, positioned on the anterior chest wall about a the mid clavicular line, infv the intercostal space.
- In most cases, with the patient supine, air can be seen in areas marked in the figure with red arrows.
- Moving the probe laterally, identifying the presence of sliding, will suggest an incomplete pneumothorax, and the presence of a lung-point allows the diagnosis of a pneumothorax with a specificity of 100%.

- **Pleural effusion (videos 7a and 7b)**: the accumulation of fluids in the pleural space is often visualized as an anechoic space between the parietal pleura and the lung. The presence of echoes in the fluid is suggestive of exudative or haemorrhagic effusion (Plankton sign) (Video 7d). In a free, non- complex effusion, a dynamic sign observed in M-mode is the 'sinusoid sign' which represent the sinusoidal movement of the visceral pleura synchronous with the respiratory cycle. Many approaches have been suggested to estimate effusion volume. A simple one is to measure interpleural distance: a distance greater than 5 cm between parietal and visceral pleura is predictive of an effusion >500 ml. Video 7c demonstrates pleural effusion, atelectasis and lung point (pneumothorax) in the same scan. LUS is superior to CXR for determining the presence of pleural fluid, predicting the characteristics of the fluid, and guiding pleural intervention. An important application of LUS is guidance during procedures such as thoracentesis or drainage placement. LUS is also used to identify intercostal vessels and aberrant vessel position that would contraindicate needle insertion (videos 7e and 7f demonstrate intercostal vessel identification before drainage tube positioning. A lung-point can be viewed in video 7e).

- **Interstitial syndrome**: three or more B lines in a longitudinal scan indicates the presence of interstitial syndrome. Interstitial syndrome in observed in cardiogenic pulmonary oedema (video 3), interstitial lung diseases, pneumonia, pulmonary contusion, acute respiratory distress syndrome (ARDS) (video 8).

- **Interstitial lung diseases**: different conditions whether primary or secondary, can cause pulmonary fibrosis. The interlobular septa are thickened, and interstitial syndrome is characteristic in these patients. The number of B lines on LUS correlates with Chest CT pattern and has a high diagnostic accuracy.

- **Pneumonia**: LUS can be considered as a *densitometer* of the lungs; the more is the alveolar air deprivation, the more is the appearance of consolidations. Consolidations can appear as small hypoechoic sub-pleural areas with peri-lesional B lines, margins may appear irregular and shredded which is better assessed with the linear transducer. When all the lung becomes totally deareated the typical appearance of 'hepatization' is characteristic of lobar consolidation. The presence of a dynamic air bronchogram has a high specificity and positive predictive value for pneumonia (Video 9), while a static air bronchogram is observed in atelectasis and rarely in pneumonia (video 5).

- **Atelectasis**: a sonographic differential diagnosis between consolidation and atelectasis may be difficult. If dynamic air bronchogram is specific for pneumonia, static air bronchogram can be seen in both conditions. The presence of large pleural effusion may suggest a compressive atelectasis (video 11), while a small pleural effusion makes pneumonia more likely (video 10).

Limitations of LUS

LUS has many advantages and a few limitations to keep in mind:

- LUS is a surface analysis; if the pulmonary disease doesn't reach the pleura or if air is interposed between the lesion and the pleura and if the lesion is covered by the bones, LUS will often fail to visualize any image.
- Rarely, lack of patient cooperation may affect the accuracy of the LUS evaluation.
- Surgical drainage and chest dressing may prevent access to areas of the thorax involved.
- Subcutaneous emphysema may affect or prevent the acquisition of a good LUS image. In the latter case, it becomes difficult to visualize the two important landmarks (i.e.: the ribs) and in between the pleural interface. Some vertical artifacts will be present, the so called 'E lines', not to be confused with the B lines. Those E lines arise from the subcutaneous tissue and not the pleural line. They are also well defined, and they erase B lines but they don't move synchronously with respiration.

Fundamentals of Diaphragmatic Ultrasound

The diaphragm is the pillar of respiratory muscles involved in the breathing function. It has a domed structure consisting of a central tendinous part and a peripheral one with a prevalent muscular component. From a functional point of view, the latter is divided into two parts: the crural part with medial localization, originating from the L2–L4 tract of lumbar spine and the associated ligaments. And the costal part which is more extended compared to crural one, located laterally, and is in apposition to the internal surface of the lower six ribs. This zone of apposition (ZOA) between the diaphragm and the ribs plays a key role in the determination of breathing because the shortening of the ZOA muscular fibers induces a lowering of the central dome with a consequent decrease in pleural pressure. The lowering of the central dome increases the abdominal pressure, resulting in an outward displacement of the anterior abdominal wall; moreover, the contraction of the muscle fibers of the costal part of the diaphragm causes a lifting of the lower portion of the thoracic cage, deforming it outwards and anteriorly. All these modifications lead to an excursion of the diaphragm in the cranio-caudal direction, with a consequent increase in the size of the thorax, a drop in the pleural pressure, and a final lung inflation. During the breath, the diaphragm activity is under the continuous control of the respiratory neural centers localized in the brainstem that transfer their output to the diaphragm through phrenic nerves arising from C3–C5 nerve roots.

In the clinical settings, diaphragmatic activity monitoring is nowadays of a widespread application in the intensive care unit (ICU), by means of the assessment of the electrical activity of diaphragm, trans-diaphragmatic pressure, and ultrasonographic assessment. However, contrary to the electrical activity of the diaphragm and trans-diaphragmatic pressure assessment, the evaluation of diaphragm function with POCUS has been increasingly investigated both in and outside the ICU in the last years. The growing popularity of POCUS in diaphragmatic assessment is due to: a non-invasive tool promptly available at bedside, does not expose the patients to ionizing radiation, provides immediate results, and is characterized by good levels of reliability as well as intra- and inter-observer agreements.

Technical Aspects and Measurements

Equipment required to perform a sonographic assessment of diaphragmatic function is easily available both in and outside the ICU. The ultrasound machine must be equipped with 2–10 MHz curvilinear probe and >10.0 MHz linear probe to assess diaphragmatic displacement and thickness throughout the whole respiratory cycle, respectively. Usually, the ultrasound imaging of the diaphragm for excursion and thickness can be obtained through ultrasound machine running the dedicated application software with the abdominal preset. Regardless of the respiratory assistance, the examination is conducted with patient in a 30°–45° semi-recumbent position, preferably on the right side because of the poor acoustic window due to the presence of the spleen and the suboptimal windows derived from gastric and/or colonic shadows on the left side, mainly in the pathway of diaphragmatic excursion assessment.

For diaphragmatic displacement (excursion) evaluation (video 13), the transducer is positioned in the subcostal region between midclavicular and anterior axillary lines (Fig. 6), and

then identify the confluence of the hepatic veins into the inferior vena cava or, alternatively, the gallbladder (Fig. 7). The diaphragm appears as a hyperechoic line surrounding the posterior and lateral portion of the liver (Fig. 7). With the ultrasound beam perpendicularly oriented towards the middle or posterior third of the diaphragm, the M-mode feature is switched on to acquire the diaphragmatic displacement over time (Fig. 7). In spontaneously breathing patients, the posterior and middle portions of the diaphragm are responsible for the greatest craniocaudal excursion. Diaphragmatic displacement is plotted over time for four consecutive breaths. Diaphragmatic excursions during inspiration are indicated by red arrows (Fig. 8). During inspiration, the diaphragm moves towards the transducer. Each inspiratory displacement is identified by two white crosses of the caliper placed at the beginning and at the end of inspiration, respectively. The vertical distance between two consecutive crosses corresponds to the diaphragmatic excursion during inspiratory phase (Fig. 8).

Diaphragmatic thickness is assessed by placing the linear transducer, perpendicularly angled

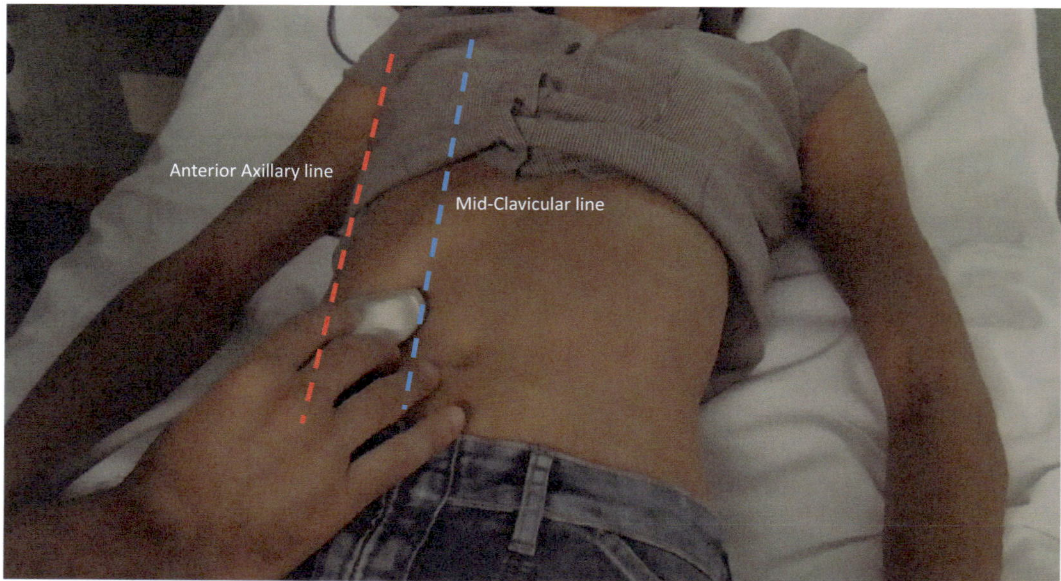

Fig. 6 Sonographic window for evaluation of diaphragm. The transducer should be placed below the costal margin between the mid-clavicular line and the anterior axillary line, oriented cranially allowing ultrasound beam to reach perpendicularly the posterior part of the diaphragm

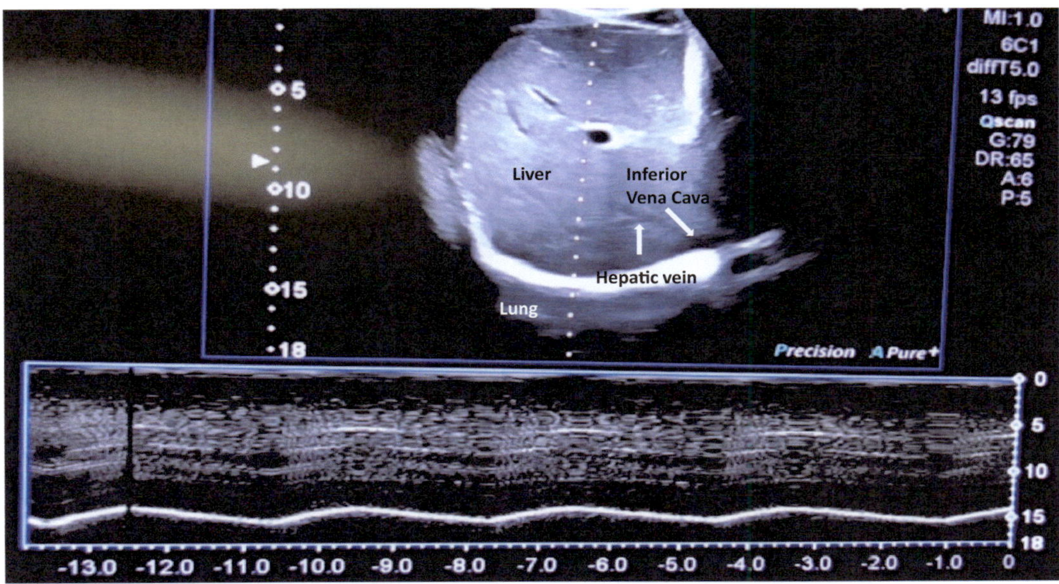

Fig. 7 The top of the figure depicts right hemi-diaphragm in B-mode, while the bottom depicts M-mode ultrasound of the diaphragm during quiet breathing

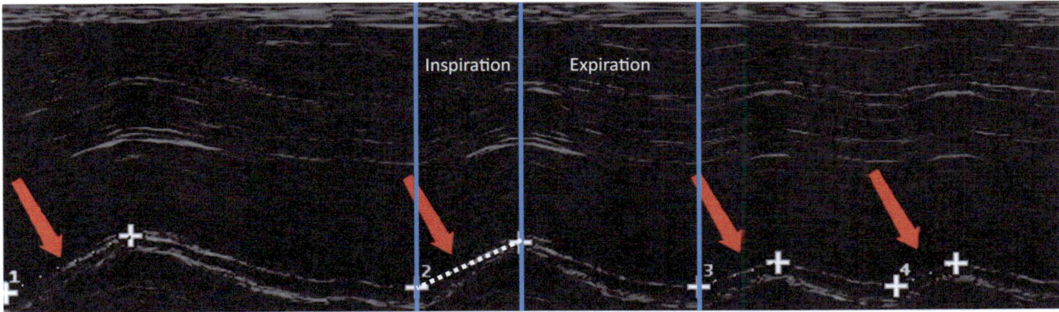

Fig. 8 Excursion is measured in M-mode: the diaphragm is visualized as an hyper-echoic line, the first caliper is placed at the beginning of inspiration slope and the second caliper at the apex of the slope

to the chest wall, between the anterior and midaxillary lines, in the ninth or tenth intercostal space (Fig. 9) (video 12). In this position, diaphragmatic ZOA is evaluated and the diaphragm appears as a three-layered structure just superficial to the liver, consisting of a relatively non-echogenic muscular layer in the middle bounded by the hyperechoic membranes of the diaphragmatic pleura and peritoneum, respectively (Fig. 10).

Once the correct insonation of the diaphragm is obtained at a depth of 1.5–3.0 cm, M-mode is then switched on to assess diaphragmatic thickness at end-inspiration and end-expiration (Fig. 11). Combining end-inspiratory and end-expiratory thickness it is also possible to compute diaphragmatic thickening fraction, according to the standard formula:

$$Diaphragmatic\ thickening\ fraction\ (\%)$$
$$= \frac{(End - inspiratory\ thickness - End - expiratory\ thickness)}{End - expiratory\ thickness} * 100$$

Diaphragmatic thickening fraction is considered an indirect estimate of diaphragmatic effort.

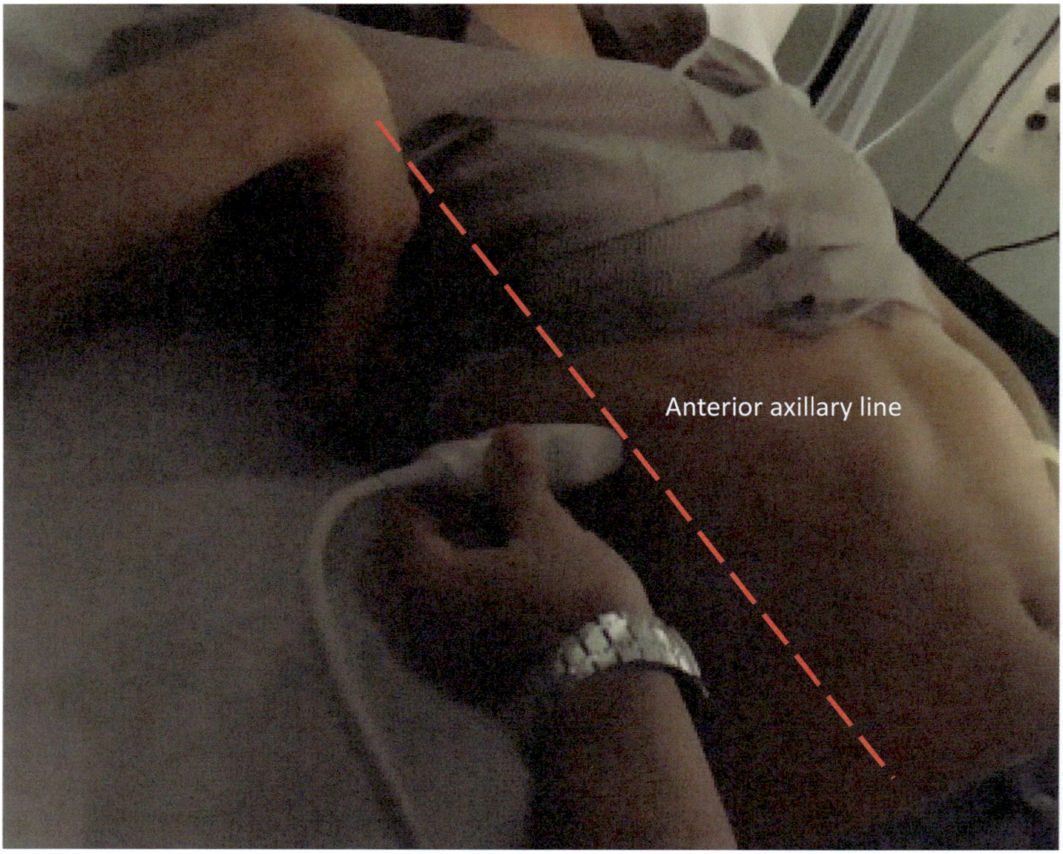

Fig. 9 Evaluation of diaphragm thickness: the transducer must be placed perpendicular to the chest wall, in the eighth or ninth intercostal space between the anterior axillary and the midaxillary lines, in the zone of apposition of the muscle

Fig. 10 The diaphragm is visualized as a structure with three distinct layers: two parallel echoic lines, the diaphragmatic pleura and the peritoneal membrane and a hypoechoic structure between them

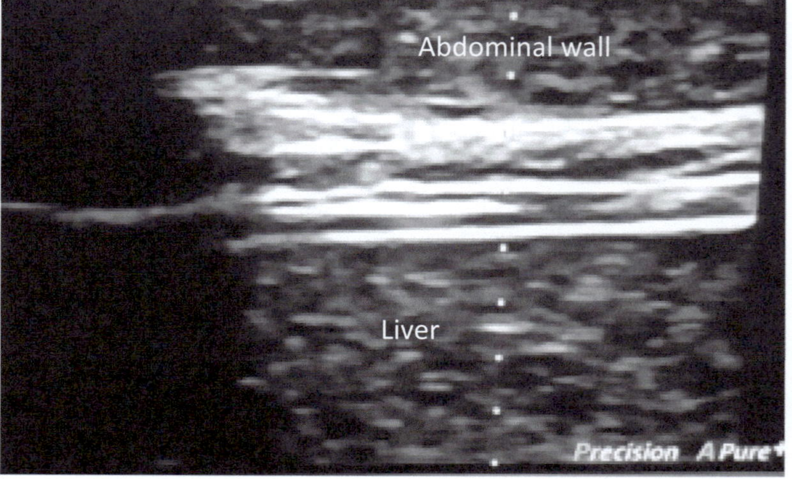

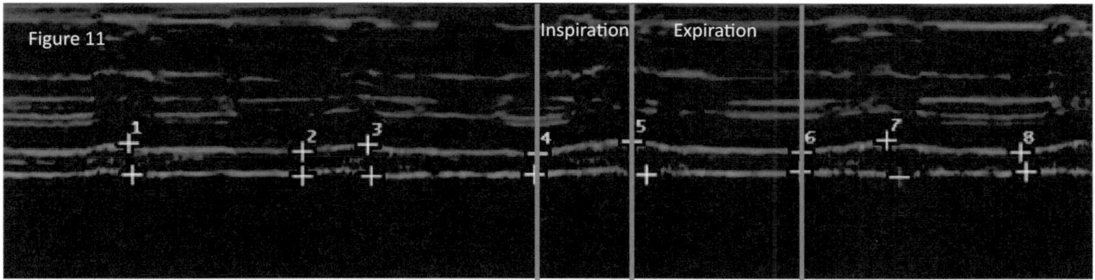

Fig. 11 Thickness measurement can be performed either in B-mode or in M-mode: the caliper must be placed as close as possible to the pleural and peritoneal line without including them in the measurement

In healthy volunteers lying in semi-recumbent position, the normal inspiratory diaphragmatic displacement has been reported ranging from 1.8 ± 0.8 cm to 2.2 ± 0.9 cm during quiet breathing and from 6.9 ± 1.4 cm to 7.9 ± 1.3 cm during deep breathing, depending on assessor's expertise. A Diaphragmatic thickness of 2.7 ± 0.5 mm with a corresponding thickening fraction of 37 ± 9% has been measured in healthy volunteers breathing at functional residual capacity.

Clinical Applications of Diaphragmatic ultrasound

Critical Care

In critically ill patients, diaphragmatic disfunction is associated to adverse outcomes such as weaning failure, prolonged mechanical ventilation duration and ICU stay, and increased mortality. In some cases, diaphragmatic dysfunction has been demonstrated on ICU admission especially in patients requiring mechanical ventilation. Also, the monitoring of diaphragmatic function is of a pivotal importance in the perspective of ensuring a lung and diaphragm protective mechanical ventilation.

A diaphragmatic displacement less than 10 mm has been suggested as a criterion for diaphragmatic dysfunction in critically ill patients. In patients undergoing prolonged mechanical ventilation, a diaphragmatic dysfunction has been reported in 34% of the cases. In subjects recovering form cardiac surgery with a prolonged mechanical ventilation, a diaphragmatic displacement less than 25 mm, acquired during a best excursion maneuver, was indicative for a poor diaphragmatic function.

In ICU patients, diaphragmatic thickness assessment has been employed to investigate diaphragmatic atrophy. In this regard, a 6.5–7.0% reduction of diaphragmatic thickness per day of mechanical ventilation was demonstrated to be a risk factor for diaphragmatic atrophy. Moreover, a linear relationship between the increasing level of ventilatory assistance and diaphragmatic atrophy was described.

Mechanical ventilation is a life-saving therapy which is widely used in the ICUs. However, it is associated to several adverse complications that could negatively affect clinical outcome. In patients undergoing invasive MV for longer than 72 h, a trend towards reduction or increase in end-expiratory diaphragmatic thickness as compared to baseline thickness assessed at ICU admission, were both associated to a prolonged mechanical ventilation duration. In this setting, a thickening fraction ranging from 15 to 30% was a good compromise to aim for the shortest period of mechanical ventilation.

The process of liberation from mechanical ventilation is a crucial step for ICU patients and identifying the risk factors responsible for weaning failure is of particular interest. To this end, diaphragmatic ultrasound has been employed to assess diaphragmatic function during weaning from invasive MV. A diaphragmatic displacement less than 11–14 mm and a thickening fraction lower than 20–36% have been suggested as predictors for weaning failure.

Diaphragmatic Paralysis

The role of diaphragmatic ultrasound in evaluating diaphragmatic paralysis has been investigated. A diaphragmatic end-expiratory thickness <2 mm and a thickening fraction <20% were observed in patients with diaphragmatic paralysis compared to healthy subjects. Moreover, in patients with a paralyzed hemidiaphragm, the thickening fraction reached negative values compared to non-pathological hemidiaphragm due to the passive stretching of the paralyzed portion of the muscle during breathing.

Expiratory diaphragmatic thickness may be unaltered in case of acute diaphragmatic paralysis, as atrophy may not have occurred yet. According to recent findings, in healthy individuals, the lower limit of expiratory diaphragmatic thickness is 1.2 mm in women and 1.3 mm in men.

In patients undergoing elective cardiac surgery, a diaphragmatic dysfunction diagnosed as a thickening fraction <20% was identified in 38% of population enrolled, and it was correlated to cardiopulmonary bypass duration. This impairment of diaphragmatic function exposed patients to a prolonged duration of mechanical ventilation and a longer ICU stay.

In order to assess diaphragmatic weakness or paralysis, ultrasonography of diaphragmatic displacement has also been obtained during quiet spontaneous breathing, deep breathing, and sniffing maneuver. Diaphragmatic paralysis was characterized by a lack of excursion during quiet breathing or by a paradoxical movement/absence of displacement during deep breathing and sniffing maneuver; the pattern of diaphragmatic weakness was characterized by a reduced diaphragmatic excursion during quiet and deep breathing, with or without paradoxical motion at sniffing maneuver.

Chronic Obstructive Pulmonary Disease (COPD)

Diaphragmatic ultrasound has been used to assess diaphragmatic function in patients with COPD [4]. In this subset of patients, diaphragmatic ultrasound was used to ascertain the diaphragmatic motility during exercise. COPD patients showed a reduced diaphragmatic displacement compared to healthy subjects. Moreover, the diaphragmatic excursion was directly correlated to distance over the course of a six-minute walk test and inversely correlated with dyspnea on exertion.

Dos Santos Yamaguti et al. investigated the relationship between lung function and diaphragmatic activity. The Authors concluded that the extent of reduction in diaphragmatic excursion and thickening fraction correlated to the severity air trapping and hyperinflation, respectively [5].

POCUS has also been used to screen for patients with COPD exacerbations undergoing non-invasive ventilation (NIV) for diaphragmatic dysfunction defined as a thickening fraction <20%.

On the one hand, the incidence of diaphragmatic dysfunction was 24% and was associated to corticosteroids use, and on the other hand, it was responsible of poor outcomes, including NIV failure, longer ICU stays, prolonged mechanical ventilation, the need for tracheostomy, and ICU mortality.

In exacerbated COPD patients admitted to emergency department for NIV support, diaphragmatic displacement was always reduced in NIV failure patients compared to NIV successes after 2 h of NIV application. In this context, diaphragmatic excursion revealed a good predictor of early NIV failure [6].

Novel Coronavirus-19 Disease (COVID-19)

Diaphragmatic function has been assessed through POCUS in COVID-19 patients admitted for acute hypoxemic respiratory failure. In the critically ill patients, a reduced diaphragmatic thickening fraction was associated to a failure of NIV and subsequent need for invasive MV. The cut–off value of diaphragmatic thickening fraction predicting CPAP failure was of 21.4% [7].

In COVID-19 patients admitted to intermediate care unit, a reduced thickness of the diaphragm (≤ 2 mm) was a risk factor for adverse outcome. In this setting, patients with a lower diaphragmatic mass or an impaired diaphragmatic function were more at risk for muscular fatigue while sustaining the respiratory workload [8].

References

1. Volpicelli G, Elbarbary M, Blaivas M, Lichtenstein DA, Mathis G, Kirkpatrick AW, et al. International evidence-based recommendations for point-of-care lung ultrasound. Intensive Care Med. 2012;38 (4):577–91.
2. Dietrich CF, Mathis G, Blaivas M, Volpicelli G, Seibel A, Wastl D, et al. Lung B-line artefacts and their use. J Thorac Dis. 2016;8(6):1356–65.
3. Piette E, Daoust R, Denault A. Basic concepts in the use of thoracic and lung ultrasound. Curr Opin Anaesthesiol. 2013;26(1):20–30.
4. Cammarota G, Sguazzotti I, Zanoni M, Messina A, Colombo D, Vignazia GL, et al. Diaphragmatic ultrasound assessment in subjects with acute hypercapnic respiratory failure admitted to the emergency department. Respir Care. 2019;respcare.06803.
5. Dos Santos WP, Paulin E, Shibao S, Chammas MC, Salge JM, Ribeiro M, et al. Air trapping: the major factor limiting diaphragm mobility in chronic obstructive pulmonary disease patients. Respirology. 2008;13 (1):138–44.
6. Cammarota G, Sguazzotti I, Zanoni M, Messina A, Colombo D, Vignazia GL, et al. Diaphragmatic ultrasound assessment in subjects with acute hypercapnic respiratory failure admitted to the emergency department. Respir Care [Internet]. 2019;64 (12):1469–77. http://rc.rcjournal.com.bvsp.idm.oclc.org/content/64/12/1469.
7. Corradi F, Vetrugno L, Orso D, Bove T, Schreiber A, Boero E, et al. Diaphragmatic thickening fraction as a potential predictor of response to continuous positive airway pressure ventilation in Covid-19 pneumonia: a single-center pilot study. Respir Physiol Neurobiol [Internet]. 2020;284(November 2020):103585. https://doi.org/10.1016/j.resp.2020.103585.
8. Corradi F, Isirdi A, Malacarne P, Santori G, Baribieri G, Romei C, et al. Low diaphragm muscle mass predicts adverse outcome in patients hospitalized for COVID-19 pneumonia: an exploratory pilot study [Internet]. Minerva Anestesiologica. 2021:432–8. https://www-minervamedica-it.bvsp.idm.oclc.org/it/riviste/minerva-anestesiologica/articolo.php?cod=R02Y2021N04A0432&acquista=1.

POCUS in Diagnosis: Acute Heart Failure

Luna Gargani and Alberto Palazzuoli

The most deadly disease truly is the failure of the heart
Oscar Arias–Former President of Costa Rica and Nobel Peace Prize Laureate (1987)

Abstract

POCUS is a real game-changer for the diagnosis of acute heart failure (AHF). It is readily available at the bedside and provides crucial information for the management of patients. The cardiac evaluation, performed with the FoCUS approach (focus cardiac ultrasound) offers an immediate assessment of cardiac morphology and function, pericardial effusion and gross valvular abnormalities, which may rapidly indicate the main cause for decompensation. Lung ultrasound can be easily integrated to FoCUS to assess pulmonary congestion by sonographic B-lines and pleural effusion, thus suggesting the degree of decompensation. The portability of this tool, whose information can be readily used at the bedside, with minimal discomfort or risk for the patient, without using of contrast material or ionizing radiation, can significantly speed up the correct diagnosis and the decision-making process, making integrated cardiopulmonary POCUS the most versatile and cost-effective imaging approach for the evaluation of patients with acute cardiovascular conditions.

Keywords

Acute heart failure · POCUS · Lung ultrasound · B-lines · Echocardiography · FoCUS

Abbreviations

POCUS	Point of care ultrasound
FoCUS	Focus cardiac ultrasound
AHF	Acute heart failure
EACVI	European Association of Cardiovascular Imaging
HFpEF	Heart failure with preserved ejection fraction
NPs	Natriuretic peptides
LV	Left ventricle
EF	Ejection fraction
RV	Right ventricle

L. Gargani (✉)
Department of Surgical, Medical and Molecular Pathology and Critical Care Medicine, University of Pisa, Pisa, Italy
e-mail: luna.gargani@unipi.it

A. Palazzuoli
Department of Internal Medicine, University of Siena, Siena, Italy
e-mail: palazzuoli2@unisi.it

© The Author(s), under exclusive license to Springer Nature Switzerland AG 2023
H. Soliman-Aboumarie et al. (eds.), *Cardiopulmonary Point of Care Ultrasound,*
https://doi.org/10.1007/978-3-031-29472-3_7

LA	Left atrium
IVC	Inferior vena cava
MR	Mitral regurgitation
AR	Aortic regurgitation
PASP	Pulmonary artery systolic pressure
HFrEF	Heart failure with reduced ejection fraction
TDI	Tissue Doppler imaging
LAVI	Left atrial volume index
TR	Tricuspid regurgitation
PCWP	Pulmonary capillary wedge pressure
RVSP	Right ventricular systolic pressure
RAP	Right atrial pressure
LUS	Lung ultrasound
CXR	Chest X-ray

Key Messages

- POCUS is a real game-changer for the diagnosis of acute heart failure (AHF).
- FoCUS (focus cardiac ultrasound) offers an immediate assessment of cardiac morphology and function, pericardial effusion and gross valvular abnormalities, which may rapidly indicate the main cause for decompensation.
- Lung ultrasound can be easily integrated to FoCUS to assess pulmonary congestion.

Focus Cardiac Ultrasound (FoCUS) and Standard Echocardiography

Transthoracic echocardiography is the most commonly used sonographic imaging in patients with acute heart failure (AHF), since it offers immediate and comprehensive assessment of cardiovascular morphology, function and hemodynamics. For these reasons, echocardiography has been defined by the American College of Cardiology/American Heart Association guidelines for the diagnosis and management of heart failure <The single most useful diagnostic test in the evaluation of patients with HF> [1]. There are

different types of echocardiographic examinations and it is important to fully understand which is the right examination for the right situation [2]. When speaking about POCUS we should clearly distinguish a *standard echocardiography*, which is a <complete and comprehensive echocardiographic examination, including morphological and functional assessment performed by an operator fully trained in echocardiography, which acquires a well-defined data set> from an *emergency echocardiogram*, which is <a standard/conventional echocardiogram performed in emergency environments in the assessment of patients with unstable cardiovascular diseases, and even more from a focus cardiac ultrasound (FoCUS), which is defined as a specific type of POCUS exam applied to the heart, as an extension of the clinical examination, by an operator not necessarily trained in comprehensive echocardiography, but appropriately trained in FoCUS, usually responsible for decision making and/or treatment> [2–4].

In patients with AHF, it is a FoCUS echo that is often performed as first assessment (i.e. in the Emergency Department or even on the ambulance, if the facilities and the expertise are available), being completed by a standard echocardiogram as soon as possible, or in ambulatory setting to identify the main reason of dyspnoea.

FoCUS is not a comprehensive evaluation: it allows the evaluation of a limited but critical number of cardiac conditions, that may be life-threatening, and may aid decision-making during cardiopulmonary resuscitation. In particular, global left and right ventricular systolic function and size, presence of pericardial effusion, intravascular volume assessment, gross signs of chronic cardiac disease, gross valvular abnormalities, large intracardiac masses. Other assessments are beyond the scope of FoCUS and should be addressed with a standard echocardiography. The characteristics of FoCUS, as standardized by the European Association of CardioVascular Imaging (EACVI) are summarized in Table 1.

Table 1 Main principles of FoCUS

• FoCUS should be used as a POCUS cardiac examination, aimed to detect a limited number of critical cardiac conditions
• FoCUS may provide key clinical information about global left and right ventricular systolic function and size, presence of pericardial effusion, intravascular volume assessment, gross signs of chronic cardiac disease, gross valvular abnormalities, large intracardiac masses
• FoCUS should never be considered or reported as echocardiographic examination
• FoCUS should be used by operators who have completed appropriate education and training programmes, and who fully understand and respect its scope and limitations
• Whenever the information about cardiovascular abnormalities provided by the FoCUS exam is insufficient for the immediate or definitive care of patients, these should be referred to a comprehensive echocardiographic examination as soon as possible

(Adapted from reference 3)

By means of FoCUS, it is often possible to suspect the main cause of AHF, although a large part of situations, in particular patients with HFpEF would need a complete standard echocardiography to confirm the diagnosis, together with the clinical picture, NPs and, possibly lung ultrasound. As soon as a more comprehensive evaluation is feasible, a more detailed assessment of cardiac morphology, function and non-invasive hemodynamics can be implemented, in order to identify the cause of decompensation. Two-dimensional and Doppler echocardiography have markedly improved our understanding of the pathophysiology of AHF, often providing a visualization of the aetiology of AHF, a hemodynamic evaluation at baseline and during treatment, and precious prognostic information to guide further management. An early understanding of the ongoing cause of the AHF syndrome is mandatory in order to initiate appropriate therapy. The main available information are schematized in Table 2.

Table 2 Comprehensive cardiopulmonary assessment in AHF

Heart		Questions to address/pitfalls
Chambers' size	• *Normal* • *Dilated*	
LV systolic function	•*Normal* •*Impaired* – Global dysfunction Regional wall motion abnormalities	What is the degree of LV systolic dysfunction? Has LV systolic function changed from a previous echo (if known)?
LV diastolic function	• Normal • Indeterminate • Impaired	E/e' ratio is not accurate as an index of LV filling pressures in normal subjects, with heavy annular calcification, surgical rings, mitral valve disease, constrictive pericarditis
Valvular heart disease	• Acute • Chronic decompensated	Is the valvular abnormality severe? Is it organic or functional? What is the cause? Is it amenable to surgical intervention? How urgent is surgical repair or replacement?
RV function	• *Normal* • *Impaired*	Is there associated PH? Is there associated tricuspid regurgitation?
Hemodynamics	• E/e' • CO • PASP, mPAP	E/e' allows only a semi-quantitative assessment of LV filling pressures.

(continued)

Table 2 (continued)

Heart		Questions to address/pitfalls
Chambers' size	• *Normal* • *Dilated*	

Pericardial effusion	• *Absent*
	• *Present*
	  – *No hemodynamic effects*
	  – *Tamponade physiology*
		Differentiate between pericardial effusion and pericardial fat. Differentiate between pericardial and pleural effusion.

Inferior vena cava	• *Normal diameter and collapsibility* • *Abnormal diameter and collapsibility* • *Indeterminate*	
Lung		
B-lines	• *Number* • *Distribution* • *Dynamicity*	B-lines are not specific for cardiogenic interstitial pulmonary edema. Cardiogenic B-lines should be multiple diffuse and bilateral, with gravity-related distribution. The pleural line should be not frankly irregualar.
Pleural effusion	• *Size* • *Position*	

In *Italic* those abnormalities assessable by FoCUS evaluation

Given the nature of POCUS, the cardiac examination is restricted to some standardized views. The basic FoCUS examination includes 5 views, illustrated in Fig. 1 (parasternal long-axis and short-axis views, apical 4-chamber view, subcostal inferior vena cava, and subcostal 4-chamber). ECG monitoring should be placed whenever possible.

It is crucial to be aware of the limitations related to this approach, including limited data set due to restricted image acquisition protocol, inferiority of the imaging devices typically used for FoCUS, limited number of detectable evidence, typically unfavourable settings (emergencies, critically ill, time constrains), subtle/complex cardiac abnormalities difficult to assess, and always be ready to refer to comprehensive echocardiography those patients with detected/suspected abnormalities.

Global Left Ventricular Systolic Function and Size

The assessment of left ventricular (LV) systolic function and size is critical to the proper evaluation and management of patients with AHF. The main targets in a POCUS/FoCUS examinations would be:

– LV dimensions, which would be mostly eyeballing at least at first assessment.
– Wall thickness, to understand if there is a significant hypertrophy.

Global LV systolic function, which would be initially estimated eyeballing with "visual" ejection fraction. As soon as possible, it is then advisable to measure LV volumes in 4-and 2-chamber views to perform a proper EF estimation according to the modified Simpson's rule.

There are some conditions that require caution with the interpretation of global LV systolic function, such as in patients with both bradycardia and tachycardia, severe hypotension and hypertension, severe mitral/aortic regurgitation or stenosis, severe left ventricular hypertrophy, hyperdynamic states, LV underfilling, left bundle branch block, paced rhythm and in patients with inotropes [3].

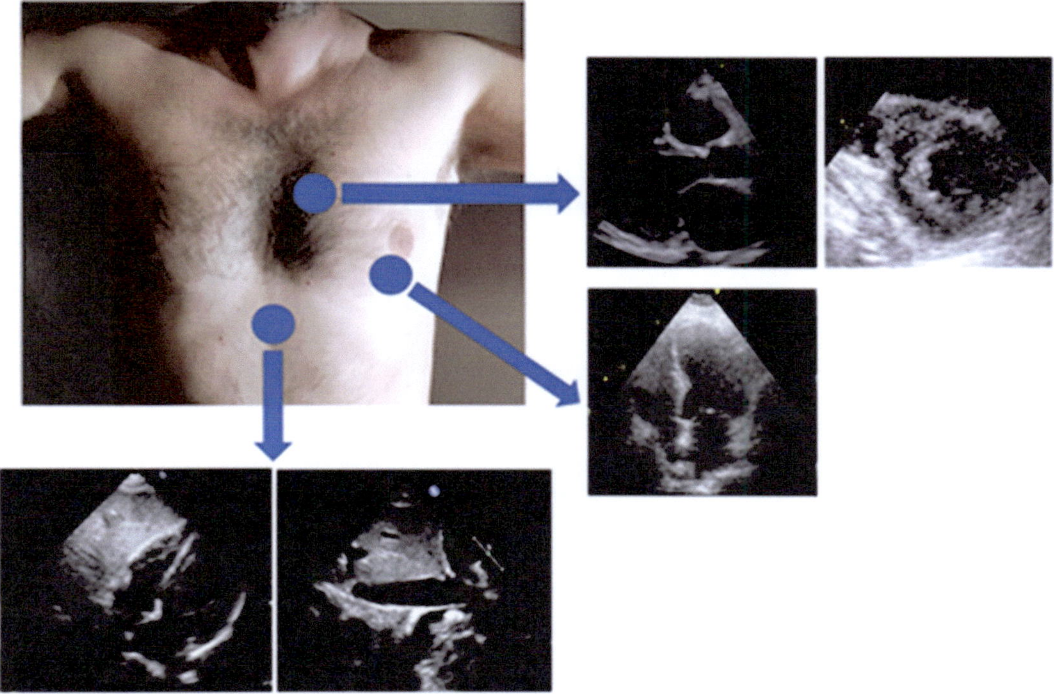

Fig. 1 Schematic of basic FoCUS examination which includes 5 cardiac views (left parasternal long-axis and short-axis views, apical 4-chamber view, subcostal inferior vena cava, and subcostal 4-chamber views)

The interventricular septum should be also evaluated for morphology and motion, i.e septal flattening (D-shape of the left ventricle) in the short-axis view: D-shape during systole suggests RV pressure overload, whereas a D-shape in diastole suggests RV volume overload. The interatrial septum should also be evaluated: its motion is influenced by the pressure gradient between the two atria (septal bowing to the left with each beat would suggest high right sided pressures and viceversa).

– Gross regional wall motion abnormalities, i.e. a clear apical akinesia. It should be noted whether the regional wall motion abnormality follows the territory of distribution of a specific coronary artery or not. A qualitative assessment between hyperkinesis, normokinesis, hypokinesis, akinesis, and dyskinesis is usually feasible when the cardiac window is appropriate. Sometimes, especially in critically-ill patients and emergency situation, it may be not so easy to differentiate a hypokinesis from a normokinesis; in these cases it is advisable to rely only on clear wall motion abnormalities showing akinesis. A thinned wall with hyperechogenicity can represent a scar.

For the assessment of LV wall motion abnormalities, the 17-segment model including the apical cap should be used [5].
In the presence of an apical akinesia, a Takotsubo cardiomyopathy could be in the differential diagnosis, although this diagnosis would become confirmed only after coronary angiography.

– LA dimensions: a dilated LA is usually a sign of pre-existing cardiac abnormalities.

Global Right Ventricular Systolic Function and Size

Similarly to the LV, the global RV systolic function should be initially assessed eyeballing. Dimensions should be compared to those of the LV to better appreciate a potential RV dilation. RV dilation can be evaluated qualitatively by TTE by identifying a larger RV compared with the LV in the standard apical 4-chamber view. RV dilation or RV free wall hypokinesia are signs of RV failure. Quantitative measurements of RV dilation should be estimated in an RV-focused apical 4-chamber view, which shows the maximal diameter of the RV without foreshortening the longitudinal axis; with gradual RV dilatation, the RV apex progressively replaces the LV as the true apex of the heart [6].

The IVS should also be evaluated as highlighted above. Presence of RV hypertrophy would suggest a chronic condition (i.e. a chronic cor pulmonale). Right atrium dimensions should also be taken into account.

Pericardial Effusion

Pericardial effusion can be present in patients with AHF. Caution should be taken not to misunderstand epicardial fat for pericardial effusion: epicardial fat is less mobile than fluid, and fat is usually more echogenic with a "granular", sparkling appearance than fluid.

Sometimes there is the need to differentiate pericardial effusion from pleural effusion: an important reference point is the ascending aorta in parasternal long axes, since fluid that is in front of the aorta (anterior to it) is a pericardial effusion, whereas fluid that is posterior to the aorta is a pleural effusion. Then, pericardial effusion reflects at the posterior atrioventricular groove in the parasternal long-axis view, whereas pleural effusion can continue under the left atrium, posterior to the descending aorta. We should then double-check in the subcostal view, where pericardial effusion is usually visible between the liver and the right ventricular wall (Fig. 2).

In patients with shock/hypotension, assessment of pericardial effusion becomes crucial to understand whether there is a cardiac tamponade. Cardiac tamponade is a clinical diagnosis, but in presence of hemodynamic instability, a pericardial effusion should promptly raise the suspicion of tamponade. There are some other echocardiographic signs, supporting the diagnosis of tamponade physiology: RA systolic collapse, RV diastolic collapse, IVC plethora, and a swinging heart. It is important to remember that the amount of pericardial effusion is quite irrelevant for the diagnosis of tamponade.

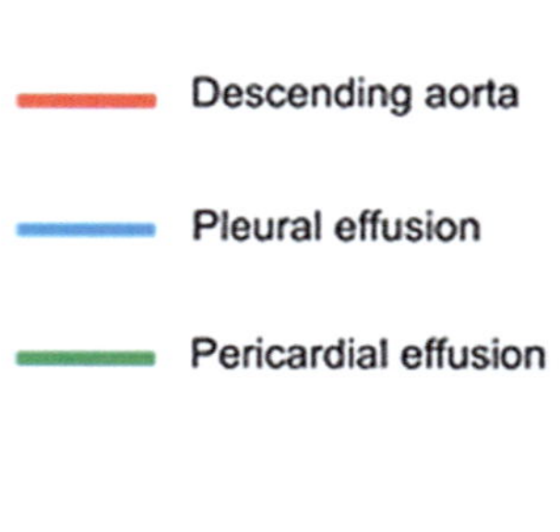

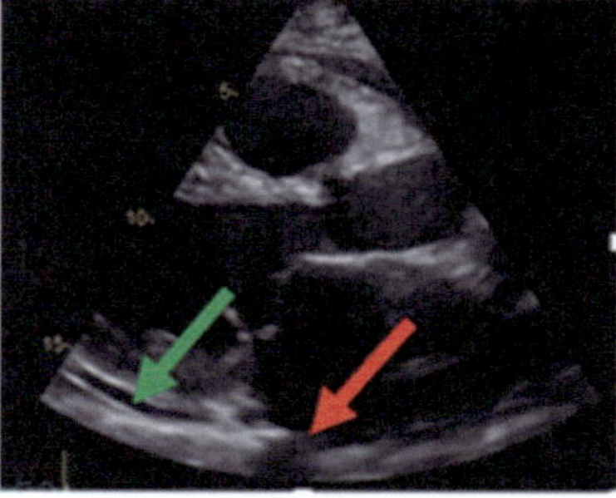

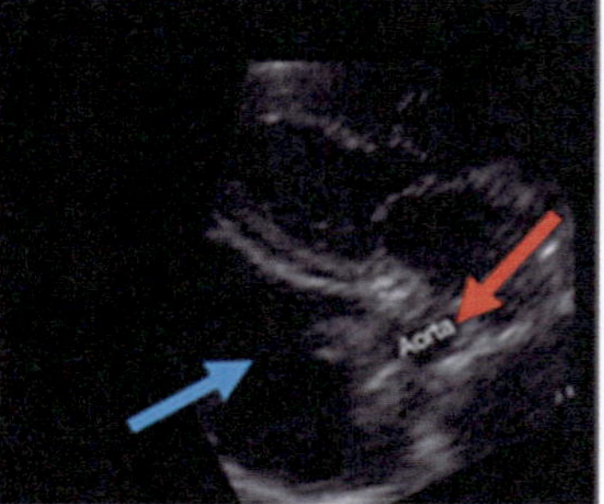

Fig. 2 Differentiating pericardial effusion from pleural effusion on echocardiography: An important reference point is the descending aorta in parasternal long axis view, since fluid that is in front of the aorta (anterior to it) is a pericardial effusion, whereas fluid that is posterior to the aorta is a pleural effusion

Intravascular Volume Assessment and Inferior Vena Cava

Echocardiography can be of help in assessing volume status, which is a crucial information in patients with AHF who often requires high doses of diuretic therapy. There are some typical echocardiographic features of severe hypovolaemia (which is usually rare in AHF) and volume responsiveness: a small, hyperkinetic LV and/or RV (by visual assessment), a small IVC (usually <10−12 mm).

The inferior vena cava should be visualized from the subcostal view, and its dimensions and collapsibility should be noted. Dimensions should be assessed at end-expiration, whereas collapsibility should be assessed during inspiration with spontaneous breathing. If patients are under mechanical ventilation, the evaluation of the IVC is more complex. The changes in IVC diameter and collapsibility can also be a sign of volume responsiveness. It is important to be able to differentiate a situation of hypovolaemia from vasodilation, because in both cases end-systolic area will be small. In case of vasodilation, however, end-diastolic area is usually normal or only slightly reduced. In case of hypovolaemia, end-diastolic area will be much more reduced.

There are some conditions that make volume status assessment more challenging, such as mechanical ventilation, the presence of chronic cardiac disease (especially valve disease, acute RV myocardial infarction, chronic cor pulmonale, dilated cardiomyopathy), and arrhythmias.

Volume overload is much more frequent in AHF. The IVC pattern would be the opposite, with increased diameter (> 21 mm) and reduced or absent collapsibility.

Major Signs of Chronic Cardiac Disease

Screening for signs of chronic pre-existing cardiac disease is part of the first echocardiographic assessment of AHF. Usually relevant LA and LV dilatation, marked LV hypertrophy, RA dilatation, RV dilatation with hypertrophy, relevant valve calcifications would suggest chronic cardiac disease, making the interpretation of POCUS findings more complex. These patients should be referred as soon as possible for a standard echocardiography.

Gross Valvular Abnormalities

Valvular dysfunction can be a cause and a consequence of AHF.

- Acute valvular heart disease can be the cause of AHF in a previously healthy patient (e.g. chordal rupture).
- Chronic valvular heart disease can be the cause of AHF in case of decompensation.
- Valvular heart disease can be the consequence of AHF, when functional mitral or tricuspid regurgitation occur in the setting of dilated cardiomyopathy or ischemic cardiac disease.

The aim of FoCUS is to trigger a comprehensive echocardiography once gross valvular abnormalities are suspected. In case of mitral or aortic regurgitation, the main issues are:

- Is the regurgitation severe?
- Is the regurgitation organic or functional?
- Is it acute MR/AR or chronic decompensated MR/AR?
- What is the cause of MR/AR?

For the mitral valve, the morphology and function should be evaluated: whether the leaflets are thin, if there is a complete opening or not, if there is a complete closure at the annulus level.

A severely dysfunctional mitral valve is usually associated to typical findings, such as marked leaflet thickening, calcifications, masses, 'holes' in the leaflets, hypermobility or hypomobility of the leaflets. Clues towards a chronic mitral valve disease are marked calcifications, LA enlargement, LV enlargement, RV dilatation and hypertrophy.

In acute severe MR, the LA and LV face a sudden volume overload, which increases LV preload, allowing for a modest increase in total stroke volume, but with reduced forward stroke volume [7]. At the same time, the LA and LV cannot accommodate the regurgitant volume, which results in pulmonary congestion. The patient has therefore both reduced forward output and pulmonary edema. TTE allows evaluating the anatomy of the mitral valve and helps to provide semiquantitative information on lesion severity. However, inadequate imaging of the color flow jet may sometimes lead to underestimation of the severity. Thus, in case of hyperdynamic LV systolic function in a patient with AHF, the suspicion of severe MR should always be raised.

A similar assessment should be done for the aortic valve. The echocardiographic findings associated with severe dysfunction include distinct cusps thickening, calcifications, masses, 'holes', or functional alterations such as hypermobility, hypomobility, prolapse into left ventricular outflow tract. Clues towards chronic aortic valve disease are marked calcifications, LV hypertrophy, LV dilation, LA enlargement.

In acute severe AR a sudden large regurgitant volume is imposed on a LV of normal size that has not had time to adapt to the sudden volume increase. With an abrupt increase in end-diastolic volume, LV end-diastolic and LA pressures may increase rapidly, resulting in pulmonary congestion and concomitant decrease in forward stroke volume.

Decompensated chronic aortic stenosis is a relatively frequent cause of AHF in the elderly population, especially with concomitant systolic dysfunction. Severe hypertension is a common precipitating factor. The valve appears severely calcified with extensive thickening, increased echogenicity and a prominent acoustic shadow.

In presence of a heavily calcified mitral valve or thickening and immobility of the leaflets, thickening and fusion of the chorda tendinae or mitral annular and commissural calcification, mitral stenosis should always be suspected. Severe mitral stenosis is characterized at TTE by a valve area <1.0 cm^2, mean gradient >10 mmHg, or PASP >50 mmHg.

Large Intracardiac Masses

Large valve vegetations or visible intracardiac or inferior vena cava masses/thrombi are less frequently causes of AHF, but can be suspected by a FoCUS examination. Unless the patient is unstable and the echo exam shows right heart thrombus, also the detection of masses should trigger formal comprehensive echocardiography.

Echocardiography in AHF Beyond POCUS

Echocardiography can provide many additional information in patients with AHF.

<u>Left ventricular diastolic function</u> can be noninvasively assessed and is definitely relevant both for patients with HFrEF and HFpEF.

The ratio of flow Doppler mitral E wave peak velocity and early diastolic velocity of the mitral annulus (E/e') obtained by Tissue Doppler Imaging (TDI) is considered a non-invasive surrogate to establish LV filling pressures [8].

In patients with depressed LV systolic function, the mitral inflow pattern can be used to estimate filling pressures with reasonable accuracy. In case of impaired relaxation patterns and peak E velocities <50 cm/s, LV filling pressures are usually normal. In patients with E/A ratios >0.8 to <2, the use of additional parameters is recommended, such as an average E/e' > 14, a TR velocity > 2.8 m/s and a LAVI >34ml/m^2 [8].

In patients with normal EF, the following parameters should be considered as abnormal: an average E/e' ratio >14, a septal e' velocity < 7 cm/s or a lateral e' velocity <10 cm/s, a TR velocity > 2.8 m/s and a LAVI >34ml/m^2. If at least 3 of these values are abnormal, it is considered that a diastolic dysfunction is present.

Some limitations should however be highlighted before interpreting these values:
(1) e' and E/e' are influenced by the mitral annular side of measurement, therefore a mean of the values obtained at the septum and the lateral wall is advisable.

(2) E/e' allows only a semi-quantitative assessment of LV filling pressures.

(3) The E/e' ratio is not accurate as an index of LV filling pressures in normal subjects, in patients with heavy annular calcification, surgical rings, mitral valve disease, basal LV wall motion abnormalities related to left bundle branch block, paced-rhythm, myocardial infarction, cardiopulmonary bypass and constrictive pericarditis.

Hemodynamics

In addition to LV filling pressures estimation, echocardiographic Doppler techniques are the modality of choice for the non-invasive evaluation of hemodynamics [9]. A non-invasive hemodynamic assessment can also be used to monitor the patients after institution of appropriate therapy.

Non-invasive hemodynamic variables that can be useful in AHF are mainly:

- Stroke volume and cardiac output by pulsed-wave Doppler of the left ventricular outflow tract.
- PCWP by the following regression equation [10]:
- PCWP = (1.24 x [E/e']) + 1.9
  where E/e' should be calculated by using the average e'.
- Right ventricular systolic pressure (RVSP), right atrial pressure (RAP) and pulmonary artery systolic pressures (PASP) from tricuspid valve velocity and inferior vena cava dimension and collapsibility.

RVSP can be easily assessed in most subjects who present some degree of tricuspid regurgitation. The velocity recorded across the regurgitant jet corresponds to the right ventricular-right atrial gradient.

RAP can be estimated from the end-expiratory diameter and respiratory changes of the inferior vena cava (IVC) as follows [11, 12]:

- Normal diameter (≤ 2.1 cm) and inspiratory collapse (>50%), RAP = 3 mmHg (range: 0–5 mmHg).

- Dilated IVC (≥ 2.1 cm) with reduced respiratory variation (<50%), RAP = 15 mmHg (range: 10–20 mmHg).

- IVC diameter and respiratory variation unfitting the previous paradigm, without resolving hepatic flow pattern (absence of prevalent systolic or diastolic flow component) or tricuspid E/e' wave ratio, RAP = 8 mmHg (range: 5–10 mmHg).

PASP can be obtained by adding RVSP to mean RAP.

Lung Ultrasound

Lung Ultrasound (LUS) is the perfect companion of FoCUS in patients with AHF. It is a quantitative, simple, and rapid method to assess pulmonary congestion [13–15]. The association of this tool with the clinical evaluation and natriuretic peptides (NPs) assessment has greatly increased the diagnostic effectiveness of heart failure [16–19]. LUS in heart failure helps with the detection of pulmonary interstitial oedema, which can be visualized through sonographic B-lines, discrete laser-like vertical hyperechoic reverberation artifacts arising from the pleural line, extending to the bottom of the screen without fading, and moving synchronously with lung sliding [20]. B-lines can be assessed by scanning along the intercostal spaces using either a phased array or curvilinear transducer.

Methodology

There are two main methods to quantify B-lines: a score-based and a count-based approach. The score-based method considers a minimum number of B-lines for each scanning area as a "positive" zone (typically at least 3 B-lines), and then the number of positive zones are added up [21, 22]. The count-based method consists in counting B-lines in each scanning area and summing them up to obtain a total score; when B-lines are confluent and cannot be easily counted one by one, their number can be estimated from the percentage of space they occupy on the screen below the pleural line, divided by 10 (i.e. if about 70% of the screen below the pleural line is occupied by B-lines, it would conventionally count as 7 B-lines, up to a maximum of 10 per zone) [14, 23, 24].

A thoracic scheme with 8 scanning areas can be considered, dividing each hemithorax into 4 areas: two anterior (from the clavicle to the diaphragm) and two lateral (from the armpit to the diaphragm) [20].

Diagnostic Role of LUS in AHF

There are many studies demonstrating the additive role of LUS in the differential diagnosis of dyspnoea. When comparing two arms of patients admitted to the emergency department with acute dyspnoea, patients evaluated with LUS had a final correct diagnosis in a shorter time compared to patients evaluated by chest X-ray (CXR) and NPs (a median of 5 min for LUS and 100 min for CXR/NPs) [16]. The accuracy was also higher in favour of the LUS arm with a sensitivity of 85.0% and a specificity of 89.4% when the clinical evaluation was integrated with CXR/NPs, and a sensitivity of 93.5% and a specificity of 95.5% when the clinical evaluation was integrated with LUS B-lines. Thus, by implementing LUS in the first assessment of dyspnoeic patients suspected to have AHF we obtain both an advantage in terms of diagnostic accuracy and time saving.

B-lines are present in AHF independently of the aetiology, with similar values in patients with HFrEF and HFpEF [19, 25], and indeed their role in AHF, after the diagnosis is established, is to provide a semi-quantification of the degree of pulmonary congestion. In particular, absence of B-lines on the supero-anterior chest bilaterally (apical zones) exclude a very severe degree of congestion n and usually these patients do not require mechanical ventilation [26, 27]. B-lines tend to accumulate at first in the dependent zones, and non-gravity-related distribution of B-lines should raise the suspicion of a different diagnosis [23], such as non-cardiogenic pulmonary oedema or interstitial pneumonia.

In the differential diagnosis of acute dyspnoea, LUS can indeed also support the physician by showing other causes of acute dyspnoea, such as lobar or interstitial pneumonia, pulmonary infarction, pneumothorax [20]. Of course, a strong integration with the clinical picture is mandatory and is the basis of POCUS philosophy [28].

The number of B-lines at AHF admission provides also prognostic stratification in terms of death and rehospitalization for AHF, both in HFrEF and HFpEF, and also in patients admitted to a cardiology department without overt signs and symptoms of AHF [29]. The typical LUS pattern in AHF is with multiple, diffuse, bilateral B-lines, where *multiple* means a "positive" area, that is more than 2 B-lines (at least 3 B-lines) in a single scanning area [20] (although in AHF B-lines are usually much more numerous than only 3 per scanning area); *diffuse* refers to at least 2 adjacent positive areas per hemithorax, and this picture must of course be *bilateral* [30]. When considering the total number of B-lines, a cut-off of 15 is usually considered enough in AHF for the diagnosis. A typical LUS pattern in AHF is shown in Fig. 3.

Prognostic Role of LUS in AHF

The role of B-lines in guiding therapy is another interesting field [12] because serial LUS examinations during hospitalization could help in tailoring diuretic therapy and grading congestion before discharge, which can help identifying persistent sublinical congestion in patients thought to be ready to be send home. A moderate or severe degree of B-lines at discharge has been proven in different observational studies to predict a new hospitalization for AHF in the following months [7, 24, 31, 32]. This topic is addressed in details in Chap. 12 (Sect. III – Monitoring).

Fig. 3 Typical LUS patterns in acute heart failure

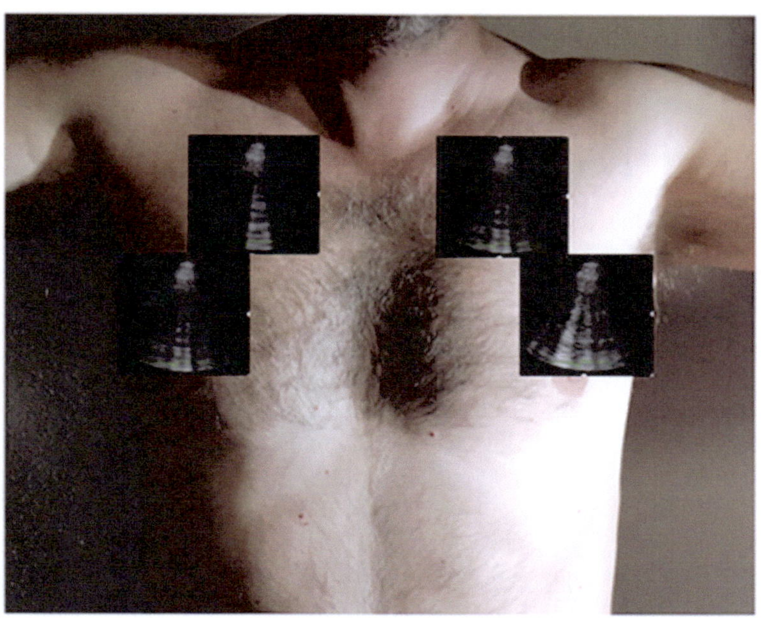

Typical LUS pattern in acute heart failure

The prognostic value of LUS is high also in out-patients. Presence of B-lines during an ambulatory office visit in patients after a hospitalization for AHF predicts a new event [33, 34], even when patients are asymptomatic and clinically stable [35]. This assessment can be done also with hand-held devices, with similar results [36]. Tailoring therapy according to LUS in HF out-patients can improve outcomes [37].

Limitations

Despite the elevated sensitivity of B-lines in the assessment of pulmonary congestion, specificity is not as high, and it must be taken into account that B-lines are not only a sign of cardiogenic interstitial pulmonary oedema, but can be present in many conditions characterized by a partial deaeration of the lung [14], including COVID-19 pneumonia [38].

B-lines number could slightly change assuming different positions [39]: the standard position for the patients during LUS scanning is supine, since it is usually enough to scan the anterolateral chest (adding the posterior chest if pleural effusion is not clearly visible otherwise).

It should be also noted that BMI is inversely related to the number of B-lines [40]. However, B-lines decline to a lesser degree than NT-proBNP with increasing BMI.

Current limitations can be usually overcome through a strong clinical integration, and by a multiparametric approach including not only B-lines, but also inferior vena cava and other non-invasive hemodynamic ultrasound parameters of congestion [41], as well as NPs. Current European Guidelines do not suggest the use of LUS and IVC diameter for the assessment of volume status; anyway, some studies have underlined the value of a complete ultrasound score including E/e' as a proxy of increased left ventricular filling pressure, tricuspid regurgitation maximal velocity for estimation of systolic pulmonary artery pressure, and inferior vena cava diameter as a marker of central vein pressure [42, 43]. Thus, the concomitant measurement of these variables may better define the effective central, pulmonary and peripheral congestion.

Integrated Cardiopulmonary Ultrasound

Bringing together the cardiac and pulmonary assessment in a patient with or suspected to have AHF provides the powerful combination of assessing the presence and degree of decompensation (by LUS) and the cause of decompensation (by echocardiography). This versatile methodology allows scanning both organs with the same machine, same probe, same setting, which makes cardiopulmonary ultrasound an extremely useful tool in the first assessment and for the monitoring of patients with AHF (Table 2). It is especially in patients with HFpEF, where the echocardiographic examination can fail to show significant abnormalities, but the presence of multiple diffuse bilateral B-lines with a regular pleural line in a symptomatic patient can strongly suggest this diagnosis; elevated NPs would of course also have a crucial role in these situations.

The FATE protocol (Focus-assessed transthoracic echocardiography) is an established protocol, proposed by Eric Sloth and his team in 1989 to provide quick guidance to interpret echocardiography information for cardiac and critical care ultrasound. The FATE protocol provides a systematic approach to the echocardiography examination and helps to guide decision making FATE partially integrates the cardiac and pleural examination, with the same TTE views of FoCUS, adding the scanning of the costo-phrenic angles for estimation of pleural effusion [44]. It doesn't include assessment of the pulmonary parenchyma with B-lines.

References

1. Jessup M, Abraham WT, Casey DE, Feldman AM, Francis GS, Ganiats TG, et al. 2009 focused update: ACCF/AHA guidelines for the diagnosis and management of heart failure in adults: a report of the American college of cardiology foundation/American heart association task force on practice guidelines: developed in collaboration with. Circulation. 2009;119(14):1977–2016.
2. Cardim N, Dalen H, Voigt J-U, Ionescu A, Price S, Neskovic AN, et al. The use of handheld ultrasound devices: a position statement of the European association of cardiovascular Imaging (2018 update). Eur Hear J Cardiovasc Imaging. 2019;20(3):245–52.
3. Neskovic AN, Skinner H, Price S, Via G, De Hert S, Stankovic I, et al. Focus cardiac ultrasound core curriculum and core syllabus of the European association of cardiovascular imaging. Eur Heart J Cardiovasc Imaging. 2018; 19(5).
4. Neskovic AN, Edvardsen T, Galderisi M, Garbi M, Gullace G, Jurcut R, et al. Focus cardiac ultrasound: the European association of cardiovascular imaging viewpoint. Eur Hear J Cardiovasc Imaging. 2014;15 (9):956–60.
5. Lang RM, Badano LP, Mor-avi V, Afilalo J, Armstrong A, Ernande L, et al. Recommendations for cardiac chamber quantification by echocardiography in adults: an update from the American society of echocardiography and the European association of cardiovascular imaging. J Am Soc Echocardiogr. 2015;28:1-39.e14.
6. Partington SL, Kilner PJ. How to image the dilated right ventricle. Circ Cardiovasc Imaging. 2017;10(5): e004688.
7. Coiro S, Rossignol P, Ambrosio G, Carluccio E, Alunni G, Murrone A, et al. Prognostic value of residual pulmonary congestion at discharge assessed by lung ultrasound imaging in heart failure. Eur J Heart Fail. 2015;17(11):1172–81.
8. Nagueh SF, Smiseth OA, Appleton CP, Byrd BF, Dokainish H, Edvardsen T, et al. Recommendations for the evaluation of left ventricular diastolic function by echocardiography: an update from the american society of echocardiography and the European association of cardiovascular imaging. J Am Soc Echocardiogr. 2016;29(4):277–314.
9. Quiñones Ma, Otto CM, Stoddard M, Waggoner A, Zoghbi Wa. Recommendations for quantification of doppler echocardiography: a report from the doppler quantification task force of the nomenclature and standards committee of the American society of echocardiography. J Am Soc Echocardiogr. 2002; 15 (2):167–84.
10. Nagueh SF, Middleton KJ, Kopelen HA, Zoghbi WA, Quiñones MA, QuiÃ±ones AM. Doppler tissue imaging: a noninvasive technique for evaluation of left ventricular relaxation and estimation of filling pressures. J Am Coll Cardiol. 1997; 30 (6):1527–33.
11. Rudski LG, Lai WW, Afilalo J, Hua L, Handschumacher MD, Chandrasekaran K, et al. Guidelines for the echocardiographic assessment of the right heart in adults: a report from the American society of echocardiography endorsed by the European association of echocardiography, a registered branch of the European society of cardiology, and t. J Am Soc Echocardiogr. 2010; 23.

12. Mozzini C, Di M, Perna D, Pesce G, Garbin U, Meschi T, et al. Lung ultrasound in internal medicine efficiently drives the management of patients with heart failure and speeds up the discharge time inferior cave vein collassability index. Intern Emerg Med. 2017.

13. Gheorghiade M, Follath F, Ponikowski P, Barsuk JH, Blair JEa, Cleland JG, et al. Assessing and grading congestion in acute heart failure: a scientific statement from the acute heart failure committee of the heart failure association of the European society of cardiology and endorsed by the European society of intensive care medicine. Eur J Heart Fail. 2010; 12:423–33.

14. Gargani L. Ultrasound of the lungs: more than a room with a view. Heart Fail Clin. 2019; 15(2).

15. Girerd N, Seronde M-F, Coiro S, Chouihed T, Bilbault P, Braun F, et al. Integrative assessment of congestion in heart failure throughout the patient journey. JACC Heart Fail. 2018;6(4):273–85.

16. Pivetta E, Goffi A, Nazerian P, Castagno D, Tozzetti C, Tizzani P, et al. Lung ultrasound integrated with clinical assessment for the diagnosis of acute decompensated heart failure in the emergency department: a randomized controlled trial. Eur J Heart Fail. 2019;21(6):754–66.

17. Gargani L, Frassi F, Soldati G, Tesorio P, Gheorghiade M, Picano E. Ultrasound lung comets for the differential diagnosis of acute cardiogenic dyspnoea: a comparison with natriuretic peptides. Eur J Heart Fail. 2008;10(1):70.

18. Liteplo AS, Marill Ka, Villen T, Miller RM, Murray AF, Croft PE, et al. Emergency thoracic ultrasound in the differentiation of the etiology of shortness of breath (ETUDES): sonographic B-lines and N-terminal pro-brain-type natriuretic peptide in diagnosing congestive heart failure. Acad Emerg Med. 2009; 16(3):201–10.

19. Palazzuoli A, Ruocco G, Beltrami M, Nuti R, Cleland JG. Combined use of lung ultrasound, B-type natriuretic peptide, and echocardiography for outcome prediction in patients with acute HFrEF and HFpEF. Clin Res Cardiol. 2018;107(7):586–96.

20. Volpicelli G, Elbarbary M, Blaivas M, Lichtenstein DADA, Mathis G, Kirkpatrick AWAW, et al. International evidence-based recommendations for point-of-care lung ultrasound. Intensive Care Med. 2012;38(4):577–91.

21. Pivetta E, Goffi A, Lupia E, Tizzani M, Porrino G, Ferreri E, et al. LUng ultrasound-implemented diagnosis of acute decompensated heart failure in the emergency department-a simeu multicenter study. Chest. 2015; 148(1).

22. Platz E, Campbell RT, Claggett B, Lewis EF, Groarke JD, Docherty KF, et al. Lung ultrasound in acute heart failure: prevalence of pulmonary congestion and short-and long-term outcomes. JACC Heart Fail. 2019;7(10):849–58.

23. Gargani L. Lung ultrasound: a new tool for the cardiologist. Cardiovasc Ultrasound. 2011;9:6.

24. Coiro S, Porot G, Rossignol P, Ambrosio G, Carluccio E, Tritto I, et al. Prognostic value of pulmonary congestion assessed by lung ultrasound imaging during heart failure hospitalisation: a two-centre cohort study. Sci Rep. 2016;20(6):39426.

25. Martindale JL, Secko M, Kilpatrick JF, Ian S, Paladino L, Aherne A, et al. Serial sonographic assessment of pulmonary edema in patients with hypertensive acute heart failure. 2017.

26. Lichtenstein DA. Lung ultrasound in acute respiratory failure an introduction to the BLUE-protocol. 2009; 75(5):31–7.

27. Volpicelli G, Noble VE, Liteplo A, Cardinale L. Decreased sensitivity of lung ultrasound limited to the anterior chest in emergency department diagnosis of cardiogenic pulmonary edema: a retrospective analysis. Crit Ultrasound J. 2010;2(2):47–52.

28. Díaz-Gómez JL, Mayo PH, Koenig SJ. Point-of-care ultrasonography. N Engl J Med. 2021;385(17):1593–602.

29. Gargani L, Pugliese NR, Frassi F, Frumento P, Poggianti E, Mazzola M, et al. Prognostic value of lung ultrasound in patients hospitalized for heart disease irrespective of symptoms and ejection fraction. ESC Hear Fail. 2021;8(4):2660–9.

30. Lancellotti P, Price S, Edvardsen T, Cosyns B, Neskovic ANN, Dulgheru R, et al. The use of echocardiography in acute cardiovascular care: recommendations of the European association of cardiovascular imaging and the acute cardiovascular care association. Eur Hear J Acute Cardiovasc Care. 2015;4(1):3–5.

31. Gargani L, Pang PSS, Frassi F, Miglioranza MH, Dini FLL, Landi P, et al. Persistent pulmonary congestion before discharge predicts rehospitalization in heart failure: a lung ultrasound study. Cardiovasc Ultrasound. 2015;13(1):40.

32. Cogliati C, Casazza G, Ceriani E, Torzillo D, Furlotti S, Bossi I, et al. Lung ultrasound and short-term prognosis in heart failure patients. Int J Cardiol. 2016; 218.

33. Miglioranza MHMH, Picano E, Badano LPLP, Sant'Anna R, Rover M, Zaffaroni F, et al. Pulmonary congestion evaluated by lung ultrasound predicts decompensation in heart failure outpatients. Int J Cardiol. 2017; 240:271–8.

34. Platz E, Lewis EF, Uno H, Peck J, Pivetta E, Merz AA, et al. Detection and prognostic value of pulmonary congestion by lung ultrasound in ambulatory heart failure patients. Eur Heart J. 2016; ehv745.

35. Pellicori P, Shah P, Cuthbert J, Urbinati A, Zhang J, Kallvikbacka-Bennett A, et al. Prevalence, pattern and clinical relevance of ultrasound indices of congestion in outpatients with heart failure. Eur J Heart Fail. 2019;21(7):904–16.

36. Gustafsson M, Alehagen U, Johansson P. Imaging congestion with a pocket ultrasound device: prognostic implications in patients with chronic heart failure. J Card Fail. 2015; 1–7.

37. Rivas-Lasarte M, Álvarez-García J, Fernández-Martínez J, Maestro A, López-López L, Solé-González E, Pirla MJ, Mesado N, Mirabet S, Fluvià P, Brossa V, Sionis A, Roig E, Cinca J. Lung ultrasound-guided treatment in ambulatory patients with heart failure: a randomized controlled clinical trial (LUS-HF study). Eur J Heart Fail. 2019;21(12):1605–1613

38. Volpicelli G, Gargani L, Perlini S, Spinelli S, Barbieri G, Lanotte A, et al. Lung ultrasound for the early diagnosis of COVID-19 pneumonia: an international multicenter study. Intensive Care Med. 2021;47(4):444–54.

39. Pivetta E, Baldassa F, Masellis S, Bovaro F, Lupia E, Maule MM. Sources of variability in the detection of B-lines, using lung ultrasound. Ultrasound Med Biol. 2018;44(6):1212–6.

40. Palazzuoli A, Ruocco G, Franci B, Evangelista I, Lucani B, Nuti R, et al. Ultrasound indices of congestion in patients with acute heart failure according to body mass index. Clin Res Cardiol. 2020;109(11):1423–33.

41. Pellicori P, Platz E, Dauw J, Ter Maaten JM, Martens P, Pivetta E, et al. Ultrasound imaging of congestion in heart failure: examinations beyond the heart. Eur J Heart Fail. 2021;23(5):703–12.

42. Carluccio E, Dini FL, Biagioli P, Lauciello R, Simioniuc A, Zuchi C, et al. The "Echo Heart Failure Score": an echocardiographic risk prediction score of mortality in systolic heart failure. Eur J Heart Fail. 2013;15(8):868–76.

43. Bonios MJ, Kyrzopoulos S, Tsiapras D, Adamopoulos SN. Ultrasound guidance for volume management in patients with heart failure. Heart Fail Rev. 2020;25(6):927–35.

44. Holm JH, Frederiksen CA, Juhl-Olsen P, Sloth E. Perioperative use of focus assessed transthoracic echocardiography (FATE). Anesth Analg. 2012;115(5):1029–32.

POCUS in Acute Myocardial Ischaemia

Anthony J. Barron and Hatem Soliman Aboumarie

"To know the movements of the heart and to know the heart . . . From the heart arise the vessels which go to the whole body ... if the physician lay the hands or his fingers to the head, to the back of the head, to the hands, to the place of the stomach, to the arms or to the feet, then he examines the heart, because all of his limbs possess its vessels, that is: the heart speaks out of the vessels of every limb ... if the heart trembles, has little power and sinks, the disease is advancing" The Papyrus Ebers, Ancient Egyptian physician (circa 1534 BC).

Abstract

Patients who present with acute myocardial ischaemia are at significant risk of death, which can be reduced with timely management including revascularisation. The ECG is typically the gate keeper for urgent revascularisation, but many patients do not have typical ST segment changes, and certain ECG patterns such as left bundle branch block can limit the utility of the ECG. Ischaemia affects the function of myocardium, so an assessment of ventricular function through POCUS could identify patients where urgent treatment is required and those where deferral is safe. Ischaemia affects the ventricles in different ways but typically through regional systolic dysfunction, something that echocardiography is optimally designed to identify. Abbreviated echocardiographic protocols can be designed to get these answers quickly, by the patient's bedside and with the ability to share with the interventionalist in the catheter lab. This chapter will explore the evidence behind how the ventricles maladapt to ischaemia, principally with systolic dysfunction but also other changes (such as diastolic dysfunction) and the sensitivity and specificity of regional dysfunction to predict a vessel-based assessment.

A. J. Barron (✉) · H. S. Aboumarie
Consultant Cardiologist, Harefield Hospital,
Harefield, UK
e-mail: A.Barron@rbht.nhs.uk

H. S. Aboumarie
e-mail: H.SolimanAboumarie@rbht.nhs.uk

Department of Anaesthetics and Critical Care,
Harefield Hospital, London, UK

Keywords

POCUS · Myocardial infarction · Ischaemia · Regional wall motion abnormalities · 17-segment model · Ischaemic cascade

© The Author(s), under exclusive license to Springer Nature Switzerland AG 2023
H. Soliman-Aboumarie et al. (eds.), *Cardiopulmonary Point of Care Ultrasound,*
https://doi.org/10.1007/978-3-031-29472-3_8

Key Messages

- Patients with acute coronary syndromes often present with atypical symptoms, often at the time of concurrent illness. Point of Care ultrasound (POCUS) is a potential tool in patients where the diagnosis is unclear via history and ECG, or where risk stratification is needed prior to referral to cardiology
- Cardiac ischaemic sets up a cascade of abnormalities, a number of which can be identified by POCUS
- Many of these changes induced by cardiac ischaemia will persist even after the cessation of pain and ECG changes, sometimes for hours
- Diastolic changes and perfusion abnormalities can be identified with echocardiography but should be considered techniques outside of the scope of most POCUS practitioners
- The typical findings during or following a period of acute ischaemia, are regional wall motion abnormalities, or more specifically a reduction or absence in the thickening of wall segments, which will adopt a territorial distribution based on the affected coronary vessel
- Care must be taken, but POCUS may be even more informative, in challenging circumstances such as LBBB, following previous cardiac surgery, and in patients with enzymatic diagnosis of myocardial infarction but non-obstructed coronary arteries.

The Patient's Presentation

Ischaemia presentations are varied. Below is a quick summary of what to look out for, but this has been detailed previously in many publications so will not be described in much detail here.

Patient Findings—Typical and Atypical

The classic presentation of acute coronary ischaemia is central chest pain with radiation to the left shoulder, neck or jaw. The description often approximates tightness, constriction or heaviness, not settling with rest (except stable angina) or activity. Breathlessness and autonomic symptoms such as sweatiness or clamminess are associated [1, 2]. However, in reality this classical presentation is often not seen, with a complete absence of pain in over 8% in one large study [3].

The definition of an acute myocardial infarction (MI) requires the presence of symptoms, ECG changes or imaging evidence of myocardial ischaemia, alongside an elevation in cardiac enzymes (almost universally troponin) [4]. ECG changes are typically divided into ST elevation (STEMI) and all others (so called non-ST elevation MIs).

STEMIs frequently present suddenly, often in patients who were previously well, due to plaque rupture within a coronary artery blocking the vessel; a Type 1 MI. In contrast to this, whilst non-ST elevation MI presentations may be due to acute atherosclerotic rupture with a chest pain presentation, they are also often diagnosed after the detection of cardiac enzymes in an acutely unwell patient. In many of these cases stable coronary disease can become haemodynamically limiting when demand is increased, for example when the patient is septic or severely anaemic; a Type 2 MI. A Type 2 MI rarely presents with ST elevation [5]. Utilising POCUS to spot regional or global systolic dysfunction could aid decision making as often there are reasons that urgent revascularisation may not be ideal, and risk stratification maybe as important as diagnosis.

What to Do if Unsure

Typical symptoms and ECG changes with ST elevation should prompt urgent revascularisation if that is appropriate for the patient [1]. However, many patients don't present so precisely. The use of risk scoring tools, such as the TIMI [6] or

GRACE [7] scores predict mortality more than aid diagnosis. Cardiac enzymes remain the most specific test to determine myocardial necrosis. A thorough history should be obtained alongside serial ECGs. If these fail to shed light bedside echocardiography can help support the diagnosis of an MI by identifying anomalies such as regional wall motion abnormalities (RWMA). In an early study of echocardiography, many more patients, later confirmed to have MI, were diagnosed on echocardiography than ECG [8]. ECG has been shown to have poor accuracy at localising non-STEMI culprit vessels [9].

In the latest international guidelines for the management of NSTE-ACSs in the ER, patients are divided into 3 categories, rule-out, rule-in or observe. In the observe group, when patients don't fit neatly into either other group, urgent echocardiography is recommended alongside a 3-h troponin measurement, still at the time point where this would commonly be performed by emergency physicians [2].

Another patient group with uncertainty are those with ECG findings where it is unknown if they are new or old. These changes typically will not be dynamic (i.e. will not change over minutes/hours in the Emergency Room). Left bundle branch block (LBBB) has long been heralded as a STEMI equivalent, but in truth is rarely acute [10]. Echocardiography can help identify areas of reduced function compared to pure dyssynchrony of LBBB (will be discussed later).

Evidence for Timely Intervention

It is important to highlight that spending time and effort to promptly diagnose coronary ischaemia benefits patients in the most meaningful way by reducing mortality [1, 2]. In early STEMI trials prompt intervention with thrombolysis led to superior outcomes [11], and this was often heralded as a marker of departmental success. With evidence that percutaneous coronary intervention (PCI) outperforms thrombolysis [12, 13] most specialist centres around the world have moved to rapid percutaneous revascularisation as first line.

In patients presenting without ST elevation time is still important. Early PCI trials showed benefit if performed early [14, 15].

Finally in patients presenting with symptoms of stable angina and no elevation in cardiac enzymes timely intervention with medical therapy (anti-platelet agents and statins) and coronary angiography can still reduce mortality and morbidity to a lesser extent. Although ischaemia should be short lived without any evidence of infarction, suggesting that POCUS will have little role in these cases, the presence of a RWMA increases the likelihood of underlying coronary disease, and could lead an experienced emergency physician to expedite further out-patient investigations and initiate medical therapy. Myocardium may remain stunned after a period of prolonged ischaemia, even in stable angina, and so echocardiographic abnormalities may persist longer than expected.

The Ischaemic Cascade and Its Utility

The ischaemic cascade was first postulated in 1987 by Nesto and Kowalchuk [16]. Our understanding of cardiac physiology, and the utilisation of echocardiography, have come a long way since then.

Figure 1 shows the ischaemic cascade as it was originally described. As shown symptoms are a late feature of ischaemia, with changes identifiable by echocardiography prior to this point. This suggests that if a patient has developed symptoms worthy of a visit to the emergency room, we should expect some abnormalities on ultrasound, certainly if symptoms persist during the examination. Can we use POCUS to detect changes in perfusion or flow, diastology and wall motion to detect subtle periods of ischaemia, or in those presenting after the event?

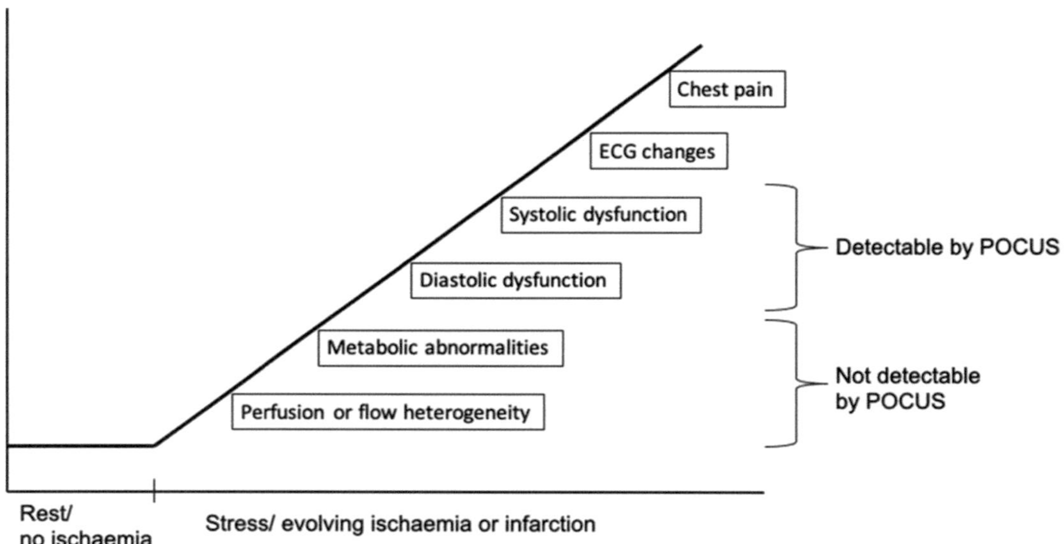

Fig. 1 The ischaemic cascade. How the original ischaemic cascade was proposed. At rest, when there is no ischaemia, all appearances are normal. With increasing time, stress and ischaemia different abnormalities occur in a predictable pattern. Here along the right-hand side, we highlight where POCUS could be useful. *Nesto RW, Kowalchuk GJ. Am J Cardiol. 1987 Mar 9;59(7):23C–30C*

How the Myocardium Differentially Responds to Ischaemia

Despite criticism of the ischaemic cascade principle [17] it is worth considering the role echocardiography can have in each of the major steps of this cascade. Even if they do not occur sequentially in all patients, being able to identify different abnormalities will be useful. A standard POCUS protocol will focus on the systolic abnormalities visible on all basic views; but for completeness these other abnormalities will be considered first.

Perfusion Abnormalities of the Left Ventricle

An early step on the ischaemic cascade is abnormal perfusion which is specifically targeted by other imaging modalities such as Single Photon Emission Computed Tomography Myocardial Perfusion Scintigraphy (SPECT MPS) or perfusion Magnetic Resonance Imaging (MRI). Neither of these are readily accessible at the point-of-care for a patient presenting emergently. Echocardiography can assess perfusion but these techniques are challenging and require advanced training. Therefore, only an overview of the concepts and potential are included here.

Technique for Contrast Echocardiographic Assessment of Myocardial Perfusion

There is extensive experience with echocardiographic contrast to improve opacification of the left ventricle, with a few products commercially available (Sonovue, Luminity, Optison). Image optimisation requires the manipulation of device settings so is suited to larger, albeit still portable machines, rather than the smallest handheld machines. If possible, use the contrast setting in the probe defaults, or alternatively (but not as effectively) turn down the Mechanical Index or power, typically to 0.4 or below (as shown in

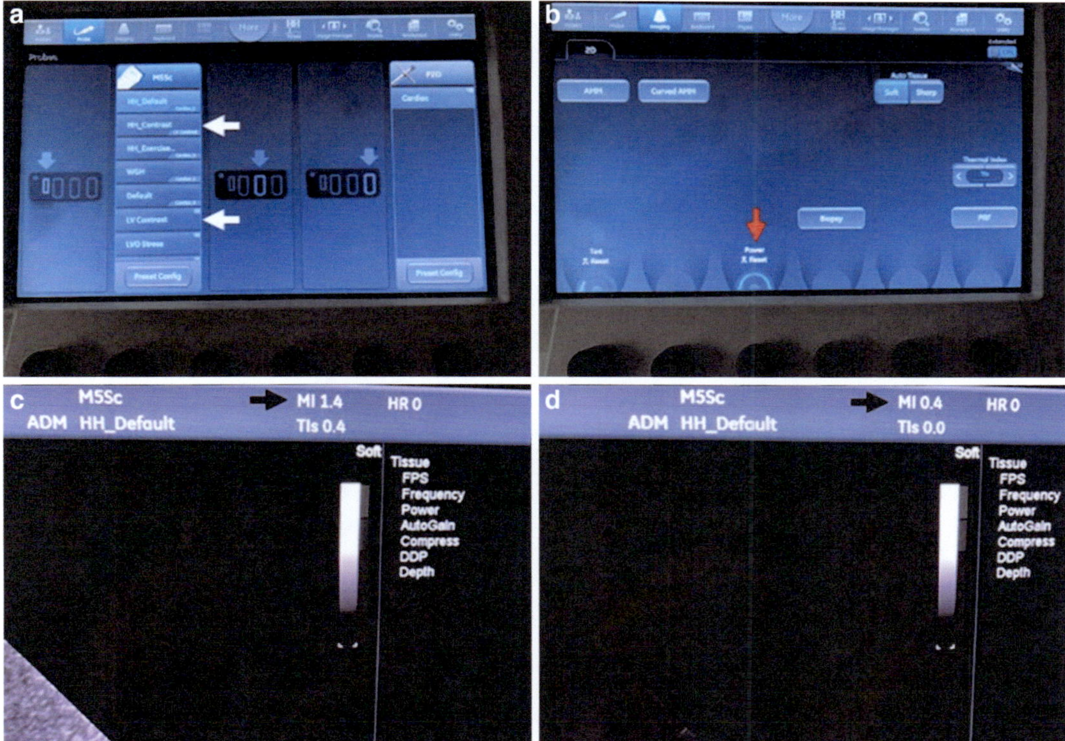

Fig. 2 Machine settings to utilise LV opacification contrast. Within each machine and manufacturer there will be a unique way to change the settings to facilitate LV opacification contrast, these examples are using the GE E95 system. The most accurate way is shown in A using the contrast presets after pressing the probe option (two options shown on this screen by large white arrows). Alternatively if these presets are not available, on the bottom screen there should be an option to reduce the power as shown in B (large red arrow), the mechanical index setting in the top right corner of the image screen (identified by large black arrow) should reduce from 1.4 —as shown in C to about 0.4—as shown in D

Fig. 2a–d). This reverses the appearances so that the myocardium becomes dark and the blood pool becomes bright when contrast is given. The first advantage is improved image quality with an increased ability to detect RWMAs (discussed in section "Left Ventricular Systolic Abnormalities"). Secondly over a small number of heart beats the muscle brightens as contrast enters the myocardium. Inadequate perfusion leads to areas where darkness persists.

Tip: It should be stressed again that this is an advanced skill, although potentially easily available and relatively quick. However, without adequate training the potential for diagnostic mistakes would be high.

Left Ventricular Diastolic Abnormalities

Left ventricular diastolic relaxation requires energy. Healthy myocardium relaxes quickly, reducing intra-ventricular diastolic pressures close to zero, maximising the pressure gradient across the mitral valve allowing good emptying of the left atrium into the left ventricle. With worsening diastolic abnormalities, and unfortunately as part of the typical ageing process, left ventricular diastolic relaxation becomes increasingly impaired, leading to changes in trans-mitral flow with typical patterns seen on trans-mitral Doppler. The four main patterns on trans-mitral Doppler are shown in Fig. 3a–d.

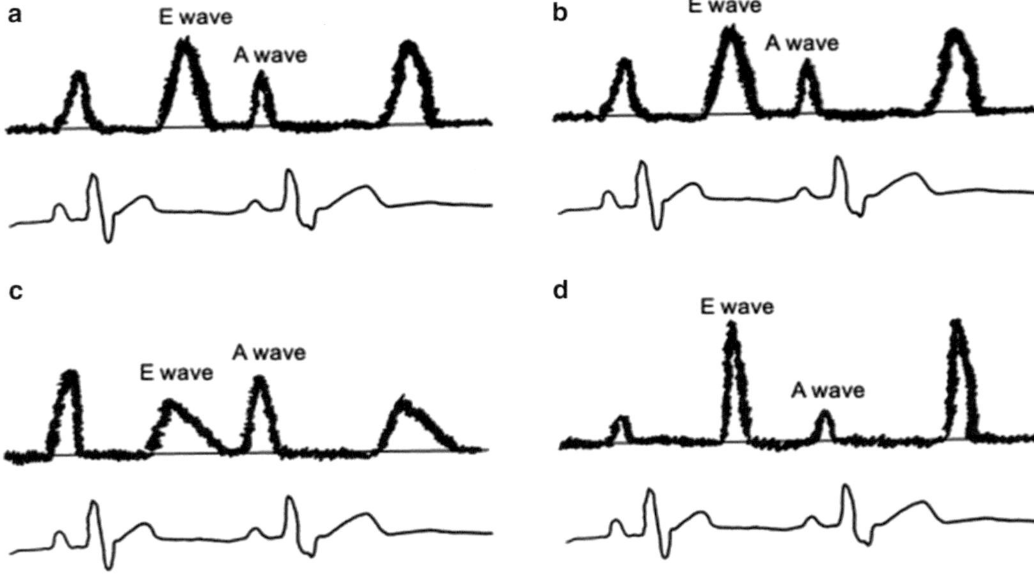

Fig. 3 Four patterns of trans-mitral Doppler flow. These four patterns, from a to d, show the evolution of increasing diastolic abnormalities and rising LV filling pressures, when using pulsed-wave Doppler at the tips of the mitral leaflets. Pattern a and c are largely identical and so are called normal and pseudo-normal and require advanced techniques to differentiate. Pattern b, abnormal, or impaired, relaxation, is the typical pattern seen in older patients, or those with significant but stable cardiac problems. Pattern d, restrictive filling where the first wave is at least twice the height of the second wave, portends the worst prognosis

An abnormal pattern is common at rest in many patients and patients in the ER would be unlikely to have had recent echocardiography to identify if this abnormality is new or old. Therefore, the clinical utility of abnormal diastolic function is significantly impaired. In one study during acute MI, left ventricular end-diastolic pressure (LVEDP) was measured invasively. Despite high mean LVEDP the predominant filling pattern was impaired relaxation [18], the pattern most likely to be encountered in older patients, and many younger patients with stable underlying cardiac disease.

Despite these limitations there is one area where diastolic dysfunction can have benefit and that is in risk stratification. A restrictive filling pattern, as defined by an E:A ratio of >2 (Fig. 3d) predicts in-hospital heart failure and mortality [19, 20]. Whilst this may not help you decide who should go straight to the catheter lab, it may help support a referral to cardiology or early use of medical therapy including diuretics. The presence of a restrictive filling pattern post-STEMI was associated with ischaemic duration in one study [21], and therefore in patients with a non-diagnostic ECG (for example LBBB) could help predict a significant episode of recent or ongoing ischaemia.

The heart's typical response to raised LV end-diastolic filling pressures is left atrial dilatation, but this will take some time. A restrictive filling pattern on trans-mitral Doppler in the presence of normal left atrial size would suggest an acute change of haemodynamics such as seen with ischaemia or infarction.

Overall diastolic abnormalities are not specific for acute coronary ischaemia and whilst some understanding of the basics can be beneficial, they are not as valuable to assess ischaemia as systolic abnormalities.

Left Ventricular Systolic Abnormalities

Regional wall motion abnormalities (RWMAs) of the left ventricle are the hallmark of point of care cardiac ultrasound to assess for current and recent ischaemia. As with all markers of myocardial performance, their sensitivity for an acute event will decline as time passes after the event, assuming flow has been restored. However, abnormalities of wall motion can persist for several days after a period of substantial ischaemia [22] with wall motion recovery inversely proportional to duration of ischaemia. This study suggested necrosis, identifiable by RWMAs on echo, occurs after 20 min of total ischaemia, and recovery can still take up to a week following just 15 min of total ischaemia [22]. In humans, shorter periods of ischaemia in patients admitted with unstable angina led to persistent RWMAs for 1–2 days [23].

It stands to reason therefore that a patient presenting with a prolonged episode of cardiac chest pain should have RWMAs persisting for hours after pain cessation and—because it is lower in the ischaemic cascade—following resolution of ECG changes.

For analysis echocardiographers typically divide the left ventricle into 17 segments (Fig. 4a), however for simplicity a 12 or 13 segment model can be employed. How these align to the 3 main coronary arteries, the left anterior descending (LAD), left circumflex (LCx) both of which come from the left main stem (LMS) and the right coronary artery (RCA) is shown in Fig. 4b.

For assessment of left ventricular wall motion the following views are recommended (Fig. 5). The relevant landmarks identifying each view are described.

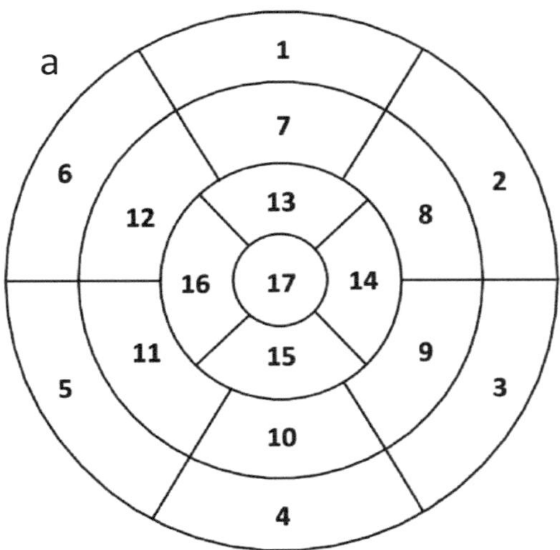
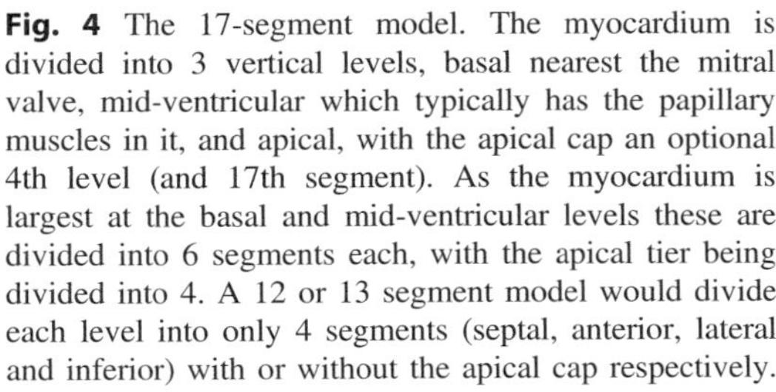

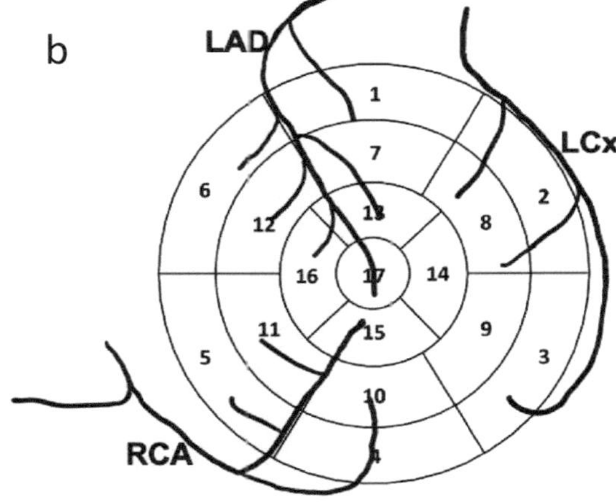

Fig. 4 The 17-segment model. The myocardium is divided into 3 vertical levels, basal nearest the mitral valve, mid-ventricular which typically has the papillary muscles in it, and apical, with the apical cap an optional 4th level (and 17th segment). As the myocardium is largest at the basal and mid-ventricular levels these are divided into 6 segments each, with the apical tier being divided into 4. A 12 or 13 segment model would divide each level into only 4 segments (septal, anterior, lateral and inferior) with or without the apical cap respectively.

In 4b the segmental model is shown alongside the most typical coronary artery distribution (RCA dominant). 1 = basal anterior, 2 = basal anterolateral, 3 = basal inferolateral, 4 = basal inferior, 5 = basal inferoseptal, 6 = basal anteroseptal, 7 = mid-ventricular anterior, 8 = mid-ventricular anterolateral, 9 = mid-ventricular inferolateral, 10 = mid-ventricular inferior, 11 = mid-ventricular inferoseptal, 12 = mid-ventricular anteroseptal, 13 = apical anterior, 14 = apical lateral, 15 = apical inferior, 16 = apical septal, 17 = apical cap

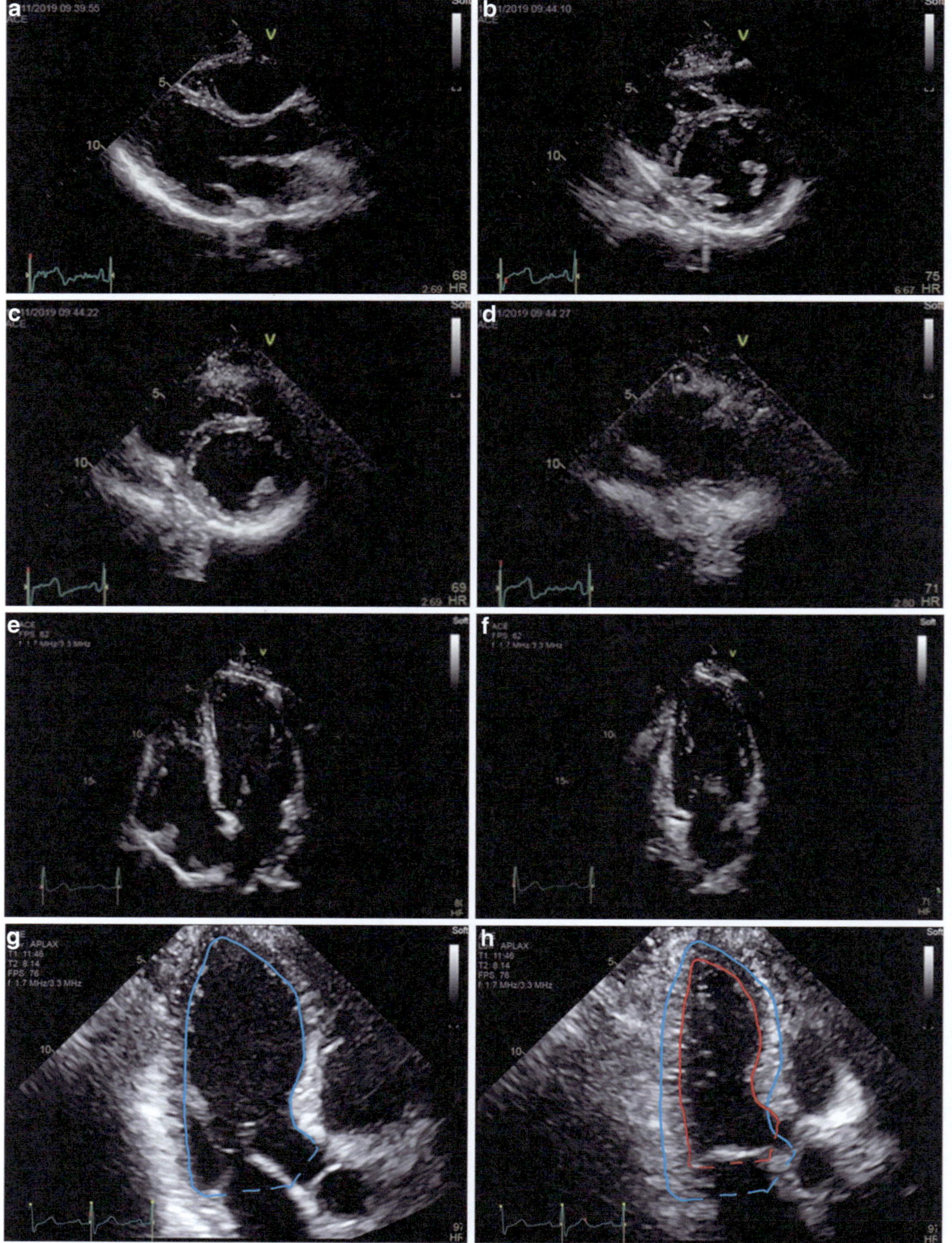

◀ **Fig. 5** The standard 2D views to assess the left ventricular myocardium. The 7 main views of the left ventricle are shown in end-diastole in the following order: Parasternal long-axis view (**a**) showing the anteroseptal and inferolateral walls of the left ventricle; parasternal short-axis view at a basal level (**b**); parasternal short-axis view at a mid-ventricular level (**c**); parasternal short-axis view at an apical level (**d**); Apical 4-chamber view (**e**) showing the inferoseptal and anterolateral walls of the left ventricle; Apical 2-chamber view (**f**) showing the anterior and inferior walls of the left ventricle; Apical 3-chamber view (**g**) showing the anteroseptal and inferolateral walls of the left ventricle; Apical 3-chamber view from G but in end-systole (**h**) showing normokinesia of the anteroseptum and inferolateral wall (blue lines indicate wall in diastole, red line systole)

- Parasternal long-axis view
- Parasternal short-axis view at 3 ventricular levels (basal, mid-ventricular and apical)
- Apical four-chamber view
- Apical two-chamber view
- Apical three-chamber (or long-axis) view.

Tip: With this approach each of the segments of the left ventricle can be viewed at least twice and most segments will be seen both parallel and perpendicular to the ultrasound beam.

Tip: It must be remembered that spatial resolution is best when the wall is perpendicular to the beam, so the inferolateral wall will be better assessed in the PLAX view than the A3C view.

Despite the description as "Wall Motion Abnormalities", the key finding is actually wall thickening, not motion, as areas of viable myocardium can still pull adjacent infarcted or stunned areas of the left ventricle towards the apex. Therefore, wall motion can happen in the absence of wall thickening—and still signify myocardial abnormalities—although the converse is unlikely. In reality, the situations where the two are divorced suggest abnormalities which may make accurate assessment of recent ischaemia almost impossible, for example with old infarcts, conduction abnormalities and right ventricular overload. When analysing each segment individually grading them 1–4 is a common convention. The scoring systems are shown in Table 1.

Hyperkinesia, the increase in wall motion and thickening, will not be considered here.

To average motion for the whole ventricle, the wall motion score index (WMSI) is calculated by adding all 17 numbers up and dividing by 17 (the total number of segments), giving a WMSI between 1 and, theoretically, 4. The WMSI correlates inversely with LV function.

Figures 6, 7, 8, 9 and 10 show images in systole and diastole of these different states in different regions within the heart.

In segments of the myocardium with normo- or hypokinesia, perfusion is generally adequate to maintain tissue viability, and wall thickness will be unchanged. This may be normal (typically 8–10 mm) or increased (>11 mm) but should be largely consistent across the associated segments. The exception will be certain conditions where the septum, especially the basal septum, preferentially hypertrophies.

In contrast dyskinetic segments of myocardium are likely to have fully infarcted, the myocardium should be thin (around 5 mm), and may appear bright to echocardiography. Akinetic myocardium may be newly infarcted, currently ischaemic (both likely to not have led to wall thinning yet) or old infarction (will lead to wall thinning). Considering segmental wall thickness, notably thinning, adds confidence to the diagnosis of significant coronary artery disease but suggests chronicity.

Table 1 How to define wall motion using a 1–4 scoring system

Wall motion segment score	Description
1	Normokinesia—>30% increase in systolic thickening
2	Hypokinesia—<30% increase in systolic thickening
3	Akinesia—absence of systolic thickening, no motion
4	Dyskinesia—paradoxical outward motion in systole

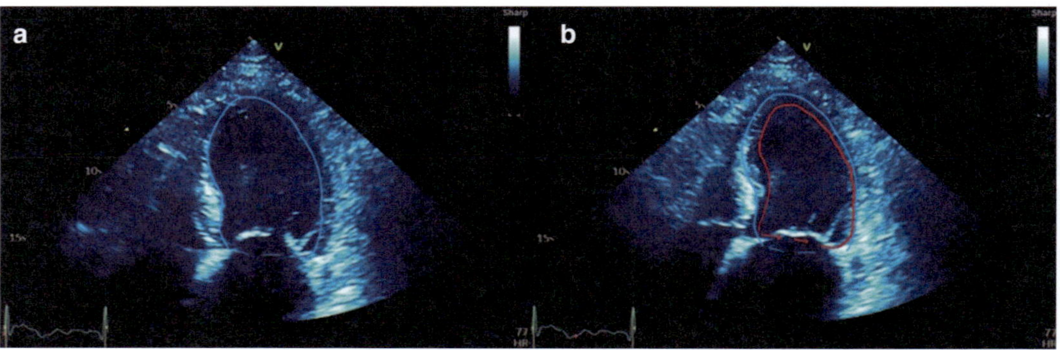

Fig. 6 Diastolic and systolic views of a left ventricle with hypokinesia of the lateral wall. This apical 4-chamber view of a patient following a circumflex infarction the septum thickens and move inwards well from end-diastole (**a**) to end-systole (**b**). In contrast the lateral wall has markedly reduced thickening (severely hypokinetic) with reduced longitudinal motion of the lateral mitral annulus compared to the septal (blue lines indicate wall in diastole, red line systole)

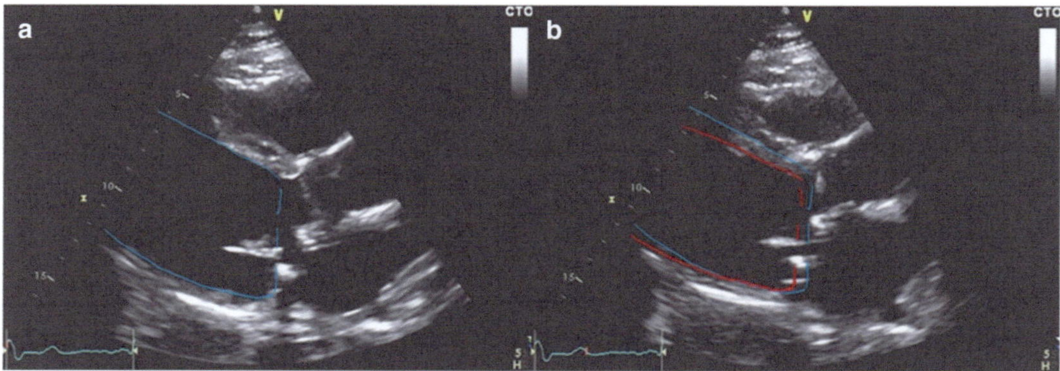

Fig. 7 Diastolic and systolic views of a left ventricle with akinesia of the inferolateral wall. In this parasternal long-axis view of a patient following a circumflex infarction the anteroseptum thickens and move inwards well from end-diastole (**a**) to end-systole (**b**). In contrast the inferolateral (previously known as posterior) wall is akinetic (blue lines indicate wall in diastole, red line systole)

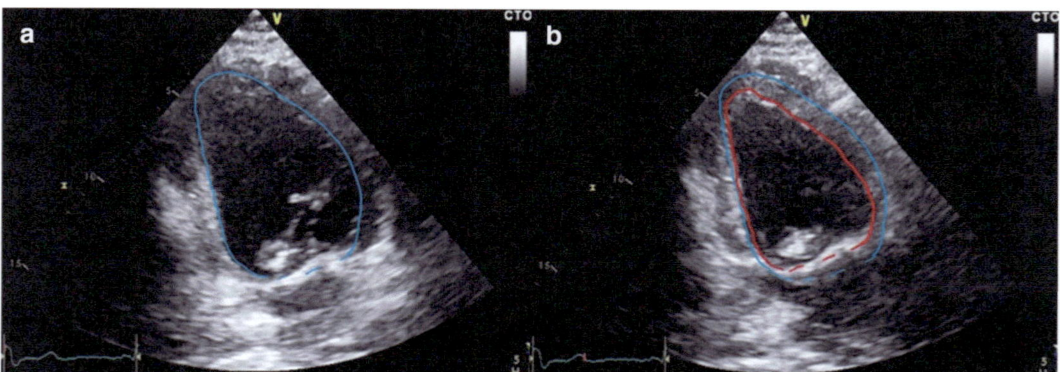

Fig. 8 Diastolic and systolic views of a left ventricle with akinesia of the inferior wall. In this apical 2-chamber view of a patient following an RCA infarction the anterior wall thickens and move inwards well from end-diastole (**a**) to end-systole (**b**). In contrast the inferior wall is akinetic (blue lines indicate wall in diastole, red line systole)

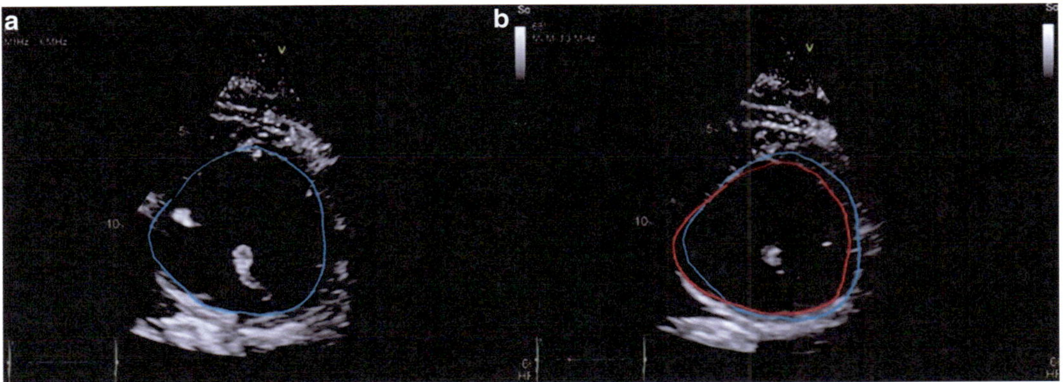

Fig. 9 Diastolic and systolic views of a left ventricle with an aneurysmal and dyskinetic inferior wall. In this parasternal short-axis view at the mid-ventricular level, the normal circular geometry is distorted at end-diastole (**a**) with an aneurysmal appearance to the inferior wall and inferoseptum. In systole (**b**) this moves outwards rather than in, dyskinesia. Note the generalised hypokinesia of the remaining walls (blue lines indicate wall in diastole, red line systole)

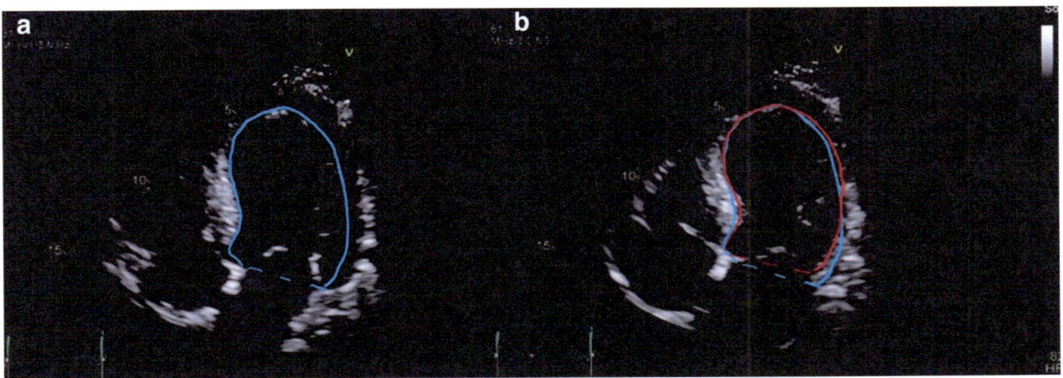

Fig. 10 Diastolic and Systolic views of a left ventricle with an akinetic anteroseptum and apex. In this apical 4-chamber view of a patient following an LAD infarction the basal to mid lateral wall thickens and move inwards well from end-diastole (**a**) to end-systole (**b**). In contrast the septum, apex and apical lateral wall are akinetic (blue lines indicate wall in diastole, red line systole)

As described in section "Perfusion Abnormalities of the Left Ventricle" contrast can be used to help the routine analysis of left ventricular segments. This has been proven to increase reproducibility, accuracy and feasibility of segmental analysis [24, 25]. The routine echocardiographic assessment should be performed prior to changing the machine's settings and administering contrast. In an echocardiography department the largest time lost is in obtaining venous access, something that should already be performed in those presenting to the ED and so the procedure should be quick. Figure 11 shows an apical 4 chamber view with the administration of Sonovue contrast.

Other Motion Abnormalities Including LBBB

Tip: In a patient with a normal ECG and without a prior cardiac history all RWMAs should be taken seriously as support for a recent event.

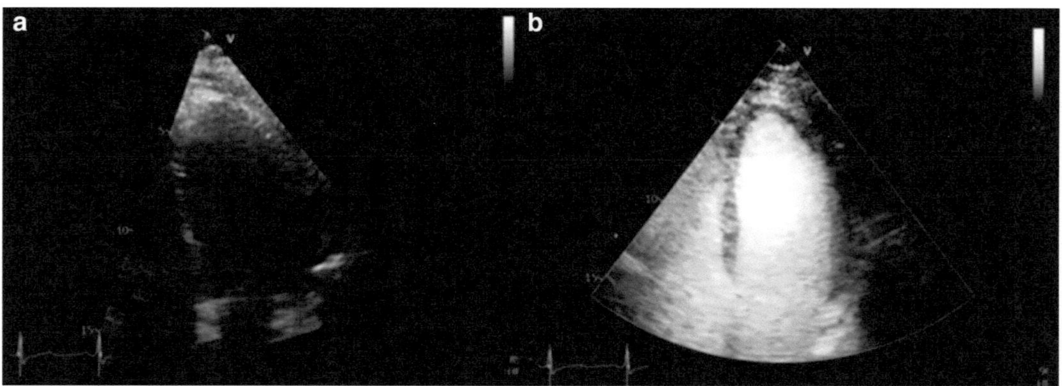

Fig. 11 Apical 4-chamber view showing poor image quality (**a**) and following contrast administration (**b**). Left ventricular opacification contrast. In this example Sonovue was used. **a**–Apical 4-chamber view without contrast showing poor wall/blood pool differentiation. **b**–Same view 20 s following contrast administration

However, in many cases the patient's heart was not normal prior to the recent event for which they have attended emergently.

Left bundle branch block (LBBB) gives particular concern as it often hinders the emergency physician's ability to utilise the ECG to make a diagnosis. Because of the time delay between septal to lateral wall contraction, this could often give the impression of RWMAs. Septal activation occurs prior to aortic valve opening, with an initial rapid inwards motion as RV pressure rises, followed by a paradoxical motion towards the right heart, without typical wall thickening. The broader the QRS complex, the more likely the paradoxical motion of the interventricular septum towards the right heart.

Tip: An M-mode line across the basal to mid-ventricle in the PLAX view will show the typical LBBB pattern explainable by the conduction abnormality, not by acute ischaemia.

Tip: RWMAs seen in the anterior, inferior and lateral walls to indicate hypo- or akinesia due to recent ischaemia are more reliable than those seen in the septum.

Tip: A patient who is paced (pacing spikes may not be seen but a LBBB pattern with "concordance"–all QRS complexes from V1-6 typically point downwards–is highly suggestive) will have similar motion abnormalities to pure LBBB.

The other groups that typically lead to septal motion abnormalities include situations of right heart overload, and in patients following cardiac surgery and cardiopulmonary bypass.

A full POCUS assessment of an unwell patient will include the right ventricle, which should normally in the A4C view appear significantly smaller than the left ventricle. If it does not, especially if the apex appears to belong to the RV rather than the LV or co-shared by both the RV and LV, it is likely the RV is dilated, and the right heart is volume or pressure overloaded. In a normal PSAX view, the LV should be circular with the RV crescent shaped around it. With a dilating and increasingly volume overloaded RV, this geometry changes so that the RV adopts a more circular appearance, with a D-shaped LV, predominantly in diastole. In contrast a pressure overloaded RV, for example due to pulmonary hypertension from a pulmonary embolus, will flatten the septum in systole.

Patients who have undergone cardiac surgery often have total paradoxical motion of the septum in systole (towards the right heart) although wall thickening should be preserved. The exact mechanism is not fully understood but probably relates to changes in pericardial restraint [26, 27].

Overall, it is the authors' opinion that whenever one of the above conditions is noted, septal (and probably apical) wall motion abnormalities must be taken with a degree of scepticism. However, it must also be remembered that the likelihood of a significant acute event is much higher in patients with a prior cardiac history, LBBB, or the other abnormalities described, and therefore the threshold to call the echocardiogram abnormal, and refer the patient, should naturally be lower.

Further Abnormalities

POCUS assessment of the heart may reveal other abnormalities that help support or refute the diagnosis. Aortic valve disease can cause ischaemia due to reduced cardiac output (and increased demand) in aortic stenosis, and low diastolic pressure in aortic regurgitation (the period when the coronaries fill with blood). Identifying an abnormal aortic valve is discussed in another chapter but significant calcific aortic stenosis presenting with chest pain should expedite a formal echocardiogram to assess severity, probably prior to angiography, unless there is ST segment elevation. Making this

diagnosis is also important to plan your anti-ischaemic strategy.

Mitral regurgitation (MR) is commonly associated with left ventricular ischaemia. This is because the valve is dependent on the functioning of the papillary muscles, which as an active part of the myocardium, are susceptible to ischaemia.

Tip: Interestingly acute ischaemia can both cause and improve mitral regurgitation.

Chronic RCA or LCx ischaemia and infarction often lead to tethering and remodelling of the posteromedial papillary muscle, leading to posteriorly directed MR. The anterolateral papillary muscle is less commonly affected due to its dual blood supply from both the LAD and LCx. Conversely acute ischaemia can lead to a lengthening of the papillary muscle, allowing greater closure of the mitral leaflets and reducing chronic MR.

The most devastating mitral consequence of myocardial infarction is a papillary muscle rupture (Fig. 12a). A large mass attached to the mitral leaflets moving into the left ventricle in diastole and left atrium in systole, with a clinical

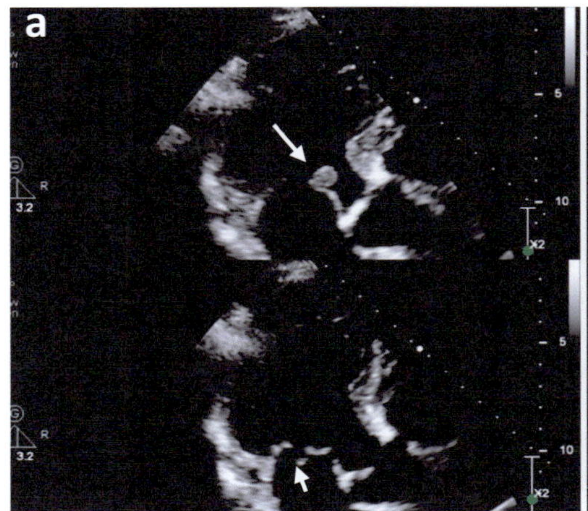
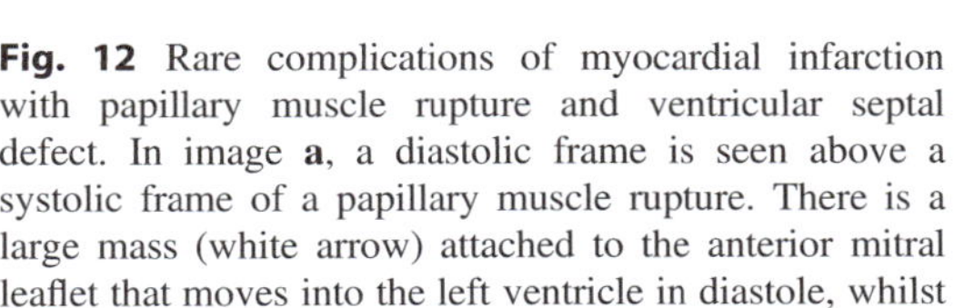
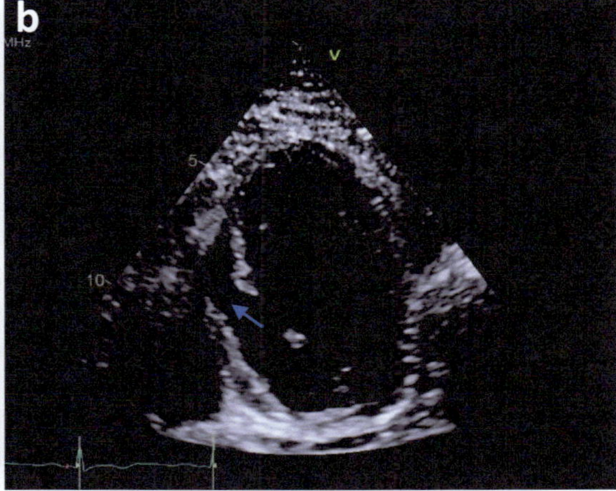

Fig. 12 Rare complications of myocardial infarction with papillary muscle rupture and ventricular septal defect. In image **a**, a diastolic frame is seen above a systolic frame of a papillary muscle rupture. There is a large mass (white arrow) attached to the anterior mitral leaflet that moves into the left ventricle in diastole, whilst in systole we can see the mass in the left atrium and the anterior leaflet is flail In image **b** a patient with an inferior myocardial infarction has presented late to hospital (after 24 h) with a defect in the inter-ventricular septum between the LV and the RV (blue arrow)

history suggestive of an acute MI rather than endocarditis, should strongly support this diagnosis. These patients will usually be in hydrostatic pulmonary oedema (Lung ultrasound will show abundance of B-lines). Urgent critical care management should be sought and the patient referred immediately for consideration of surgery.

Another rare complication of infarction is a ventricular septal defect (Fig. 12b). This may happen in the inferoseptum after a right coronary artery infarct. A gap will be seen, most easily imaged in the PSAX view.

As described in other sections, a full assessment including the aorta, right ventricle and left atrium should be undertaken which will help identify other causes for acute chest pain. Whilst it wouldn't be expected for an uncomplicated episode of myocardial ischaemia to cause acute changes to the other cardiac chambers, identifying abnormalities such as significant left atrial or right ventricular dilatation strongly support chronic cardiac conditions, but make the assessment of the left ventricle segments potentially harder.

Prognosis

Quite simply put the greater the total wall motion score index the worse the prognosis.

Tip: Areas of akinesia and dyskinesia more reliably predict completed infarction where revascularisation has come too late with the increased risk of post-infarction heart failure and arrhythmia.

Generally, the two greatest predictors of a poor outcome are the number of affected segments and left ventricular dysfunction. Therefore, an assessment for ischaemia should always include the LV ejection fraction. Whether predicting prognosis from abnormalities should influence decision making is debatable but almost certainly those with the most impaired hearts have the most to gain from therapy, even if the opportunity for revascularisation has passed and their overall prognosis is worse.

The most devastating myocardial infarctions typically involve the left main stem or proximal LAD, with a greater likelihood of death, cardiogenic shock or heart failure [28, 29]. Therefore, patients displaying signs of ischaemia within these territories, assuming no ST segment elevation, could be prioritised for referral to cardiology. Isolated RCA or Cx ischaemia (or distal LAD), in the absence of ST elevation, could initially be managed more safely medically, especially in a patient who is acutely unwell for other reasons, for example sepsis or acute anaemia, allowing time to treat the underlying condition exacerbating the ischaemia. Given that ECG is poorly able to diagnose a NSTEMI [8] or localise culprit vessels [9] makes the use of POCUS even more vital.

Regionality and Benefit in Identifying Culprit Vessel Ischaemia

A summary of the typical coronary arteries, and how they commonly align to the 17-segment model of the left ventricle, is shown in Fig. 4b. There is a variation across adults as to the myocardial segments they each perfuse; however, some typical rules apply. The LAD typically supplies the most segments including the apex, with its branches, the diagonals, perfusing the anterior wall. LAD ischaemia should affect the apex, although if the ischaemia is within a diagonal only the apex could be spared. The RCA, when dominant—as in the majority of the population (80–85%)—becomes the posterior descending artery (PDA), meeting the LAD at the apex. Unlike the LAD where the most distal (apical) myocardial segments are typically the most affected, in RCA ischaemia, the basal and mid segments of the inferior wall and inferoseptum can be affected together or separately, often with sparing of the inferoapical region, as the LAD wraps around the apex supplying collateral flow. Unless the LCx is dominant, ischaemia here should be confined to the lateral wall.

Specificity for diagnosing ischaemia is low when only a single segment is believed to be abnormal. The basal inferior wall is frequently inaccurately identified as abnormal. This is due to two phenomena; firstly incomplete counter-clockwise rotation from the A4C to the A2C view with foreshortening. Ideally basal inferior wall motion abnormalities should be confirmed in the PSAX view, however this is susceptible to the second phenomenon; in systole, atrial myocardium, or the fibrotic area of the mitral annulus, may translocate to a point occupied by ventricular myocardium in diastole, seen as absent thickening. Therefore, the authors feel that basal inferior abnormalities should be confirmed in both the PSAX and A2C views, and even then, if not associated with any other abnormalities, should be viewed with a high probability of artefact. Isolated basal anterior or anterolateral wall motion abnormalities are also susceptible to attenuation from the overlying anterolateral papillary muscle but should be reliably imaged in the PSAX view.

Because proximal LAD and LMS lesions are associated with the worst prognosis, the RWMAs that when seen together should encourage rapid action include the anterior wall, anteroseptum and apex. The apex and anteroseptum strongly suggest the LAD, and the anterior wall localises this before the first diagonal, i.e. proximal LAD or above in the LMS.

In critically ill patients their resting haemodynamics may approximate conditions that would be considered stress when well. Undoubtably ischaemia during deliberate stress portends a worse prognosis than no ischaemia at all, but prognosis is far superior to those with acute, unprovoked, ischaemia. Prognosis is also influence by the degree of stress, for example RWMAs appearing at only 2 min at 25W on a bicycle are far more concerning than the same RWMAs appearing after 15 min at 150W. However when the stressor is critical illness these patients often have a worse prognosis than those presenting just with acute ischaemia. The difficulty lies in establishing whether the RWMAs are a direct consequence of the ongoing stress for example sepsis, anaemia or vasopressors where the underlying coronary disease is likely to be mild, versus critical coronary disease tipped over the edge by the abnormal haemodynamics. An accurate assessment should make a note of any influencing factors and entering the blood pressure on the screen is always a useful addition.

Myocardial Infarction with Non-obstructed Coronary Arteries (MINOCA)

With angiography being offered to increasing numbers of patients emergently, unsurprisingly increasing numbers of patients are being discovered without a clear cause for the ACS. Some of these will have spontaneous plaque rupture that resolved prior to angiography. Typical RWMAs would still be expected with significant ischaemia duration.

Spontaneous coronary artery dissection is another relatively frequent cause of MINOCA. Whilst the identification and treatment of this angiographically differs from a normal MI, again we would expect to see a typical regionality to RWMAs on echocardiography.

An example of Takotsubo, or apical ballooning syndrome (although there are variants with ballooning elsewhere) is shown in Fig. 13. This has appearances similar to a mid-LAD infarction, but appears more symmetrical than a true LAD infarction with all mid-ventricular to apical wall segments involved (compared with a mid-LAD infarct where the mid-ventricle to apical septum is typically affected but the corresponding lateral wall is not). Because the apex can be one of the hardest areas of the heart to image this can often be a difficult diagnosis to make. Attempts at a PSAX view should always include an apical cross-section; dropping down a rib-space often facilitates this.

The final diagnosis to consider is myocarditis. Like Takotsubo this is probably more myocardial injury than infarction. Crucially with myocarditis a typical regional pattern consistent with a single coronary artery isn't typically seen. The whole ventricle can be reduced in function, often with increased wall thickness due to oedema rather

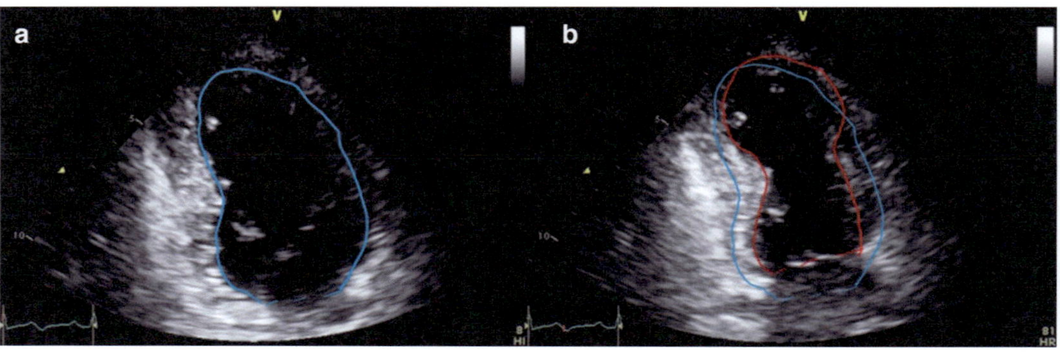

Fig. 13 Takotsubo Syndrome with typical apical ballooning which could be confused with an acute LAD infarction. Apical 2 chamber view of a patient day 1 post admission with acute chest pain, ST elevation, raised cardiac enzymes but normal coronary arteries diagnosed with Takotsubo syndrome. The apex shows the characteristic pattern of akinesia. Image **a** is the ventricle in diastole, image **b** at end-systole. Whilst the basal to mid-ventricular segments contract well, the apex can be seen to be of similar geometry at both time points, thus appearing to "balloon" in systole (blue lines indicate wall in diastole, red line systole)

than thinning. Global hypokinesia with an associated pericardial effusion should always raise the possibility of myocarditis.

Ultimately the diagnosis of MINOCA is made following angiography confirming non-obstructive coronary disease. Whilst there might be clues that suggest to the echocardiographer one of these rarer situations, angiography almost always remains essential at the earliest opportunity.

Conclusions

Patients presenting with chest pain to the emergency room are common, but frequently this pain is not myocardial ischaemia. The ECG remains an excellent test, but its value limited in patients with long-standing abnormalities such as LBBB, and may well be the first anomaly to normalise following cessation of chest pain. Biomarkers such as troponin are specific for infarction, but poorly sensitive for milder ischaemic events and can take time to be processed.

In contrast, a POCUS examination can be performed immediately and it is likely that abnormalities of myocardial regional function will persist well after ECG normalisation if the pain was truly ischaemic. Patterns of abnormalities can be identified that indicate, with reasonable accuracy, the affected coronary artery. This could be invaluable in patients where the MI is believed secondary to another acute illness, allowing the underlying cause to be treated, or in certain cases, priority given to the heart.

Ischaemic segments will initially be hypokinetic, with reduced motion and thickening. As ischaemia evolves to infarction areas will become akinetic, with no motion or thickening, and sometimes become dyskinetic, with paradoxical motion outwards in systole.

An understanding of how the heart should behave in certain conditions, such as LBBB, allows the POCUS operator to look for alternative abnormalities to aid diagnosis. A thorough look at the other cardiac chambers can help assess for alternative diagnoses and inform the assessment of the left ventricle in challenging cases as well as the integration with pulmonary ultrasound which has high sensitivity and ability to detect the increase in extravascular lung water early in the ischaemia cascade [30]. Finally, POCUS assessment of myocardial ischaemia should take into account the operator experience and the need for expert referral in complex situations.

References

1. Ibanez B, James S, Agewall S, Antunes MJ, Bucciarelli-Ducci C, Bueno H, Caforio ALP, Crea F, Goudevenos JA, Halvorsen S, Hindricks G, Kastrati A, Lenzen MJ, Prescott E, Roffi M, Valgimigli M, Varenhorst C, Vranckx P, Widimský P; ESC Scientific Document Group. 2017 ESC Guidelines for the management of acute myocardial infarction in patients presenting with ST-segment elevation: The Task Force for the management of acute myocardial infarction in patients presenting with ST-segment elevation of the European Society of Cardiology (ESC). Eur Heart J. 2018;39(2):119–177.

2. Collet JP, Thiele H, Barbato E, Barthélémy O, Bauersachs J, Bhatt DL, Dendale P, Dorobantu M, Edvardsen T, Folliguet T, Gale CP, Gilard M, Jobs A, Jüni P, Lambrinou E, Lewis BS, Mehilli J, Meliga E, Merkely B, Mueller C, Roffi M, Rutten FH, Sibbing D, Siontis GCM; ESC Scientific Document Group. 2020 ESC Guidelines for the management of acute coronary syndromes in patients presenting without persistent ST-segment elevation. Eur Heart J. 2020:ehaa575.

3. Brieger D, Eagle KA, Goodman SG, Steg PG, Budaj A, White K, Montalescot G; GRACE Investigators. Acute coronary syndromes without chest pain, an underdiagnosed and undertreated high-risk group: insights from the Global Registry of Acute Coronary Events. Chest. 2004;126(2):461–9.

4. Thygesen K, Alpert JS, Jaffe AS, Chaitman BR, Bax JJ, Morrow DA, White HD; Executive Group on behalf of the Joint European Society of Cardiology (ESC)/American College of Cardiology (ACC)/American Heart Association (AHA)/World Heart Federation (WHF) Task Force for the Universal Definition of Myocardial Infarction. Fourth Universal Definition of Myocardial Infarction (2018). Circulation. 2018;138(20):e618–e651.

5. Sandoval Y, Thygesen K. Myocardial infarction type 2 and myocardial injury. Clin Chem. 2017;63(1):101–7.

6. Antman EM, Cohen M, Bernink PJ, McCabe CH, Horacek T, Papuchis G, Mautner B, Corbalan R, Radley D, Braunwald E. The TIMI risk score for unstable angina/non-ST elevation MI: A method for prognostication and therapeutic decision making. JAMA. 2000;284(7):835–42.

7. Granger CB, Goldberg RJ, Dabbous O, Pieper KS, Eagle KA, Cannon CP, Van De Werf F, Avezum A, Goodman SG, Flather MD, Fox KA, Global Registry of Acute Coronary Events Investigators. Predictors of hospital mortality in the global registry of acute coronary events. Arch Intern Med 2003;163:2345–2353.

8. Sabia P, Afrookteh A, Touchstone DA, Keller MW, Esquivel L, Kaul S. Value of regional wall motion abnormality in the emergency room diagnosis of acute myocardial infarction. A prospective study using two-dimensional echocardiography. Circulation. 1991;84(3 Suppl):I85–92.

9. Gifft K, Ghadban R, Assefa N, Luebbering Z, Allaham H, Enezate T. The accuracy of distribution of non-ST elevation electrocardiographic changes in localising the culprit vessel in non-ST elevation myocardial infarction. Arch Med Sci Atheroscler Dis. 2020;10(5):e226–9.

10. Chang AM, Shofer FS, Tabas JA, Magid DJ, McCusker CM, Hollander JE. Lack of association between left bundle-branch block and acute myocardial infarction in symptomatic ED patients. Am J Emerg Med. 2009;27(8):916–21.

11. Anderson JL, Marshall HW, Bray BE, Lutz JR, Frederick PR, Yanowitz FG, Datz FL, Klausner SC, Hagan AD. A randomized trial of intracoronary streptokinase in the treatment of acute myocardial infarction. N Engl J Med. 1983;308(22):1312–8.

12. Zijlstra F, Hoorntje JC, de Boer MJ, Reiffers S, Miedema K, Ottervanger JP van 't Hof AW, Suryapranata H. Long-term benefit of primary angioplasty as compared with thrombolytic therapy for acute myocardial infarction. N Engl J Med. 1999;341(19):1413–9.

13. Andersen HR, Nielsen TT, Rasmussen K, Thuesen L, Kelbaek H, Thayssen P, Abildgaard U, Pedersen F, Madsen JK, Grande P, Villadsen AB, Krusell LR, Haghfelt T, Lomholt P, Husted SE, Vigholt E, Kjaergard HK, Mortensen LS; DANAMI-2 Investigators. A comparison of coronary angioplasty with fibrinolytic therapy in acute myocardial infarction. N Engl J Med. 2003;349(8):733–42.

14. Invasive compared with non-invasive treatment in unstable coronary-artery disease: FRISC II prospective randomised multicentre study. FRagmin and Fast Revascularisation during InStability in Coronary artery disease Investigators. Lancet. 1999;354(9180):708–15.

15. Cannon CP, Weintraub WS, Demopoulos LA, Vicari R, Frey MJ, Lakkis N, Neumann FJ, Robertson DH, DeLucca PT, DiBattiste PM, Gibson CM, Braunwald E; TACTICS (Treat Angina with Aggrastat and Determine Cost of Therapy with an Invasive or Conservative Strategy)–Thrombolysis in Myocardial Infarction 18 Investigators. Comparison of early invasive and conservative strategies in patients with unstable coronary syndromes treated with the glycoprotein IIb/IIIa inhibitor tirofiban. N Engl J Med. 2001;344(25):1879–87.

16. Nesto RW, Kowalchuk GJ. The ischemic cascade: temporal sequence of hemodynamic, electrocardiographic and symptomatic expressions of ischemia. Am J Cardiol. 1987;59(7):23C-30C.

17. Maznyczka A, Sen S, Cook C, Francis DP. The ischaemic constellation: an alternative to the ischaemic cascade-implications for the validation of new ischaemic tests. Open Heart. 2015;2(1).

18. Prasad SB, See V, Tan T, Brown P, McKay T, Kovoor P, Thomas L. Serial Doppler

echocardiographic assessment of diastolic dysfunction during acute myocardial infarction. Echocardiography. 2012;29(10):1164–71.

19. Poulsen SH, Jensen SE, Gøtzsche O, Egstrup K. Evaluation and prognostic significance of left ventricular diastolic function assessed by Doppler echocardiography in the early phase of a first acute myocardial infarction. Eur Heart J. 1997;18 (12):1882–9.

20. Oh JK, Ding ZP, Gersh BJ, Bailey KR, Tajik AJ. Restrictive left ventricular diastolic filling identifies patients with heart failure after acute myocardial infarction. J Am Soc Echocardiogr. 1992;5:497–503.

21. Prasad SB, See V, Brown P, McKay T, Narayan A, Kovoor P, Thomas L. Impact of duration of ischemia on left ventricular diastolic properties following reperfusion for acute myocardial infarction. Am J Cardiol. 2011;108(3):348–54.

22. Braunwald E, Kloner RA. The stunned myocardium: prolonged, postischemic ventricular dysfunction. Circulation. 1982;66(6):1146–9.

23. Nixon JV, Brown CN, Smitherman TC. Identification of transient and persistent segmental wall motion abnormalities in patients with unstable angina by two-dimensional echocardiography. Circulation. 1982;65(7):1497–503.

24. Hoffmann R, von Bardeleben S, Kasprzak JD, Borges AC, Ten Cate F, Firschke C, Lafitte S, Al-Saadi N, Kuntz- Hehner S, Horstick G, Greis C, Engelhardt M, Vanoverschelde JL, Becher H. Analysis of regional left ventricular function by cineventriculography, cardiac magnetic resonance imaging, and unenhanced and contrast-enhanced echocardiography: a multicenter comparison of methods. J Am Coll Cardiol. 2006;47(1):121–8.

25. Moir S, Shaw L, Haluska B, Jenkins C, Marwick TH. Left ventricular opacification for the diagnosis of coronary artery disease with stress echocardiography: an angiographic study of incremental benefit and cost-effectiveness. Am Heart J. 2007;154(3):510–8.

26. Reynolds HR, Tunick PA, Grossi EA, Dilmanian H, Colvin SB, Kronzon I. Paradoxical septal motion after cardiac surgery: a review of 3,292 cases. Clin Cardiol. 2007;30(12):621–3.

27. Choi SH, Choi SI, Chun EJ, Chang HJ, Park KH, Lim C, Kim SJ, Kang JW, Lim TH. Abnormal motion of the interventricular septum after coronary artery bypass graft surgery: comprehensive evaluation with MR imaging. Korean J Radiol. 2010;11 (6):627–31.

28. Klein LW, Weintraub WS, Agarwal JB, Schneider RM, Seelaus PA, Katz RI, Helfant RH. Prognostic significance of severe narrowing of the proximal portion of the left anterior descending coronary artery. Am J Cardiol. 1986;58(1):42–6.

29. Elsman P, van't Hof AW, Hoorntje JC, de Boer MJ, Borm GF, Suryapranata H, Ottervanger JP, Gosselink AT, Dambrink JH, Zijlstra F. Effect of coronary occlusion site on angiographic and clinical outcome in acute myocardial infarction patients treated with early coronary intervention. Am J Cardiol. 2006;97(8):1137–41.

30. Soliman-Aboumarie H, Miglioranza MH. J Am Coll Cardiol Case Rep. 2020;2(10):1550–2.

POCUS in Diagnosis: Acute Pulmonary Embolism

Peiman Nazerian and Matteo Castelli

In 1987, I was in Edinburgh doing my first one-man show. I took part in a kickabout with some fellow comedians and tripped over my trousers and heard this cracking sound in my leg. A couple of days later I went into a coma and was diagnosed with a pulmonary embolism.

Paul Merton, Contemporary English write and comedian.

Abstract

Lung, cardiac and veins point of care ultrasound (POCUS) are rapid, safe and bedside tools that can be integrated with traditional clinical examination. In patients with suspected pulmonary embolism, multiorgan ultrasound can improve the accuracy of validated diagnostic algorithms and is useful in terms of prognosis and monitoring of response to therapy.

Keywords

Pulmonary embolism · Lung ultrasound · Focused cardiac ultrasound · Compression ultrasound · Point of care ultrasound · Multiorgan ultrasound

Key Messages

- Prompt diagnosis of pulmonary embolism is challenging, mainly due to multiform clinical presentation
- Lung, cardiac and veins POCUS is a rapid bedside tool that can be easily integrated with traditional clinical examination
- POCUS is particularly useful in the evaluation of unstable patients, allowing rapid diagnosis of pulmonary embolism when other diagnostic tests are not feasible

Supplementary Information The online version contains supplementary material available at https://doi.org/10.1007/978-3-031-29472-3_9.

P. Nazerian (✉) · M. Castelli
Department of Emergency Medicine, Careggi University Hospital, Largo Brambilla 3, 50134 Florence, Italy
e-mail: nazerianp@aou-careggi.toscana.it

M. Castelli
e-mail: matte.castelli@inwind.it

Introduction

Pulmonary thromboembolism (PE) is the third most frequent acute cardiovascular syndrome [1].

PE consists of migration of blood clots - usually from lower limbs veins—to the pulmonary arteries. This interferes with both pulmonary circulation and gas exchange, leading to a broad range of clinical pictures. Increased Right ventricle (RV) acute afterload with subsequent RV dilatation and dysfunction is the main cause of hemodynamic collapse and death.

Correct diagnosis of PE is a challenge, mainly due to not specific clinical manifestations (i.e.: sudden cardiac arrest, shock, dyspnea, chest pain, syncope). Mortality is high, around 30% without therapy; and that decreases to 3–8% with prompt diagnosis and therapy [2].

Differential diagnosis is broad and includes pneumonia, pleurisy, pneumothorax, acute coronary syndromes, heart failure, syncope, shock from many other causes and musculoskeletal chest pain.

The gold-standard diagnostic test for PE is computed tomography pulmonary angiography (CTPA) [1]. In clinical practice, there is a tendency to overuse CTPA with consequent risks due to radiation and iodine contrast exposure. Besides costs, clinical implications and limitations (i.e., pregnancy, chronic kidney disease and iodine allergy), CTPA can be unavailable around the clock in many hospitals and in rural settings.

International guidelines suggest the use of a combination of clinical scores (i.e., Wells score) and D-dimer test to optimize the diagnostic pathway and the selection of patients needing CTPA [1]. Planar ventilation/perfusion (V/Q) lung scintigraphy is an alternative exam, however, it is not available in the majority of settings, is often inconclusive and unable to provide alternative diagnosis if PE is excluded.

Lung, cardiac, and veins point of care ultrasound (POCUS) are bedside, real-time tools that can be easily integrated with traditional bedside physical examination. POCUS is useful in the diagnostic pathway of almost all patients with suspected PE; it is an additional resource to better identify patients needing CTPA and in selected cases can be used to diagnose or exclude PE without further testing. At the same time, POCUS can identify an alternative diagnosis and can be used to monitor response to therapy and stratify prognosis in patients with PE.

Lung Ultrasound (LUS)

Lung ultrasound (LUS) has been found useful in the evaluation of patients with suspected PE and for the differential diagnosis of acute dyspnea or chest pain due to other causes: pneumonia, pleural effusion, pleurisy, pneumothorax and diffuse interstitial syndromes (i.e., congestive heart failure and interstitial pneumonia).

LUS can be performed using a curvilinear transducer or a linear transducer with longitudinal and oblique scans on the anterior, lateral and posterior intercostal spaces. The examination is targeted to the detection of pulmonary subpleural infarcts. Ultrasonographic distinctive features of subpleural infarcts are pleural-based, well-demarcated and hypoechoic sub-pleural consolidations, typically 5–20 mm in size and presenting a triangular (>85%), round (11%) or polygonal (3%) shape; a mild pleural effusion can be associated (Video 1) [3]. From the histological point of view, they correspond to occlusion of secondary pulmonary arteries with subsequent congestion of alveolar spaces due to inflow of interstitial fluid and erythrocytes with full preservation of lung structure. The identification of such consolidations with a mostly central roundish hyperechoic area, due to the presence of residual aerated tissue within infarcted lung parenchyma, are highly specific of PE-related pulmonary infarctions, corresponding to the typical "bubbly consolidation" described on CTPA [4].

A whole lung examination (anterior, lateral and posterior fields) is needed in suspected PE patients. Subpleural infarcts can be find in any lung segment; however, they are more frequently located in the posterior basal segments of the lungs (65%) as pulmonary arteries have a large axial trunk that branches off at an angle and terminates in the posterior segments. An average of two subpleural infarctions are usually detected in the same patient [5].

A metanalysis showed that LUS target to the detection of subpleural infarcts have an overall sensitivity of 87% and specificity of 82% for pulmonary embolism diagnosis [6].

The presence of pleuritic chest pain—defined as an acute localized sharp, stabbing pain exacerbated by respiration - is present in about 30% of PE patients. In patients with pleuritic chest pain, scanning of the most painful area is important to increase diagnostic accuracy as a subpleural infarct due to PE that causes pleural irritation and pain can be detected with LUS.

Focused Cardiac Ultrasound (Focus)

PE acutely increase RV afterload, leading in severe cases to RV dilatation and dysfunction with consequent decrease in RV output, reduced left ventricle preload and systemic hypoperfusion.

Focused cardiac ultrasound (FOCUS) in patients with suspected PE is aimed to identify signs of acute RV pressure overload or dysfunction. FOCUS is also recommended in prognostic stratification of patients with intermediate to high-risk PE and can be used in real-time to monitor the clinical response to treatment (i.e., thrombolytic administration) [1].

In a patient with shock and high clinical probability of PE, bedside FOCUS showing signs of acute RV dysfunction, especially if associated to more specific findings (see later), can justify emergency reperfusion treatment, also without the need for a CTPA confirmation [1] (i.e., patients in a critically unstable condition). On the other hand, a negative examination virtually excludes PE in a patient with hemodynamic instability [1], allowing at the same time the detection of other causes of shock, for example left ventricular or valvular dysfunction, pericardial tamponade, hypovolemia and sometimes acute aortic syndromes.

If we consider all patients with suspected PE, due to the wide range of etiologies of cardiac involvement, a normal FOCUS has a negative predictive value not superior to 40–50%, too low to exclude PE without other tests [7]. Conversely, misleading signs of RV overload or dysfunction can be found in patients with pre-existing or acute cardiac and/or respiratory diseases different from PE (i.e., chronic cor pulmonale, RV acute coronary syndromes, sepsis, acute respiratory distress syndrome): more specific echocardiographic findings have been showed to retain a high positive predictive value for PE also in this setting, distinguishing acute from preexisting RV failure.

FOCUS is generally performed with a phased-array transducer. Recommended views are the subcostal, parasternal and apical four-chamber views. Main PE-related echocardiographic findings are:

- *Right ventricular dilatation* (Video 2): this is the main finding in patients with PE (>25% of patients). It is defined as a right/left ventricular end-diastolic diameter ratio ≥ 1 (apical four-chambers or subcostal view) and a RV end-diastolic diameter > 30 mm (parasternal long axis view). This finding showed a sensitivity of 31% to 72% and a specificity of 87% to 98% for PE diagnosis [1, 5].
- *Flattened interventricular septum (D-shaped LV sign)* (Video 2): is defined as the flattening of the intraventricular septum, during end-systolic phase, due to RV pressure overload.
- *McConnell sign* (Video 2): is defined as a RV free wall hypokinesia with apical sparing. McConnell sign has a low-sensitivity and high-specificity (94–100%) for PE [1].
- *Mobile right heart thrombi* (Video 3): is defined as the presence of in-transit or mobile thrombi in the right heart cavities. This is a direct POCUS sign of PE and has a very high specificity but is present in less than 5% of patients with PE [1].
- *Decreased tricuspid annular plane systolic excursion (TAPSE)* defined as <16 mm.
- *Pulmonary hypertension,* defined as a tricuspid regurgitation pressure gradient >30 mmHg in the absence of RV hypertrophy (normal RV wall thickness: 2–5 mm).

All these POCUS signs are not only useful for diagnosis but also for prognostication of PE: a RV/LV diameter ratio $\geq$ 1, TAPSE < 16 mm are the findings most frequently associated to unfavorable prognosis [1].

Compression Ultrasound (CUS)

In the majority of cases, PE originates from lower limbs deep vein thrombosis (DVT) and only rarely from upper limbs DVT (mostly following catheterization).

Lower limb veins compression ultrasound (CUS) is the most used non-invasive bedside test for the diagnosis of proximal DVT and can detect DVT in 30–50% of patients with PE [1].

Normal veins of the limbs appear easily compressible on a transverse view using a linear probe (2D mode imaging). Blood clots generally appears as hyperechoic structures, but recently formed clots can be anechoic. Consequently, the only accepted diagnostic criterion for DVT is incomplete compressibility, indicating the presence of a clot in the vessel (Video 4). Longitudinal views are not recommended because efforts for longitudinal compression can lead to a wrong perception of incomplete compressibility. Color Doppler can be useful in the same cases but is not routinely recommended in this setting.

In case of a patient with suspected PE, examination can be limited to common femoral and popliteal veins (*two-points CUS*), respectively located in the groin and popliteal fossa. A *three-point* approach, including the evaluation of the superficial femoral vein, can increase the sensitivity of the exam [1]. Sequential compression of the whole proximal venous system scanning compressing the vein every 2–3 cm (common femoral vein, saphenofemoral junction, superficial femoral and popliteal vein up to the popliteal trifurcation) is more accurate but requires greater technical skills.

The extension of CUS to calf veins is a time-consuming test needing particular expertise and is not routinely recommended in this setting.

Additional skills are required to explore the iliac or inferior vena cava district, using a linear or curvilinear probes and color Doppler. Upper extremities venous thrombosis, although rarely a cause of symptomatic PE, can be diagnosed at the same manner in particular cases.

For the diagnosis of proximal DVT, CUS showed a sensitivity > 90% and a specificity around 95% in patients with signs or symptoms of DVT (i.e., edema or lower limb pain). The sensitivity is lower in asymptomatic patients (<55%) and when CUS is used for diagnosing distal DVT [7, 8].

Regarding the diagnosis of PE, CUS showed a high specificity (around 95%) and a low sensitivity (around 40%) in patients with suspected symptoms [7, 8]. The diagnosis of proximal DVT by CUS in patients with clinical suspicion of PE is sufficient for the diagnosis, allowing specific therapy with no further diagnostic exams (i.e., computed tomography pulmonary angiography, CTPA) especially when they are not easily feasible or contraindicated.

Guidelines recommend CUS as the first diagnostic imaging test to avoid unnecessary irradiation in pregnant patients with suspected PE. A positive CUS is sufficient to diagnose PE, avoiding CTPA or ventilation/perfusion lung scintigraphy in such patients [1].

Multiorgan Point of Care Ultrasound

Lung, cardiac and veins POCUS can be performed in few minutes by the same operator, as a multiorgan approach, in suspected PE patients. The sensitivity of multiorgan POCUS, aimed to identify subpleural infarctions, RV impairment, mobile right heart thrombi and lower limbs DVT of PE is significantly superior to that of lung, cardiac, or veins POCUS alone. Moreover, multiorgan POCUS can disclose other acute diseases (i.e., pneumothorax, pleural effusion, pneumonia, cardiac tamponade, acute heart failure) with similar clinical presentation (chest pain, dyspnea, shock).

A multiorgan POCUS approach showed a sensitivity of 90% in patients with suspected PE; at the same time, a completely negative exam has a negative predictive value of 95%, even higher when an alternative US diagnosis is evident [5].

In the emergency setting, multiorgan POCUS can improve the potential of clinical score and D-dimer assay for optimal selection of patients who should undergo CTPA. Integrated in a traditional diagnostic algorithm, multiorgan POCUS can decrease the demand for CTPA or can be even an alternative to CTPA when it is contraindicated or unavailable. Figure 1 illustrates a diagnostic algorithm based on the integration of Wells score plus D-dimer with lungs, cardiac and veins POCUS [5].

A simpler approach is proposed in Fig. 2. It integrates traditional Wells score (Ws) with LUS and CUS, to better select patients requiring D-dimer assay and/or CTPA. In the so-called *US-modified Wells score* (USWs) the first two items of the Ws are modified using lung and veins POCUS results. Supporting a clinical judgement *—alternative diagnosis less likely than PE—*with LUS findings and the identification of DVT with CUS can increase the accuracy of pre-test evaluation. The USWs $\leq$ 4 showed a better diagnostic accuracy and rule out sensitivity than traditional Ws [9].

Finally, the particular features of multiorgan POCUS (rapid, safe and bedside) are particularly helpful in the emergency evaluation of unstable patients with shock or cardiac arrest. Patients with PE develop hemodynamic instability in less than 10% of cases, but risk for death in the short term is high (>30%) [1].

Consequently, to expedite diagnosis and reperfusion treatment, international guidelines [1] recommend FOCUS to identify signs of RV failure. Findings consistent with PE allow emergency reperfusion treatment, avoiding or postposing confirmation by CTPA. In this critical

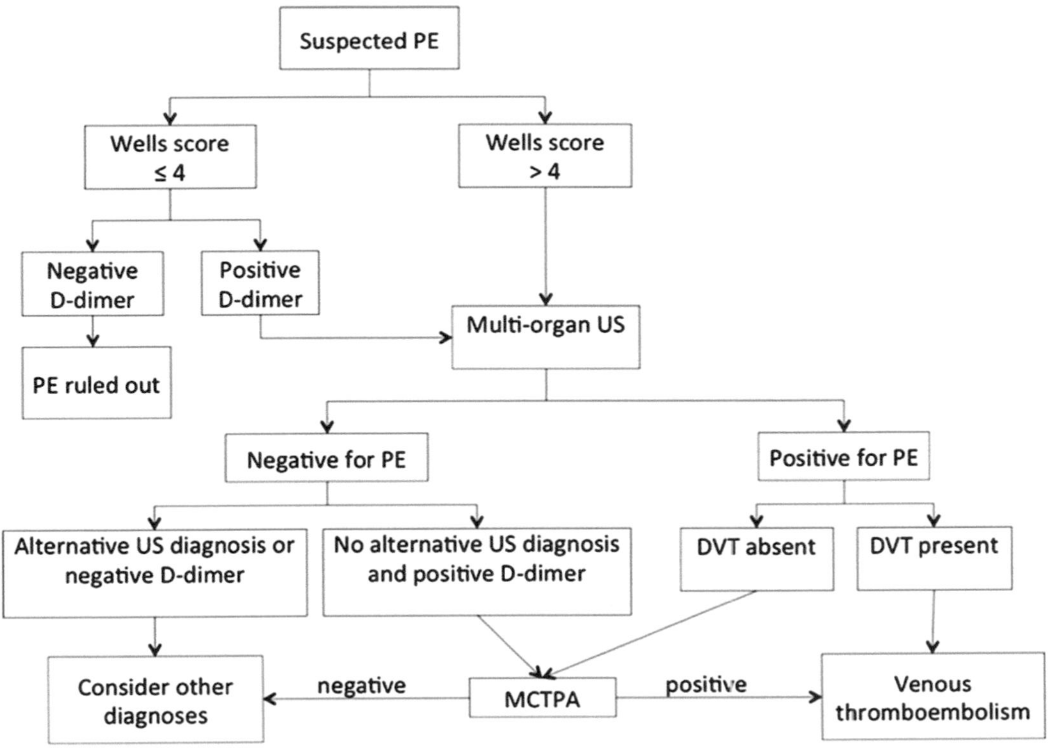

Fig. 1 Diagnostic algorithm based on the integration of Wells score plus multiorgan POCUS

Fig. 2 Items of the Wells score and of the ultrasound-modified Wells score

Ws	USWs	Points
Signs and symptoms of DVT	Venous ultrasound positive for DVT	+3
Alternative diagnosis less likely than PE	Alternative diagnosis less likely than PE after lung ultrasound	+3
Heart rate > 100 beats/min		+1.5
Immobilization > 3 d or surgery in the previous 4 wk		+1.5
Previous, objectively diagnosed PE or DVT		+1.5
Hemoptysis		+1
Malignancy on treatment, treated within 6 mo, or in palliative therapy		+1

DVT = deep venous thrombosis; PE = pulmonary embolism.

setting,the combination of FOCUS and simultaneous CUS were found to increase the diagnostic accuracy offered by FOCUS alone, with a positive predictive value of 100% in the presence of both positive FOCUS and CUS and a negative predictive value > 95% when both exams were negative [10].

References

1. 2019 ESC Guidelines for the diagnosis and management of acute pulmonary embolism developed in collaboration with the European Respiratory Society (ERS): The Task Force for the diagnosis and management of acute pulmonary embolism of the European Society of Cardiology (ESC). Konstantinides SV, Meyer G, Becattini C, Bueno H, Geersing GJ, Harjola VP et al. Eur Respir J. 2019 Oct 9;54 (3):1901647.
2. Clinical features and short term outcomes of patients with acute pulmonary embolism. The Italian Pulmonary Embolism Registry (IPER). Casazza F, Becattini C, Bongarzoni A, Cuccia C, Roncon L, Favretto G et al. Thromb Res. 2012 Dec;130(6):847–52.
3. Sonography of lung and pleura in pulmonary embolism: sonomorphologic characterization and comparison with spiral CT scanning. Reissig A, Heyne JP, Kroegel C.Chest. 2001 Dec;120(6):1977–83.
4. The "Survived Lung:" An Ultrasound Sign of "Bubbly Consolidation" Pulmonary Infarction. Copetti R, Cominotto F, Meduri S, Orso D. et al. Ultrasound Med Biol. 2020 Sep;46(9):2546–2550.
5. Accuracy of point-of-care multiorgan ultrasonography for the diagnosis of pulmonary embolism. Nazerian P, Vanni S, Volpicelli G, Gigli C, Zanobetti M, Bartolucci M et al. Chest. 2014 May;145(5):950–957.
6. Diagnostic accuracy of lung ultrasound for pulmonary embolism: a systematic review and meta-analysis. Squizzato A, Rancan E, Dentali F, Bonzini M, Guasti L, Steidl L et al. J Thromb Haemost. 2013 Jul;11(7):1269–78.
7. Systematic review and meta-analysis of strategies for the diagnosis of suspected pulmonary embolism. Roy PM, Colombet I, Durieux P, Chatellier G, Sors H, Meyer G. BMJ 2005;331:259.
8. Diagnostic characteristics of lower limb venous compression ultrasonography in suspected pulmonary embolism: a meta-analysis. Da Costa Rodrigues J, Alzuphar S, Combescure C, Le Gal G, Perrier A et al. J Thromb Haemost 2016; 14:1765–1772.
9. Diagnostic Performance of Wells Score Combined With Point-of-care Lung and Venous Ultrasound in Suspected Pulmonary Embolism. Nazerian P, Volpicelli G, Gigli C, Becattini C, Sferrazza Papa GF, Grifoni S et al; Ultrasound Wells Study Group.Acad Emerg Med. 2017 Mar;24 (3):270–280.
10. Diagnostic accuracy of focused cardiac and venous ultrasound examinations in patients with shock and suspected pulmonary embolism. Nazerian P , Volpicelli G , Gigli C, Lamorte A, Grifoni S, Vanni S. et al. Intern Emerg Med 2018 Jun;13 (4):567–574.

Lung Ultrasound in Pneumonia Diagnosis

Francesco Corradi, Francesco Forfori, Giada Cucciolini, and Danila Trunfio

If you don't look, you won't know!
Anonymous

Abstract

Interest in lung ultrasound (LUS) has been growing over time, thanks also to the COVID-19 outbreak. Clinical aspects such as fever, cough and purulent sputum are fundamental for diagnosing pneumonia, along with laboratory exams (leucocytosis and procalcitonin elevation). An imaging technique is however required for diagnosis, and the gold standard has been represented for a long time by a chest X-ray (CXR) or a CT scan. Nevertheless, LUS is useful in diagnosis, monitoring of the response to therapy and follow up. These features have demonstrated to be very useful in various settings, such as emergency departments, wards and intensive care units. Multiple scanning protocols of the thorax have been proposed; at the moment, the most advantageous in terms of diagnostic accuracy and time-consume is the one considering six scanning fields for each side. POCUS findings correspond to anatomo-pathologic modifications found in pneumonia. Among the most common POCUS signs we found B lines, pleural abnormalities (thickness and irregularity), meta-pneumonic effusions and consolidations with either static or dynamic air bronchogram. For what concerns assessment and follow up of the severity of illness, it is useful to adopt the lung ultrasound aeration score, assigning a score from 0 to 3 for each field explored; the sum of the points obtained ranges from 0 to 36 (see chapter for more details). During the pandemic era LUS has been very useful for mass screening of patients attending the emergency departments allowing identification of potentially positive patients, even if the findings

Supplementary Information The online version contains supplementary material available at https://doi.org/10.1007/978-3-031-29472-3_10.

F. Corradi (✉) · F. Forfori · G. Cucciolini · D. Trunfio
Department of Surgical, Medical, Molecular Pathology and Critical Care Medicine, University of Pisa, via Savi 10, 56126 Pisa, Italy
e-mail: francesco.corradi@unipi.it

F. Forfori
e-mail: francesco.forfori@unipi.it

G. Cucciolini
e-mail: giada.cucciolini@phd.unipi.it

D. Trunfio
e-mail: danilatrunfio@yahoo.it

were not illness-specific. For this reason, usefulness of LUS for COVID-19 diagnosis will need to be re-evaluated at the end of the pandemic.

Keywords

POCUS · Ventilator-associated pneumonia · Community acquired pneumonia · CAD– Computer aided diagnosis · COVID-19

Abbreviations

BLUE	Bedside Lung Ultrasound in Emergency
CAD	Computer aided diagnosis
CAP	Community Acquired Pneumonia
COVID 19	Coronavirus Disease 19
CT	Computed tomography
CXR	Chest x-ray
ED	Emergency department
ICU	Intensive care unit
LUS	Lung Ultrasound
PCT	Procalcitonin
POCUS	Point of care ultrasound
PSI	Pneumonia severity index
VAP	Ventilator Associated Pneumonia

Key Messages

- LUS is however useful in diagnosis, monitoring the response to therapy and follow up of patients with pneumonia
- POCUS findings correspond to anatomo-pathologic modifications found in pneumonia. Among the most common POCUS signs we found B lines, pleural abnormalities (thickness and irregularity), meta-pneumonic effusions and consolidations with either static or dynamic air bronchogram
- For assessment and the follow up of the severity of illness, it is useful to adopt the lung ultrasound aeration score.

Introduction

Pneumonia is a common infective disease, involving patients from childhood to old age, with a wide range of clinical presentations with a notable morbidity and mortality [1].

In the last few decades, there has been increasing interest in LUS application for the diagnosis and monitoring in numerous cardiopulmonary conditions, as well as pneumonia.

In this chapter we will try to discuss and summarize the evidence about the use of LUS in pneumonia and elucidate the role of this exam for the diagnosis and follow up of pneumonic patients (Fig. 1).

Clinical Aspects of Pneumonia

Pneumonia is a lower respiratory tract infection that represents the most common infection worldwide, associated with high morbidity and mortality [1]. Its presentation varies from mild symptoms such as fever, cough and sputum production, to severe forms characterised by increased work of breath, respiratory distress and sepsis. Severity scores can be helpful tools to stratify the severity of illness together with the clinical judgment, in order to define the most appropriate level of care. Commonly used assessment tools are the "Pneumonia Severity Index" (PSI or PORT) and the CURB-65 [2].

Classification of pneumonia is based on the place where the patient contracted the infection, and in particular:

Community-acquired pneumonia (CAP) refers to an acute infection of the pulmonary parenchyma acquired outside of the hospital.

Nosocomial pneumonia refers to a pneumonia that occurs 48 h or more after admission and does not appear to be incubating at the time of admission. It includes *ventilator-associated pneumonia (VAP)* if acquired ≥ 48 h after endotracheal intubation.

The suspicion of pneumonia requires a compatible clinical presentation with suggestive signs

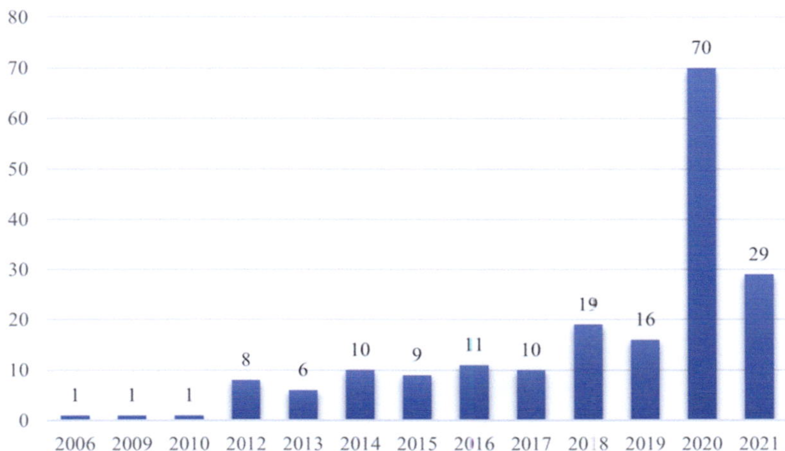

Fig. 1 Search results in Pubmed for "Pneumonia" and "Lung Ultrasound"—published articles increased in time, and COVID-19 was a clear source of interest for researching and publishing in LUS

and symptoms, with a consistent radiographical finding as a fundamental component of the diagnosis [3]. Indeed, the latest guidelines consider chest X-ray (CXR) the gold standard technique, yet the role of thoracic ultrasound was not mentioned despite it being routinely applied in clinical practice [4, 5].

The patterns found on CXR are usually related to the causative agent. We can distinguish between a lobar pneumonia, a bronchopneumonia or lobular pneumonia and an interstitial pneumonia.

Lobar pneumonia involves single or multiple lobes and is the most common radiographic pattern of CAP, usually caused by typical bacteria as *S. pneumoniae*. Bronchopneumonia is most commonly caused by *S. aureus, H. influenzae*, and fungi, and is characterised by multiple small nodular or reticulonodular opacities which tend to be patchy and/or confluent. Interstitial pneumonia presents itself as diffuse bilateral peri-bronchial thickening and ill-defined reticulonodular opacities. The prevalent pathogens of interstitial pneumonia are viruses and *M. pneumoniae* [6].

Chest radiography can sometimes be normal, especially in the early phases of the disease process or in interstitial pneumonia, that has a preference for lower lung areas behind the heart and the diaphragm; in this case chest CT can be a useful alternative thanks to its higher sensitivity [7]. However, CT has only a limited role in the everyday practice due to its costs, radiation exposure, needing to move the patient to the

radiology unit and low time-resolution. Therefore, CT is commonly preferred in the most severe forms, to better characterize pneumonia and its complications, and to rule out other diagnoses.

As mentioned above, clinical applications of LUS have increased in the last decades. It has become part of the clinical management in several pulmonary conditions, and in many different settings, such as in the emergency departments, intensive care units (ICUs), internal medicine wards and even in outpatient evaluation. In 2008 Lichtenstein and Mezière published one of the first protocols, called the BLUE Protocol (Bedside Lung Ultrasound in Emergency, Fig. 2), which assesses the use of LUS in diagnosing the most frequent causes of acute respiratory failure [8]. Since then, many experimental and clinical studies protocols and rating systems have been presented, mostly regarding the ability of LUS to detect loss of aeration or gain of extravascular lung water [7, 9–12].

Many studies compared LUS to CXR in terms of sensitivity and specificity in pneumonia diagnosis; in the emergency room, LUS is considered a valid alternative for early diagnosis of pneumonia in adults [8, 13–16]. In this setting, consolidations have 93% sensitivity and 98% specificity for the diagnosis of community-acquired pneumonia [16]. For Reissig et al. combination of LUS and auscultation findings resulted in a positive likelihood-ratio of diagnosis of 42.9 (CI 10.8, 17.0) and a negative likelihood-ratio of 0.04 (CI 0.02, 0.09) [17]. The high

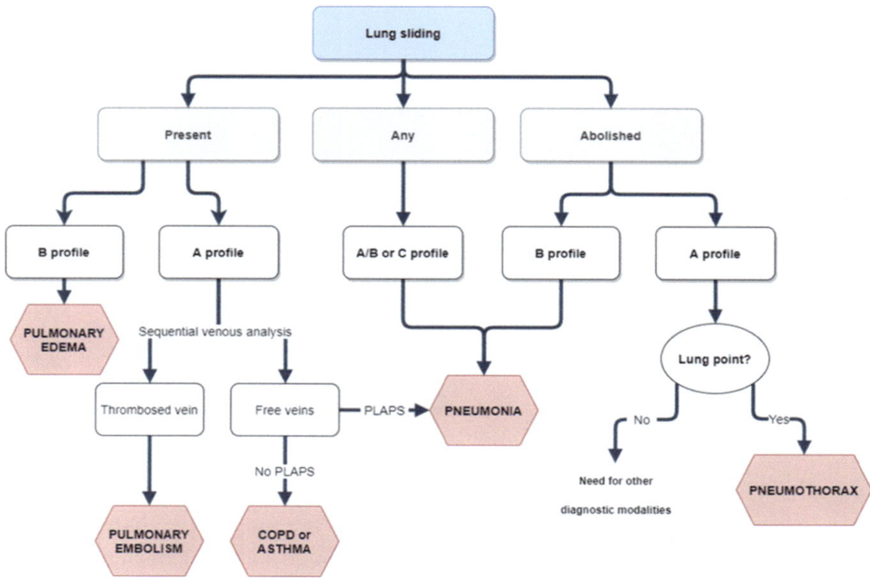

Fig. 2 The Blue Protocol. Modified from Lichtenstein et al. [8]. COPD: chronic obstructive pulmonary disease. PLAPS: posterolateral alveolar and/or pleural syndrome

reliability of LUS for detection of consolidations was confirmed when compared to chest CT imaging as well [18, 19].

Moreover, LUS tends to detect pulmonary infiltrates more often than CXR; the same applies to Covid-19 pneumonia where more than half of the patients had an initially normal CXR [20].

For what concerns VAP diagnosis, clinical and microbiological information are fundamental and should always be considered together with the imaging findings. The 'Chest Echography and Procalcitonin Pulmonary Infection Score' (CEPPIS) encompasses all these components in order to improve the diagnostic accuracy of POCUS, which included for the first time the presence of infiltrates on LUS, in addition to other clinical and laboratory parameters (type of tracheal secretions, cultures of tracheal secretions, procalcitonin levels, fever or hypothermia, and worsening of oxygenation index PaO_2/FiO_2). This tool seems to have higher sensitivity, specificity, positive and negative predictive value when compared with LUS alone or LUS plus procalcitonin (Table 1) [22].

Table 1 Chest Echography and Procalcitonin Pulmonary Infection Score (CEPPIS). Modified from Zagli et al. [22]. A value > 5 showed to be effective in increasing the diagnostic accuracy of VAP. ARDS: Acute respiratory distress syndrome

	0	1	2
Tracheal secretions	Non purulent	–	Purulent
Procalcitonin	< 0.5	≥ 0.5 and < 1	≥ 1
Culture of tracheal aspirate	Negative	–	Positive
Temperature	≥ 36 and < 38.4	38.5 and < 38.9	< 36 or 39
Infiltrates on chest ultrasound	Negative	–	Positive for subpleural poor echogenity regions or tissue-like texture
Oxygenation: PaO_2/FiO_2	> 240 or ARDS	–	240 and no evidence of ARDS

How to Perform Lung Ultrasound

As Mayo et al. [21] wrote in their review, "There is no best way to perform image acquisition for thoracic ultrasonography".

Linear, curvilinear abdominal or cardiac probes can all be used, based on the physician preference and the clinical need. The high frequency probe is mostly used to acquire a detailed image of the pleural line. The cardiac phase array probe has a small footprint that allows to better scan the intercostal space.

Regarding the scanning technique, two anterior zones can be sufficient to formulate a rough differential diagnosis between a cardiogenic pulmonary oedema and a primary parenchymal respiratory dyspnoea (e.g. chronic obstructive pulmonary disease exacerbation), but this should not be recommended for the systematic examination of the lungs in order to detect infectious consolidations [23].

The BLUE Protocol [8] proposed an examination method that included three scanning points per chest side, anterior, lateral and posterolateral, in a supine position and consists in scanning each rib interspace moving the probe longitudinally and transversally. The international recommendations for point-of-care LUS [24] described other possible techniques. The basic eight-region sonographic technique [25] for antero-lateral field examination considers four areas per side, upper and lower anterior, upper lateral and basal lateral and has been suggested to be used in the emergency department. In critically ill patients, a more comprehensive examination is often applied, that considers six scans per side: superior and inferior regions for the anterior, lateral and posterior fields [26, 27] (Fig. 3). In this case, placing the probe as posteriorly as possible, even in the supine critically ill patients is important to explore the posterior areas of the thorax which are frequently involved in the critically ill patients. Whenever possible, it

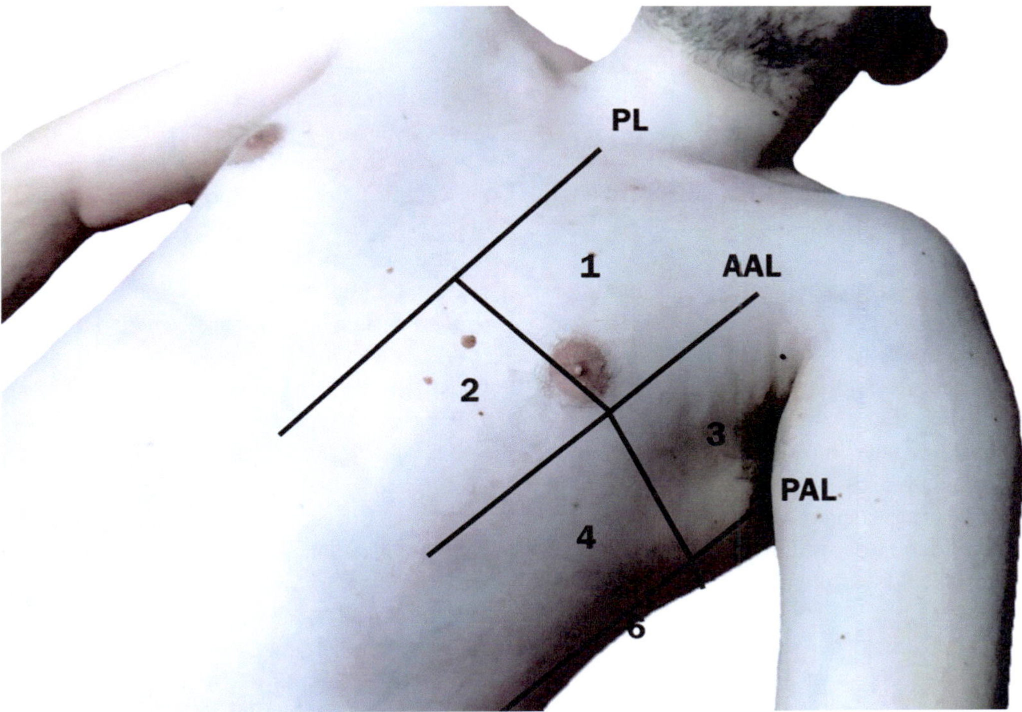

Fig. 3 Suggested scans in LUS examination. ML: midline. AAL: anterior axillary line. PAL: posterior axillary line

is recommended to place the patient in the lateral decubitus position to fully explore these fields. This approach has been recently used in the evaluation of LUS aeration scores as well as in the evaluation of COVID-19 pneumonia and it has the advantage of providing a complete exam in a short time period time, ranging from 8 min (for experts) to 10 min (for trainees) [28–30].

In our experience, we suggest to follow a mental algorithm called the "SAFED approach" in order to interpret LUS findings and achieve a diagnosis regardless of the chosen scanning protocol and depending on different clinical contexts and the level of urgency [31].

"S" for anatomical Size to measure subpleural consolidations whenever present.

"A" for Air, to detect and characterize air bronchograms.

"F" for Fluids, looking for meta-pneumonic effusion.

"E" for Excursion, looking for "lung pulse" suggesting atelectasis with pleural involvement.

"D" for Doppler, because a highly perfused lung consolidation with loss of aeration will likely correspond to intrapulmonary shunt suggesting a significant contribution of the consolidation to arterial hypoxemia.

Anatomopathological Modifications in Pneumonia

Understanding anatomopathological modifications of lung parenchyma in pneumonia is crucial to comprehend sonographic alterations. In fact, POCUS reveals nothing but alterations in the mode of reflecting and absorbing US waves; the variations in tissue impedance causes reflection of waves, creating images.

Modifications occurring in pneumonia are typically different depending on the pathogenetic mechanisms and aetiologic agent [32].

In lobar pneumonia, an entire lobe is involved, and there are subsequent phases with different involvement of the parenchyma:

- *Congestion phase*: the lung has high water content, is heavy and oedematous; this stage is characterised by vascular congestion, so anatomically the tissues appear red. The alveoli are still partially aerated.
- *Red hepatization phase*: this second stage is characterized by a fibrinous exudate in the alveoli, rich in proteins, red and white cells. Alveoli are almost not aerated, and the parenchyma appears to be red and stiff.
- *Grey hepatization phase*: the lung is no longer wet, but a fibrinous purulent exudate is still present; the lobe appears to be grey-brownish.
- *Resolution phase*: in this phase there is a granulomatous reaction mediated by immune cells (macrophages), gradual enzymatic digestion and reabsorption of semifluid substances produced during inflammation phases. Fibroblasts contribute in this phase to organizing the pulmonary parenchyma and reconstitution of tissue [33].

Pleural involvement is seldom detected, but when it is, it results in pleural thickening, purulent and fibrinous reaction.

Another type of lung involvement is the bronchopneumonia. In this case a diffuse patchy multilobar and often bilateral involvement of lungs is seen. Lesions appear to be granular, prominent, not well defined, and there is always an airway inflammation with abundant secretions. These latter are often purulent and accumulate in the lower regions; fibrin rich exudate can fill the alveoli.

In some cases, we can find complications of pneumonia such as abscesses, meta-pneumonic pleural effusion, or empyema.

Based on the host-causal agent interaction, the tissue response patterns are quite different. However, patterns of lobar, interstitial, and bronchopneumonia can overlap, and are not mutually exclusive.

It is mandatory to keep in mind all the macroscopic modifications of the lung parenchyma as well as the location of consolidations in the lung parenchyma to be able to match these with LUS patterns and modification of echogenicity. Indeed, LUS is a key to interpret the changes in tissue impedance, thus an anatomical parenchymal consolidation can be visualized by LUS either as an ultrasonographic consolidation or as an ultrasonographic alveolo-interstitial syndrome depending on the distance from the pleural line (Fig. 4). Knowledge of tissue modification in lung disease is crucial to understand LUS images and provide their interpretation.

Sonographic Findings in Pneumonia

Pneumonia can appear with different images, depending on the severity, the diffusion in the parenchyma and the underlying pathogenetic mechanism.

B-lines are vertical hyperechoic artifacts that arise from the pleural line, move with lung sliding, spread to the edge of the screen without fading, and erase A lines [24]. First described in 1982 in relation to an intra-hepatic gunshot, they were associated to alveolar-interstitial syndrome in 1997 by Lichtenstein [34] and only recently have been proved to occur due to the different acoustic impedances between an object and its surroundings, such as the presence of liquid filled areas next to alveolar air and thus a direct representation of air-to-water ratio. B-lines artifacts are associated, among other conditions, with pneumonia, due to the increased extravascular lung water or partial loss of aeration of the lung, probably as consequences of the neutrophil rich exudate that floods peripheral alveoli as an inflammatory reaction [7].

For this reason, B-lines represent the fundamental components of the LUS aeration score, that is used to determine the rate of involvement of lung parenchyma. Score 0 corresponds to A-lines or two or fewer B-lines and identifies a normally aerated parenchyma. Score 1 is defined by three or more B-lines involving 50% or less of the pleural line; in score 2 B-lines involve more than 50% of the imaged pleural line, as they represent a worsening of lung aeration. The last one, score 3, is characterised by a tissue-like pattern and corresponds to a complete loss of aeration (Fig. 5). The final aeration score is given by the sum of the maximum score visualized in each area, ranging from 0 to 36 if the

twelve regions protocol is adopted [9] (see Chapter "POCUS in Monitoring: How Monitor Pulmonary Aeration/Deaeration?" for more details).

In pneumonia, the changes in the characteristics, number, coalescence, intensity and persistence of B-lines may help to define the characteristics of the pneumonia, including its severity, residual aeration with potential recruitment, bronchial patency and response to treatments [28].

A pneumonia consolidation is usually visualized by LUS as a subpleural hypoechoic area with irregular margins sometimes with reduced or absent lung sliding. The lower and deeper irregular margins of the consolidation constitute the so called "shred sign" (Fig. 6). Frequently, from the shredded boundaries of consolidations, multiple spreading B-lines can be seen, representing the transition zone caused by the presence of perilesional oedema surrounding the focus of pneumonia [35].

Sometimes, in the context of consolidations, we can recognize hyperechoic intraparenchymal images consisting of few millimetres spots or tree-shaped structures: the so called "air bronchograms". They can be either dynamic, when moving synchronous with tidal ventilation, or static, when no movement is detected. Dynamic behavior indicates patency of airways as it seems to be generated by the movement of air within the bronchi, while an absent or static bronchogram indicates that there is no gas transit in the corresponding airway. (Figs. 7 and 8, video v2–3 in online supplement material).

Bronchograms may help distinguish infective consolidation from resorptive atelectasis. The dynamic bronchogram, in fact, is a specific sign of pneumonia, with a 94% specificity and a 97% positive predictive value for the diagnosis and helps rule out atelectasis as the movement of air, by definition, cannot be detected in atelectasis. Nevertheless, a static or absent bronchogram can be present in both conditions, and is detected in most cases of late resorptive atelectasis, and in one third of cases of pneumonia [36].

Less frequently, we can also recognize a "fluid bronchogram" within the consolidated

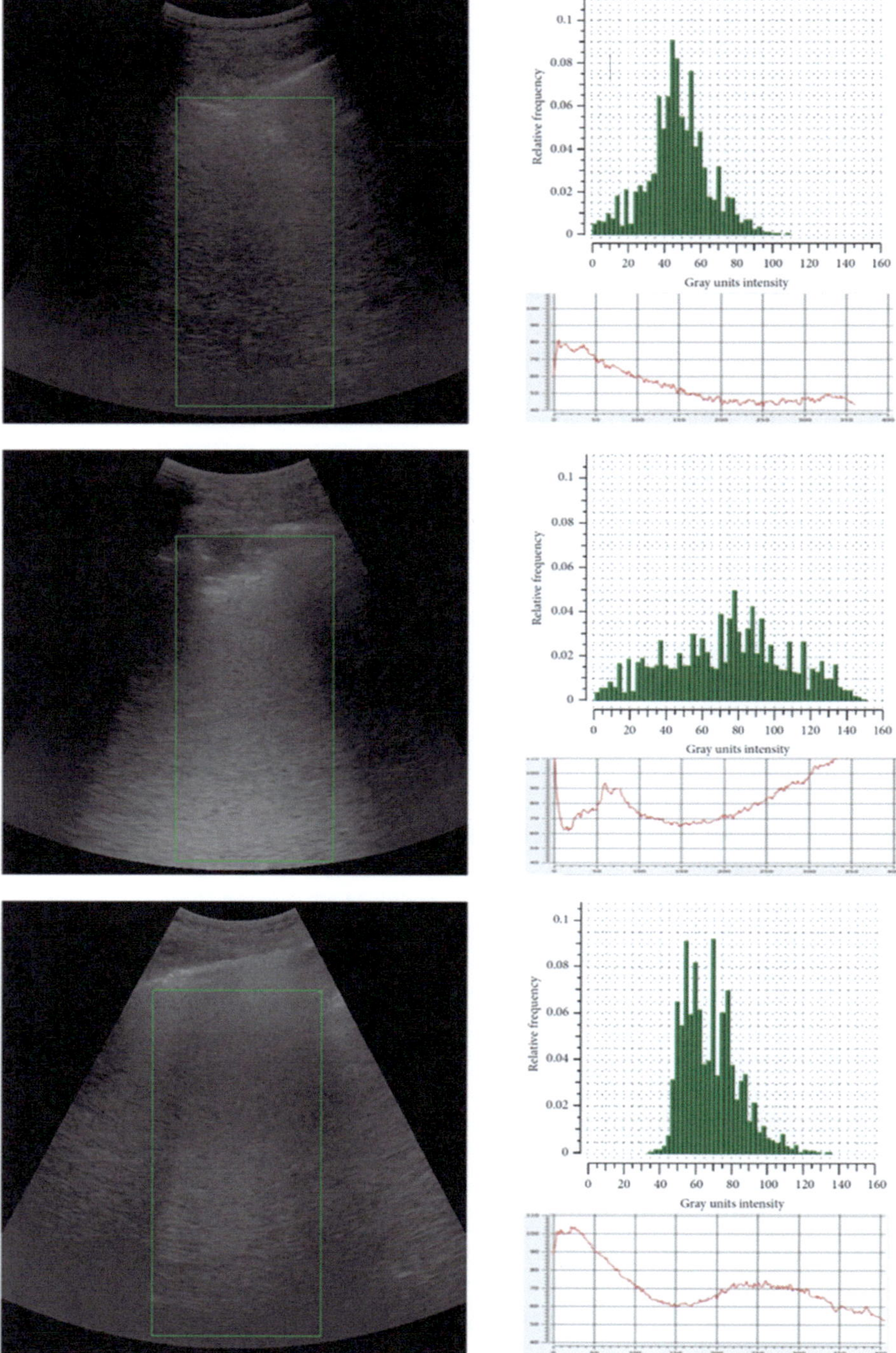

◄ **Fig. 4** Representative echo images (left) and quantitative lung ultrasonography analysis (right) for three patients with normal hemi-thorax (upper panels), sub-pleural consolidation (middle panels), and non-sub-pleural consolidation (lower panels). Upper panels show the echo intensities against distance from the pleural line; in the middle panels, notice the frequency distribution of echo intensities for the whole image. Note the progressive attenuation of the echo intensity going deep into the lung in the normal hemi-thorax as compared with the increasing echo intensity in the sub-pleural consolidation (indicating acoustic enhancement artifact), and the biphasic pattern in the non-sub-pleural consolidation (suggesting acoustic scattering). Computer aided techniques allow to detect signal pattern distribution of a consolidative lesion in the deep lung that does not reach the pleural line [7]

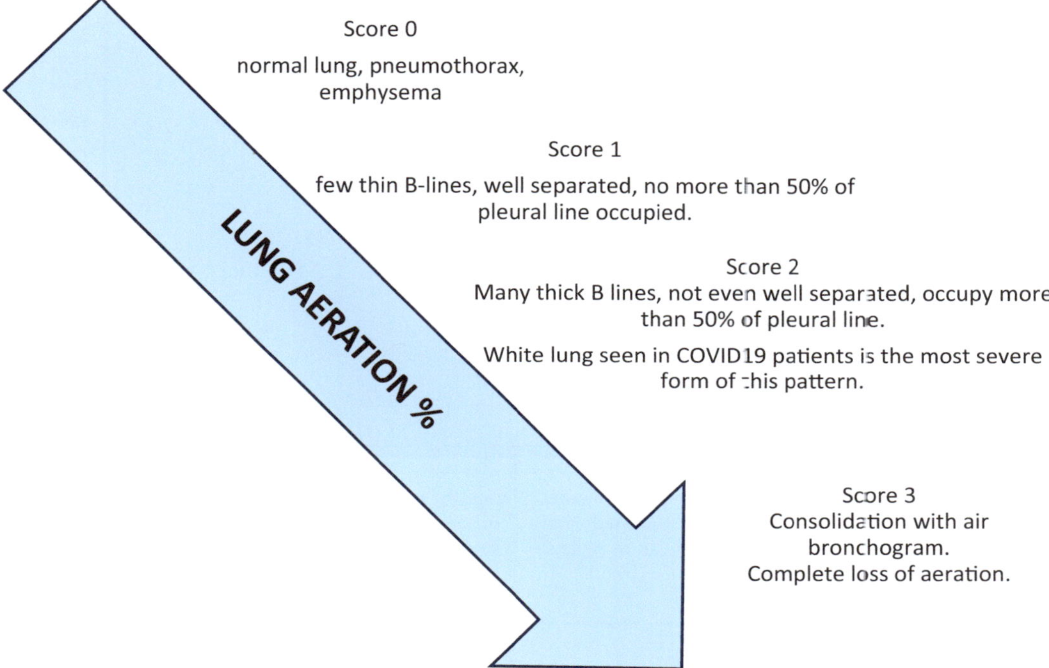

Fig. 5 Lung ultrasound aeration score based on lung aeration. See text for details

parenchyma, which is seen as a tubular, echo-free structure, that reflects a stenotic airway filled with exudate, and that can be differentiated from vascular structures using color Doppler [35].

Sonographic findings in interstitial pneumonia reflect the underlying inflammatory process; this is characterised by thickened subpleural inter-lobular septa, as a result of fibroblast proliferation and increased number of collagen fibres. B-lines are the principal sonographic artifacts seen in interstitial pneumonia and their number corre-lates with the extent of fibrosis and reticular pattern. They are generally diffuse in both lungs, with a non-homogeneous distribution; areas of B lines alternate with spared areas of A-lines, and are likely non-gravity distributed, feature that help differentiate interstitial pneumonia from pulmonary congestion in heart failure or end stage renal disease (where B-lines are diffuse, homogeneous, bilateral and gravity distributed) (Fig. 9).

Pleural involvement is typical in interstitial pneumonia. It demonstrates alterations of the sonographic pleural line, which looks thick (more than 2 mm), irregular and fragmented, with multiple spots of small subpleural consoli-dation and abolished lung sliding, resulting from pleural layers adherences [37].

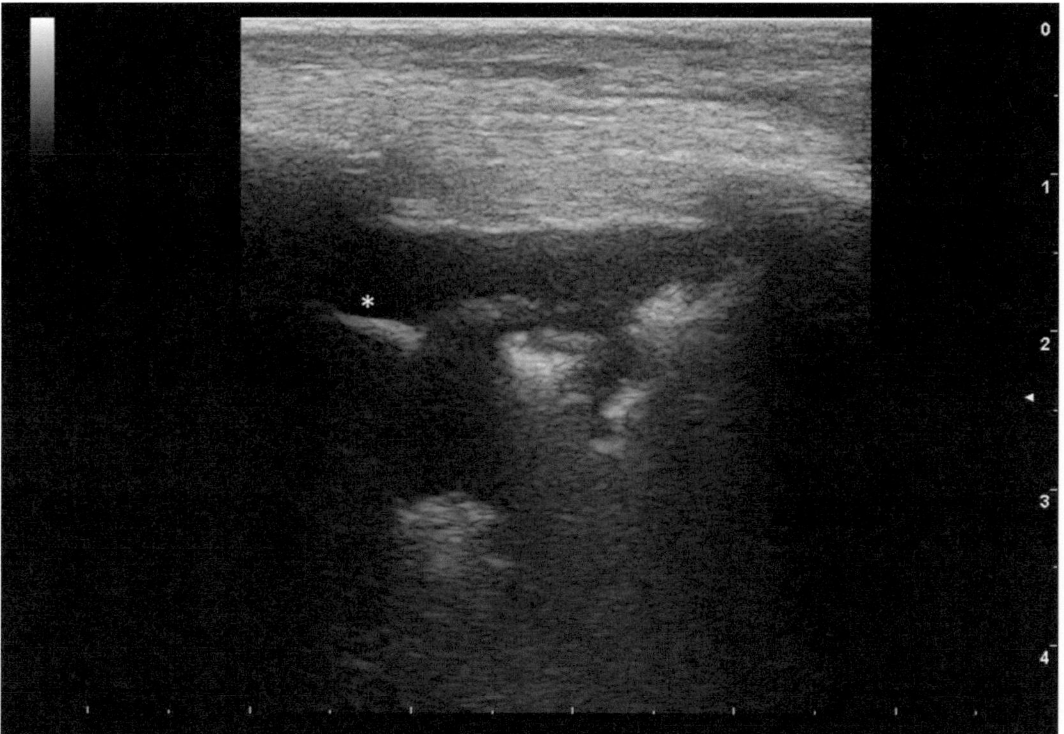

Fig. 6 Image acquired with the linear probe. Subpleural consolidation; Pleural line (*) results distorted and retracted. It is possible to see a minimal quote of pleural effusion, probably reactive to the inflammatory process. For a dynamic image check the online supplement video, v1

Ultrasound in COVID-19

Coronavirus disease 19 (COVID-19) is the viral pneumonia caused by severe acute respiratory syndrome coronavirus 2 (SARS-CoV-2), that, starting as an epidemic cluster in Wuhan, a city in the Hubei Province of China, in November 2019, spreaded worldwide and became a pandemic emergency with 109.068.745 confirmed cases and 2.409.011 deaths, at the time of writing [45].

It has a wide range of clinical presentations, from asymptomatic or mild disease with fever, cough, loss of smell and taste and fatigue, to severe forms of pneumonia or even critical forms of respiratory and multiorgan failure.

In the context of a pandemic infective disease, lung ultrasound has become a valuable tool in diagnosis, evaluation of severity and monitoring in every setting: from home to emergency department and ICU. As previously mentioned, LUS was already part of the everyday clinical practice, thanks to its characteristics of rapidity, point-of-care feasibility and short learning curve; moreover, during the pandemic the possibility of performing a complete examination of the chest without moving the patient reduced the number of healthcare providers exposed [46].

To describe COVID-19 behavior, Gattinoni et al. [47] proposed two phenotypes: "Type L, characterized by Low elastance (i.e., high compliance), Low ventilation-to-perfusion ratio, Low lung weight and Low recruitability", with predominant groundglass opacities; "Type H, characterized by High elastance, High right-to-left shunt, High lung weight and High recruitability", where lobar consolidations may be evidenced. This pattern seems to correspond to a more advanced stage of the disease, with a decrease in gas volume and increased oedema.

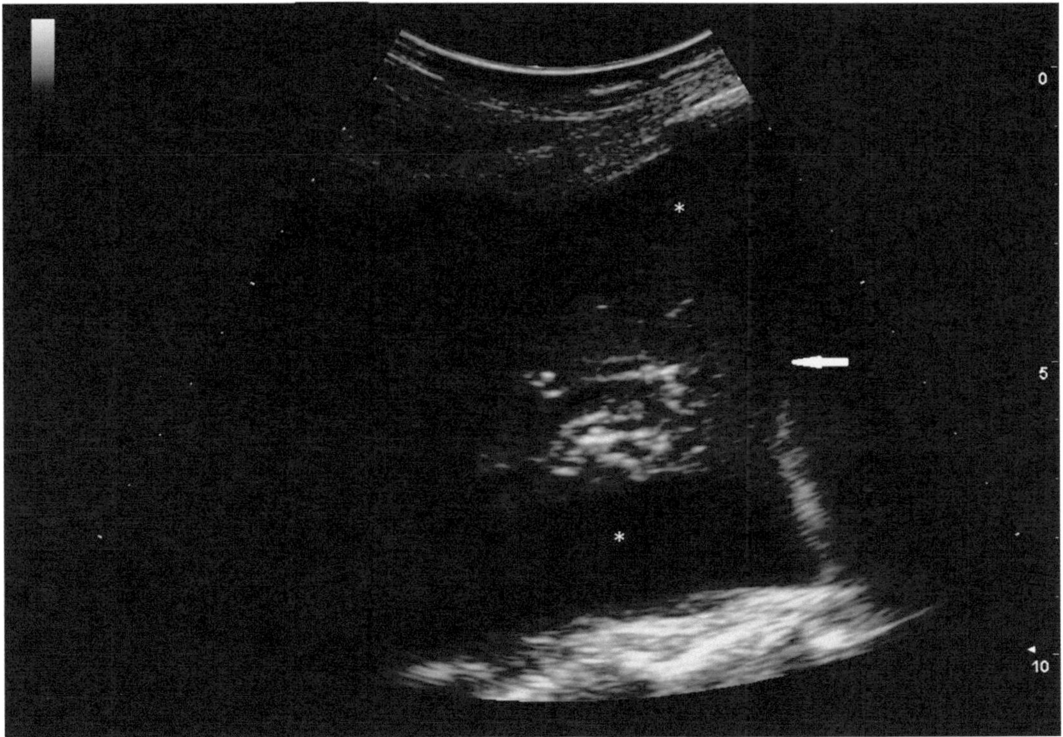

Fig. 7 Image acquired with curvilinear probe, in a patient with nosocomial pneumonia. The image shows right inferior lobe, completely consolidated. It is possible to note some static air bronchogram in the context. In the lower and upper region pleural effusion (star keys). Probably there is a fibrinous effusion that makes consolidated parenchyma with the parietal pleura adhere to the diaphragm (arrow). This image is part of the online supplement video v2

In COVID-19 we can describe all LUS findings typical of pneumonia: B-lines may be separated, coalescent, with areas of white lung and spared areas of A-lines. Pleural line can be regular in some regions, but often it is irregular, thick and fragmented (Fig. 10), with subpleural consolidations and abolished lung sliding, or with large consolidations, typical of phenotype H [48–50].

An artifact firstly described in COVID-19 pneumonia, that seems to be typical of it, is a shining vertical band arising from a large portion of pleural line, that appears and disappears with respiration, sometimes with a normal A-pattern visible on the background. This image has been called the "light beam" [38] and seems the result of an acute phase of groundglass opacity, as it reflects the presence of lesions next to preserved areas of parenchyma [48].

Usefulness of Lung Ultrasonography in Pneumonia

LUS is a non-invasive technique that is very advantageous for a lot of reasons. It is readily available almost everywhere and in different clinical settings (emergency departments, intensive care units, wards, and also in out of hospital settings); it can be practiced by members of

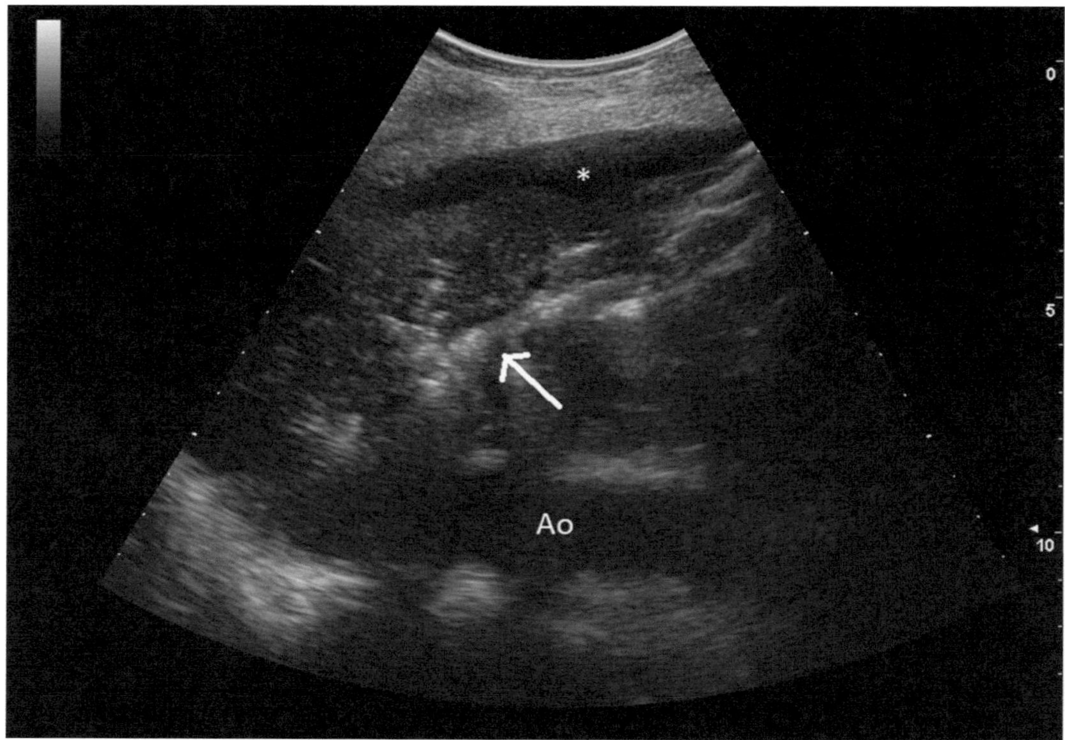

Fig. 8 Image acquired with curvilinear probe The left lung scanned in coronal plane at its base. Lobar pneumonia caused by Enterobacter aerogenes. A static arboriform air bronchogram is visible (arrow). Star key: pleural effusion. Ao: Aorta. Look for the online supplement video v3 to note the completely loss of aeration of parenchyma. Lung pulse (sinchronous movement of parenchyma with the heart pulse) is also present

various medical specialties and is characterized by a steep learning curve with minimal costs and biological impact.

In addition, POCUS is typically performed at the bedside without the need to move the patient to the radiology department, and this is particularly notable for ICU patients, especially those with severe respiratory failure and hemodynamic instability.

LUS is often chosen for its rapidity and ability to provide rapid answers to clinical questions and confirm or exclude alternative diagnostic hypothesis in a few minutes. An expert operator can perform the exam in 5–15 min [30] and this rapidity of execution makes it available for following up pathologic processes, and checking the response to therapies.

Daily LUS monitoring has been successfully applied to estimate antibiotic-induced reaeration in ventilator-associated pneumonia (VAP) [45].

Limitations of Lung Ultrasonography in Pneumonia

While there are advantages offered by LUS, there are some limits clinicians must be aware of:

- Physicians should always be aware that LUS is a layer technique, therefore it can only detect consolidations that reach the pleural line. Therefore, visualization of consolidations is dependent on their distance from the pleura and the size of consolidations. Hence, LUS

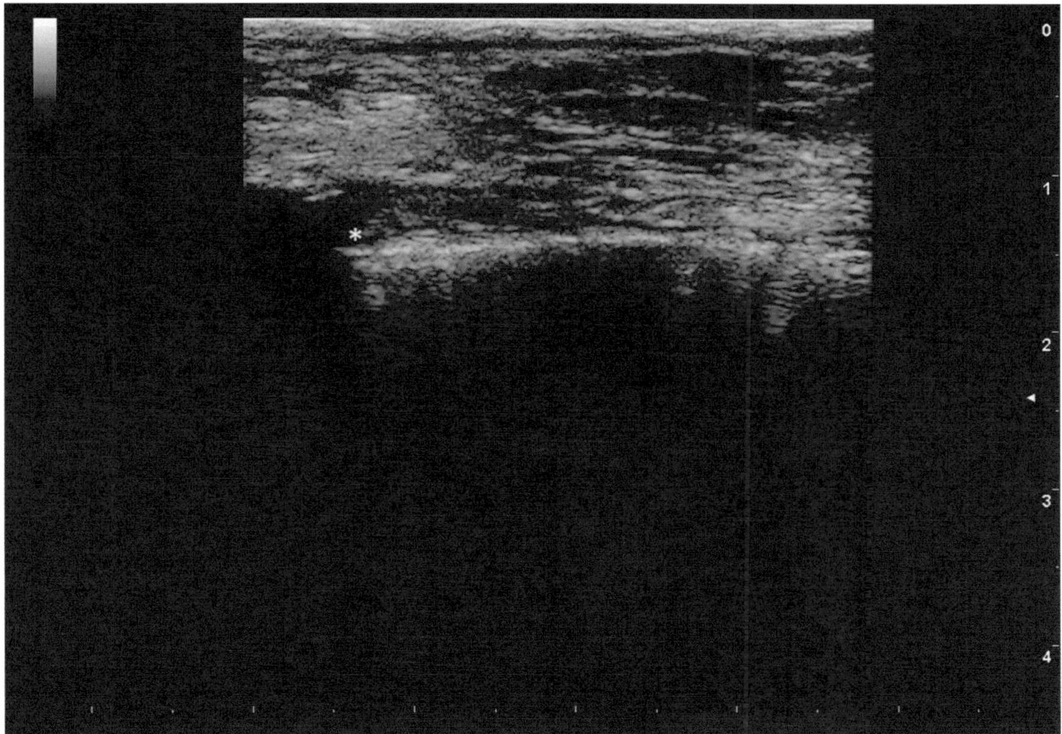

Fig. 9 Image acquired with linear probe. B-lines in a patient with community acquired pneumonia. Star key: pleural line. This image is part of video v4 in the online supplement material

may miss findings with minimal or no extension to the peripheral field (e.g. pneumonias located centrally, deep within the lung) [7]

- POCUS is an operator-dependent examination, and the co-existence of different scoring systems and scanning protocols to grade lung aeration may be confusing for the non-experts. Thus, novel automated ultrasound techniques could be considered as 'a second opinion' in order to create a unique quantification system, standardize diagnostic and monitoring scores and reduce inter and intra-observer variability, especially when LUS is handled by novice operators [11, 46–49].

- Pneumonia is a frequent complication in patients with COPD, but it is not always easy to distinguish it from a COPD exacerbation. Moreover, in COPD, POCUS has not been widely used as the acoustic window is believed to be unfavourable due to the large air content, particularly in patients with lung hyperinflation [50].

- Lung consolidation with massive aeration loss is a differential diagnoses between atelectasis and pneumonia. In mechanically ventilated patients, the presence of atelectasis is very common. During examination, we can observe some clues that can guide us towards the correct diagnosis. For example, the presence of abundant pleural effusion can imply a compression atelectasis; generally, the presence of a dynamic air bronchogram excludes obstructive atelectasis, however, its absence doesn't rule out pneumonia. In fact, a study involving examination of ICU patients with alveolar consolidation and bronchograms, demonstrated that static air bronchograms were seen in most resorptive atelectasis but

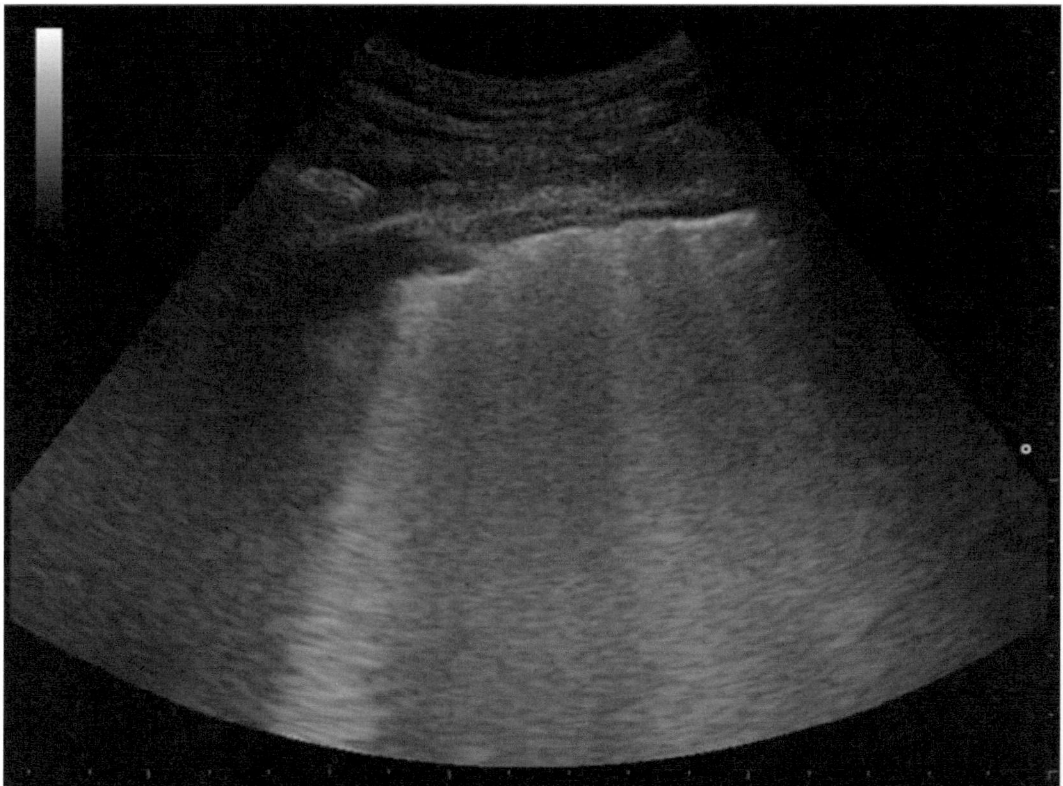

Fig. 10 Image from a COVID 19 patient, acquired with a curvilinear probe. Note the pleural thickness and irregularity, with few B-lines. Search for video v5 on online supplement material

also in almost 30% of cases of pneumonia [36]. Interpretation of POCUS findings within the clinical context is thus fundamental in POCUS practice.

Conclusions

Pneumonia can be diagnosed and followed up by LUS that has been shown to have an excellent diagnostic accuracy in most cases. In the critically ill patients, especially those on invasive mechanical ventilation, the physician should be aware that positive end expiratory pressure may hamper the visualization of some subpleural consolidations or B-lines. LUS represents a layer technique, thus a CT scan should be performed if the clinical suspicious of non-subpleural pulmonary consolidation is suspected or in order to characterize a pulmonary consolidation with complete loss of aeration; indeed air bronchograms become less pronounced with time in case of pneumonias treated with antibiotic therapy, and atelectasis and cancers usually do not reveal any air bronchogram; these consolidations are thus indistinguishable. Interpretation of images within the clinical context is mandatory.

References

1. WHO|Revised Global Burden of Disease (GBD) estimates [Internet]. 2002. https://www.who.int/healthinfo/global_burden_disease/estimates_regional_2002_revised/en/. Accessed 10 Feb 2021
2. Noguchi S, Yatera K, Kawanami T, Fujino Y, Moro H, Aoki N, et al. Pneumonia severity assessment tools for predicting mortality in patients with

healthcare-associated pneumonia: a systematic review and meta-analysis. Respiration [Internet]. 2017;93(6):441–50. https://www.karger.com/Article/FullText/470915. Accessed 7 Feb 2021

3. Metlay JP, Waterer GW, Long AC, Anzueto A, Brozek J, Crothers K, et al. Diagnosis and treatment of adults with community-acquired pneumonia. Am J Respir Crit Care Med [Internet]. 2019;200(7):E45–67. https://doi.org/10.1164/rccm.201908-1581ST. Accessed 7 Feb 2021

4. Mandell LA, Wunderink RG, Anzueto A, Bartlett JG, Campbell GD, Dean NC, et al. Infectious Diseases Society of America/American Thoracic Society Consensus Guidelines on the management of community-acquired pneumonia in adults [Internet]. Vol. 44, Clinical Infectious Diseases. Clin Infect Dis; 2007. https://pubmed.ncbi.nlm.nih.gov/17278083/. Accessed 12 Jan 2021

5. Torres A, Niederman MS, Chastre J, Ewig S, Fernandez-Vandellos P, Hanberger H, et al. International ERS/ESICM/ESCMID/ALAT guidelines for the management of hospital-acquired pneumonia and ventilator-associated pneumonia [Internet]. Vol. 50, European Respiratory Journal. European Respiratory Society; 2017. p. 1700582. http://ow.ly/dGhv30dAVoa. Accessed 9 Feb 2021

6. Franquet T. Imaging of Community-Acquired Pneumonia. In: Journal of Thoracic Imaging [Internet]. Lippincott Williams and Wilkins; 2018. p. 282–94. https://pubmed.ncbi.nlm.nih.gov/30036297/. Accessed 8 Jan 2021

7. Corradi F, Brusasco C, Garlaschi A, Paparo F, Ball L, Santori G, et al. Quantitative analysis of lung ultrasonography for the detection of community-acquired pneumonia: A pilot study. Biomed Res Int [Internet]. 2015;2015. https://pubmed.ncbi.nlm.nih.gov/25811032/. Accessed 7 Feb 2021

8. Lichtenstein DA, Mezière GA. Relevance of lung ultrasound in the diagnosis of acute respiratory failure the BLUE protocol. Chest [Internet]. 2008;134(1):117–25. https://pubmed.ncbi.nlm.nih.gov/18403664/. Accessed 12 Jan 2021

9. Silvia Mongodi A, Bouhemad B, Orlando A, Stella A, Tavazzi G, Via G, et al. Modified Lung Ultrasound Score for Assessing and Monitoring Pulmonary Aeration Modifizierter Lungen-US-Score zur Bewertung und Überwachung der Belüftung der Lunge. Modif Lung Ultrasound Ultraschall Med [Internet]. 2017;37:530–7. https://doi.org/10.1055/s-0042-120260. Accessed 8 Feb 2021

10. Chiumello D, Mongodi S, Algieri I, LucaVergani G, Orlando A, Via G, et al. Assessment of lung aeration and recruitment by CT scan and ultrasound in acute respiratory distress syndrome patients. Crit Care Med [Internet]. 2018;46(11):1761–8. https://pubmed.ncbi.nlm.nih.gov/30048331/. Accessed 8 Feb 2021

11. Corradi F, Brusasco C, Vezzani A, Santori G, Manca T, Ball L, et al. Computer-Aided Quantitative Ultrasonography for Detection of Pulmonary Edema in Mechanically Ventilated Cardiac Surgery Patients. Chest [Internet]. 2016;150(3):640–51. https://doi.org/10.1016/j.chest.2016.04.013

12. Corradi F, Ball L, Brusasco C, Riccio AM, Baroffio M, Bovio G, et al. Assessment of extravascular lung water by quantitative ultrasound and CT in isolated bovine lung. Respir Physiol Neurobiol [Internet]. 2013;187(3):244–9. https://pubmed.ncbi.nlm.nih.gov/23584050/. Accessed 19 Mar 2021

13. Reissig A, Copetti R, Mathis G, Mempel C, Schuler A, Zechner P, et al. Lung ultrasound in the diagnosis and follow-up of community-acquired pneumonia: A prospective, multicenter, diagnostic accuracy study. Chest. 2012;142(4):965–72.

14. Cortellaro F, Colombo S, Coen D, Duca PG. Lung ultrasound is an accurate diagnostic tool for the diagnosis of pneumonia in the emergency department. Emerg Med J [Internet]. 2012;29(1):19–23. https://pubmed.ncbi.nlm.nih.gov/21030550/. Accessed 12 Jan 2021

15. Laursen CB, Sloth E, Lassen AT, Christensen R de P, Lambrechtsen J, Madsen PH, et al. Point-of-care ultrasonography in patients admitted with respiratory symptoms: A single-blind, randomised controlled trial. Lancet Respir Med [Internet]. 2014;2(8):638–46. https://pubmed.ncbi.nlm.nih.gov/24998674/. Accessed 19 Mar 2021

16. Ye X, Xiao H, Chen B, Zhang S. Accuracy of Lung Ultrasonography versus Chest Radiography for the Diagnosis of Adult Community-Acquired Pneumonia: Review of the Literature and Meta-Analysis. Chalmers JD, editor. PLoS One [Internet]. 2015;10(6):e0130066. https://doi.org/10.1371/journal.pone.0130066. Accessed 19 Mar 2021

17. Reissig A, Gramegna A, Aliberti S. The role of lung ultrasound in the diagnosis and follow-up of community-acquired pneumonia. Eur J Intern Med [Internet]. 2012;23(5):391–7. https://doi.org/10.1016/j.ejim.2012.01.003

18. Nazerian P, Volpicelli G, Vanni S, Gigli C, Betti L, Bartolucci M, et al. Accuracy of lung ultrasound for the diagnosis of consolidations when compared to chest computed tomography. Am J Emerg Med [Internet]. 2015;33(5):620–5. https://pubmed.ncbi.nlm.nih.gov/25758182/. Accessed 13 Jan 2021

19. Lichtenstein DA, Lascols N, Mezière G, Gepner A. Ultrasound diagnosis of alveolar consolidation in the critically ill. Intensive Care Med [Internet]. 2004;30(2):276–81. https://pubmed.ncbi.nlm.nih.gov/14722643/. Accessed 11 Feb 2021

20. Mateos González M, García de Casasola Sánchez G, Muñoz FJT, Proud K, Lourdo D, Sander J-V, et al. Comparison of Lung Ultrasound versus Chest X-ray for Detection of Pulmonary Infiltrates in COVID-19. Diagnostics (Basel, Switzerland) [Internet]. 2021;11(2). http://www.ncbi.nlm.nih.gov/pubmed/33671699. Accessed 19 Mar 2021

21. Mayo PH, Copetti R, Feller-Kopman D, Mathis G, Maury E, Mongodi S, et al. Thoracic ultrasonography: a narrative review [Internet]. Vol. 45, Intensive Care Medicine. Springer Verlag; 2019. p. 1200–11. https://doi.org/10.1007/s00134-019-05725-8. Accessed 8 Jan 2021

22. Zagli G, Cozzolino M, Terreni A, Biagioli T, Caldini AL, Peris A. Diagnosis of Ventilator-Associated Pneumonia: A Pilot, Exploratory Analysis of a New Score Based on Procalcitonin and Chest Echography. Chest [Internet]. 2014;146(6):1578–85. https://pubmed.ncbi.nlm.nih.gov/25144666/. Accessed 14 Feb 2021

23. Lichtenstein D, Mezière G. A lung ultrasound sign allowing bedside distinction between pulmonary edema and COPD: The comet-tail artifact. Intensive Care Med [Internet]. 1998;24(12):1331–4. https://pubmed.ncbi.nlm.nih.gov/9885889/. Accessed 19 Mar 2021

24. Volpicelli G, Elbarbary M, Blaivas M, Lichtenstein DA, Mathis G, Kirkpatrick AW, et al. International evidence-based recommendations for point-of-care lung ultrasound. In: Intensive Care Medicine [Internet]. Springer; 2012. p. 577–91. https://doi.org/10.1007/s00134-012-2513-4. Accessed 13 Jan 2021

25. Volpicelli G, Mussa A, Garofalo G, Cardinale L, Casoli G, Perotto F, et al. Bedside lung ultrasound in the assessment of alveolar-interstitial syndrome. Am J Emerg Med [Internet]. 2006;24(6):689–96. https://pubmed.ncbi.nlm.nih.gov/16984837/. Accessed 19 Mar 2021

26. Mongodi S, Via G, Girard M, Rouquette I, Misset B, Braschi A, et al. Lung ultrasound for early diagnosis of ventilator-associated pneumonia. Chest [Internet]. 2016;149(4):969–80. https://doi.org/10.1016/j.chest.2015.12.012

27. Soummer A, Perbet S, Brisson H, Arbelot C, Constantin JM, Lu Q, et al. Ultrasound assessment of lung aeration loss during a successful weaning trial predicts postextubation distress. Crit Care Med [Internet]. 2012;40(7):2064–72. https://pubmed.ncbi.nlm.nih.gov/22584759/. Accessed 19 Mar 2021

28. Mojoli F, Bouhemad B, Mongodi S, Lichtenstein D. Lung ultrasound for critically ill patients. Am J Respir Crit Care Med. 2019;199(6):701–14.

29. Volpicelli G, Lamorte A, Villén T. What's new in lung ultrasound during the COVID-19 pandemic. Intensive Care Med [Internet]. 2020;46(7):1445–8. https://www.ncbi.nlm.nih.gov/pmc/articles/PMC7196717/. Accessed 21 Jan 2021

30. Rouby JJ, Arbelot C, Gao Y, Zhang M, Lv J, An Y, et al. Training for lung ultrasound score measurement in critically ill patients [Internet]. Vol. 198, Am J Respir Critical Care Med. American Thoracic Society; 2018. p. 398–401. https://doi.org/10.1164/rccm.201802-0227LE. Accessed 19 Mar 2021

31. Ball L, Corradi F, Pelosi P. Ultrasonography in Critical Care Medicine: The WAMS Approach. ICU Manag Pract [Internet]. 2012;12(2):30–3. https://healthmanagement.org/c/icu/issuearticle/ultrasonography-in-critical-care-medicine-the-wams-approach

32. Kumar V, Abbas A, Aster J. Robbins & Cotran Pathologic Basis of Disease [Internet]. 10th ed. 2020. 1392 https://www.elsevier.com/books/robbins-and-cotran-pathologic-basis-of-disease/kumar/978-0-323-53113-9

33. Ware LB, Matthay MA. The Acute Respiratory Distress Syndrome. N Engl J Med [Internet]. 2000;342(18):1334–49. https://doi.org/10.1056/NEJM200005043421806. Accessed 19 Mar 2021

34. Lichtenstein D, Mézière G, Biderman P, Gepner A, Barré O. The comet-tail artifact: An ultrasound sign of alveolar-interstitial syndrome. Am J Respir Crit Care Med. 1997;156(5):1640–6.

35. Reissig A, Kroegel C. Sonographic diagnosis and follow-up of pneumonia: A prospective study. Respiration. 2007;74(5):537–47.

36. Lichtenstein D, Mézière G, Seitz J. The dynamic air bronchogram: A lung ultrasound sign of alveolar consolidation ruling out atelectasis. Chest. 2009;135(6):1421–5.

37. Asano M, Watanabe H, Sato K, Okuda Y, Sakamoto S, Hasegawa Y, et al. Validity of ultrasound lungcomets for assessment of the severity of interstitial pneumonia. J Ultrasound Med [Internet]. 2018;37(6):1523–31. https://pubmed.ncbi.nlm.nih.gov/29194717/. Accessed 13 Jan 2021

38. WHO Coronavirus Disease (COVID-19) Dashboard [Internet]. https://covid19.who.int/?gclid=CjwKCAiAmrOBBhA0EiwArn3mfCJKUEDBXkdjAKKQZ1bvekFSiEwZrJnF2O_K1SJhy_2ampQQBKPtcRoC2RMQAvD_BwE. Accessed 17 Feb 2021

39. Gargani L, Soliman-Aboumarie H, Volpicelli G, Corradi F, Pastore MC, Cameli M. Why, when, and how to use lung ultrasound during the COVID-19 pandemic: Enthusiasm and caution [Internet]. Vol. 21, Eur Heart J Cardiovasc Imaging. Oxford University Press; 2020. p. 941–8. https://pubmed.ncbi.nlm.nih.gov/32515793/. Accessed 13 Jan 2021

40. Gattinoni L, Chiumello D, Caironi P, Busana M, Romitti F, Brazzi L, et al. COVID-19 pneumonia: different respiratory treatments for different phenotypes? [Internet]. Vol. 46, Intensive Care Medicine. Springer; 2020. p. 1099–102. https://pubmed.ncbi.nlm.nih.gov/32291463/. Accessed 17 Feb 2021

41. Guarracino F, Vetrugno L, Forfori F, Corradi F, Orso D, Bertini P, et al. Lung, heart, vascular, and diaphragm ultrasound examination of COVID-19 patients: a comprehensive approach [Internet]. J Cardiothorac Vasc Anesth. W.B. Saunders; 2020;35(6):1866–1874. Accessed 7 Feb 2021

42. Gargani L, Soliman-Aboumarie H, Volpicelli G, Corradi F, Pastore MC, Cameli M. Why, when, and how to use lung ultrasound during the COVID-19 pandemic: enthusiasm and caution. Eur Heart J Cardiovasc Imaging [Internet]. 2020;21(9):941–8. https://academic.oup.com/ehjcimaging/article/21/9/941/5855021

43. Hussain A, Via G, Melniker L, Goffi A, Tavazzi G, Neri L, et al. Multi-organ point-of-care ultrasound for COVID-19 (PoCUS4COVID): international expert consensus [Internet]. Vol. 24, Critical Care. BioMed Central Ltd; 2020. https://pubmed.ncbi.nlm.nih.gov/33357240/. Accessed 21 Mar 2021

44. Volpicelli G, Gargani L. Sonographic signs and patterns of COVID-19 pneumonia. Ultrasound J [Internet]. 2020;12(1):22. https://doi.org/10.1186/s13089-020-00171-w. Accessed 21 Jan 2021

45. Bouhemad B, Liu ZH, Arbelot C, Zhang M, Ferarri F, Le-Guen M, et al. Ultrasound assessment of antibiotic-induced pulmonary reaeration in ventilator-associated pneumonia. Crit Care Med [Internet]. 2010;38(1):84–92. https://pubmed.ncbi.nlm.nih.gov/19633538/. Accessed 9 Feb 2021

46. Mongodi S, Santangelo E, De Luca D, Rovida S, Corradi F, Volpicelli G, et al. Quantitative Lung Ultrasound: Time for a Consensus? [Internet]. Vol. 158, Chest. Elsevier Inc; 2020. p. 469–70. https://pubmed.ncbi.nlm.nih.gov/32768066/. Accessed 11 Jan 2021

47. Brusasco C, Santori G, Tavazzi G, Via G, Robba C, Gargani L, et al. Second-order grey-scale texture analysis of pleural ultrasound images to differentiate acute respiratory distress syndrome and cardiogenic pulmonary edema. J Clin Morit Comput [Internet]. 2020. https://pubmed.ncbi.nlm.nih.gov/33313979/. Accessed 21 Mar 2021

48. Corradi F, Via G, Forfori F, Brusasco C, Tavazzi G. Lung ultrasound and B-lines quantification inaccuracy: B sure to have the right solution [Internet]. Vol. 46, Intensive Care Medicine. Springer; 2020. p. 1081–3. https://www.rcbi.nlm.nih.gov/pmc/articles/PMC7087507/. Accessed 7 Feb 2021

49. Brusasco C, Santori G, Bruzzo E, Trò R, Robba C, Tavazzi G, et al. Quantitative lung ultrasonography: a putative new algorithm for automatic detection and quantification of B-lines. Crit Care [Internet]. 2019;23(1):288. https://doi.org/10.1186/s13054-019-2569-4. Accessed 7 Feb 2021

50. Corradi F, Brusasco C, Brusasco V. Cuándo, dónde y cómo utilizar la ecografía en pacientes con enfermedad pulmonar obstructiva crónica? Arch Bronconeumol [Internet]. 2017;53(5):229–30. https://pubmed.ncbi.nlm.nih.gov/28024665/. Accessed 11 Jan 2021

Pneumothorax

Giovanni Volpicelli

The knowledge of anything, since all things have causes, is not acquired or complete unless it is known by its causes.

Ibn Sina (Avicenna)—Persian Medieval Physician and Polymath (980–1037 AD)

Keywords

Pneumothorax · POCUS · Point of care ultrasound · Lung point · Pleural sliding

Key Messages

- Bedside lung ultrasound is useful in the diagnostic work-up for pneumothorax in the extreme emergencies and it is superior to bedside chest radiography.
- Absence of lung sliding is not specific to pneumothorax as can be found in several other pathologies
- When the operator places the probe on the chest wall and does not visualize pleural sliding, B-lines or lung pulse, the diagnosis of pneumothorax is highly probable
- Lung point is the most specific lung ultrasound sign of pneumothorax

Supplementary Information The online version contains supplementary material available at https://doi.org/10.1007/978-3-031-29472-3_11.

G. Volpicelli (✉)
Emergency Medicine, San Luigi Gonzaga University Hospital, Torino, Italy
e-mail: giovi.volpicelli@gmail.com

Introduction

Air in the pleural space cannot be imaged by lung ultrasound due to intrinsic properties of the interaction between the ultrasound beam and the human tissues. However, although this assumption is true, thanks to the intuition of some clinicians nowadays bedside lung ultrasound is considered a fundamental tool to expedite the diagnostic work-up and diagnose safely pneumothorax in several critical conditions.

'A 51-year-old woman was ejected from the vehicle during a high-speed car accident. She was hypotensive on arrival to the emergency department with signs of severe head injury. She was orally intubated shortly after arrival, and she had a E-FAST exam which included evaluation for pneumothorax. The rest of the FAST exam was unremarkable, but she had absence of sliding bilaterally. The caring physicians did not believe in the possibility of a bilateral pneumothorax and decided to perform a chest radiography before any intervention. Chest radiography showed the oral tube correctly positioned above the carina and clear signs of left-side pneumothorax. Thus, a left chest tube was immediately placed. The radiography did not show clear right-side pneumothorax. So, despite the patient continued hypotension and

"

lack of lung sliding on the right side, a chest tube was not immediately placed. This turned out to be a bad decision. A chest CT scan was performed by moving to the radiology facility a patient in conditions of severe instability. CT demonstrated the residual pneumothorax on the left side and a large pneumothorax on the right side'

This simple and not so rare trauma case demonstrates the important role of bedside lung ultrasound in the diagnostic work-up for pneumothorax in the extreme emergencies and its superiority to bedside chest radiography.

Imaging Process in Pneumothorax

How has this new role of lung ultrasound for pneumothorax been recognized? The change in the consideration of the importance of lung ultrasound was a long scientific process that started from the concept that ultrasound cannot allow visualization of the intra-pleural air. It is well known that the presence of air inside or outside the lung blocks the propagation of the ultrasound beam when the chest wall is insonated. Indeed, the strong acoustic interface, due to the opposite values of impedance of the chest wall tissues on one side and the alveolar or intrapleural air on the other, blocks the route of the ultrasound emission and does not allow the visualization of structures that lie deeper to the parietal pleura. The effect of this phenomenon is the visualization of an image of the lung that is only artefactual, due to a mixture of reflection and reverberation of the beam back to the transducer [1]. The image obtained will be a mirroring of the same chest wall reflected below the parietal pleural line, which repeats through a phenomenon of multiple reverberation (Fig. 1). The pleura, the site of maximum acoustic interface, is like a mirror that reflects down the image of the chest wall and prevents the visualization of the real lung. Then, the echoic pleural line reverberates down into the lung image, repeating the same distance between the probe and the pleura, which is the phenomenon that creates the A-lines [2]. The static image of the lung will be

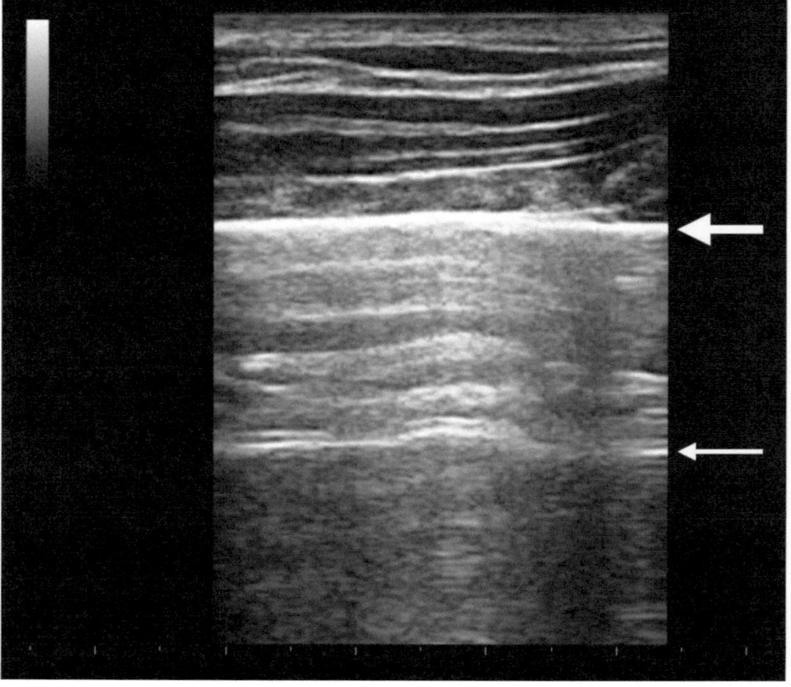

Fig. 1 Presence of air inside the alveolar spaces or in the pleural space (pneumothorax) creates the same artifactual ultrasound image, due to the strong acoustic interface with the tissue of the chest wall. The effect is a mirroring of the image of the chest wall below the pleural line (*thick arrow*), with repetitions due to reverberations (A-lines, *thin arrow*)

the same both when the air is inside the lung parenchyma, in a condition of normal aeration, and when it is in the pleural space in a condition of pneumothorax. However, lung ultrasound also allows the evaluation of the dynamic movements of the lung during the respiratory phases and, eventually, also the movements transmitted from the heart beats. Because of the presence of air between the two pleural layers, in the condition of pneumothorax there is not any possibility to observe those movements. Thus, the main difference between the two conditions with or without pneumothorax is the dynamic evaluation of the artifactual image of the lung [3].

This introductory description of the main principles of lung ultrasound is valid for any pathology that is at the origin of pneumothorax. It is true that most of the literature supporting the usefulness of lung ultrasound for pneumothorax have been produced in pneumothorax secondary to trauma and invasive procedures, but the same ultrasound principles can be translated to spontaneous pneumothorax, either primary or secondary to chronic pulmonary diseases [3]. However, we will see that the clinical condition of the patient during the examination and the setting where the operator needs to diagnose pneumothorax, have an influence on the technique that should be applied and even on the accuracy of the ultrasound signs. Indeed, this variability is typical of the philosophy of a point-of-care diagnostic tool [4].

Ultrasound Signs

Lung Sliding

As said, when air is in the interpleural space the propagation of the beam down to the visceral pleura is blocked, and any movement of the lung in the ultrasound scan disappears. Thus, even if the anatomy of the aerated lung cannot be imaged by ultrasound, the artefactual image with A-lines that moves with respiration indicates the absence of pneumothorax, while the same A-lines pattern not moving during ventilation has a probability of being due to pneumothorax. The respiratory movement of the lung image at ultrasound is called *lung sliding* (Video 1) [5]. The intensity of this movement is variable because it depends on the area of the chest that is examined, the ventilatory effort done by the patient, and the elastic compliance of the lung parenchyma. For instance, when the transducer is placed at the apex of the lung in a patient scarcely collaborating with shallow breathing, and affected by a chronic emphysematous disease, lung sliding may become hardly visible. However, lung sliding responds to the all-or-nothing rule and the quantification of the respiratory movement of the lung detected by ultrasound has no diagnostic meaning when assessed in B-mode. Thus, even the mildest visible movement allows to rule-out pneumothorax in the same way as when the sliding is more consistent. However, it must be said that there are some attempts to allow quantification of lung sliding by additional ultrasound techniques. One possibility is using the speckle tracking [6]. Quantifying lung sliding may be useful to differentiate hyperinflation or chronic diseases with reduced pulmonary compliance, besides being useful in increasing the sensitivity in the diagnosis of pneumothorax. The real usefulness and impact in practice of these new techniques remain to be investigated.

Importance of Additional Signs

One main consideration limits the role of lung sliding in the process for diagnosing pneumothorax. Absence of lung sliding is not only a basic characteristic of pneumothorax, but also of several other conditions [3]. For instance, in conditions of apnea, selective intubation and in respiratory arrest, there is no ventilation, and the lung sliding will be absent. Other pathologic conditions, like ARDS, pneumonia, contusions, may be characterized by absence of lung sliding [7]. Thus, while the presence of lung sliding allows the operator to rule-out pneumothorax with a very high sensitivity, its absence cannot be considered enough specific to finalize the diagnostic decision and rule-in pneumothorax. After the first ultrasound studies based uniquely on the consideration of lung sliding, it became evident that specificity could not be considered sufficient to confirm safely the diagnosis of pneumothorax in any condition [8–10]. The studies using only lung sliding to confirm pneumothorax were strongly limited, and this limitation should be always considered when the literature is analyzed for the validity of ultrasound [11, 12]. Further research demonstrated that some additional ultrasound signs are extremely important to increase the diagnostic accuracy of lung ultrasound when lung sliding is absent [13–15]. Namely, in a condition when lung sliding is not visualized, there are some parenchymal signs and movements of the lung image that may help to rule-out pneumothorax, and one other sign that can be helpful in confirming with high specificity the diagnosis. The correct interpretation of lung ultrasound for pneumothorax may only be the result of the analysis of a combination of signs [7].

Parenchymal Signs

When air interposes between the transducer and the lung it is not possible to see the respiratory movements down to the parietal pleura, but also it hides any ultrasound sign that could emerge from the lung parenchyma. These are interstitial vertical artifacts (*B-lines*) and alveolar patterns (*consolidations*) (Fig. 2). Keen readers will note that in the literature the B-lines were previously called *comet tail* artifacts; they are synonymous. Thus, visualization of B-lines and/or consolidations, even in the absence of lung sliding, allows to exclude with great sensitivity the diagnosis of pneumothorax [13]. In a situation when lung sliding is absent and B-lines or a consolidation are visualized, the operator can confidently rule-out pneumothorax and is also authorized to conclude about a pathologic lack of ventilation in the area examined. Another sign that may be helpful in ruling out pneumothorax is the sonographic visualization of a space between the two pleural layers. This happens in case of effusion, both anechoic and complex. Of course, when present, the effusion will occupy the interpleural space ruling-out pneumothorax. For convenience, we will call "B-lines" any visible sign, including consolidations, that origins from the parenchyma and rules-out pneumothorax.

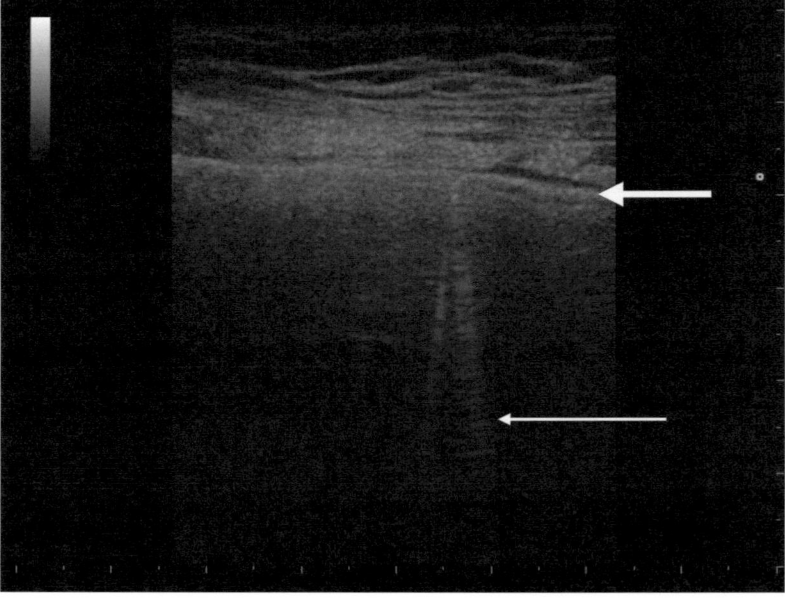

Fig. 2 In a condition of absence of lung sliding, visualization of even one isolated B-line allows to rule-out pneumothorax in the scan area. The *thick arrow* indicates the pleural line, while the *thin arrow* indicates the B-line

Lung Pulse

Most often, the parenchymal signs at lung ultrasound are the effect of a pathology of the lung. However, not always the lung of a patient examined for pneumothorax is pathologic. In the normal lung there are no significant B-lines and no consolidations. Thus, even in the absence of B-lines or consolidations, the image of a lung that does not slide can still be due to other conditions than pneumothorax. In this case, another important sign to evaluate is the *lung pulse* [15]. This latter is again a fine movement of the image of the lung. However, while lung sliding is synchronous with respiration, lung pulse is synchronized with the heart beats (Video 2). When the lung is normally attached to the parietal pleura but does not ventilate for any reason, the cardiac movements will be transmitted through the parenchyma to the chest wall and a pulsation of the lung image will become evident at lung ultrasound. In some conditions, this movement is crucial to rule-out pneumothorax, again with very high sensitivity. Of course, this is only valid when there is at least a minimal cardiac activity. Indeed, lung ultrasound can visualize even the minimum cardiac movement, and a lung pulse is visible even in conditions of cardiac arrest in PEA. However, when the cardiac arrest is in asystole the movement is not detectable and cannot be used to discriminate absence of pneumothorax [16].

Lung Point

So far, we described signs that are useful to rule-out pneumothorax with high sensitivity. There is only one sign at lung ultrasound that is decisive and highly specific to confirm pneumothorax. It is the *lung point* [14]. This sign is visible when the pneumothorax does not cause a complete collapse of the lung and the position of the ultrasound probe corresponds to the border between the intrapleural air on one side and the lung still attached to the parietal pleura on the other. This situation creates an interface pneumothorax/lung between, giving sliding versus absence of sliding. The visual effect in the ultrasound scan is a sliding that interposes rhythmically, following the lung expansion, over the side showing absence of sliding (Video 3). The lung point identifies a point on the thoracic wall that corresponds to the edge of the intrapleural air and is also useful for mapping and measuring the extension of pneumothorax [17].

Combination of Signs

We described the combination of lung sliding, lung pulse and parenchymal signs, to exclude with high sensitivity pneumothorax. Thus, in the conditions of either (a) a visible lung sliding, or (b) absence of lung sliding but visible B-lines, or (c) absence of lung sliding and B-lines but visible lung pulse, the pneumothorax can be excluded, in the area where the probe is placed, with high sensitivity. When the operator places the probe on the chest wall and does not visualize sliding, B-lines or pulse, the diagnosis of pneumothorax is highly probable. In this combination, only the visualization of a lung point can definitively confirm pneumothorax. However, we will see that in some circumstances even in the absence of a lung point, the final confirmation of pneumothorax is authorized.

Ultrasound Technique

The lungs are wide organs and the technique for lung ultrasound can be performed in many areas, including the anterior, the lateral, and the posterior chest. When the probe is positioned on the thorax, the evaluation for the ultrasound signs for pneumothorax will be valid only in the place where they are investigated. If, for example, the operator positions the probe on the lateral chest and a regular lung sliding is visualized, the conclusion will be that there is no intrapleural air in that area, but it is not possible to conclude that there is no pneumothorax. Thus, it is important that a correct technique is applied, consisting mainly in the correct sequence of positioning the probe and combining the signs [3, 7].

To understand the technique for pneumothorax, the operator should consider that air inside the pleural space naturally moves for gravity in the less dependent area of the chest. Because of this observation, it is important to care the position of the patient. When the patient is in the supine position, pneumothorax should be investigated first in the anterior inferior area of the chest, that is also said the less dependent zone (Fig. 3) [7]. If lung sliding is found there, pneumothorax can be ruled-out with high sensitivity because even the smallest quantity of air inside the pleural space would move in that area.

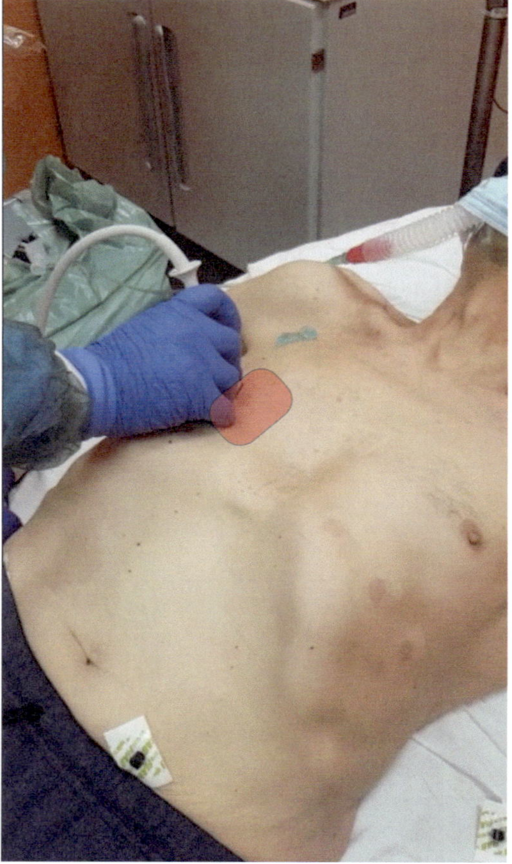

Fig. 3 The correct lung ultrasound examination for pneumothorax should start from the anterior inferior chest (*red box*), with the patient in the supine position. This area is the "hot zone", corresponding to the less dependent area, where even the smallest amount of intrapleural air can be detected

Thus, when the operator works in the hospital, the patient should always lie down in the supine position to perform a correct examination. When the patient is forced in another decubitus, like for instance in case of intervention in a trauma scenario due to car accidents or casualties, the position of the probe should be adapted accordingly, in a manner that the most superior chest area is scanned first. The probe will be oriented longitudinally to observe the echoic ribs and the echoic pleural line in between and below them. If the pattern is positive for at least one between lung sliding/B-lines/lung pulse, pneumothorax can be ruled-out with high sensitivity. In this case the next step will be extending the examination to the other chest side and repeating the maneuver. As a second possibility, if the pattern does not show lung sliding, B-lines, and lung pulse, then there is a high probability that the patient has pneumothorax. When the patient is in stable condition, the next step that follows visualization of a pattern negative for sliding/B-lines/pulse in the anterior chest, is searching for the lung point. This maneuver consists in moving the probe from the anterior chest to the lateral base of the lung. The probe should be oriented in oblique, thus rotated transversely between the ribs to bring the echogenic pleural stripe into profile; the movement should be done by following the laterality of the intercostal space and passing from one space to the next inferior until the lateral base is fully scanned. This maneuver can be considered a stepping down movement that follows all the intercostal spaces (Fig. 4) [17]. When a lung point is detected, the diagnosis of pneumothorax is confirmed, and it is also possible a measure of its extension of the chest surface. If a lung point cannot be visualized, there is the possibility that the lung is completely collapsed, but further imaging is needed to confirm the diagnosis (usually chest radiography or CT in complicated cases) [18].

In extreme emergency situations, when the patient is hemodynamically unstable or in cardiac arrest, the technique of lung ultrasound is simplified because there is no need to identify the lung point to conclude and decide for a lifesaving intervention [7]. In extreme emergencies the

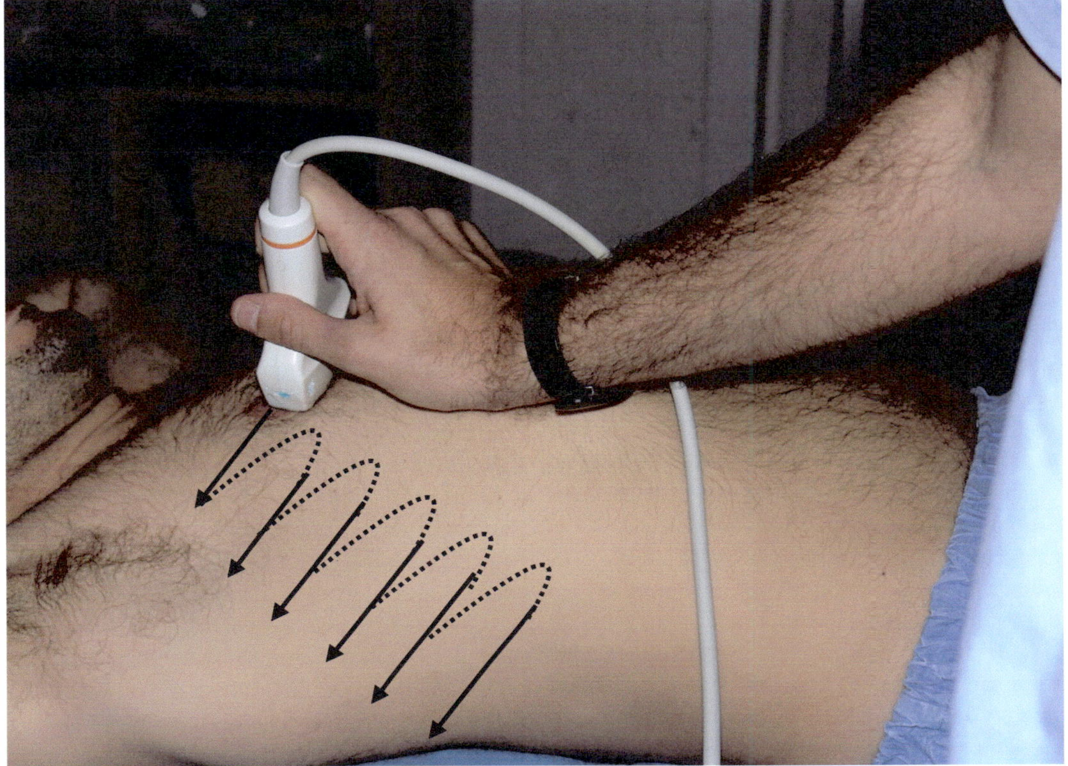

Fig. 4 Starting from the "hot zone" on the chest wall, the movement of the probe to search for the *lung point* should be done by following the laterality of the intercostal space in oblique scan (*black arrows*) and then passing to the next inferior space (*dotted lines*), until the whole lateral chest is scanned

procedure to rule-out pneumothorax remains the same, and when a regular sliding is detected in the anterior-inferior chest on both sides, the next step will be to look for alternative critical pulmonary conditions.

Ultrasound Probes

The standard probe to perform the ultrasound examination for pneumothorax in stable patients is commonly the linear high frequency probe. This probe allows high-definition imaging of the pleural line and maximum sensitivity for detecting the respiratory and cardiac movements of the lung [3]. In case the linear probe is not available or when lung ultrasound is part of a general and more panoramic point-of-care ultrasound examination of the patient, a convex low-frequency probe is also indicated. The convex abdominal is particularly suitable in conditions of extreme emergency in unstable patients, because in these conditions there is the necessity to quickly extend the ultrasound examination to other organs and obtain a more panoramic view [3, 7]. The microconvex low-frequency probe may also be used when available, with the advantage of slipping more readily between the ribs with easier handling but the limitation of a worse image resolution of the pleural line [2, 3]. The cardiac sectorial probe is the less indicated in the images of the pleural line but should be used without hesitation in case it is the only probe available.

Regarding the position of the probe, we already reported that the examination of pneumothorax can be limited and simplified to few "hot zones", where the ultrasound signs should be investigated. However, there are some complex conditions in which the ultrasound scans should be extended to the whole chest. We will see in a following paragraph that, in some complex situations, it is mandatory to extend the examination also to the lateral and even posterior chest before taking a diagnostic conclusion.

Clinical Conditions and Settings

The setting of examination and the clinical condition of the patient have both great influence on the diagnostic power of each lung ultrasound sign for pneumothorax and indicate the technique that should be applied. Bedside lung ultrasound for pneumothorax fits very well with the philosophy of Point-of-Care ultrasound. For instance, while the combination of absence of sliding, B-lines and pulse has a low specificity in the confirmation of pneumothorax in a stable patient, the same ultrasound pattern during the examination in emergency of a trauma patient severely unstable allows definitive confirmation and demands for immediate drainage [7]. In the stable patient the role of lung ultrasound is guiding only the first diagnostic approach that precedes a more complete examination, whereas in the extreme emergency situations the simplicity and promptness of the ultrasound approach make the difference, because it may become sufficient to confirm the diagnosis and guide appropriate lifesaving interventions. In some other situations, lung ultrasound may reveal an unexpected diagnosis of pneumothorax in conditions of undifferentiated respiratory failure and/or hemodynamic compromise [19]. For this reason, it is always valid the rule of starting the general lung ultrasound examination from the analysis of the respiratory sliding [18]. It is also important to note that even the smallest pneumothorax in complex patients who need emergency surgery or helicopter transportation, should be promptly diagnosed, and treated or monitored. Lung ultrasound represents the ideal tool to examine complex patients, orientate the differential diagnoses at bedside and guide further diagnostic and therapeutic approaches.

Comparison with Chest Radiography and CT

Besides lung ultrasound, chest imaging for pneumothorax also includes chest radiography and chest CT. While CT scan remains the imaging gold standard for the diagnosis of pneumothorax, it is beyond any reasonable doubt that lung ultrasound represents the bedside tool of choice in emergency. When a lung point is visualized, the specificity of lung ultrasound for the diagnosis of pneumothorax is extremely high and comparable to the equally high specificity of chest radiography. The lung point is a new diagnostic language having the same confirming power of the old and conventional radiology language represented by the visualization of a space between the pleural layers at chest radiography.

However, while specificities of lung ultrasound and chest radiography for pneumothorax are similarly high, there are some critical differences in their diagnostic performances. (1) Regarding sensitivity, lung ultrasound is far superior to bedside chest radiography [20–22]. Solid evidence in dedicated literature supports this superiority. In trauma patients, it is common to encounter discrepancy between false negative supine chest radiography and true positive lung ultrasound for pneumothorax. (2) Even if chest radiography can be performed at bedside, the time expenditure and the need for additional personnel are losing factors when compared to the promptness and ease of use of lung ultrasound, especially when ultrasound is performed by the same clinician caring the patient. (3) Even if chest radiography is still the commonest bedside imaging tool applied when pneumothorax is suspected, there are no research trials published in literature demonstrating its diagnostic accuracy compared to CT scan. On the contrary, lung ultrasound is largely validated in several trials in trauma and post-procedure pneumothoraxes. Thus, the argument that lung ultrasound is not enough validated, which gives strength to the maintenance of chest radiography as standard of care, is at least specious and should be re-discussed in the future societal guidelines [12]. (4) When compared to volumetric CT scan, lung ultrasound performs better than chest radiography in the gross estimation of the size of pneumothorax [17]. This is highly impactful in the decision-making process for juvenile spontaneous pneumothorax and may also have a great influence in the possibility to monitor the evolution of pneumothorax in trauma patients. This last consideration introduces the topic of quantification and monitoring pneumothorax by lung ultrasound.

Quantification and Monitoring

In the daily clinical practice, the clinician may encounter the necessity to quantify the severity of pneumothorax. Even if quantification of pneumothorax is often only a marginal aspect to decide management, in some situations this information may become decisive. For instance, in the societal guidelines for juvenile spontaneous pneumothorax, classification of pneumothorax in large and small by chest radiography reading is the main indication to decide conservative treatment or drainage [12]. Even in stable patients, drainage should be performed when the size of pneumothorax exceeds a certain limit because the time to spontaneous resorption would be too long and expose the patient to risks. Using lung ultrasound, it is possible to semi-quantify the severity of pneumothorax through the evaluation of the laterality of the lung point. Indeed, the more lateral is located the lung point the more extended and severe is pneumothorax [2, 20]. Data from literature demonstrate that when the lung point is anterior to the mid axillary line, the volume of pneumothorax is inferior to 15% of lung collapse, which corresponds to the classification of small pneumothorax [17]. The same data show that in the semi-quantification of pneumothorax, lung ultrasound performs better than chest radiography, when they are compared to volumetric CT scan.

The concept of semi-quantification paved the way to another important application of lung ultrasound for pneumothorax, that is monitoring the time course of its severity to prognosticate and to observe the effect of a treatment. For instance, the possibility to monitor the change in the laterality of the lung point at bedside in critically ill trauma patients with pneumothorax, allows to maintain a safe conservative approach, avoiding drainage even during positive pressure ventilation [23]. Indeed, lung ultrasound is the ideal bedside tool to monitor patients in intensive care setting. Furthermore, any change in the location of the lung point may become an adjunctive tool in the hands of the clinician, to follow the trend after removal of a drainage, but also after thoracoscopy or any other invasive intervention [24].

Pitfalls and Complex Pneumothorax

There are some known complex conditions in which the lung ultrasound exam for pneumothorax may become particularly challenging. All these conditions have been discovered and described in literature quite recently [25]. The reader should consider that lung ultrasound for pneumothorax is a relatively new diagnostic technique, still open to new experiences and refinements. We cannot exclude that in the next future, substantial changes in the main principles of the technique will appear and change the standard practice.

Double Lung Point

The main feature of a double lung point is the appearance of two lung points that interpose to an area of absence of sliding, moving in opposite direction [25, 26]. Sometimes, the two lung points appear on the same scan (Video 4). Most of the times, the air inside the pleural space of a pneumothorax is free of moving following the change in decubitus of the patient. In this case, when the patient is supine, the air will move to the superior part of the chest and will extend from the sternum to a zone that will be more lateral the larger is pneumothorax. Thus, the visible lung point will be only one at the interface air/lung. In some other conditions, most of the time in case of pleural adherences, the air remains trapped in some area of the chest. In these cases, the lung ultrasound examination will show two edges lung/air/lung and two opposite lung points will appear at the extremities of a non-sliding zone. Thus, when pleural adherences are suspected, it is mandatory to extend the examination to the whole chest before ruling-out pneumothorax, to exclude the possibility of even a small quantity of loculated intrapleural air.

Septated Pneumothorax

In recurrent pneumothorax after pleurodesis, there is the possibility to visualize the concomitance of B-lines with absence of sliding [25, 27]. When B-lines are observed in a condition of pneumothorax, they may become confounding. In general, B-lines are parenchymal signs that exclude pneumothorax. Visualization of even one isolated B-line has the power to rule-out the presence of interpleural air. However, when there are septa still connecting the lung to the parietal pleura inside the area of a pneumothorax, some B-lines may become visible (Video 5). Septa may typically be the result of a previous invasive intervention, like pleurodesis. This pattern is misleading and may induce the operator to exclude pneumothorax wrongly. When a pneumothorax is suspected in patients already treated by pleurodesis, the operator should consider this eventuality.

Hydropneumothorax

When pleural effusion is combined with pneumothorax and there is no contact between the lung and the chest wall, it is not possible to observe a common lung point; instead, an interface between the air and the fluid becomes evident. In ultrasound this condition is demonstrated by an air/fluid pattern that appears as a motionless lung (A-lines and no sliding) on one side of the scan and the anechoic fluid image on the other side (Video 6) [25, 28–30]. Usually, the fluid shows a slight waving movement at the interface with air [31–33]. This condition is typical of thoracic trauma with concomitance of hemothorax and pneumothorax, or in a condition of iatrogenic pneumothorax that may occur during drainage of an effusion. This air/fluid interface has been named "hydropoint" and has the same diagnostic meaning of the lung point because it is also highly specific for pneumothorax [28, 34].

False Lung Sliding and False Lung Pulse

A common pitfall in lung ultrasound is the visualization of a false movement of the lung image that may be misinterpreted as sliding or pulsation and be confounding even to the most expert operators. The false sliding or pulse are quite common conditions in cases of pneumothorax, which happen when some part of the thoracic wall moves independently from the lung and gives to the whole image the effect of a respiratory or pulsatory movement [32]. It happens when, in a condition of pneumothorax, the patient breathes and contracts the intercostal muscles synchronous with respiration, or when an intercostal artery pulses and bumps the parietal pleura synchronous with the cardiac activity. To avoid misdiagnoses, it is crucial to observe if the movement that the operator visualizes is of the whole image. Only when it is evident that the lung image under the pleura moves against the chest wall, the operator can diagnose with certainty lung sliding or lung pulse and rule out pneumothorax.

References

1. Volpicelli G. Lung sonography. J Ultrasound Med. 2013;32(1):165–71. https://doi.org/10.7863/jum.2013.32.1.165.
2. Lichtenstein DA. Ultrasound in the management of thoracic disease. Crit Care Med. 2007;35(5 Suppl): S250–61. https://doi.org/10.1097/01.CCM.0000260674.60761.85.
3. Volpicelli G, Elbarbary M, Blaivas M, Lichtenstein DA, Mathis G, Kirkpatrick AW, Melniker L,

Gargani L, Noble VE, Via G, Dean A, Tsung JW, Soldati G, Copetti R, Bouhemad B, Reissig A, Agricola E, Rouby JJ, Arbelot C, Liteplo A, Sargsyan A, Silva F, Hoppmann R, Breitkreutz R, Seibel A, Neri L, Storti E, Petrovic T. International liaison committee on lung ultrasound (ILC-LUS) for international consensus conference on lung ultrasound (ICC-LUS). International evidence-based recommendations for point-of-care lung ultrasound. Intensive Care Med. 2012;38(4):577–91. https://doi.org/10.1007/s00134-012-2513-4.

4. Gargani L, Volpicelli G. How I do it: lung ultrasound. Cardiovasc Ultrasound. 2014;4(12):25. https://doi.org/10.1186/1476-7120-12-25.

5. Lichtenstein DA, Menu Y. A bedside ultrasound sign ruling out pneumothorax in the critically ill. Lung sliding. Chest. 1995;108(5):1345–8. https://doi.org/10.1378/chest.108.5.1345.

6. Duclos G, Bobbia X, Markarian T, Muller L, Cheyssac C, Castillon S, Resseguier N, Boussuges A, Volpicelli G, Leone M, Zieleskiewicz L. Speckle tracking quantification of lung sliding for the diagnosis of pneumothorax: a multicentric observational study. Intensive Care Med. 2019;45(9):1212–8. https://doi.org/10.1007/s00134-019-05710-1.

7. Volpicelli G. Sonographic diagnosis of pneumothorax. Intensive Care Med. 2011;37(2):224–32. https://doi.org/10.1007/s00134-010-2079-y.

8. Goodman TR, Traill ZC, Phillips AJ, Berger J, Gleeson FV. Ultrasound detection of pneumothorax. Clin Radiol. 1999;54(11):736–9. https://doi.org/10.1016/s0009-9260(99)91175-3.

9. Targhetta R, Bourgeois JM, Chavagneux R, Coste E, Amy D, Balmes P, Pourcelot L. Ultrasonic signs of pneumothorax: preliminary work. J Clin Ultrasound. 1993;21(4):245–50. https://doi.org/10.1002/jcu.1870210406.

10. Kirkpatrick AW, Sirois M, Laupland KB, Liu D, Rowan K, Ball CG, Hameed SM, Brown R, Simons R, Dulchavsky SA, Hamiilton DR, Nicolaou S. Hand-held thoracic sonography for detecting post-traumatic pneumothoraces: the extended focused assessment with sonography for trauma (EFAST). J Trauma. 2004;57(2):288–95. https://doi.org/10.1097/01.ta.0000133565.88871.e4.

11. Agricola E, Arbelot C, Blaivas M, Bouhemad B, Copetti R, Dean A, Dulchavsky S, Elbarbary M, Gargani L, Hoppmann R, Kirkpatrick AW, Lichtenstein D, Liteplo A, Mathis G, Melniker L, Neri L, Noble VE, Petrovic T, Reissig A, Rouby JJ, Seibel A, Soldati G, Storti E, Tsung JW, Via G, Volpicelli G. Ultrasound performs better than radiographs. Thorax. 2011;66(9):828–9; author reply 829. https://doi.org/10.1136/thx.2010.153239.

12. Havelock T, Teoh R, Laws D, Gleeson F; BTS Pleural Disease Guideline Group. Pleural procedures and thoracic ultrasound: British thoracic society pleural disease guideline 2010. Thorax. 2010;65 Suppl 2:ii61–76. https://doi.org/10.1136/thx.2010.137026.

13. Lichtenstein D, Mezière G, Biderman P, Gepner A. The comet-tail artifact: an ultrasound sign ruling out pneumothorax. Intensive Care Med. 1999;25(4):383–8. https://doi.org/10.1007/s001340050862.

14. Lichtenstein D, Mezière G, Biderman P, Gepner A. The, "lung point": an ultrasound sign specific to pneumothorax. Intensive Care Med. 2000;26(10):1434–40. https://doi.org/10.1007/s001340000627.

15. Lichtenstein DA, Lascols N, Prin S, Mezière G. The, "lung pulse": an early ultrasound sign of complete atelectasis. Intensive Care Med. 2003;29(12):2187–92. https://doi.org/10.1007/s00134-003-1930-9.

16. Breitkreutz R, Seibel A, Zechner PM. Ultrasound-guided evaluation of lung sliding for widespread use? Resuscitation. 2012;83(3):273–4. https://doi.org/10.1016/j.resuscitation.2011.12.034.

17. Volpicelli G, Boero E, Sverzellati N, Cardinale L, Busso M, Boccuzzi F, Tullio M, Lamorte A, Stefanone V, Ferrari G, Veltri A, Frascisco MF. Semi-quantification of pneumothorax volume by lung ultrasound. Intensive Care Med. 2014;40(10):1460–7. https://doi.org/10.1007/s00134-014-3402-9.

18. Lichtenstein DA, Mezière GA. Relevance of lung ultrasound in the diagnosis of acute respiratory failure: the BLUE protocol. Chest. 2008;134(1):117–25. https://doi.org/10.1378/chest.07-2800.

19. Volpicelli G, Lamorte A, Tullio M, Cardinale L, Giraudo M, Stefanone V, Boero E, Nazerian P, Pozzi R, Frascisco MF. Point-of-care multiorgan ultrasonography for the evaluation of undifferentiated hypotension in the emergency department. Intensive Care Med. 2013;39(7):1290–8. https://doi.org/10.1007/s00134-013-2919-7.

20. Soldati G, Testa A, Sher S, Pignataro G, La Sala M, Silveri NG. Occult traumatic pneumothorax: diagnostic accuracy of lung ultrasonography in the emergency department. Chest. 2008;133(1):204–11. https://doi.org/10.1378/chest.07-1595.

21. Rowan KR, Kirkpatrick AW, Liu D, Forkheim KE, Mayo JR, Nicolaou S. Traumatic pneumothorax detection with thoracic US: correlation with chest radiography and CT–initial experience. Radiology. 2002;225(1):210–4. https://doi.org/10.1148/radiol.2251011102.

22. Blaivas M, Lyon M, Duggal S. A prospective comparison of supine chest radiography and bedside ultrasound for the diagnosis of traumatic pneumothorax. Acad Emerg Med. 2005;12(9):844–9. https://doi.org/10.1197/j.aem.2005.05.005.

23. Clements TW, Sirois M, Farry N, Roberts DJ, Trottier V, Rizoli S, Ball CG, Xiao ZJ, Kirkpatrick AW. OPTICC: a multicentre trial of occult pneumothoraces subjected to mechanical ventilation: the final report. Am J Surg 2021;221(6):1252–8. https://doi.org/10.1016/j.amjsurg.2021.02.012.

24. Galbois A, Ait-Oufella H, Baudel JL, Kofman T, Bottero J, Vienrot S, Rabate C, Jabbouri S, Bouzeman A, Guidet B, Offenstadt G, Maury E. Pleural ultrasound compared with chest radiographic detection of pneumothorax resolution after drainage.

Chest. 2010;138(3):648–55. https://doi.org/10.1378/chest.09-2224.

25. Volpicelli G, Boero E, Stefanone V, Storti E. Unusual new signs of pneumothorax at lung ultrasound. Crit Ultrasound J. 2013;5(1):10. https://doi.org/10.1186/2036-7902-5-10.

26. Volpicelli G, Audino B. The double lung point: an unusual sonographic sign of juvenile spontaneous pneumothorax. Am J Emerg Med. 2011;29(3):355. e1-2. https://doi.org/10.1016/j.ajem.2010.03.020.

27. Volpicelli G, Garofalo G, Lamorte A, Frascisco MF. Images in emergency medicine. Young man with left thoracic pain. Recurrent pneumothorax after failed pleurodesis. Ann Emerg Med. 2012;60(2):e3–4. https://doi.org/10.1016/j.annemergmed.2012.03.002.

28. Volpicelli G, Lamorte A, Tullio M, Boero E, Stefanone V. Worsening dyspnea and cough following thoracentesis. Chest. 2013;144(2):e1–3. https://doi.org/10.1378/chest.13-0674.

29. Mahalingam S, Rajendran G, Nathan B, Kugan E, Sadasivam A. 'Hydro-point' - The forgotten and unspoken entity in hydropneumothorax. Australas J Ultrasound Med. 2021;24(4):246–8. https://doi.org/10.1002/ajum.12278.

30. Reissig A, Kroegel C. Accuracy of transthoracic sonography in excluding post-interventional pneumothorax and hydropneumothorax. Comparison to chest radiography. Eur J Radiol. 2005;53(3):463–70. https://doi.org/10.1016/j.ejrad.2004.04.014.

31. Laursen CB, Graumann O, Davidsen JR, Madsen PH. Pitfall in lung ultrasound: 'pseudo B-line' seen in both hydropneumothorax and in a cup of coffee. BMJ Case Rep. 2014;2014:bcr2013201341. https://doi.org/10.1136/bcr-2013-201341.

32. Blanco P, Volpicelli G. Common pitfalls in point-of-care ultrasound: a practical guide for emergency and critical care physicians. Crit Ultrasound J. 2016;8(1):15. https://doi.org/10.1186/s13089-016-0052-x.

33. Volpicelli G, Mayo P, Rovida S. Focus on ultrasound in intensive care. Intensive Care Med. 2020;46(6):1258–60. https://doi.org/10.1007/s00134-020-06027-0.

34. Targhetta R, Bourgeois JM, Chavagneux R, Marty-Double C, Balmes P. Ultrasonographic approach to diagnosing hydropneumothorax. Chest. 1992;101(4):931–4. https://doi.org/10.1378/chest.101.4.931.

POCUS in Monitoring: Cardiogenic Pulmonary Oedema

Pierpaolo Pellicori and Luna Gargani

'Misura ciò che è misurabile, e rendi misurabile ciò che non lo è.'
'Measure what can be measured, and make measurable what is not so.'

Galileo Galilei-Italian astronomer and polymath (Pisa 1564–Arcetri 1642)

Abstract

Cardiogenic pulmonary oedema is a life-threatening condition that reflects a rapid elevation in left atrial pressure. There are solid data about the usefulness of point of care ultrasound (POCUS) for the diagnosis of cardiogenic pulmonary oedema, whereas there is little evidence supporting use of POCUS to monitor its clinical evolution. Ongoing and future trials will clarify whether serial assessment of cardiac hemodynamics, inferior vena cava diameter and lung ultrasound in patients admitted with cardiogenic pulmonary oedema will improve in-hospital management and guide decongestive therapy or the timing of discharge in this population.

Keywords

Pulmonary oedema · Lung ultrasound · B-lines · POCUS · Inferior vena cava · Decongestion

Abbreviations

POCUS	Point of care ultrasound
HF	Heart failure
ARDS	Acute respiratory distress syndrome
LV	Left ventricle
LAP	Left atrial pressure
NPs	Natriuretic peptides
PASP	Pulmonary artery systolic pressure
LUS	Lung ultrasound
AHF	Acute heart failure
HFrEF	Heart failure with reduced ejection fraction
HFpEF	Heart failure with preserved ejection fraction
IVC	Inferior vena cava
LVEF	Left ventricular ejection fraction

P. Pellicori (✉)
Robertson Centre for Biostatistics, University of Glasgow, Glasgow, Scotland
e-mail: pierpaolo.pellicori@glasgow.ac.uk

L. Gargani
University of Pisa, Pisa, Italy

© The Author(s), under exclusive license to Springer Nature Switzerland AG 2023
H. Soliman-Aboumarie et al. (eds.), *Cardiopulmonary Point of Care Ultrasound*,
https://doi.org/10.1007/978-3-031-29472-3_12

147

Key Messages

- B Lines are the sonographic biomarker of extravascular lung water
- There are solid data about the usefulness of point of care ultrasound (POCUS) for the diagnosis of cardiogenic pulmonary oedema, whereas there is little evidence supporting use of POCUS to monitor its clinical evolution.
- Integration of LUS with echocardiography is recommended in the evaluation of patients with cardiogenic pulmonary oedema.

Introduction

Heart failure (HF) is a common hospital diagnosis, worldwide. The main HF symptoms are breathlessness on exertion and peripheral oedema, usually in combination, at least to some extent. Many registries suggest that acute onset of breathless at rest and cardio-respiratory distress, in other words, cardiogenic pulmonary oedema, is the chief complaint of around 50% of those admitted with HF. On the other hand, many patients hospitalised with HF who receive large doses of intravenous diuretics for extensive peripheral oedema might breathe quite comfortably at rest.

Cardiogenic pulmonary oedema is a medical emergency that develops quickly, when a rapid increase in the left atrial and pulmonary capillaries pressure causes transudation of fluids into the lung interstitium, and then in the alveoli, limiting gas exchange and decreasing lung compliance. Timely identification and treatment of the precipitant causes (for instance an acute coronary syndrome, especially when complicated by mitral regurgitation or a ventricular septal defect, severe hypertension, or a tachyarrhythmia, commonly atrial fibrillation) [1–3], and of their adverse haemodynamic consequences with vasodilators and diuretics, is lifesaving. Cardiogenic pulmonary oedema should be distinguished from acute respiratory distress syndrome (ARDS), as management, treatments and outcomes differ. The main etiological precipitants of ARDS are usually an infection, aspiration of toxic substances or, more rarely, a traumatic chest injury, which might damage the alveolar–capillary barrier and lead to a rapid leakage of fluids into the pulmonary interstitium or alveolar space; in these circumstances, left atrial and pulmonary capillary pressure are usually normal [4].

Point-of-care ultrasound (POCUS) is increasingly being used at the patient's bedside in emergency departments, providing that both equipment and expertise are available, and it complements clinical history and other diagnostic tests to identify the reasons for breathlessness, to stratify the risk and to formulate an initial management plan. Guidelines do not recommend to monitor patients with cardiogenic pulmonary oedema with echocardiography, unless cardiogenic shock develops. However, serial assessment of cardiac haemodynamics with POCUS could be a non-invasive, easy to deploy method to assess response to therapy and predict the short-term risk of developing adverse cardiovascular complications. In the next paragraphs, we will discuss evidence that supports routine use of POCUS in monitoring patients with cardiogenic pulmonary oedema. Table 1 provides a simplified overview of cardiopulmonary parameters that might be monitored by ultrasound in patients with cardiogenic pulmonary oedema [5].

What Should I Monitor?

The Heart: Structure, Function and Hemodynamics

A severely ill patient in respiratory distress, coughing and struggling to breathe whilst sat in the middle of a hospital bed, is often unable to cope with detailed instructions and is at risk of death: therefore, the acquisition or interpretation of echocardiographic images has to be rapid and it can be complex [6]. Cardiogenic pulmonary oedema can occur with either a preserved or an impaired left ventricular systolic function, the

Table 1 Cardio-pulmonary parameters that might be monitored by ultrasound in patients with pulmonary oedema

	Dinamicity	What to look for	
Left atrial volume index	+	Reduction of LA dimensions	
Functional mitral regurgitation (A)	++	Reduction of MR severity	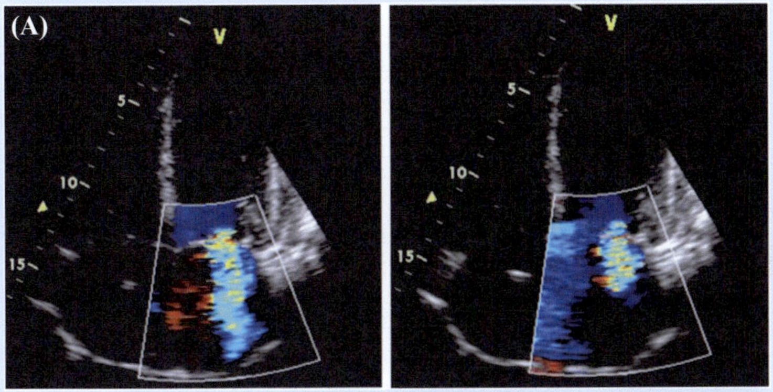

(continued)

Table 1 (continued)

	Dinamicity	What to look for	
E/e' (B)	++	Reduction of E/e'	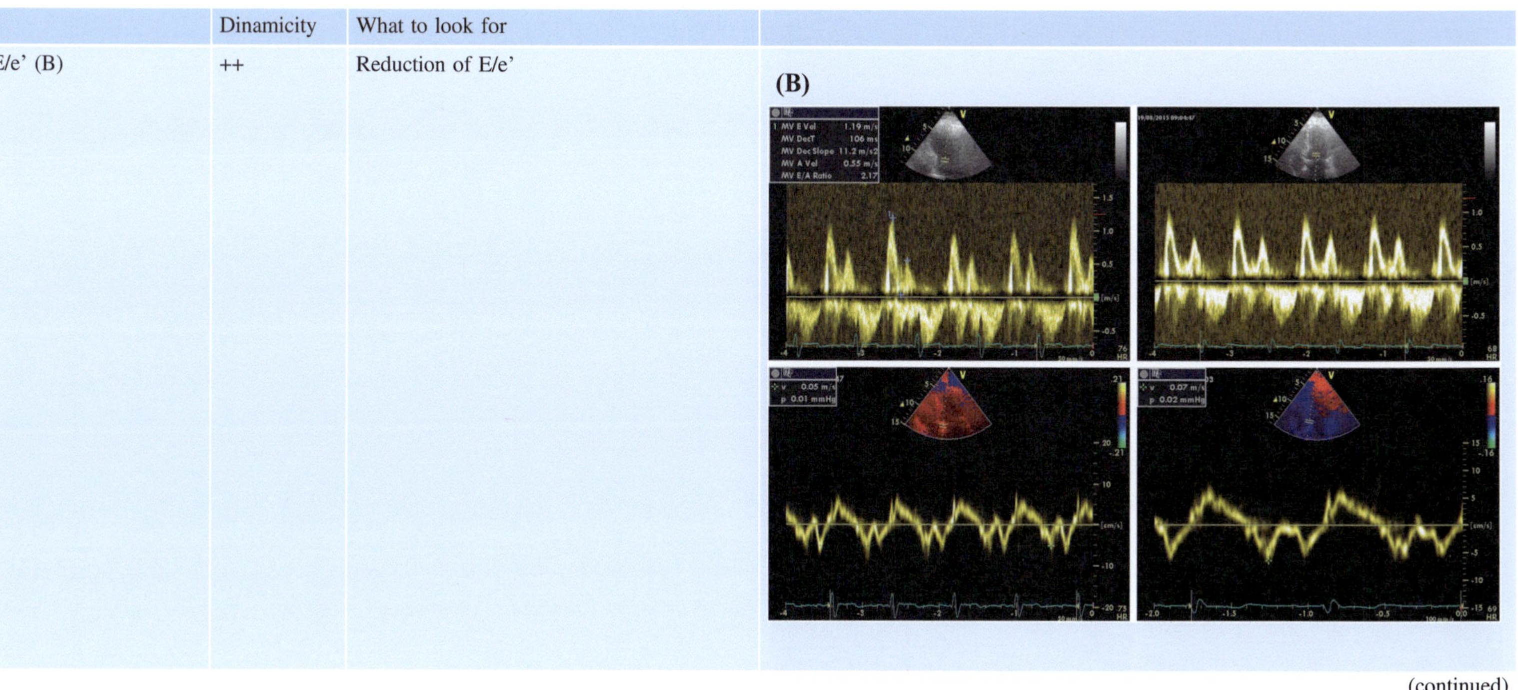

(continued)

Table 1 (continued)

	Dinamicity	What to look for	
Pulmonary artery systolic pressure (C)	++	Reduction of pressure gradient	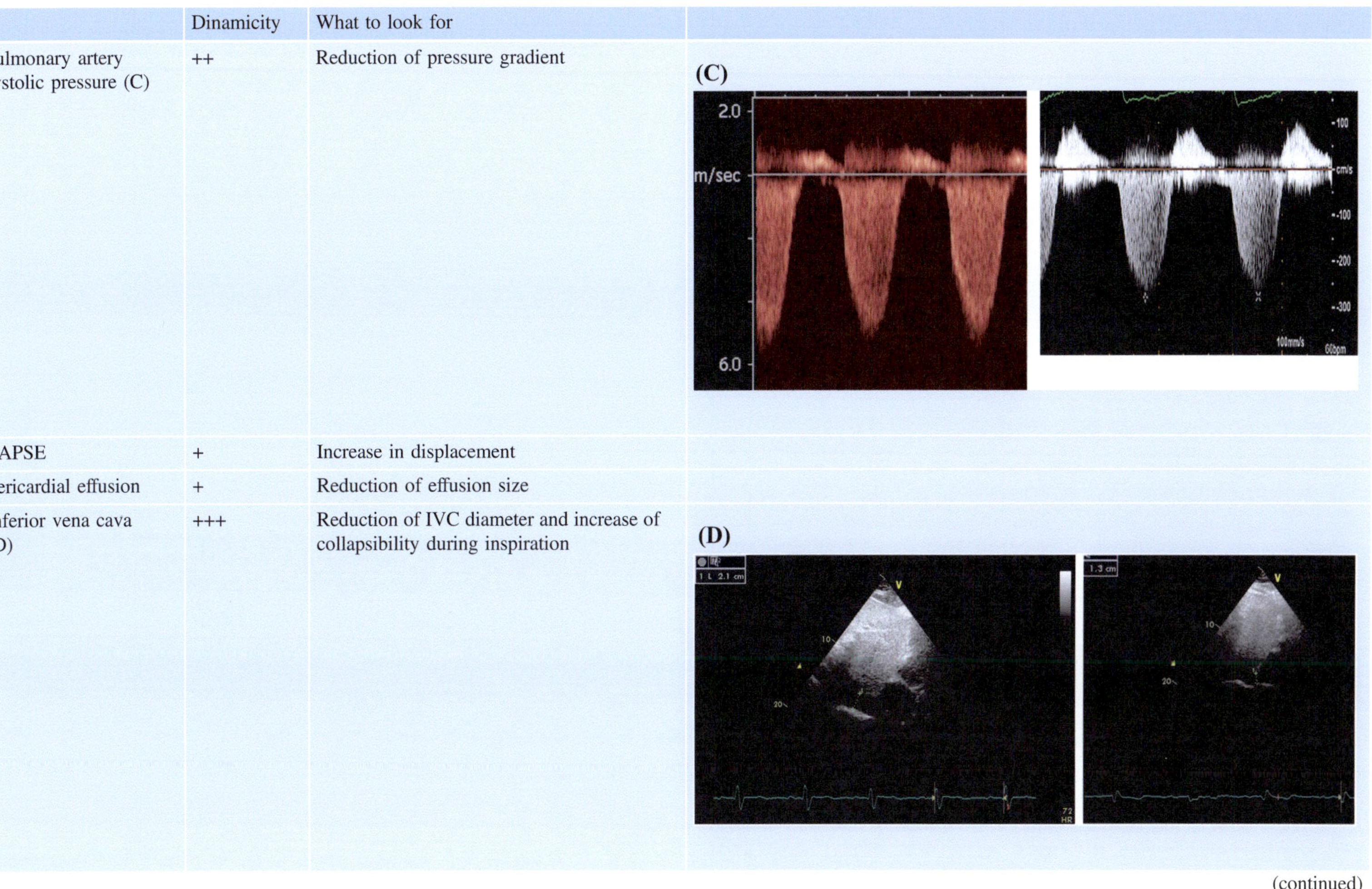
TAPSE	+	Increase in displacement	
Pericardial effusion	+	Reduction of effusion size	
Inferior vena cava (D)	+++	Reduction of IVC diameter and increase of collapsibility during inspiration	

(continued)

Table 1 (continued)

	Dinamicity	What to look for	
B-lines (E)	++++	Reduction of B-lines number	(E)
Pleural effusion	++	Reduction of effusion size	

identification of which has important diagnostic and therapeutic consequences. Evidence of new regional wall motion abnormalities would point towards an acute ischaemic insult, whilst a globally dysfunctional left ventricle (LV) would suggest a cardiomyopathy. POCUS can also raise the suspicion of severe valvular abnormalities and suggest their likely aetiology; presence of cardiac tamponade, ventricular outflow tract obstruction or a takotsubo cardiomyopathy are other rarer causes of cardiogenic pulmonary oedema that should be also ruled out. If LV systolic function is normal, determination of left atrial pressure (LAP) is key to distinguish between cardiogenic pulmonary oedema and ARDS. A restrictive mitral inflow pattern at Doppler suggests high LAP and abnormal LV relaxation, correlates with elevated natriuretic peptides (NPs) plasma levels, a known marker of cardiac stress, and has a high diagnostic accuracy in those presenting with acute dyspnoea of cardiac origin [7]. The left atrium, a thin wall cardiac chamber, is very sensitive to changes in cardiac haemodynamics [8]. A dilated and dysfunctional left atrium reflects chronic elevation of LAP, associates with more severe symptoms and increases chances of developing atrial fibrillation [9]. Atrial fibrillation, a common finding in patients with pulmonary oedema, complicates interpretation of the Doppler indices but, at the same time, it would suggest a high likelihood of elevated left atrial pressure. Elevated LAP will eventually result in development of pulmonary hypertension [10]. An increased right ventricular afterload in the absence of signs suggesting elevated LAP should orientate towards a diagnosis of pulmonary embolism, ARDS, or other respiratory conditions.

There is no consensus on the usefulness of monitoring patients with acute pulmonary oedema using hemodynamic echocardiographic parameters, such as E/e' (which is also a proxy for elevated LAP) or pulmonary artery systolic pressure (PASP). However, a decrease in PASP and a reduction in the severity of functional mitral regurgitation during an episode of pulmonary oedema may suggest the return to a compensated state [11]. Performing serial multiorgan POCUS exams might assist clinicians to identify patients with acute HF at greater risk of developing pulmonary hypertension [12]: for those who develop signs of hemodynamic instability, an echocardiographic examination is required for an immediate differential diagnosis and tailored therapy [13–15].

The Lungs: B-Lines and Pleural Effusion

Lung ultrasound (LUS) is easy and quick to perform [16], can be learned by medics and other healthcare personnel [17, 18] with little training and has a high inter- and intra-operator reproducibility [19, 20]. LUS identifies fluids replacing aerated lung parenchyma or their accumulation in the pleural space, therefore it facilitates diagnosis in patients with acute dyspnoea [21], outperforming lung auscultation and chest-X-ray [22, 23]. In an aerated lung, below the pleural line, only hyperechoic horizontal artefacts (called "A-lines") should be noticed. With increasing interstitial fluids, vertical comet tail-like artefacts, or B-lines, would eventually originate from the pleura and traverse the ultrasound screen, singly or fused together. When multiple (i.e.: ≥ 3 in a single intercostal space, or "chest zone"), diffuse (i.e.: in more than one intercostal space) and bilateral, in a patients with dyspnoea, B-lines would suggest a diagnosis of heart failure [24] and reduce time to diagnosis [23, 25, 26], although they are not specific for this condition [27].

Different protocols for assessment of B-lines have been proposed, and technical aspects can be found elsewhere in more details. An increasing number of B-lines is associated with greater extravascular water in the lungs [28, 29], faster respiratory rate [30], higher NPs plasma levels [31], the presence of LV systolic or diastolic dysfunction [32] and with impaired right ventricular function [33]. In patients admitted with AHF, an increasing number of B-lines is associated with poorer outcomes, both in HFpEF and HFrEF, even when clinical signs of congestion are no longer detectable [34, 35]. However, an

Table 2 Main applications of lung ultrasound (LUS) in patients with heart failure

	AIM	LUS picture	Advantages
Diagnosis	Rule in and rule out AHF in patients with dyspnoea	Multiple, diffuse, bilateral B-lines rule in AHF Absence of multiple, diffuse, bilateral B-lines rules out AHF	LUS improves diagnostic accuracy compared to standard strategy (chest X-ray + NTproBNP) LUS reduces time to correct diagnosis LUS detects subclinical pulmonary congestion in patients with HF who have mild or absent signs and symptoms
Monitoring	Monitoring dynamic changes during AHF hospitalization Titrate diuretic therapy after discharge	Reduction of the number of B-lines Reduction of the size of pleural effusion, if any	Bedside monitoring to support decision-making in diuretic therapy and fluid management A significant reduction of B-lines during hospitalization is associated with a lower risk of rehospitalization for AHF and death at 6 months LUS-guided therapy might reduce risk of urgent HF visits and hospital admission for AHF
Prognosis	Identification of patients at higher risk of rehospitalisation for AHF or death (i.e.: end of life care)	Persistent B-lines at discharge, even with resolved signs and symptoms of HF	A high number of B-lines at discharge predicts rehospitalization for AHF and death at 3 months An elevated number of B-lines in outpatients predicts hospitalisation for AHF and death at 6 months

inverse correlation exists between body mass index and B-lines [36], and additional care must be taken when interpreting their number and distribution in patients with obesity who fight to breathe.

Up to 70% of those admitted with heart failure have pleural effusion [37], which can be easily appreciated by LUS posteriorly, at the base of the chest, or laterally, placing a transducer a few centimeters below the axilla. When severe, pleural effusion is often accompanied by a collapsed homolateral lung. As pericardial and pleural effusion might coexist, they should not be confused.

There are preliminary data demonstrating that B-lines can be useful in monitoring patients with AHF. The number of B-lines is extremely dynamic and, for patients who respond to diuretic therapy and other treatments, B-lines decrease rapidly [38–40], regardless of the HF aetiology [41]. Preliminary experience suggests that LUS might guide titration of diuretic therapy and reduce congestion and the length of hospital stay [42, 43]. Resolution of pulmonary congestion by ultrasound during a heart failure hospitalisation is associated with better outcomes [44, 45], whilst for those with a high number of B-lines at discharge, the risk of readmission or premature death is substantial [30, 46–49].

The severity of pleural effusion is typically monitored by chest X-ray in patients with AHF, but serial ultrasound is also effective in quantifying changes in the size of pleural effusion associated with decongestive therapy [50]. The main applications of LUS in patients with HF are summarized in Table 2.

Intravascular Fluids: Inferior Vena Cava

A failing heart would inevitably cause intravascular congestion [51] and venous hypertension. Assessment of the inferior vena cava (IVC) diameter and of its respiratory changes with POCUS is feasible in the majority of patients with heart failure, even when they are acutely ill, to estimate intravascular volumes and central venous pressure. A large proportion of patients with cardiogenic pulmonary oedema have a dilated IVC (>2 cm) that collapses <50% on inspiration [52–54]. In patients with heart failure, a dilated IVC is associated with elevated NT-proBNP, more severe pulmonary hypertension and right ventricular dysfunction, but not with LVEF or measures of body size, such as body mass index [55]. Combining assessment of LVEF, B-lines and IVC in patients with acute dyspnoea increases diagnostic specificity for heart failure and helps differentiating pulmonary oedema from ARDS [56–58].

Future Perspectives

POCUS provides information at the bedside quickly, at little costs, and without exposing patients to radiations; in other words, it is safe, time- and cost-efficient, and can be repeated whenever it is clinically required. There is now evidence to suggest that, in expert hands, handheld scanners are likely to be as good as standard machines to identify a large variety of cardiac disorders [59, 60]. Importantly, images can be interpreted as seen, prompting immediate and lifesaving therapeutic actions and avoiding exposure to treatments that are not required. An accurate diagnosis necessitates of the right diagnostic tests. Surprisingly, not all patients discharged with a diagnosis of heart failure would receive an echocardiogram whilst in hospital [61], particularly when they are not admitted under cardiologists. With the commercialisation of affordable and miniaturised devices, or transducers that can scan the entire body whilst connected to a tablet or a smartphone, or even communicating via WiFi with a central unit, POCUS is likely to replace soon stethoscopes and improve heart failure diagnosis and management not only in cardiology, but also in other medical specialties. There is an ongoing process to include POCUS in the core curriculum of medical student, as well as in residency programs; ideally, in the next 5–10 years, many doctors should be able

to perform a standardized POCUS exam to diagnose and treat life-threatening conditions early, and with more precision. This development will be successful if POCUS users will firmly keep in mind that the main asset of this revolutionary approach is the integration with clinical reasoning, judgment and other existing resources [62, 63] supported by robust evidences.

References

1. Bentancur AG, Rieck J, Koldanov R, Dankner RS. Acute pulmonary edema in the emergency department: clinical and echocardiographic survey in an aged population. Am J Med Sci. 2002;323(5): 238–43.
2. Gandhi SK, Powers JC, Nomeir AM, Fowle K, Kitzman DW, Rankin KM, et al. The pathogenesis of acute pulmonary edema associated with hypertension. N Engl J Med. 2001;344(1):17–22.
3. Stone GW, Griffin B, Shah PK, Berman DS, Siegel RJ, Cook SL, et al. Prevalence of unsuspected mitral regurgitation and left ventricular diastolic dysfunction in patients with coronary artery disease and acute pulmonary edema associated with normal or depressed left ventricular systolic function. Am J Cardiol. 1991;67(1):37–41.
4. Ware LB, Matthay MA. The acute respiratory distress syndrome. N Engl J Med. 2000;342 (18):1334–49.
5. Pellicori P, Platz E, Dauw J, Ter Maaten JM, Martens P, Pivetta E, et al. Ultrasound imaging of congestion in heart failure: examinations beyond the heart. Eur J Heart Fail. 2021;23(5):703–12.
6. Cook CH, Praba AC, Beery PR, Martin LC. Transthoracic echocardiography is not cost-effective in critically ill surgical patients. J Trauma. 2002;52 (2):280–4.
7. Logeart D, Saudubray C, Beyne P, Thabut G, Ennezat P-V, Chavelas C, et al. Comparative value of Doppler echocardiography and B-type natriuretic peptide assay in the etiologic diagnosis of acute dyspnea. J Am Coll Cardiol. 2002;40(10):1794–800.
8. Dovancescu S, Pellicori P, Mabote T, Torabi A, Clark AL, Cleland JGF. The effects of short-term omission of daily medication on the pathophysiology of heart failure. Eur J Heart Fail. 2017.
9. Bisbal F, Baranchuk A, Braunwald E, Bayés de Luna A, Bayés-Genís A. Atrial failure as a clinical entity: JACC review topic of the week. J Am Coll Cardiol. 2020;75(2):222–32.
10. Park J, Joung B, Uhm J-S, Young Shim C, Hwang C, Hyoung Lee M, et al. High left atrial pressures are associated with advanced electroanatomical remodeling of left atrium and independent predictors for

clinical recurrence of atrial fibrillation after catheter ablation. Hear Rhythm. 2014;11(6):953–60.

11. Ennezat PV, Maréchaux S, Bouabdallaoui N, Le Jemtel TH. Dynamic nature of pulmonary artery systolic pressure in decompensated heart failure with preserved ejection fraction: role of functional mitral regurgitation. J Card Fail. 2013;19(11):746–52.

12. Torres-Arrese M, García de Casasola-Sánchez G, Méndez-Bailón M, Montero-Hernández E, Cobo-Marcos M, Rivas-Lasarte M, et al. Usefulness of serial multiorgan point-of-care ultrasound in acute heart failure: results from a prospective observational cohort. Medicina (Kaunas). 2022;58(1).

13. Walley PE, Walley KR, Goodgame B, Punjabi V, Sirounis D. A practical approach to goal-directed echocardiography in the critical care setting. Crit Care. 2014;18(6):681.

14. Neskovic AN, Skinner H, Price S, Via G, De Hert S, Stankovic I, et al. Focus cardiac ultrasound core curriculum and core syllabus of the European Association of Cardiovascular Imaging. Eur Heart J Cardiovasc Imaging. 2018;19(5).

15. Soliman-Aboumarie H, Pastore MC, Galiatsou E, Gargani L, Pugliese NR, Mandoli GE, et al. Echocardiography in the intensive care unit: an essential tool for diagnosis, monitoring and guiding clinical decision-making. Physiol Int. 2021.

16. Gargani L. Lung ultrasound: a new tool for the cardiologist. Cardiovasc Ultrasound. 2011;9:6.

17. Mumoli N, Vitale JJ, Giorgi-Pierfranceschi M, Cresci A, Cei M, Basile V, et al. Accuracy of nurse-performed lung ultrasound in patients with acute dyspnea: a prospective observational study. Medicine (Baltimore). 2016;95(9): e2925.

18. Vignon P, Dugard A, Abraham J, Belcour D, Gondran G, Pepino F, et al. Focused training for goal-oriented hand-held echocardiography performed by noncardiologist residents in the intensive care unit. Intensive Care Med. 2007;33(10):1795–9.

19. Bedetti G, Gargani L, Corbisiero A, Frassi F, Poggianti E, Mottola G. Evaluation of ultrasound lung comets by hand-held echocardiography. Cardiovasc Ultrasound. 2006;4:34.

20. Gargani L, Sicari R, Raciti M, Serasini L, Passera M, Torino C, et al. Efficacy of a remote web-based lung ultrasound training for nephrologists and cardiologists: a LUST trial sub-project. Nephrol Dial Transplant. 2016;31(12):gfw329.

21. Cibinel GA, Casoli G, Elia F, Padoan M, Pivetta E, Lupia E, et al. Diagnostic accuracy and reproducibility of pleural and lung ultrasound in discriminating cardiogenic causes of acute dyspnea in the Emergency Department. Intern Emerg Med. 2012;7: 65–70.

22. Cox EGM, Koster G, Baron A, Kaufmann T, Eck RJ, Veenstra TC, et al. Should the ultrasound probe replace your stethoscope? A SICS-I sub-study comparing lung ultrasound and pulmonary auscultation in the critically ill. Crit Care. 2020;24(1):14.

23. Pivetta E, Goffi A, Nazerian P, Castagno D, Tozzetti C, Tizzani P, et al. Lung ultrasound integrated with clinical assessment for the diagnosis of acute decompensated heart failure in the emergency department: a randomized controlled trial. Eur J Heart Fail. 2019;21(6):754–66.

24. Lancellotti P, Price S, Edvardsen T, Cosyns B, Neskovic ANN, Dulgheru R, et al. The use of echocardiography in acute cardiovascular care: recommendations of the European association of cardiovascular imaging and the acute cardiovascular care association. Eur Hear J Acute Cardiovasc Care. 2015;4(1):3–5.

25. Zanobetti M. Point-of-care ultrasonography for evaluation of acute dyspnea in the emergency department. Chest. 2017.

26. Laursen CB, Sloth E, Lassen AT, Christensen R dePont, Lambrechtsen J, Madsen PH, et al. Point-of-care ultrasonography in patients admitted with respiratory symptoms: a single-blind, randomised controlled trial. Lancet Respir Med. 2015;2(8):638–46.

27. Volpicelli G, Elbarbary M, Blaivas M, Lichtenstein DADA, Mathis G, Kirkpatrick AWAW, et al. International evidence-based recommendations for point-of-care lung ultrasound. Intensive Care Med. 2012;38(4):577–91.

28. Agricola E, Bove T, Oppizzi M, Marino G, Zangrillo A, Margonato A, et al. "Ultrasound comet-tail images": a marker of pulmonary edema: a comparative study with wedge pressure and extravascular lung water. Chest. 2005;127:1690–5.

29. Enghard P, Rademacher S, Nee J, Hasper D, Engert U, Jörres A, et al. Simplified lung ultrasound protocol shows excellent prediction of extravascular lung water in ventilated intensive care patients. Crit Care. 2015;19(1).

30. Palazzuoli A, Ruocco G, Beltrami M, Nuti R, Cleland JG. Combined use of lung ultrasound, B-type natriuretic peptide, and echocardiography for outcome prediction in patients with acute HFrEF and HFpEF. Clin Res Cardiol. 2018;107(7):586–96.

31. Gargani L, Frassi F, Soldati G, Tesorio P, Gheorghiade M, Picano E. Ultrasound lung comets for the differential diagnosis of acute cardiogenic dyspnoea: a comparison with natriuretic peptides. Eur J Heart Fail. 2008;10(1):70.

32. Frassi F, Gargani L, Gligorova S, Ciampi Q, Mottola G, Picano E. Clinical and echocardiographic determinants of ultrasound lung comets. Eur J Echocardiogr. 2007;8(6):474.

33. Kobayashi M, Gargani L, Palazzuoli A, Ambrosio G, Bayés-Genis A, Lupon J, et al. Association between right-sided cardiac function and ultrasound-based pulmonary congestion on acutely decompensated heart failure: findings from a pooled analysis of four cohort studies. Clin Res Cardiol. 2021;110(8): 1181–92.

34. Gargani L, Pugliese NR, Frassi F, Frumento P, Poggianti E, Mazzola M, et al. Prognostic value of lung ultrasound in patients hospitalized for heart

disease irrespective of symptoms and ejection fraction. ESC Hear Fail. 2021;8(4):2660–9.

35. Rastogi T, Bozec E, Pellicori P, Bayes-Genis A, Coiro S, Domingo M, et al. Prognostic value and therapeutic utility of lung ultrasound in acute and chronic heart failure: a meta-analysis. JACC. Cardiovascular Imaging. United States; 2022.

36. Palazzuoli A, Ruocco G, Franci B, Evangelista I, Lucani B, Nuti R, et al. Ultrasound indices of congestion in patients with acute heart failure according to body mass index. Clin Res Cardiol. 2020;109(11):1423–33.

37. Pan D, Pellicori P, Dobbs K, Bulemfu J, Sokoreli I, Urbinati A, et al. Prognostic value of the chest X-ray in patients hospitalised for heart failure. Clin Res Cardiol. 2021;110(11):1743–56.

38. Volpicelli G, Caramello V, Cardinale L, Mussa A, Bar F, Frascisco MF. Bedside ultrasound of the lung for the monitoring of acute decompensated heart failure. Am J Emerg Med. 2008;26(5):585–91.

39. Platz E, Campbell RT, Claggett B, Lewis EF, Groarke JD, Docherty KF, et al. Lung ultrasound in acute heart failure: prevalence of pulmonary congestion and short- and long-term outcomes. JACC Heart Fail. 2019;7(10):849–58.

40. Cortellaro F, Ceriani E, Spinelli M, Campanella C, Bossi I, Coen D, et al. Lung ultrasound for monitoring cardiogenic pulmonary edema. Int Emerg Med. 2016;1–7.

41. Martindale JL, Secko M, Kilpatrick JF, Ian S, Paladino L, Aherne A, et al. Serial sonographic assessment of pulmonary edema in patients with hypertensive acute heart failure. 2017.

42. Mozzini C, Di M, Perna D, Pesce G, Garbin U, Meschi T, et al. Lung ultrasound in internal medicine efficiently drives the management of patients with heart failure and speeds up the discharge time Inferior Cave Vein Collassability index. Intern Emerg Med. 2017.

43. Pang PS, Russell FM, Ehrman R, Ferre R, Gargani L, Levy PD, et al. Lung ultrasound-guided emergency department management of acute heart failure (BLUSHED-AHF): a randomized controlled pilot trial. JACC Heart Fail. 2021;9(9):638–48.

44. Öhman J, Harjola V-P, Karjalainen P, Lassus J. Focused echocardiography and lung ultrasound protocol for guiding treatment in acute heart failure. ESC Hear Fail. 2018;5(1):120–8.

45. Öhman J, Harjola V-P, Karjalainen P, Lassus J. Assessment of early treatment response by rapid cardiothoracic ultrasound in acute heart failure: cardiac filling pressures, pulmonary congestion and mortality. Eur Hear J Acute Cardiovasc Care. 2018;7(4):311–20.

46. Gargani L, Pang PSS, Frassi F, Miglioranza MH, Dini FLL, Landi P, et al. Persistent pulmonary congestion before discharge predicts rehospitalization in heart failure: a lung ultrasound study. Cardiovasc Ultrasound. 2015;13(1):40.

47. Al Coiro et S, Coiro S, Rossignol P, Ambrosio G, Carluccio E, Alunni G, et al. Prognostic value of residual pulmonary congestion at discharge assessed by lung ultrasound imaging in heart failure. Eur J Heart Fail. 2015;17(11):1172–81.

48. Cogliati C, Casazza G, Ceriani E, Torzillo D, Furlotti S, Bossi I, et al. Lung ultrasound and short-term prognosis in heart failure patients. Int J Cardiol. 2016;218.

49. Coiro S, Porot G, Rossignol P, Ambrosio G, Carluccio E, Tritto I, et al. Prognostic value of pulmonary congestion assessed by lung ultrasound imaging during heart failure hospitalisation: a two-centre cohort study. Sci Rep. 2016;20(6):39426.

50. Brogi E, Gargani L, Bignami E, Barbariol F, Marra A, Forfori F, et al. Thoracic ultrasound for pleural effusion in the intensive care unit: a narrative review from diagnosis to treatment. Crit Care. 2017;21(1).

51. Cleland JGF, Pfeffer MA, Clark AL, Januzzi JL, McMurray JJV, Mueller C, et al. The struggle towards a universal definition of heart failure—how to proceed? Eur Heart J. 2021;42(24):2331–43.

52. Kajimoto K, Madeen K, Nakayama T, Tsudo H, Kuroda T, Abe T. Rapid evaluation by lung-cardiac-inferior vena cava (LCI) integrated ultrasound for differentiating heart failure from pulmonary disease as the cause of acute dyspnea in the emergency setting. Cardiovasc Ultrasound. 2012;10(1):49.

53. Nagdev AD, Merchant RC, Tirado-Gonzalez A, Sisson CA, Murphy MC. Emergency department bedside ultrasonographic measurement of the caval index for noninvasive determination of low central venous pressure. Ann Emerg Med. 2010;55(3):290–5.

54. Blehar DJ, Dickman E, Gaspari R. Identification of congestive heart failure via respiratory variation of inferior vena cava diameter. Am J Emerg Med. 2009;27(1):71–5.

55. Pellicori P, Carubelli V, Zhang J, Castiello T, Sherwi N, Clark AL, et al. IVC diameter in patients with chronic heart failure: relationships and prognostic significance. JACC Cardiovasc Imaging. 2013;6(1):16–28.

56. Anderson KL, Jerq KY, Fields JM, Panebianco NL, Dean AJ. Diagnosing heart failure among acutely dyspneic patients with cardiac, inferior vena cava, and lung ultrasonography. Am J Emerg Med. 2013;31(8):1208–14.

57. Sekiguchi H, Schenck LA, Horie R, Suzuki J, Lee EH, McMenomy BP, et al. Critical care ultrasonography differentiates ARDS, pulmonary edema, and other causes in the early course of acute hypoxemic respiratory failure. Chest. 2015;148(4).

58. Öhman J, Harjola V-P, Karjalainen P, Lassus J. Rapid cardiothoracic ultrasound protocol for diagnosis of acute heart failure in the emergency department. Eur J Emerg Med Off J Eur Soc Emerg Med. 2019;26(2):112–7.

59. Kitada R, Fukuda S, Watanabe H, Oe H, Abe Y, Yoshiyama M, et al. Diagnostic accuracy and cost-effectiveness of a pocket-sized transthoracic echocardiographic imaging device. Clin Cardiol. 2013;36 (10):603–10.
60. Prinz C, Voigt J-U. Diagnostic accuracy of a hand-held ultrasound scanner in routine patients referred for echocardiography. J Am Soc Echocardiogr Off Publ Am Soc Echocardiogr. 2011;24(2):111–6.
61. NICOR. National Heart Failure Audit (NHFA) 2020 Summary Report (2018/2019 data). https://www. nicor.org.uk/wp-content/uploads/2020/12/National-Heart-Failure-Audit-2020-FINAL.pdf. 2020.
62. Gargani L, Volpicelli G. How I do it: lung ultrasound. Cardiovasc Ultrasound. 2014;12(1):1–10.
63. Díaz-Gómez JL, Mayo PH, Koenig SJ. Point-of-care ultrasonography. N Engl J Med. 2021;385(17):1593–602.

POCUS in Monitoring: Non-cardiogenic Pulmonary Oedema

Erminio Santangelo, Silvia Mongodi,
and Bélaid Bouhemad

Immediately, ...I rolled a quire of paper into a kind of cylinder and applied one end of it to the region of the heart and the other to my ear and was not a little surprised and pleased to find that I could thereby perceive the action of the heart in a manner much more clear and distinct than I had ever been able to do by the immediate application of my ear.

[René Laennec, "De l'Auscultation Médiate"]-French physician, inventor and musician (1781–1826)

Abstract

Pulmonary oedema is caused by an excessive accumulation of fluids into the alveolar space leading to water-thickened interlobular septa and altered air/tissue ratio. In cardiogenic pulmonary oedema, the cause of fluid accumulation is high pulmonary capillary pressure. On the contrary, non-cardiogenic pulmonary oedema may be determined by various disorders—e.g., ARDS, pneumonia, pulmonary contusion, etc.—ultimately leading to alveolar fluid accumulation. POCUS is a widely accepted technique for the assessment of critically ill patients, and it can be used as a tool for the diagnosis of these conditions. Non-cardiogenic pulmonary oedema is characterized by non-homogeneous ultrasound findings all over the thorax: spared areas mixed with areas showing multiple coalescent B-lines and consolidation. As a readily available, easily accessible and radiation-free bedside tool, LUS is also repeatable over the time giving both a therapeutical guidance for the treatment choice (mechanical ventilation setting, antimicrobial treatment) and a monitoring tool to follow up the patient response.

E. Santangelo · B. Bouhemad (✉)
Department of Anesthesiology and Critical Care Medicine, Centre Hospitalier Universitaire Dijon, Dijon, France
e-mail: belaid_bouhemad@hotmail.com

E. Santangelo
Department of Translational Medicine, University of Eastern Piedmont, Novara, Italy

S. Mongodi
Department of Anaesthesia and Intensive Care, Istituto di Ricovero e Cura a Carattere Scientifico, Policlinico San Matteo Foundation, Pavia, Italy

B. Bouhemad
Université Bourgogne Franche-Comté, Dijon, France

Keywords

Non cardiogenic pulmonary oedema · B-lines · Lung ultrasound · Lung aeration · Lung ultrasound score

© The Author(s), under exclusive license to Springer Nature Switzerland AG 2023
H. Soliman-Aboumarie et al. (eds.), *Cardiopulmonary Point of Care Ultrasound,*
https://doi.org/10.1007/978-3-031-29472-3_13

Key Messages

- Pulmonary oedema is caused by an excessive accumulation of fluids into the interstitial-alveolar space.
- Non cardiogenic pulmonary edema has various etiologies.
- Non cardiogenic pulmonary edema is characterized by non-homogeneously distributed ultrasound findings throughout the thorax.
- The distinction between cardiogenic and non-cardiogenic edema is often challenging and requires an integrated multimodal approach and clinical correlation.
- Lung ultrasound score allows a reliable quantification of lung aeration.

Introduction

Pulmonary oedema is defined as fluid accumulation into the interstitial-alveolar space, derived from one or more alterations in the mechanisms regulating the movements of water across the pulmonary capillaries. Unlike cardiogenic pulmonary oedema where the leading force of fluid accumulation is the elevated pulmonary capillary pressure, non-cardiogenic pulmonary oedema may be due to several underlying disorders ultimately leading to protein and fluid accumulation in the alveoli. Hence, the diagnosis of non-cardiogenic pulmonary oedema is often challenging and the treatments may differ depending on various physio-pathological mechanisms (Table 1).

POCUS is a useful tool to assess these conditions and to support clinicians in the decision-making process to decide the proper treatment. Furthermore, as radiation-free and readily bedside available tool, POCUS can be easily repeated over the time allowing to follow up the patient's clinical condition. This chapter provides an overview on the main ultrasonographic signs of non-cardiogenic pulmonary and the ultrasound monitoring of patient's response to treatment.

Main LUS Findings

B-Lines

The ultrasonographic pattern of pulmonary oedema derives from the histopathological changes of lung tissue occurring during the disease onset. Regardless the underlying cause of pulmonary edema, these changes are characterized by alveolar fluid accumulation, water-thickened interlobular septa and altered air/tissue ratio. Due to the resonance phenomenon, the co-presence of tissues with different ultrasound impedance—i.e. air, water and tissues—generates an altered ultrasound transmission through the pulmonary parenchyma: when the ultrasound beam reaches the thickened interlobular septa and the surrounding air-filled spaces, they are reflected to the ultrasound probe with a time-lag depending on the acoustic impedance of each interface [1]. Thus, the different reflection times of the various tissues are visualized as a persistent source of ultrasound reflection on the pleural line, generating an

Table 1 Main causes of noncardiogenic pulmonary oedema

- Acute respiratory distress syndrome (ARDS)
- Neurogenic pulmonary oedema
- High altitude pulmonary oedema
- Pulmonary contusion
- Transfusion-related acute lung injury
- Re-expansion pulmonary oedema
- Pulmonary embolism-related pulmonary oedema
- Overdose-related pulmonary oedema
- Chemical pneumonia
- Viral pneumonia

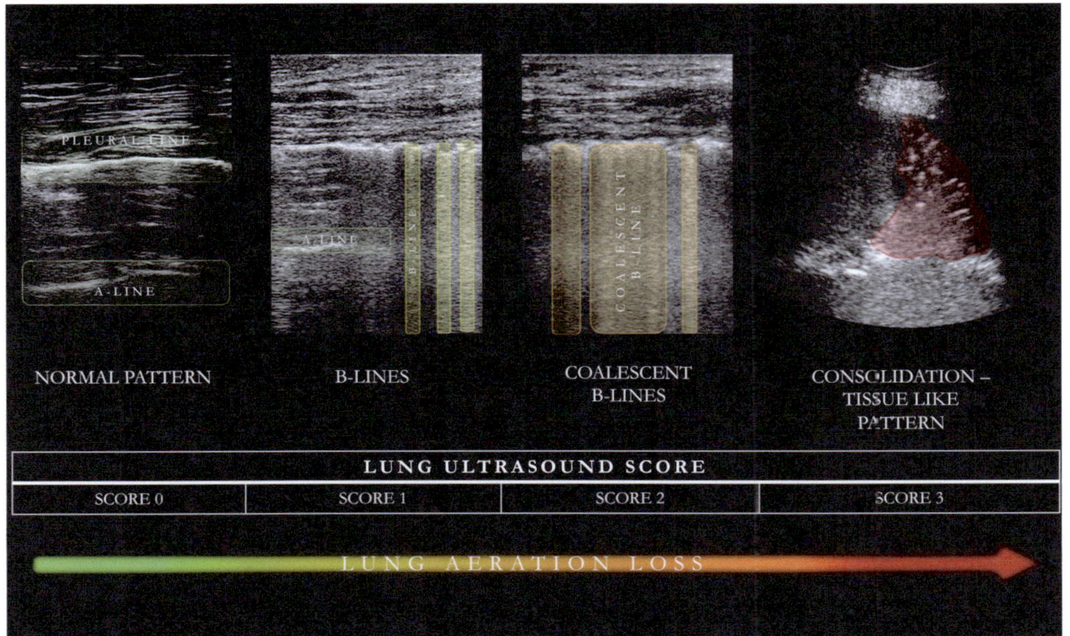

Fig. 1 B-line visualization. The B-line appears as a hyperechoic vertical line arising from the pleural line. Notably, it reaches the bottom of the screen erasing the A lines. The distance between the pleural line and the A-line is the same as that existing from the skin and the pleural line

artifact, also known as "B-line". The B-lines are visualized like a hyperechoic vertical lines from the pleural line to the bottom of the screen, moving synchronously with lung sliding and erasing the A lines [2, 3] (Fig. 1).

A maximum of 2 B-lines per intercostal space is compatible with healthy lungs. Three or more B-lines are considered artifacts of abnormal lung aeration and correlated to thickened interlobular septa [4]. More than five B-lines have been correlated with ground-glass areas and interstitial syndrome [3].

Pleural Effusion and Consolidations

Pleural effusion appears as a hypo/anechoic area that surrounds the pulmonary parenchyma floating within the effusion and moving synchronously with respiratory movements. It can be visualized in the longitudinal view with the probe aligned with the intercostal spaces exploring the costophrenic angle. The inter-pleural space (between visceral and parietal pleura) can be measured allowing a reliable quantification of pleural effusion: the maximal inter-pleural distance measured in the inferior fields at the end expiration is related to the amount of drained fluid and it allows an easy quantification of the effusion in order to decide whether performing thoracentesis is indicated in high-risk patients [5, 6].

Sub-pleural consolidation are visualized as irregularities of the pleural line extending below the pleura without well-defined boundaries. They have been associated with various parenchymal lung diseases (fibrosis, sarcoidosis, interstitial pneumonia, silicosis, etc.) and pulmonary infarcts [7, 8]. Usually, the sub-pleural consolidation is visualized with a coalescence of B-lines extending below the pleural consolidation itself.

Lung consolidations can be visualized as a 'tissue-like pattern'. They correspond to a complete loss of lung aeration and may be accompanied by the presence of air bronchograms (hyperechoic spots within consolidation). The visualization of dynamic linear/arborescent

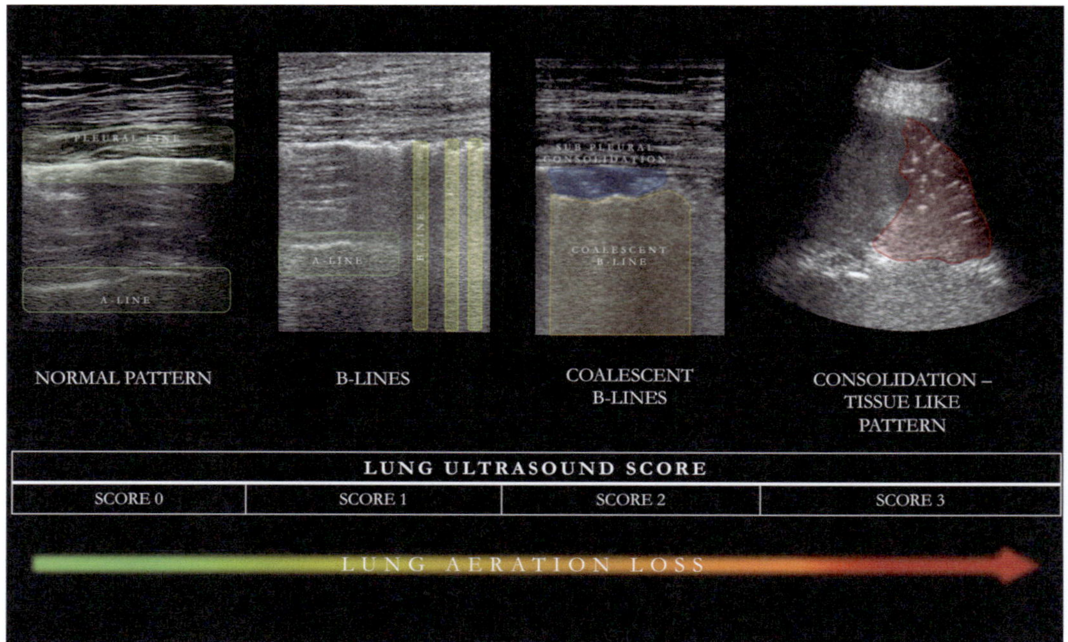

Fig. 2 Main ultrasonographic findings and the LUS score. The score identifies four progressive steps of aeration (score 0: A-lines—no aeration loss; score 1: three or more well-spaced B-lines—moderate aeration loss; score 2: coalescent B-lines—severe aeration loss; score 3: consolidation/tissue-like pattern—complete aeration loss). The distinction between score 1 and score 2 can be estimated by the percentage of the pleura affected by B-lines or subpleural consolidations (less or greater than 50%), as suggested by the recent literature

air-bronchogram within a consolidation has been related to ventilator associated pneumonia. Even though lung consolidations are not specific signs for non-cardiogenic pulmonary edema, their visualization provides additional information about the visualized ultrasound pattern, helping to identify the aetiology of the underlying pathological condition (Fig. 2).

Cardiogenic Pulmonary Oedema and Non-cardiogenic Pulmonary Oedema: The Differences

The ultrasound artifacts visualized in each field during lung examination, vary in number and type as a function of the regional lung aeration loss. The normal pattern of lung aeration is described as a lung sliding associated with the visualization of the A-lines all over the lungs. As the aeration loss increases, a progressive number of B-lines up to coalescent B-lines are visualized on the respective lung field. Once the lung aeration loss is complete, a tissue-like pattern is shown.

However, even though the visualization of these signs is pathognomonic for impaired air/tissue ratio, they are not related to a specific disease or condition. Thus, the type and the distribution of lung ultrasound findings as well as their integration with other clinical and instrumental information are detrimental for the correct interpretation of sonographic findings (Table 2).

Theoretically, since the cardiogenic pulmonary oedema results from increased intravascular hydrostatic pressure, the distribution of alveolar flooding is homogeneously distributed in the lung parenchyma. The resulting lung ultrasound pattern is characterized by bilateral symmetrical visualization of B-lines homogenously distributed throughout the lungs [9]. Even though they are not specific, simple scores based

Table 2 Main POCUS findings for non-cardiogenic pulmonary oedema

- B-lines
- Pleural effusion
- Subpleural consolidation
- Non homogenous distribution of abnormal findings
- No altered echocardiographic parameters or anatomical morphology

on the number of B-lines correlate with surrogate markers of pulmonary oedema [10–12]. B-lines visualization is strongly correlated with Extravascular Lung water (EVLW): higher the amount of EVLW, higher the number of visualized B-lines. In addition, in patients undergoing renal replacement therapy (haemofiltration), the number of B-lines progressively decreases as pulmonary oedema resolves [13, 14]. Furthermore, the visualization of B-pattern also helps to distinguish cardiogenic pulmonary oedema from other non-parenchymal lung disease lung such as acute COPD decompensation [15, 16].

Conversely, non-cardiogenic pulmonary oedema is characterized by heterogeneous ultrasonographic pattern where regions with multiple B-lines can be in close proximity to regions with A-lines (spared areas) or lung consolidations. Consolidated lung areas predominate in the dependent lung regions, coexisting with interstitial–alveolar edema (B-lines) present in the anterior and lateral lung regions. Often, the lung sliding can be also reduced and associated with thickened pleura and subpleural consolidations. In acutely hypoxemic patients, this latter pattern can be used to differentiate cardiogenic pulmonary edema from ARDS [9] (Table 3).

The non-homogeneous distribution of lung consolidations and interstitial–alveolar oedema along with the presence of spared areas have been confirmed by CT scan data from ARDS patients [17, 18]. Recently, it has been shown that LUS is a valid technique in the diagnosis of ARDS in limited resource settings, where the availability of advanced and resource-consuming radiological imaging is limited [19].

Mixed Pulmonary Edema

Increased interstitial lung permeability may derive from the increased intravascular pressure, decreased interstitial hydrostatic pressure or capillary endothelial injury. It may be seen typically in various conditions such as high-altitude pulmonary oedema, neurogenic pulmonary oedema, reperfusion/re-expansion, post-transplantation, post-pneumonectomy or post-volume reduction pulmonary oedema. It can be also found in patients with who initially developed non-cardiogenic oedema with a subsequent increase in intravascular pressure.

Therefore, a rigorous distinction between cardiogenic and non-cardiogenic oedema is not

Table 3 Main LUS findings of cardiogenic pulmonary oedema and non-cardiogenic pulmonary oedema

Cardiogenic pulmonary oedema	Non cardiogenic pulmonary oedema
• Normal lung sliding	• Reduced lung sliding
• Regular and thin pleural line	• Irregular pleural line
• B-lines bilaterally and symmetrically distributed	• B-lines asymmetrically distributed
• Posterior bilateral pleural effusion	• Subpleural consolidation
	• Posterior lung consolidation
	• Spared areas

always possible in clinical practice. Often, in the critically ill patients both the hemodynamic and respiratory alterations occur simultaneously, and a clear differentiation between hydrostatic pulmonary oedema and alterations in interstitial lung permeability might be challenging.

In order to confirm the cardiogenic pulmonary edema instead of the non-cardiogenic one, the examination can be completed by looking for a moderate bilateral pleural effusion, and a large inferior vena cava diameter [9]. Furthermore, a detailed echocardiographic examination is suggested in order to exclude cardiac causes of pulmonary edema.

Non-cardiogenic Pulmonary Oedema and LUS Monitoring

As mentioned above, LUS findings correlate well with the degree of lung aeration. Furthermore, as a rapidly available and radiation-free tool, LUS can be easily repeated over the time. These characteristics make LUS examination a reliable technique for monitoring lung aeration changes when a standardized approach is applied. Therefore, different scoring systems have been proposed to quantify lung aeration. In this context, the best-known score is the lung ultrasound score (LUS score). It is computed over 6-areas per each hemithorax. Each hemithorax is divided into anterior, lateral, and posterior regions by the anterior and posterior axillary lines respectively. Each region is then divided in a superior and an inferior zone. Depending on the visualized artifacts, a score ranging from 0 to 3 is assigned to each field (Fig. 2). The global LUS score results from the sum of the scores assigned in each field, ranging from 0 to 36 (where 0 corresponds to normal aerated lungs, and 36 corresponds to fully non aerated lungs). As a result, the LUS score enables the quantification of the lung aeration at the time of examination. If the LUS score is computed periodically, an increasing score indicates a decrease in lung aeration over time (Fig. 3).

Accordingly, LUS score allows the clinician to monitor the recovery from the disease. To grade the improvements in lung aeration, a LUS re-aeration score can also be computed as the difference in LUS score between two time points. LUS re-aeration score has been validated in different clinical contexts, such as ARDS patients and ventilator associated pneumonia [20, 21].

In this context, bedside evaluation of lung morphology is also helpful for choosing the most appropriate therapeutic strategy and for titrating the mechanical ventilation. Here, we describe two examples of further applications of LUS as a monitoring tool to guide mechanical ventilation management.

Positive End Expiratory Pressure (PEEP) Setting

Since the distribution of lung aeration in ARDS patients is heterogeneous (i.e. consolidated lungs areas are mainly distributed in the dependent lung regions, coexisting with other oedematous or normally aerated lung areas), the choice of mechanical ventilation settings is challenging. In particular, the setting of optimum level of PEEP to improve the aeration of the consolidated lung avoiding lung overdistention, requires a careful evaluation of lung morphology and a periodical assessment of lung aeration changes.

The first assessment of PEEP with LUS has been made through the assessment of lung consolidated areas in lower lobes using transesophageal echocardiography [22–25]. Although these studies were limited to the non-aerated dependent regions, significant correlations have been found between the decrease in the consolidated area dimensions and oxygenation improvement.

However, these applications focused only on the dependent lung regions without considering the entire distribution of aeration in the lungs. As a result, an approach based on a complete lung examination and LUS re-aeration score (previously described) has been proposed to accurately

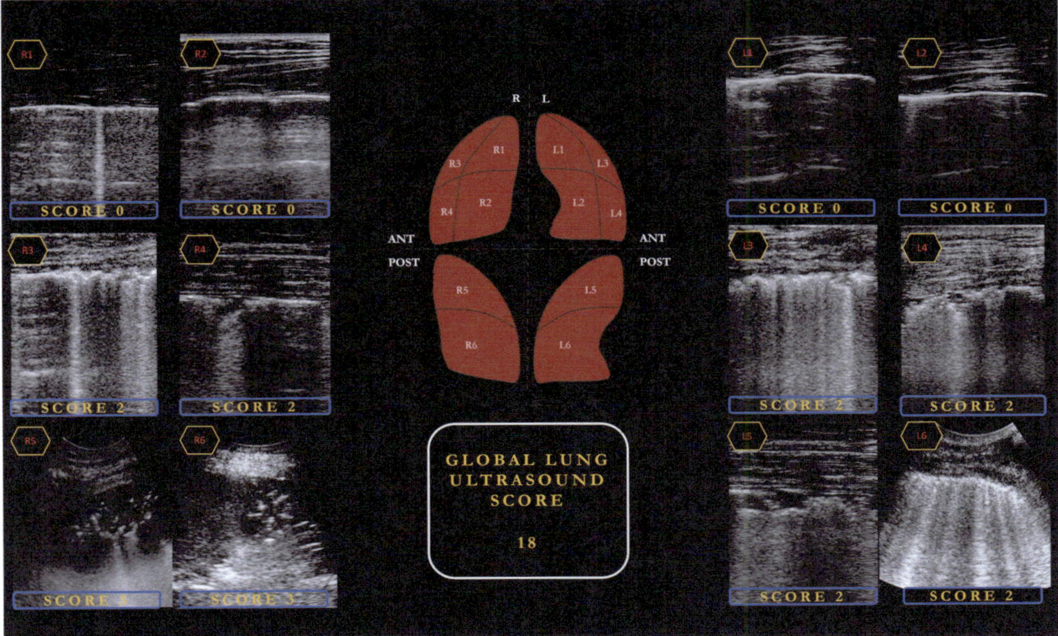

Fig. 3 LUS findings and LUS aeration score computation during ARDS. The figure shows the ultrasonographic findings and global LUS aeration score computed in 12 standard thoracic regions in a patient with ARDS from SARS-Cov-2 infection. The patient shows normal aeration with spared areas in the anterior field, moderate/severe loss of aeration in the lateral fields with irregular pleural line and scattered subpleural consolidations and complete loss of aeration in the right posterior fields with consolidation and tissue-like pattern. No evidence of pleural effusion is shown

assess PEEP-induced reaeration. Notably, it has also been demonstrated that the lung recruitment derives from the reaeration of poorly aerated lung regions (LUS score 2) instead from fully non-aerated ones (LUS score 3). On the contrary, lung consolidation are rarely reopened in response to PEEP increasing [20, 26].

Furthermore, this approach based on the assessment of 12 zones also allows a regional estimation of lung recruitment.

Recently, it has been demonstrated that ARDS is a complex syndrome involving different phenotypes with different clinical outcomes. Therefore, the evaluation of lung morphology is useful to correctly identify the ARDS phenotypes and to identify patients who may respond to both high levels of PEEP and recruitment maneuvers avoiding the risk of overdistention [17, 27]. High PEEP levels and recruitment manoeuvres might be more suitable in non-focal rather than focal ARDS phenotype, whereas patients with focal ARDS could poorly respond to high PEEP levels and recruitment manoeuvres. In this context, a pratical approach has been proposed to titrate PEEP in ARDS patients.

This can be done by LUS examination of the anterior areas of chest wall at low levels of PEEP (5 cm H_2O or less): a normal pattern in the anterior areas of the chest wall characterizes focal aeration loss [28]. On the contrary, in diffuse lung loss aeration loss, well-separated or coalescent B-lines are found in the anterior fields. A PEEP trial could be performed in the latter group and the aeration changes in response to each increase of PEEP level may be monitored using LUS. For patients with focal loss of aeration, low level of PEEP (≤ 10 cm H_2O) can be tested. In these patients, higher levels of PEEP rarely result in recruitment of consolidated areas with an increased risk of overdistension [29].

Unfortunately, lung overdistension cannot be reliably detected by LUS and further respiratory monitoring tools are required.

Prone Positioning

Ability of LUS to predict the oxygenation response to prone positioning has been investigated with contradictory results. In patients with ARDS, a normal LUS pattern of antero-basal lung regions in supine position may predict a significant PaO2/FIO2 ratio improvement [28]. On the other hand, according to others previous CT studies, LUS did not predict the prone-positioning oxygenation response [30, 31]. However, LUS can be used to assess the aeration changes during prone positioning. In patients with focal ARDS with only a transient improvement in oxygenation during prone positioning, LUS accurately detects a significant reaeration of the posterior areas and a loss of aeration in the anterior ones. On the contrary, in patients with non-focal ARDS, prone positioning significantly improved the aeration of the anterior regions [31]. In the same way, LUS can monitor aeration changes of the lung-dependent areas during prone position [31]. Although no significant correlation has been found between global aeration and oxygenation during prone position, these findings suggest that LUS examination might be useful in the management of ARDS patients helping physicians to discriminate the different phenotypes and therefore choosing the most suitable treatments [32].

Conclusion

As described above, lung ultrasound and POCUS provide useful information to achieve a rapid diagnosis and promptly set up the correct treatment. However, despite the easily access of the echo machine, a dedicated training in the technique as well as an integrated approach with other clinical and instrumental information is suggested.

Conflict of Interest None of the authors have any financial interest in the subject matter, materials, or equipment discussed and in competing materials.

Images have not been previously published.

References

1. Jambrik Z, Monti S, Coppola V, Agricola E, Mottola G, Miniati M, et al. Usefulness of ultrasound lung comets as a nonradiologic sign of extravascular lung water. Am J Cardiol. 2004;93(10):1265–70. http://www.ncbi.nlm.nih.gov/pubmed/15135701
2. Lichtenstein D, Mézière G, Biderman P, Gepner A, Barré O. The comet-tail artifact. Am J Respir Crit Care Med. 1997;156(5):1640–6. http://www.atsjournals.org/doi/abs/10.1164/ajrccm.156.5.96-07096
3. Lichtenstein D, Mézière G, Biderman P, Gepner A, Barré O. The comet-tail artifact: an ultrasound sign of alveolar-interstitial syndrome. Am J Respir Crit Care Med. 1997;156(5):1640–6.
4. Lichtenstein DA, Mezière GA. Relevance of lung ultrasound in the diagnosis of acute respiratory failure the BLUE protocol. Chest. 2008;134 (1):117–25.
5. Vignon P, Chastagner C, Berkane V, Chardac E, François B, Normand S, et al. Quantitative assessment of pleural effusion in critically ill patients by means of ultrasonography. Crit Care Med. 2005;33 (8):1757–63. http://www.ncbi.nlm.nih.gov/pubmed/16096453
6. Balik M, Plasil P, Waldauf P, Pazout J, Fric M, Otahal M, et al. Ultrasound estimation of volume of pleural fluid in mechanically ventilated patients. Intensive Care Med. 2006;32(2):318. http://www.ncbi.nlm.nih.gov/pubmed/16432674
7. Nazerian P, Vanni S, Volpicelli G, Gigli C, Zanobetti M, Bartolucci M, et al. Accuracy of point-of-care multiorgan ultrasonography for the diagnosis of pulmonary embolism. Chest. 2014;145 (5):950–7. http://www.ncbi.nlm.nih.gov/pubmed/24092475
8. Reissig A, Kroegel C. Transthoracic sonography of diffuse parenchymal lung disease: the role of comet tail artifacts. J Ultrasound Med. 2003;22(2):173–80. http://www.ncbi.nlm.nih.gov/pubmed/12562122
9. Copetti R, Soldati G, Copetti P. Chest sonography: a useful tool to differentiate acute cardiogenic pulmonary edema from acute respiratory distress syndrome. Cardiovasc Ultrasound. 2008;6(1):16. https://cardiovascularultrasound.biomedcentral.com/articles/10.1186/1476-7120-6-16
10. Volpicelli G, Skurzak S, Boero E, Carpinteri G, Tengattini M, Stefanone V, et al. Lung ultrasound

predicts well extravascular lung water but is of limited usefulness in the prediction of wedge pressure. Anesthesiology. 2014;121(2):320–7. https://pubs.asahq.org/anesthesiology/article/121/2/320/11926/Lung-Ultrasound-Predicts-Well-Extravascular-Lung

11. Jambrik Z, Monti S, Coppola V, Agricola E, Mottola G, Miniati M, et al. Usefulness of ultrasound lung comets as a nonradiologic sign of extravascular lung water. Am J Cardiol. 2004;93(10):1265–70. https://linkinghub.elsevier.com/retrieve/pii/S0002914904002279

12. Enghard P, Rademacher S, Nee J, Hasper D, Engert U, Jörres A, et al. Simplified lung ultrasound protocol shows excellent prediction of extravascular lung water in ventilated intensive care patients. Crit Care. 2015;19(1):36. http://ccforum.com/content/19/1/36

13. Mallamaci F, Benedetto FA, Tripepi R, Rastelli S, Castellino P, Tripepi G, et al. Detection of pulmonary congestion by chest ultrasound in dialysis patients. JACC Cardiovasc Imaging. 2010;3(6):586–94. https://linkinghub.elsevier.com/retrieve/pii/S1936878X10002007

14. Noble VE, Murray AF, Capp R, Sylvia-Reardon MH, Steele DJR, Liteplo A. Ultrasound assessment for extravascular lung water in patients undergoing hemodialysis. Chest. 2009;135(6):1433–9. https://linkinghub.elsevier.com/retrieve/pii/S0012369209603445

15. Lichtenstein D, Mezière G. A lung ultrasound sign allowing bedside distinction between pulmonary edema and COPD: the comet-tail artifact. Intensive Care Med. 1998;24(12):1331–4. http://link.springer.com/10.1007/s001340050771

16. Lichtenstein DA, Mezière GA. Relevance of lung ultrasound in the diagnosis of acute respiratory failure*: the BLUE protocol. Chest. 2008;134(1):117–25. https://linkinghub.elsevier.com/retrieve/pii/S0012369208601555

17. Gattinoni L, Caironi P, Cressoni M, Chiumello D, Ranieri VM, Quintel M, et al. Lung recruitment in patients with the acute respiratory distress syndrome. N Engl J Med. 2006;354(17):1775–86. http://www.nejm.org/doi/abs/10.1056/NEJMoa052052

18. Vieira Srr, Puybasset L, Richecoeur J, Lu Q, Cluzel P, Gusman Pb, et al. A lung computed tomographic assessment of positive end-expiratory pressure–induced lung overdistension. Am J Respir Crit Care Med. 1998;158(5):1571–7. http://www.atsjournals.org/doi/abs/10.1164/ajrccm.158.5.9802101

19. Riviello ED, Kiviri W, Twagirumugabe T, Mueller A, Banner-Goodspeed VM, Officer L, et al. Hospital incidence and outcomes of the acute respiratory distress syndrome using the Kigali modification of the Berlin definition. Am J Respir Crit Care Med. 2016;193(1):52–9. http://www.atsjournals.org/doi/10.1164/rccm.201503-0584OC

20. Bouhemad B, Brisson H, Le-Guen M, Arbelot C, Lu Q, Rouby J-J. Bedside ultrasound assessment of positive end-expiratory pressure–induced lung recruitment. Am J Respir Crit Care Med. 2011;183(3):341–7. http://www.atsjournals.org/doi/abs/10.1164/rccm.201003-0369OC

21. Bouhemad B, Liu ZH, Arbelot C, Zhang M, Ferarri F, Le-Guen M, et al. Ultrasound assessment of antibiotic-induced pulmonary reaeration in ventilator-associated pneumonia. Crit Care Med. 2010;38(1):84–92.

22. Tsubo T, Yatsu Y, Suzuki A, Iwakawa T, Okawa H, Ishihara H, et al. Daily changes of the area of density in the dependent lung region – evaluation using transesophageal echocardiography. Intensive Care Med. 2001;27(12):1881–6. http://link.springer.com/10.1007/s00134-001-1115-3

23. Tsubo T, Yatsu Y, Tanabe T, Okawa H, Ishihara H, Matsuki A. Evaluation of density area in dorsal lung region during prone position using transesophageal echocardiography. Crit Care Med. 2004;32(1):83–7. http://journals.lww.com/00003246-200401000-00011

24. Tsubo T, Sakai I, Suzuki A, Okawa H, Ishihara H, Matsuki A. Density detection in dependent left lung region using transesophageal echocardiography. Anesthesiology. 2001;94(5):793–8. https://pubs.asahq.org/anesthesiology/article/94/5/793/41744/Density-Detection-in-Dependent-Left-Lung-Region

25. Stefanidis K, Dimopoulos S, Tripodaki E-S, Vitzilaios K, Politis P, Piperopoulos P, et al. Lung sonography and recruitment in patients with early acute respiratory distress syndrome: a pilot study. Crit Care. 2011;15(4):R185. http://ccforum.biomedcentral.com/articles/10.1186/cc10338

26. Bouhemad B, Liu Z-H, Arbelot C, Zhang M, Ferarri F, Le-Guen M, et al. Ultrasound assessment of antibiotic-induced pulmonary reaeration in ventilator-associated pneumonia*. Crit Care Med. 2010;38(1):84–92. http://journals.lww.com/00003246-201001000-00014

27. Puybasset L, Cluzel P, Gusman P, Grenier P, Preteux F, Rouby JJ. Regional distribution of gas and tissue in acute respiratory distress syndrome. I. Consequences for lung morphology. Intensive Care Med. 2000;26(7):857–69.

28. Costamagna A, Pivetta E, Goffi A, Steinberg I, Arina P, Mazzeo AT, et al. Clinical performance of lung ultrasound in predicting ARDS morphology. Ann Intensive Care. 2021;11(1):51. https://annalsofintensivecare.springeropen.com/articles/10.1186/s13613-021-00837-1

29. Bouhemad B, Mongodi S, Via G, Rouquette I. Ultrasound for "lung monitoring" of ventilated patients. Anesthesiology. 2015;122(2):437–47.

30. Papazian L, Paladini M-H, Bregeon F, Thirion X, Durieux O, Gainnier M, et al. Can the tomographic aspect characteristics of patients presenting with acute respiratory distress syndrome predict improvement in oxygenation-related response to the prone

position? Anesthesiology. 2002;97(3):599–607. https://pubs.asahq.org/anesthesiology/article/97/3/599/40256/Can-the-Tomographic-Aspect-Characteristics-of

31. Haddam M, Zieleskiewicz L, Perbet S, Baldovini A, Guervilly C, Arbelot C, et al. Lung ultrasonography for assessment of oxygenation response to prone position ventilation in ARDS. Intensive Care Med. 2016;42(10):1546–56. http://link.springer.com/10.1007/s00134-016-4411-7

32. Wang X, Ding X, Zhang H, Chen H, Su L, Liu D. Lung ultrasound can be used to predict the potential of prone positioning and assess prognosis in patients with acute respiratory distress syndrome. Crit Care. 2016;20(1):385. http://ccforum.biomedcentral.com/articles/10.1186/s13054-016-1558-0

POCUS in COVID-19 Pneumonia

Hatem Soliman-Aboumarie, Luna Gargani, and Giovanni Volpicelli

'When we all think alike, then no one is thinking'
Walter Lippmann, American Writer (1889–1974 AD)

Abstract

Lung ultrasound is a useful and reliable tool in the assessment, triaging, and monitoring of patients with SARS CoV2 infection with COVID-19 pneumonia. The higher sensitivity of the modality compared to chest radiography has led to an increasing use by frontline clinicians at the bedside. Integrating LUS probability with the clinical suspicion would simplify the decision-making process, providing a clear guidance to the healthcare personnel allowing to rule-in or rule-out the possibility of COVID-19.

Keywords

COVID-19 · SARS CoV2 · ARDS · POCUS

Key Messages

- Bedside real-time lung ultrasound (LUS) for the assessment of COVID-19 pneumonia could support and integrate lung imaging with several advantages and can detect typical features of COVID-19 pneumonia.
- The high sensitivity of LUS for the detection of pulmonary involvement allows it to be a reliable monitoring tool for the regular assessment of patients with COVID-19.
- Integrating LUS probability with the clinical suspicion would simplify the decision-making process, providing a clear guidance to the healthcare personnel allowing to rule-in or rule-out the possibility of COVID-19.

Supplementary Information The online version contains supplementary material available at https://doi.org/10.1007/978-3-031-29472-3_14.

H. Soliman-Aboumarie (✉)
Department of Anaesthetics and Critical Care, Harefield Hospital. Royal Brompton and Harefield Hospitals, London, UK
e-mail: h.solimanaboumarie@rbht.nhs.uk

L. Gargani
University of Pisa, Pisa, Italy

G. Volpicelli
Emergency Medicine, San Luigi Gonzaga University Hospital, Torino, Italy

Introduction

The coronavirus disease-2019 (COVID-19) pandemic has become a major global health issue, due to its high rate of infection and increasing morbidity and mortality. SARS CoV2 is a novel coronavirus that spreads easily from symptomatic and asymptomatic patients through close contact and respiratory droplets, causing a severe acute respiratory infection in a certain percentage of cases [1]. It represented a challenge for clinicians to provide early diagnosis to identify patients and prevent the most severe forms of respiratory failure and acute distress respiratory syndrome (ARDS), which represent a serious burden even for the most advanced medical systems [2, 3].

Diagnosis of COVID-19 is based on the real-time reverse transcription PCR (rRT–PCR) analysis of respiratory tract specimens. However, rRT–PCR has a low sensitivity, translating in a subgroup of patients admitted to the hospital with the typical clinical aspects of the diseases but with false negative specimens. Chest computed tomography (CT) has a high sensitivity for the diagnosis of COVID-19 pneumonia, so it is considered the reference imaging method [4, 5]. Chest CT analysis of patients with COVID-19 pneumonia typically shows bilateral, and peripheral ground-glass opacities, crazy paving, and consolidations in a patchy distribution, that worsen with the progression of the disease [6]. Nevertheless, the feasibility of CT can be limited by its availability, the need to mobilize the patient, and the long-term risks related to ionizing radiation [7]. Bedside real-time lung ultrasound (LUS) for the assessment of COVID-19 pneumonia could support and integrate lung imaging with several advantages [8–10]. In fact, beyond its consolidated importance as a diagnostic and prognostic tool in heart failure and critically ill patients [11–13]. LUS can detect some typical characteristics of COVID-19 pneumonia [8–10, 14].

The Revolution of POCUS in COVID-19

The pandemic has led to an ever-increasing use of POCUS for cardiac, lung, fluid, vascular and other organ assessment. POCUS has shown a growing value in everyday clinical practice, especially in the emergency and intensive care settings. This imaging modality is portable, quick, repeatable, easy to learn, as compared with other ultrasonographic techniques, and with high inter-observer and intra-observer reproducibility [15, 16]. It can reduce a patient's exposure to ionizing radiation and contribute to the safety of the healthcare providers by minimizing the need for moving the patient, therefore reducing the incidence of cross-contamination and the number of healthcare professionals exposed to the patient. Moreover, the growing use of small and portable handheld devices is running in parallel with the wider integration of POCUS in daily practice as an extension to bedside clinical examination [17, 18]. The high sensitivity of LUS for the detection of pulmonary involvement allows it to be a reliable monitoring tool for the regular assessment of patients with COVID-19 [19].

LUS in COVID-19 Pneumonia

LUS in the Diagnosis of COVID-19 Pneumonia

LUS Signs of COVID-19

In COVID-19 pneumonia we can find many different LUS signs, in particular:

- **Separated B-lines**, especially in the first phases (Video 7).
- **Coalescent B-lines**, sometimes giving the appearance of a shining white lung (Video 8). They can arise from one point of the pleural line and from small peripheral consolidations

and spread down like rays maintaining their brightness until the edge of the screen without fading. In the early phases of COVID-19 pneumonia, we often observe a shining band-form artifact spreading down from a large portion of a, usually, regular pleural line, often appearing and disappearing with an on–off effect in the context of a normal A-lines pattern visible on the background. This sign has been defined "the light beam". This sign is usually visible in the very acute phase of ground glass lesions during the early spread of the active disease, when limited diseased areas are juxtaposed to preserved lung parenchyma. The name "light beam" reminds of a large beam of light sometimes appearing and disappearing during respiration (Video 2). The curvilinear (convex) probe is the most suitable to identify the light beam. It is also advisable to position the focus at the level of the pleural line to improve the visualization of the vertical artifacts.

These artifacts represent the typical signs of the disease but can be also observed in other interstitial diseases of different etiologies.

- **Spared areas**, which are typically seen in non-cardiogenic pulmonary edema, such as in ALI/ARDS, whereas they are not usually present in cardiogenic pulmonary edema, where B-lines are more homogeneously distributed over the chest. Spared areas are zones of sonographically normal parenchyma in close continuity to diseased parenchyma (Videos 1 and 2).
- **Alterations of the pleural line** are another ultrasound feature that may help in the differential diagnosis between cardiogenic and non-cardiogenic edema. In cardiogenic edema, even in the eldest population, the pleural line is usually thin and regular with multiple diffuse bilateral B-lines spreading from it. In non-cardiogenic pulmonary edema, the pleural line has an irregular appearance with sub-pleural hypo/anechoic spaces (Videos 3 and 4), which may represent the alveolar involvement that in this condition is

present, together with the interstitial involvement. It is important to note, that it is not the anatomical *pleura* that is irregular and "thickened", but it is its sonographic depiction as the '*pleural line*' which appear thickened, fragmented and irregular. In COVID-19 pneumonia the pleural line looks often irregular but can also be found smooth and thin in the early phases.
- **Small peripheral consolidations** are, similarly to the irregular pleural line, a sonographic characteristic that is rarely seen in cardiogenic pulmonary edema, but quite frequent in non-cardiogenic edema (Videos 4, 5 and 6). It can be considered an advanced version of the irregular pleural line, indicating an alveolar involvement. Usually, these small (<15–10 mm in the largest diameter) consolidations are multiple, although still with a patchy distribution.
- **Larger consolidations** are not so frequent in COVID-19 pneumonia. They can be seen in the advanced phases of the disease, and it is still not clear whether they represent a bacterial superinfection or they are part of the progression of this condition. Large consolidations are more frequently observed at the lung bases.
- **Pleural effusion** is also not very frequent in COVID-19 pneumonia. Usually, when present, it is trivial or mild, whereas larger pleural effusion should raise the suspicion of a different etiology.

Two different phenotypes have been described in COVID-19, at least in a theoretical model [21]. The more frequent phenotype 'L' typically presents with normal to mildly reduced lung compliance, albeit with a level of hypoxaemia disproportionate to the relatively preserved lung compliance, in which chest CT typically shows predominantly peripheral ground-glass opacifications that worsens with the progression of the disease. On the other hand, the less frequent phenotype 'H' is more similar to the classic ARDS presentation with reduced lung compliance and evidence of dense lobar consolidations on chest CT.

LUS is potentially able to distinguish these two phenotypes, based on the different signs and patterns.

How to Scan

Machine Setting

The convex or microconvex transducers are the most universally used for LUS, as they allow a good visualization of the parenchymal alterations while also providing a reasonable view of the pleural line. The examination should start by adjusting the machine on the lung pre-set (or abdominal pre-set if lung pre-set is not available), with a depth of 8–10 cm (6–8 cm for slim patients, 10–12 cm or more for obese subjects); gain should be optimized on the whole image, and the focus should be adjusted to the area of interest (e.g. the pleural line). The probe could be placed vertically perpendicular to the ribs (longitudinal approach) or horizontally along the intercostal spaces (transverse/oblique approach). Phased array transducers could also be used to visualize the parenchyma, albeit with more limited visualization of the pleura. Each point should be examined for at least one complete respiratory cycle (5–6 s).

Scanning Scheme

At the moment, there is no validated scanning scheme for COVID-19 patients. Therefore, it is advisable to rely on previously validated schemes that have already proven to be useful, although in different conditions, such as ARDS [14], which represents a good balance between being simple and comprehensive. Whenever possible, we recommend including the scanning of the posterior zones, where lung lesions are more commonly seen in these patients. If the patient cannot move from the supine position, the posterolateral part of the chest can usually be scanned by turning the patient to his/her side.

For these reasons, LUS scanning in COVID-19 patients should be as thorough as possible, and even if different schemes and areas are considered, in a given area, all available thoracic space should be checked, and the worst LUS picture should be considered.

How to Interpret LUS Signs in the Clinical Context

LUS patterns of probability (Table 1) [20]:

To practically integrate LUS in the management of patients with a suspicion of COVID-19 pneumonia, it is advisable to rely on 4 different LUS patterns of probability of COVID-19 pneumonia. This approach would simplify the decision-making process, providing a clear guidance to the healthcare personnel.

– *High probability pattern*

This pattern is determined by the presence of bilateral and multifocal clusters of separated and/or coalescent B-lines, large hyperechoic bands (light beams), multifocal small peripheral consolidations, with both regular and irregular pleural line, and with or without large consolidations. These clusters should appear in patchy distribution, abruptly alternating with normal A-line patterns ("spared areas").

Table 1 LUS patterns of probability (N = 1462 patients)

Clinical setting	Best LUS pattern to be used	AIM
Overall population	HighLUS/IntLUS (sensitivity 90.2%)	Rule-out COVID-19 pneumonia
Mild phenotype	HighLUS (sensitivity 94.4%)	Rule-in COVID-19 pneumonia
Mixed phenotype	HighLUS/IntLUS (sensitivity 94.7%)	Rule-out COVID-19 pneumonia
Severe phenotype	HighLUS/IntLUS (sensitivity 97.1%)	Rule-out COVID-19 pneumonia
Respiratory failure	HighLUS/IntLUS (sensitivity 99.3%)	Rule-out COVID-19 pneumonia

– *Intermediate probability pattern*

A less typical pattern with isolated or unilateral clusters of B-lines and light beams or focal multiple B-lines, with or without small peripheral consolidations.

– *Low probability pattern*

A normal or near-normal LUS pattern characterized by bilateral A-lines with lung sliding and without significant B-lines (less than 3 B-lines per scanning site).

– *Alternative probability pattern*

A LUS pattern more consistent with an alternative diagnosis such as an isolated large consolidation with dynamic air bronchograms (suggesting bacterial pneumonia) or without bronchograms (suggesting obstructive atelectasis), a large pleural effusion (suggesting either hydrostatic or inflammatory etiology), multiple diffuse homogeneously distributed bilateral B-lines (suggesting cardiogenic edema).

LUS in Monitoring COVID-19 Pneumonia

Lung Ultrasound Aeration Score (Further Details in Chap. 24)

Using a standardized scanning scheme enables us to assign a score to each lung zone and, therefore, assess the overall lung aeration. As for the scanning scheme, in the absence of a standardized score for COVID-19 patients, it is reasonable to rely on a previously validated Score [22].

Score 0: predominant A-lines or <3 separated B-lines.
Score 1: at least three B-lines or coalescent B-lines occupying </ = 50% of the screen without a clearly irregular pleural line.
Score 1p: at least three B-lines or coalescent B-lines occupying </ = 50% of the screen with a clearly irregular pleural line.

Score 2: coalescent B-lines occupying >50% of the screen without a clearly irregular pleural line.
Score 2p: coalescent B-lines occupying >50% of the screen with a clearly irregular pleural line.
Score 3: large consolidations (at least >1 cm). It is useful to characterize the consolidation (hypoechoic, tissue-like, air or fluid bronchogram, etc.),

Presence of pleural effusion should always be reported as well. The final score is obtained by summing up the scores of each area. The letters 'p' are not counted in the score: this is a more qualitative information, which is anyway useful because they are very frequent in COVID-19, which is compatible with the pathophysiology of the condition. It is, however, not demonstrated yet that this kind of pure 'deaeration score'— often used in other conditions such as pneumonia and ARDS—can be enough to characterize these patients. On the one hand, it is established that a higher sonographic deaeration score indicates a less aerated lung, thus a worse pulmonary involvement; on the other hand, in COVID-19 patients, the different LUS patterns and their distribution may be more relevant to guide the clinicians' choice on different approaches, especially when characterizing patients into the aforementioned theoretical phenotypes [21, 23].

Clinical Scenarios

It is necessary to combine the LUS probability pattern with the initial clinical presentation of the patient. For simplicity, we can summarize three main clinical presentations:

– *Mild phenotype*: patients without dyspnea and/or desaturation (no symptoms or signs of respiratory failure), i.e. patients presenting to the Emergency Department with fever, cough or other symptoms;
– *Severe phenotype*: patients with dyspnea and/or desaturation (dyspnea and/or signs of respiratory failure);
– *Mixed phenotype*: in patients with pre-existing cardiopulmonary comorbidities, irrespective

of the clinical condition at presentation. The presence of a history of chronic pulmonary and/or cardiac disease is a confounding element, which could reduce in particular the specificity of LUS.

Clinical—Ultrasound Integration for the Diagnosis of COVID-19 Pneumonia

The integration between the LUS probability pattern and the clinical presentation of the patient is key to a correct understanding and interpretation of the ultrasound picture, and to establish the accuracy of our findings.

A large multicentric study, including 20 Hospitals from Europe and 2 from the US, has tested this approach with interesting results (see Table 1).

In patients with the mild phenotype, LUS was particularly useful to rule in COVID-19 pneumonia: the specificity is 94.4% when finding the High probability pattern, whereas LUS is not particularly valuable for the rule-out of this condition (sensitivity is 67.6% when combining the High probability and the Intermediate probability patterns).

In patients with the mixed phenotype, LUS is particularly useful to rule out COVID-19 pneumonia: the sensitivity is 94.7% when not finding either the High probability or the Intermediate probability patterns, whereas specificity is 88.3% when finding the High probability pattern.

In patients with the severe phenotype, LUS is particularly useful to rule out COVID-19 pneumonia: the sensitivity is 97.1% when not finding either the High probability or the Intermediate probability patterns, whereas specificity is 81.8% when finding the High probability pattern. Among the sever phenotype, the subgroup of patients with overt signs of respiratory failure (saturation <94%), LUS shows the higher degree of sensitivity, which is 99.3% when not finding either the High probability or the Intermediate probability patterns, whereas specificity

is 82.3% when finding the High probability pattern.

A standardized LUS protocol combining ultrasound probability pattern with clinical phenotypes in patients suspected of COVID-19 pneumonia is then feasible and reproducible. In patients with suspected COVID-19, LUS is very sensitive in *ruling out* interstitial pneumonia, with increasing sensitivity with increasing symptoms, whereas, in patients with mild symptoms LUS is very specific in *ruling in* interstitial pneumonia. This approach may be useful to rapidly guide management and allow for wiser use of hospital resources during a pandemic surge and may even represent the only available diagnostic tool in limited resource areas.

Risk of Spreading Infection

Performing LUS in COVID-19 patients is different from other conditions, because this poses a biological risk of infection for the operator, as well as not negligible logistic issues for the management of the echo machines. The risk of infection can be significantly limited by a proper protection of the operator, and a correct cleaning of the probes and machine, for which there are specific published indications [25]. However, we should consider that colleagues are often working in very stressful and challenging situations, where the distance between the 'ideal' world of optimum personal protective equipment and procedures has to be matched with clinical needs, time constraints, and intense fatigue. Procedural errors can be numerous and highly risky for the operators and the overall system.

Future Perspectives

Deep learning (DL) and artificial intelligence may play important role in the application of POC LUS in the future. A study by Arntfield et al. on 243 patients from two tertiary centers looked at the performance of convoluted neural networks (CNN) in comparison with the human interpretation in differentiating COVID-19 from non-COVID-19 non-cardiogenic pulmonary oedema patterns [24]. The study found that CNN ability to differentiate COVID-19 from non-COVID 19 LUS patterns far exceeded the human ability which means that DL methods can identify subvisible biomarkers within LUS images.

Conclusions

The COVID-19 pandemic has further highlighted the usefulness of LUS in different clinical scenarios, underlining its advantages in terms of availability, operator- and patient-friendliness, relatively low cost and expertise needed, and high sensitivity. COVID-19 pulmonary involvement can benefit from LUS scanning at all steps of its management, from home monitoring to mechanical ventilation management and weaning. Operators who largely employ LUS in the clinical decision-making should be aware of the potential pitfalls of the technique, especially contextualized in this very peculiar situation, where robust evidence is still missing due to the time contingency. A proper acknowledgement of LUS advantages and limitations is needed to fully benefit from this undoubtedly game-changer bedside imaging approach [17].

References

1. Guan WJ, Ni ZY, Hu Y, Liang WH, Ou CQ, He JX, Liu L, Shan H, Lei CL, Hui DSC, Du B, Li LJ, Zeng G, Yuen KY, Chen RC, Tang CL, Wang T, Chen PY, Xiang J, Li SY, Wang JL, Liang ZJ, Peng YX, Wei L, Liu Y, Hu YH, Peng P, Wang JM, Liu JY, Chen Z, Li G, Zheng ZJ, Qiu SQ, Luo J, Ye CJ, Zhu SY, Zhong NS. China medical treatment expert group for Covid-19. Clinical characteristics of coronavirus disease 2019 in China. N Engl J Med. 2020;382:1708–1720.
2. Rodriguez-Morales AJ, Cardona-Ospina JA, Gutierrez-Ocampo E, Villamizar- Pe~na R, Holguin-Rivera Y, Escalera-Antezana JP, Alvarado-Arnez LE, Bonilla- Aldana DK, Franco-Paredes C, Henao-Martinez AF, Paniz-Mondolfi A, Lagos- Grisales GJ, Ramı rez-Vallejo E, Sua rez JA, Zambrano LI, Villamil-Go mez WE, Balbin-Ramon GJ, Rabaan AA, Harapan H, Dhama K, Nishiura H, Kataoka H, Ahmad T, Sah R. Latin American network of coronavirus disease 2019—COVID-19 Research (LANCOVID-19). Clinical, laboratory and imaging features of COVID-19: a systematic review and meta-analysis. Travel Med Infect Dis. 2020;34:101623.
3. Marini JJ, Gattinoni L. Management of COVID-19 respiratory distress. JAMA. 2020. https://doi.org/10.1001/jama.2020.6825.
4. Fang Y, Zhang H, Xie J, Lin M, Ying L, Pang P, Ji W. Sensitivity of chest CT for COVID-19: comparison to RT–PCR. Radiology. 2020. https://doi.org/10.1148/radiol.2020200432.
5. Ai T, Yang Z, Hou H, Zhan C, Chen C, Lv W, Tao Q, Sun Z, Xia L. Correlation of chest CT and RT–PCR testing in coronavirus disease 2019 (COVID-19) in China: a report of 1014 cases. Radiology 2020. https://doi.org/10.1148/radiol.2020200642.
6. Bernheim A, Mei X, Huang M, Yang Y, Fayad ZA, Zhang N, Diao K, Lin B, Zhu X, Li K, Li S, Shan H, Jacobi A, Chung M. Chest CT findings in coronavirus disease-19 (COVID-19): relationship to duration of infection. Radiology. 2020. https://doi.org/10.1148/radiol.2020200463.
7. Gargani L, Picano E. The risk of cumulative radiation exposure in chest imaging and the advantage of bedside ultrasound. Crit Ultrasound J. 2015;7:4.
8. Millington SJ, Koenig S, Mayc P, Volpicelli G. Lung ultrasound for patients with coronavirus disease 2019 pulmonary disease. Chest. 2021;159(1):205–11. https://doi.org/10.1016/j.chest.2020.08.2054.
9. Volpicelli G, Lamorte A, Ville n T. What's new in lung ultrasound during the COVID-19 pandemic. Intensive Care Med. 2020. https://doi.org/10.1007/s00134-020-06048-9.
10. Volpicelli G, Gargani L. Sonographic signs and patterns of COVID-19 pneumonia. Ultrasound J. 2020;12:22.
11. Gargani L. Ultrasound of the lungs: more than a room with a view. Heart Fail Clin. 2019;15:297–303.
12. Mojoli F, Bouhemad B, Mongodi S, Lichtenstein D. Lung ultrasound for critically ill patients. Am J Respir Crit Care Med. 2019;199:701–14.
13. Volpicelli G, Elbarbary M, Blaivas M, Lichtenstein DA, Mathis G, Kirkpatrick AW, Melniker L, Gargani L, Noble VE, Via G, Dean A, Tsung JW, Soldati G, Copetti R, Bouhemad B, Reissig A, Agricola E, Rouby JJ, Arbelot C, Liteplo A, Sargsyan A, Silva F, Hoppmann R, Breitkreutz R, Seibel A, Neri L, Storti E, Petrovic T; International Liaison Committee on Lung Ultrasound (ILC-LUS) for International Consensus Conference on Lung Ultrasound (ICC-LUS). International evidence based recommendations for point-of-care lung ultrasound. Intensive Care Med. 2012;38:577–591.
14. Gargani L, Soliman-Aboumarie H, Volpicelli G, Corradi F. Maria Concetta Pastore, Matteo Cameli, Why, when, and how to use lung ultrasound during

the COVID-19 pandemic: enthusiasm and caution. Eur Hear J Cardiovasc Imaging. 2020;21(9):941–8. https://doi.org/10.1093/ehjci/jeaa163.

15. Anderson KL, Fields JM, Panebianco NL, Jenq KY, Marin J, Dean AJ. Inter-rater reliability of quantifying pleural B-lines using multiple counting methods. J Ultrasound Med. 2013;32:115–20.

16. Gargani L, Sicari R, Raciti M, Serasini L, Passera M, Torino C, Letachowicz K, Ekart R, Fliser D, Covic A, Balafa O, Stavroulopoulos A, Massy ZA, Fiaccadori E, Caiazza A, Bachelet T, Slotki I, Shavit L, Martinez-Castelao A, Coudert-Krier MJ, Rossignol P, Kraemer TD, Hannedouche T, Panichi V, Wiecek A, Pontoriero G, Sarafidis P, Klinger M, Hojs R, Seiler-Mu ler S, Lizzi F, Onofriescu M, Zarzoulas F, Tripepi R, Mallamaci F, Tripepi G, Picano E, London GM, Zoccali C. Efficacy of a remote web-based lung ultrasound training for nephrologists and cardiologists: a LUST trial sub-project. Nephrol Dial Transplant. 2016;31:1982–1988.

17. Narula J, Chandrashekhar Y, Braunwald E. Time to add a fifth pillar to bedside physical examination: inspection, palpation, percussion, auscultation, and insonation. JAMA Cardiol. 2018;3:346–50.

18. Cardim N, Dalen H, Voigt JU, Ionescu A, Price S, Neskovic AN, Edvardsen T, Galderisi M, Sicari R, Donal E, Stefanidis A, Delgado V, Zamorano J, Popescu BA. The use of handheld ultrasound devices: a position statement of the European Association of Cardiovascular Imaging (2018 update). Eur Heart J Cardiovasc Imaging. 2019;20:245–52.

19. Pivetta E, Goffi A, Tizzani M, Locatelli SM, Porrino G, Losano I, Leone D, Calzolari G, Vesan M, Steri F, Ardito A, Capuano M, Gelardi M, Silvestri G, Dutto S, Avolio M, Cavallo R, Bartalucci A, Paglieri C, Morello F, Richiardi L, Maule MM, Lupia E. Molinette MedUrg Group on lung ultrasound. Lung ultrasonography for the diagnosis of SARS-CoV-2 pneumonia in the emergency department. Ann Emerg Med. 2021;77(4):385–94. https://doi.org/10.1016/j.annemergmed.2020.10.008. Epub 2020 Oct 13. PMID: 33461884; PMCID: PMC7552969.

20. Volpicelli G, Gargani L, Perlini S, Spinelli S, Barbieri G, Lanotte A, Casasola GG, Nogué-Bou R, Lamorte A, Agricola E, Villén T, Deol PS, Nazerian P, Corradi F, Stefanone V, Fraga DN, Navalesi P, Ferre R, Boero E, Martinelli G, Cristoni L, Perani C, Vetrugno L, McDermott C, Miralles-Aguiar F, Secco G, Zattera C, Salinaro F, Grignaschi A, Boccatonda A, Giostra F, Infante MN, Covella M, Ingallina G, Burkert J, Frumento P, Forfori F, Ghiadoni L. on behalf of the International Multicenter Study Group on LUS in COVID-19. Lung ultrasound for the early diagnosis of COVID-19 pneumonia: an international multicenter study. Intensive Care Med. 2021;47(4):444–54. https://doi.org/10.1007/s00134-021-06373-7. Epub 2021 Mar 20. PMID: 33743018; PMCID: PMC7980130.

21. Gattinoni L, et al. COVID-19 pneumonia: different respiratory treatments for different phenotypes?. Intensive Care Med. 2020;46.6:1099–102.

22. Bouhemad B, Mongodi S, Via G, Rouquette I. Ultrasound for "lung monitoring" of ventilated patients. Anesthesiology. 2015;122(2):437–47. https://doi.org/10.1097/ALN.0000000000000558. PMID: 25501898.

23. Gattinoni L, Chiumello D, Caironi P, et al. COVID-19 pneumonia: different respiratory treatments for different phenotypes? Intensive Care Med. 2020;46:1099–102. https://doi.org/10.1007/s00134-020-06033-2.

24. Arntfield R, VanBerlo B, Alaifan T, et al. Development of a convolutional neural network to differentiate among the etiology of similar appearing pathological B lines on lung ultrasound: a deep learning study. BMJ Open. 2021;11:e045120. https://doi.org/10.1136/bmjopen-2020-045120.

25. Skulstad H, et al. COVID-19 pandemic and cardiac imaging: EACVI recommendations on precautions, indications, prioritization, and protection for patients and healthcare personnel Eur Hear J Cardiovasc Imaging. 2020; 21.6:592–598.

POCUS in Monitoring: Volume Responsiveness

Xavier Monnet and Jean-Louis Teboul

"However I did mention it hoping to see among people, practitioners who are good at it; having enough skill, experience and training. Indeed no one should consider doing it unless he has practiced it as a student under the direct supervision of his teacher for a long time. Then practiced it on his own for sometime". -Ibn Zuhr (Avenzoar) Medieval Arab physician, surgeon and pioneer (1094–1162 AD Seville, Andalusia)

Abstract

In the critically ill patients with acute circulatory failure, fluid administration should be cautiously undertaken. First, except in case of obvious hypovolemia or very early septic shock, it leads to an increase in cardiac output in only half of the cases. Second, the risk of excessive fluid administration has been clearly established. This encourages the administration of fluids only after ensuring the presence of fluid responsiveness. For this purpose, static indices of cardiac preload (e.g.: left ventricular end-diastolic dimensions of the E/e' ratio), are useless. By contrast, a dynamic approach consists of observing the effects on stroke volume of changes in cardiac preload that are either spontaneous (for indices) or provoked (for tests). The respiratory variation of the velocity time integral (VTI) in the left ventricular outflow tract (LVOT) under positive pressure ventilation is a surrogate for pulse pressure variation. It reliably indicates fluid responsiveness but cannot be used in many instances. This is also the case for the respiratory variation in the diameter of superior or inferior vena cava which, in addition, is the least reliable of fluid responsiveness tests and indices. The changes in the LVOT VTI during a passive leg raising test are much more reliable. The effects of a mini-fluid challenge, made of 100–150 mL of fluid, can be assessed in the same way. However, the changes are near the reproducibility limit of echocardiography. The effects on the LVOT VTI of successive end-inspiratory and end-expiratory pauses can be used in mechanically ventilated patients provided that their respiratory activity allows a respiratory occlusion of a few seconds.

X. Monnet (✉) · J.-L. Teboul
Groupe de Recherche Clinique CARMAS,
Université Paris-Saclay, AP-HP, Hôpital de Bicêtre,
DMU CORREVE, Inserm UMR S_999, FHU
SEPSIS, Service de Médecine
Intensive-Réanimation, Le Kremlin-Bicêtre, France
e-mail: xavier.monnet@aphp.fr

J.-L. Teboul
e-mail: jean-louis.teboul@aphp.fr

© The Author(s), under exclusive license to Springer Nature Switzerland AG 2023
H. Soliman-Aboumarie et al. (eds.), *Cardiopulmonary Point of Care Ultrasound*,
https://doi.org/10.1007/978-3-031-29472-3_15

Keywords

Fluids · Volume expansion · Passive leg raising · Fluid challenge · End-expiratory occlusion

Abbreviations

CVP	Central venous pressure
IVC	Inferior vena cava
LV	Left ventricular
LVOT	Left ventricular outflow tract
LVOTVV	Respiratory variation of the maximal velocity in the left ventricular outflow tract
PLR	Passive leg raising
PPV	Pulse pressure variation
Vt	Tidal volume
VTI	Velocity time integral

Key messages

- Static markers of cardiac preload, such as left ventricular end-diastolic dimensions or the E/e' ratio, do not reliably predict whether cardiac output will increase in response to fluid infusion
- The respiratory variations in the peak velocity of the left ventricular outflow under mechanical ventilation predict fluid responsiveness but many conditions of use limit their applicability
- The respiratory variations of venae cavae diameter are the least reliable indices of fluid responsiveness
- Passive leg raising test can be performed guided by echocardiography by assessing the induced changes in the velocity time integral of the left ventricular outflow tract
- In patients under mechanical ventilation, fluid responsiveness can also be assessed by measuring the effects of successive end-inspiratory and end-expiratory occlusions performed a few seconds apart.

Introduction

Fluid administration is the first therapeutic option in almost all cases of acute circulatory failure. It is intended to increase cardiac preload and, in response, cardiac output [1]. However, this beneficial effect of volume expansion does not occur in many cases. Apart from cases of profound hypovolemia, the response to fluid loading occurs in only half of the patients for whom it is carried out. Given the side effects of fluid administration in many situations, it appears as reasonable to test preload responsiveness before exposing patients to these potentially dangerous drugs [2].

For this purpose, a physiology-based approach should rely on dynamic tests and indices, rather than static indices of cardiac preload. In this chapter, we will review those tests and indices that are assessed by POCUS. After briefly reviewing the concept of fluid responsiveness, we will detail their physiological background, the way they should be measured or performed in practice, their reliability and their limitations.

The Concept of Fluid Responsiveness

When making the decision to infuse fluids in a patient with acute circulatory failure, one will face a therapeutic dilemma. On the one hand, the fluid-induced increase in cardiac preload might increase cardiac output, and on the other one, it may contribute to fluid overload, a condition that has been clearly demonstrated to be associated with poor outcome, especially in patients with sepsis and acute respiratory distress syndrome (ARDS) [2].

The administration of a fluid bolus increases the mean systemic pressure, which is the upstream pressure of the systemic venous return [3]. The resulting increase in cardiac preload influences cardiac output according to the physiological relationship between these two variables. The Frank-Starling relationship is curvilinear, and the slope of the curve depends on the systolic function of both ventricles [4] (Fig. 1). Thus, the

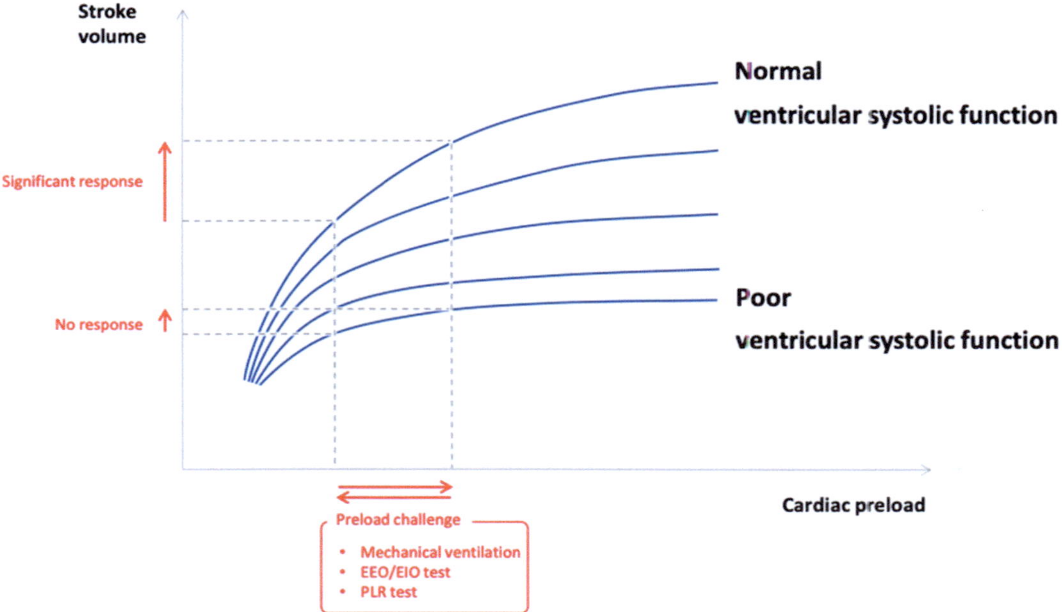

Fig. 1 Frank-Starling relationship and principles of the dynamic prediction of fluid responsiveness. The slope of the Frank-Starling curve reflects the degree of preload responsiveness. It is indicated by the response of stroke volume to changes in cardiac preload, either spontaneous during mechanical ventilation or induced by end-expiratory occlusion (EEO), end-inspiratory occlusion (EIO) or passive leg raising (PLR)

same volume of fluid administered can result in either a significant or a negligible increase in stroke volume and cardiac output. Apart from the extreme cases of profound hypovolaemia (absolute hypovolaemia in the event of hypovolemic shock, relative hypovolaemia at the initial phase of septic shock before resuscitation), this increase in cardiac output only occurs on average in half of the cases [5].

If effective on cardiac output, provided the haemodilution it induces is not too significant, volume expansion induces an increase in arterial oxygen delivery [1]—tissue oxygenation may eventually improve. Moreover, if this increase in cardiac output consequently increases the mean arterial pressure, the organs perfusion pressure is increased.

However, this effectiveness is counterbalanced by notable side effects: haemodilution (except if volume expansion if made with red blood cells) [6], interstitial oedema, hydrostatic pulmonary oedema and worsening of inflammatory pulmonary oedema in case of increased pulmonary permeability, increased intra-abdominal pressure etc. [2]. Of course, if fluid infusion has not been effective on cardiac output, it exerts only deleterious effects without causing any hemodynamic benefit.

This is the reason why some methods have been investigated in order to assess fluid responsiveness at the bedside. Some of these methods can be used with POCUS, which may be especially useful when other cardiac output monitoring tools are not available at the bedside.

Before describing these methods, two major points should be emphasised. First, the question of assessing fluid responsiveness only arises in case of acute circulatory failure, that is to say when the decision to increase cardiac output is necessary because of an obvious imbalance between the oxygen supply and requirements. Second, the tests and indices described below are useless in the conditions detailed above in which hypovolemia is strong and obvious, since fluid responsiveness is certain in these cases (Fig. 1).

Static Indices of Cardiac Preload

For years, fluid administration has been based on "static" cardiac preload indices, like for example the central venous pressure (CVP). Echocardiographic static measures of preload include the left ventricular (LV) end-diastolic dimensions and all indices derived from the mitral flow and mitral annulus motion at Doppler analysis (E/e' ratio for instance).

However, all these indices do not allow one to predict before administering it whether fluids will be effective or not. The observation of the Frank-Starling relationship clearly shows that, since the slope of the Frank-Starling curve varies from one patient to another, the same given level of preload corresponding to preload unresponsiveness or responsiveness (Fig. 1). As a matter of fact, it has been clearly demonstrated that a given value of LV end-diastolic area or diameter, of E/A or E/e' ratios, does not make it possible to predict the response to volume expansion, except perhaps for extreme values [7, 8].

In contrast to this "static" method, the detection of preload responsiveness should be based on a "dynamic" approach. Its principle is to vary the cardiac preload (for dynamic *tests*), or to observe spontaneous variations in the cardiac preload (for dynamic *indices*), and to observe the effects induced on stroke volume, cardiac output or their substitutes (Fig. 1). The superiority of this dynamic approach over the static approach is very clearly established today [4].

Respiratory Variations in LV Outflow Tract Flow Velocity

Phenomena Causing the Respiratory Variability of Stroke Volume

In brief, the principle is that the more the two ventricles are preload responsive, the more stroke volume increases during inspiration and decreases during expiration under positive pressure ventilation [9, 10].

At inspiration, the intrathoracic pressure increases in the pleural space which gets transmitted to the right atrium, and the resulting increase in right atrial pressure decreases the pressure gradient of systemic venous return. The right ventricular preload decreases. If this ventricle is preload responsive, its stroke volume decreases [11]. This decrease is transmitted to the left ventricle, whose preload also decreases. Because of the pulmonary transit time, this decrease occurs at expiration. If, in turn, the left ventricle is preload responsive, the drop in preload results in a decrease in its stroke volume [11] (Fig. 1).

Other phenomena also likely to play a role in this process. In addition to the decrease in right ventricular preload, positive pressure insufflation decreases the pressure gradient between the inside and outside of the left ventricle, which facilitates its ejection and decreases its afterload. This contributes to the expiratory increase in the LV stroke volume [10]. Also, the increase in intrathoracic pressure increases the transpulmonary pressure (alveolar pressure—intrathoracic pressure). The resulting stretch of the pulmonary vessels propels blood toward the left ventricle, contributing to increase in its preload [11]. In total, all of these phenomena explain that in the case of preload responsiveness of both ventricles, stroke volume increases on expiration and decreases on inspiration.

Stroke Volume Surrogates Used to Measure Its Respiratory Variation

Several surrogates of stroke volume have been used to assess preload responsiveness through their respiratory variation. The first that has been described is arterial pulse pressure, as it is proportional to stroke volume [11]. Pulse pressure variation (PPV) is the index of preload responsiveness that has received the highest level of evidence [12].

Echocardiography estimates the LV stroke volume through the velocity–time integral

(VTI) of the systolic pulsed Doppler signal when the pulsed wave Doppler sampling volume is placed in the LV outflow tract (LVOT). The signal area, i.e. the product of time and velocity, is proportional to LV stroke volume. Then, the respiratory variation of the LV outflow, reflected by the variation in its maximal velocity (LVOT velocity variation, LVOTVV), has been shown to detect preload responsiveness [8] (Fig. 2).

This might be interesting in practice when no monitoring technique is in place and when POCUS is the only means to assess the haemodynamic status. However, measuring the LVOTVV is difficult, especially through the transthoracic route since the ultrasound beam must be kept within the outflow despite its motion during respiration. At least, when an arterial catheter is present, assessing PPV is much easier.

It has been suggested that the phasic changes in the peak velocity in peripheral arteries reflect the respiratory change in stroke volume in mechanically ventilated patients. This may help predicting fluid responsiveness and might be easier to assess than the variation in the LVOT VTI. The diagnostic ability is likely better for carotid than for brachial artery respiratory variation [13].

Limitations of the LVOTVV

As stated above, assessing LVOTVV might be difficult as it requires that the ultrasound beam is kept in the middle of the LV outflow despite the respiratory movements. Also, like all indices which detect preload responsiveness by estimating the respiratory changes in stroke volume,

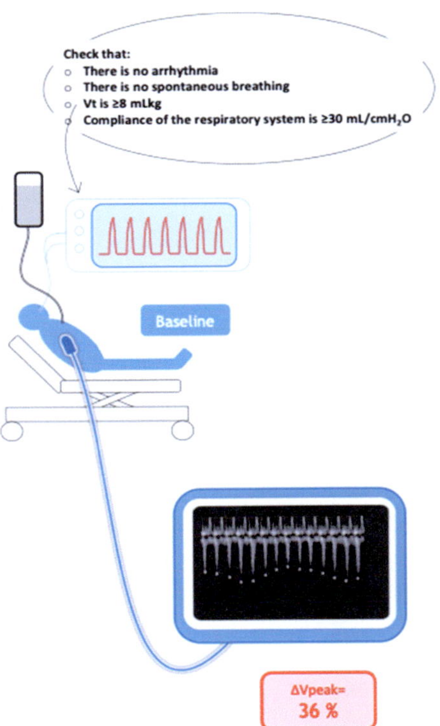

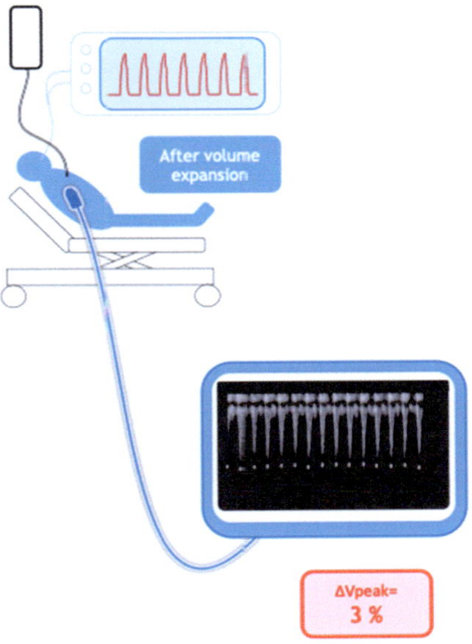

Fig. 2 Respiratory variation in the peak velocity in the left ventricular outflow tract. Under mechanical ventilation, the respiratory variation of the peak velocity in the left ventricular outflow tract (ΔVpeak) is high at baseline, indicating preload responsiveness. Fluid infusion leads to an increase in stroke volume, as reflected by the velocity time integral in the left ventricular outflow tract, and a reduction in ΔVpeak. Preload responsiveness is likely ΔVpeak before fluid infusion is $\geq 12\%$

LVOTVV suffers from the fact that it cannot be used in many clinical conditions (Fig. 2).

Spontaneous Ventilation

Spontaneous ventilation, even in patients on mechanical ventilation, induces irregular respiratory efforts, either in rate or in amplitude, which may result in changes in stroke volume which are not related to preload responsiveness. This is thus responsible for some false positives to PPV and LVOTVV.

Acute Respiratory Distress Syndrome

In the case of ARDS, two factors contribute to creating false negatives for the indices of stroke volume respiratory variations. First, the low tidal volume (Vt) means that, for the same degree of preload responsiveness, the cyclic variation of stroke volume is less. This condition creates some false negatives to LVOTVV. The second factor limiting the reliability of stroke volume respiratory variations in ARDS is the decrease in pulmonary compliance [14]. In this case, the alveolar pressure variations during ventilation are transmitted to the cardiac cavities and intrathoracic vessels to a lesser extent. It has been shown that when the pulmonary compliance was ≤ 30 mL/cmH$_2$O, the prediction was poor, essentially due to false negatives [14]. Of course, similar limitations likely occur for LVOTVV.

In case of a small Vt, it is still possible to use LVOTVV to test the preload responsiveness thanks to the "Vt challenge" [15]. This test consists of temporarily increasing Vt from 6 to 8 mL/kg of predicted body weight and observing the effects induced on the respiratory changes in stroke volume. It has been initially investigated by using PPV for assessing these changes. If PPV increases by more than 3.5%, preload responsiveness can be strongly suspected [15]. Similarly, it has been shown that if the respiratory changes in LVOTVV decreases during a Vt challenge by more than one point in absolute value, or 20% in relative change, preload responsiveness is likely [16].

Cardiac Arrhythmias

It is easy to understand that in the event of atrial fibrillation or frequent extrasystoles, the variability of the volume of systolic ejection is not only due to preload responsiveness. This is responsible for some false positives for PPV and LVOTVV.

Very High Respiratory Rate

In case of high respiratory rate, the small number of cardiac cycles occurring during a respiratory cycle does not enable the variation of stroke volume to reach its extreme values. A clinical study showed that this may occur for PPV when the heart rate/respiratory rate ratio is lower than 3.6 [17]. Again, LVOTVV is affected by the same limitation. Nevertheless, this corresponds to very high respiratory rates (28 cycles/min for heart rate at 100 beats/min, for instance) [17].

Right Ventricular Dysfunction

It has been suggested that right ventricular dysfunction may induce false positive values of stroke volume variation due to the predominant effect of mechanical insufflation on the right ventricular afterload through the compression of intra-alveolar microvessels by the transpulmonary pressure. As the failing right ventricle is very sensitive to its afterload, the decrease in right ventricular stroke volume during insufflation would be more related to right ventricular afterload-dependence than to right ventricular preload-dependence [18, 19]. This limitation likely affects LVOTVV as well. However, in the latter studies, Vt was greater than 8 mL/kg, and it is possible that right ventricular afterload dependence is attenuated at a lower Vt.

Intra-Abdominal Hypertension

An animal study suggests that in cases of intra-abdominal hypertension, PPV can still predict fluid responsiveness, but with a higher threshold value than that in the case of normal intra-abdominal pressure [20]. Nevertheless, the increase in intra-abdominal pressure was extreme in this experimental study. Conversely, in a clinical study in acute liver failure, PPV predicted fluid responsiveness, whereas the respiratory changes in the velocity–time integral did not [21].

In Summary

The respiratory changes in stroke volume reflect preload responsiveness. They are easily assessed through PPV in patients with an arterial line in place. Even though it is not easy to measure, LVOTVV measured by echocardiography can be used as a surrogate of PPV in the absence of continuous arterial pressure monitoring. Nevertheless, such indices cannot be used in many common circumstances, especially in critically ill patients.

Variability of the Diameter of the Venae Cavae

Phenomena Causing Respiratory Variability in the Diameter of Venae Cavae

Several phenomena are involved in these variations. Regarding those of the inferior vena cava (IVC), mechanical ventilation leads to a variability in CVP which is greater in the case of preload dependence than in the case of preload unresponsiveness [22]. In other words, the intramural pressure of the IVC varies. In addition, the transmission of variations in intrathoracic pressure to the abdominal cavity explains cyclic variations in the extramural pressure of the vein. The resulting variations in the diameter of the IVC are possibly greater if the compliance of the vein is high, which is more likely to occur in hypovolaemia than in case of large blood volume. With regard to the superior vena cava, the phenomena are likely identical, except of course that the extramural pressure is the intrathoracic pressure.

Thus, variations in the dimensions of the inferior or superior vena cava are not explained by the changes in stroke volume induced by changes in cardiac preload. These variabilities do not reflect the slope of the Frank-Starling relationship as do PPV or LVOTVV, for instance.

Reliability

This may be the reason why the reliability of these indices to reflect preload responsiveness is generally poor. Despite initial positive studies, several subsequent publications have reported moderate or poor diagnostic capabilities. Several meta-analyses confirmed these results [23, 24]. In a large multicentre study including 540 patients, the area under the receiver operating characteristics curve (ROC) was only 0.65 for variations in the IVC and 0.74 for those in the superior one [25].

Limitations

In addition to their lack of reliability, the indices based on the diameter of the cava veins suffer from not being able to be used in several clinical circumstances.

In the same way as PPV and LVOTVV, these indices experience false negatives in the event of low Vt [16] and, probably, of low pulmonary compliance. Spontaneous respiratory activity induces false positives, for the same reasons as for PPV and LVOTVV. On the other hand, because the variations are independent of the cardiac cycle, the indices remain valid in the event of cardiac arrhythmias. For the inferior vena cava, intra-abdominal hypertension is another condition in which reliability is reduced [25].

In Summary

The variability of the diameter of the superior or inferior venae cavae do not directly reflect the relationship between stroke volume and cardiac preload, as they are also influenced by the extramural pressures of the vessels. It is now established that these indices of fluid responsiveness are the ones with the lowest reliability. In addition, they share many conditions of use with PPV and LVOTVV.

Mini Fluid Challenge

The most obvious way to detect preload responsiveness dynamically is to administer fluid and measure the response of cardiac output. With echocardiography, this response can be assessed through the relative changes in LVOT VTI, which reflect simultaneous changes in LV stroke volume. De facto, the method of injecting 300 to 500 mL of fluid to guide fluid strategy has been used for many years [26]. Nevertheless, the fluid "challenge" is not a diagnostic test, but the treatment itself. It is not certain that a patient who has just responded to a fluid challenge by a significant increase in cardiac output will still do so during the next one since the 300 or 500 mL of the first challenge may have made the patient already preload independent.

This is the reason why some authors have suggested to administer smaller quantities of fluid to challenge cardiac preload. It has been demonstrated that the response to volume expansion could be detected by measuring changes in the VTI of the LVOT when 100 mL of colloid were administered [27].

Nevertheless, cardiac output changes induced by a mini-fluid challenge can only be small. Therefore, the method requires a very precise measurement of cardiac output. From this point of view, echocardiography may not be the ideal method [28], especially in non-expert's hands. It has been established that the smallest change in VTI of the LVOT that can be detected with echocardiography is 12% [28].

In Summary

The mini fluid challenge can be used to predict fluid responsiveness in patients for whom the risk of fluid overload is not excessive. When echocardiography is used to assess its effects

through the VTI in the LVOT, it must be kept in mind that the threshold defining the test positivity is near the reproducibility limit of ultrasound.

Respiratory Occlusion Tests

Principle

During mechanical ventilation, each insufflation increases the intrathoracic pressure and, consequently, the right atrial pressure, which opposes the systemic venous return. When mechanical ventilation is interrupted by end-expiration for a few seconds, the cyclical decrease in cardiac preload is interrupted. Cardiac preload increases transiently. If, in response, cardiac output increases, it means that both ventricles are preload responsive. Conversely, an end-inspiratory pause should decrease cardiac output in case of preload-dependence. Importantly, the duration of the ventilator occlusion should be long enough for the "preload bolus" to pass through the pulmonary circulation. Five seconds is insufficient [29], and the studies reported a reliable test when occlusions of 12–30 s were performed [29–32].

End-Expiratory Occlusion Test

It has been shown that if cardiac output increases by more than 5% in the last few seconds of an expiratory pause of at least 15 s, the response to volume expansion could be predicted with good reliability [30]. The test has the advantage of being easy to perform, especially when compared with the passive leg raising (PLR) test [33].

Combination of End-Inspiratory and End-Expiratory Occlusions

The increase in the VTI of the LV outflow tract measured by echocardiography during an end-expiratory occlusion may predict the response to volume expansion [31, 34]. Nevertheless, the diagnostic threshold might be low compared to the accuracy of echocardiography [28].

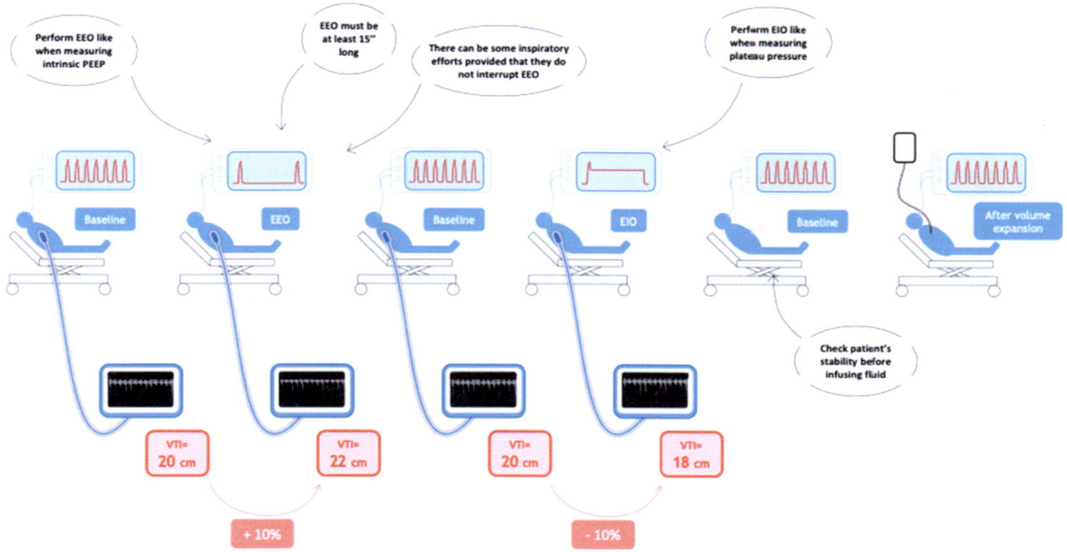

Fig. 3 **The end-expiratory and end-inspiratory occlusion tests.** Under mechanical ventilation, preload responsiveness is associated with a significant increase in the velocity time integral (VTI) in the left ventricular outflow tract during a 15-s end-expiratory occlusion (EEO) and with a significant decrease in VTI during a 15-s end-inspiratory occlusion (EIO). Preload responsiveness is likely if the sum of both changes (in absolute value) is $\geq 15\%$

Therefore, we proposed to combine a 15-s end-inspiratory pause with a 15-s end-expiratory pause, performed a few seconds apart [35] (Fig. 3). We have shown that end-inspiratory occlusion decreased the LVOT VTI more in preload responsive patients than in the other ones. Interestingly, if we considered the sum of the effects on the VTI of the end-expiratory and the end-inspiratory occlusions, the prediction of fluid responsiveness was made with sensitivity and a specificity identical to those obtained with end-expiratory occlusion alone, but with a diagnostic threshold of 13% [35], which is more compatible with the precision of echocardiography [28].

Limitations

Respiratory occlusion tests can only be performed, of course, in patients under mechanical ventilation. In addition, patients must be able to support relatively long breathing occlusions. This is not a problem in the operating room during anaesthesia but may be a significant limitation in some critically ill patients.

The level of positive end-expiratory pressure might be theoretically important, since it is the level to which the airway pressure is reduced during end-expiratory occlusion. However, in a previous study in which two levels of positive end-expiratory pressure were compared in the same patients, the diagnostic accuracy of the end-expiratory occlusion test was unchanged [36] and this has been confirmed in a meta-analysis [30].

Another factor that might theoretically affect the end-expiratory occlusion test reliability is Vt. Two studies reported that diagnostic accuracy of the end-expiratory occlusion test was correct with a Vt of 8 mL/kg but poorer if it was 6 mL/kg [15, 37]. However, even if they did not directly compare different Vt levels, some of the other studies which reported excellent diagnostic accuracy had included some patients with low Vt values, as indicated by the mean and standard deviation reported in their whole population [30].

Moreover, the effect of Vt on the end-expiratory occlusion test reliability has not been confirmed in a meta-analysis [30].

In Summary

The reliability of the expiratory occlusion test is established today [30]. Performing it by means of echocardiography is more restrictive and likely requires both end-inspiratory and end-expiratory occlusions (Fig. 3).

Passive Leg Raising

Principle

The transition from the semi-recumbent position to a position in which the lower limbs are raised to 45° and the trunk is horizontal induces the transfer of venous blood from the lower limbs, but also from the splanchnic territory, toward the heart chambers. This results in a significant increase in mean systemic pressure, the upstream systemic venous return pressure [3], and in right and left cardiac preload. Therefore, PLR can be used as a preload dependence challenge. If cardiac output increases in response to the preload increase, both ventricles are likely preload-dependent and fluid responsiveness is likely. The advantage over pulse pressure or stroke volume variations is that it can be used even in case of spontaneous breathing or cardiac arrhythmias, even in case of low Vt and lung compliance in patients under mechanical ventilation. Compared to the standard fluid challenge, the PLR test does not induce haemodilution. As it is reversible, it is not at risk of inducing hydrostatic pulmonary oedema. It has been shown that a PLR test was equivalent to about 300 mL of fluid challenge [38], but this is an average value as this volume might highly vary depending on the patient.

Reliability

Many studies have shown that the PLR test can reliably detect preload dependence. The diagnostic threshold for increasing cardiac output during PLR is 10% [39]. A great advantage of the test is that it remains valid even in clinical circumstances where PPV or stroke volume variation cannot be used. In particular, the PLR test retains all its diagnostic value in case of spontaneous breathing, cardiac arrhythmia [14], ventilation at low Vt or low lung compliance [14].

Two meta-analyses confirmed the diagnostic value of the PLR test [39, 40]. It has been included in the most recent version of the Surviving Sepsis Campaign's guidelines [41] and in the statements of a consensus conference on haemodynamic monitoring and shock of the European Society of Intensive Care Medicine [42].

Cardiac Output Measurement Techniques

The effects of the PLR test should be measured directly on cardiac output [43]. Indeed, if these effects are assessed on arterial pressure, the sensitivity of the test is lower, and the number of false-negatives is greater [39, 40].

Several cardiac output measurement techniques can be used for this purpose. They must meet the requirement to measure flow continuously and in real time, in order to capture the maximum effect of the test. In fact, when the PLR test is positive, the increase in cardiac output occurs during the first minute [44]. Nevertheless, it may occur that cardiac output decreases after reaching this maximum. This effect is particularly observed in patients with severe septic shock, whose vasodilatation is marked. This is, for example, not possible to detect with thermodilution, neither classic pulmonary nor transpulmonary.

Echocardiography is perfectly suitable to assess the PLR-induced changes in stroke volume in real time, through the changes in VTI in the LVOT (Fig. 4). Some studies have suggested that the effects of PLR can be followed by changes in the maximum velocity of systemic arterial flow, measured at the carotid [45, 46] or femoral [47] level. However, disappointing results have been reported with this method [48], so it cannot be reasonably recommended. It has also been suggested that PLR-induced changes in the duration of the carotid flow (corrected carotid flow time) could be used to assess the volume status [49, 50].

Limitations

As stated above, the main limitation of the PLR test is that it requires a direct measurement of cardiac output. Also, the test is difficult or impossible to use during a surgical procedure and is reasonably contra-indicated in case of intracranial hypertension. It is probably less sensitive in patients with venous compression stocking. Finally, in case of intra-abdominal hypertension, the volume of the splanchnic compartment is reduced, and this condition is responsible for false negatives to the PLR test [51].

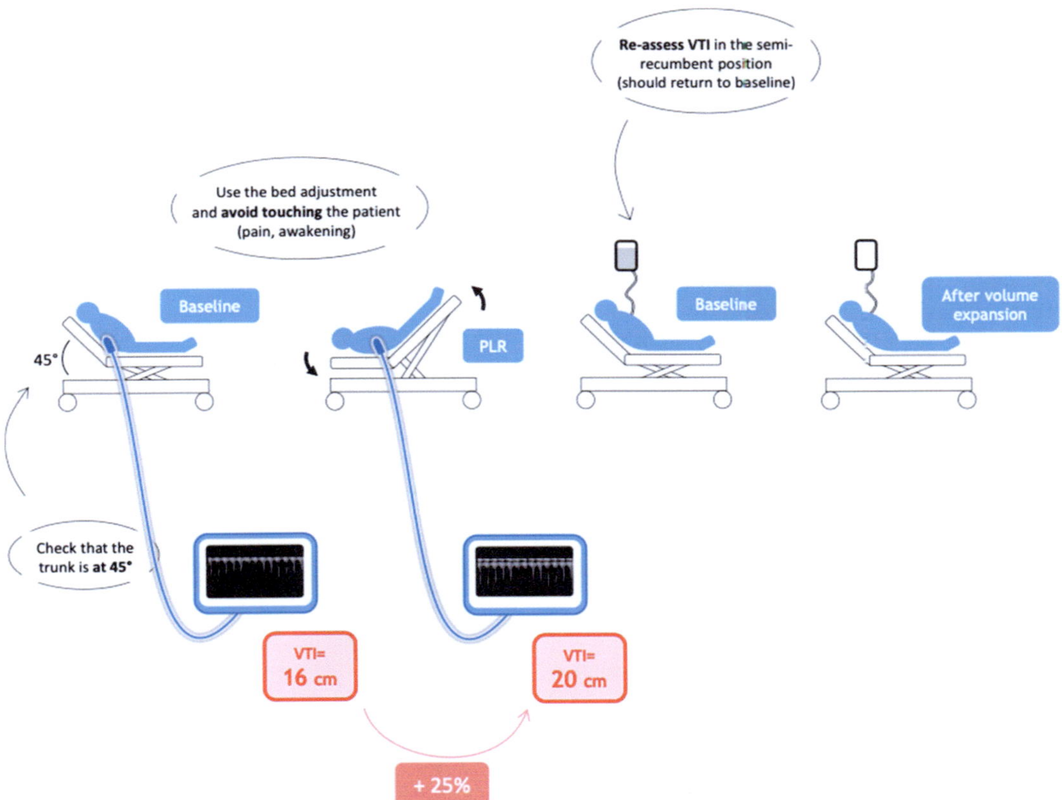

Fig. 4 The passive leg raising test. The increase in the velocity time integral (VTI) in the left ventricular outflow tract during passive leg raising (PLR) indicates preload responsiveness. Preload responsiveness is likely if the PLR-induced increase in VTI is $\geq 10\%$

In Summary

In adults, the PLR test is a way of predicting fluid responsiveness which reliability is well established. It has the advantage of supplementing PPV and stroke volume variation under the conditions where these heart–lung interaction indices cannot be used. With POCUS, its effects are assessed through relative changes in the LVOT VTI.

Conclusion

With POCUS, several tests or indices are available to predict fluid responsiveness before performing volume expansion. The respiratory variation of the LVOT peak velocity cannot be used in many circumstances. The respiratory variation in the diameter of the inferior of superior venae cavae are likely the least reliable indices or fluid responsiveness. The mini-fluid challenge is reliable, but its diagnostic threshold is near the reproducibility threshold of echocardiography. Successive end-inspiratory and expiratory occlusions can be used only in ventilated patients. Passive leg raising has received a very large level of evidence. Its effects are easily measured through changes in the VTI in the LVOT, but it is doubtful whether changes in arterial femoral or carotid velocity are reliable enough.

References

1. Monnet X, Teboul JL. My patient has received fluid. How to assess its efficacy and side effects? Ann Intensive Care. 2018; 8(1):54.
2. Malbrain M, Van Regenmortel N, Saugel B, De Tavernier B, Van Gaal PJ, Joannes-Boyau O, Teboul JL, Rice TW, Mythen M, Monnet X. Principles of fluid management and stewardship in septic shock: it is time to consider the four D's and the four phases of fluid therapy. Ann Intensive Care. 2018;8 (1):66.
3. Guerin L, Teboul JL, Persichini R, Dres M, Richard C, Monnet X. Effects of passive leg raising and volume expansion on mean systemic pressure and venous return in shock in humans. Crit Care. 2015;19:411.
4. Monnet X, Marik P, Teboul JL. Prediction of fluid responsiveness: an update. Ann Intensive Care. 2017;6(1):111.
5. Michard F, Teboul JL. Predicting fluid responsiveness in ICU patients: a critical analysis of the evidence. Chest. 2002;121(6):2000–8.
6. Monnet X, Julien F, Ait-Hamou N, Lequoy M, Gosset C, Jozwiak M, Persichini R, Anguel N, Richard C, Teboul JL. Lactate and venoarterial carbon dioxide difference/arterial-venous oxygen difference ratio, but not central venous oxygen saturation, predict increase in oxygen consumption in fluid responders. Crit Care Med. 2013;41(6):1412–20,
7. Feissel M, Michard F, Faller JP, Teboul JL. The respiratory variation in inferior vena cava diameter as a guide to fluid therapy. Intensive Care Med. 2004;30 (9):1834–7.
8. Feissel M, Michard F, Mangin I, Ruyer O, Faller JP, Teboul JL. Respiratory changes in aortic blood velocity as an indicator of fluid responsiveness in ventilated patients with septic shock. Chest. 2001;119(3):867–73.
9. Michard F, Teboul JL. Using heart-lung interactions to assess fluid responsiveness during mechanical ventilation. Crit Care. 2000;4(5):282–9.
10. Teboul JL, Monnet X, Chemla D, Michard F. Arterial pulse pressure variation with mechanical ventilation. Am J Respir Crit Care Med. 2019;199 (1):22–31.
11. Teboul JL, Monnet X, Chemla D, Michard F. Arterial Pulse Pressure Variation with Mechanical Ventilation. Am J Respir Crit Care Med. 2018.
12. Yang X, Du B. Does pulse pressure variation predict fluid responsiveness in critically ill patients? A systematic review and meta-analysis. Crit Care. 2014;18(6):650.
13. Yao B, Liu JY, Sun YB. Respiratory variation in peripheral arterial blood flow peak velocity to predict fluid responsiveness in mechanically ventilated patients: a systematic review and meta-analysis. BMC Anesthesiol. 2018;18(1):168.
14. Monnet X, Bleibtreu A, Ferré A, Dres M, Gharbi R, Richard C, Teboul JL. Passive leg raising and end-expiratory occlusion tests perform better than pulse pressure variation in patients with low respiratory system compliance. Crit Care Med. 2012;40:152–7.
15. Myatra SN, Prabu SR, Divatia JV, Monnet X, Kulkarni AP, Teboul JL. The changes in pulse pressure variation or stroke volume variation after a "tidal volume challenge" reliably predict fluid responsiveness during low tidal volume ventilation. Crit Care Med. 2016;45:415–21.
16. Taccheri T, Gavelli F, Teboul JL, Shi R, Monnet X. Do changes in pulse pressure variation and inferior vena cava distensibility during passive leg raising

and tidal volume challenge detect preload responsiveness in case of low tidal volume ventilation? Crit Care. 2021;25(1):110.

17. De Backer D, Taccone FS, Holsten R, Ibrahimi F, Vincent JL. Influence of respiratory rate on stroke volume variation in mechanically ventilated patients. Anesthesiology. 2009;110(5):1092–7.

18. Mahjoub Y, Pila C, Friggeri A, Zogheib E, Lobjoie E, Tinturier F, Galy C, Slama M, Dupont H. Assessing fluid responsiveness in critically ill patients: false-positive pulse pressure variation is detected by Doppler echocardiographic evaluation of the right ventricle. Crit Care Med. 2009;37(9):2570–5.

19. Wyler von Ballmoos M, Takala J, Roeck M, Porta F, Tueller D, Ganter CC, Schroder R, Bracht H, Baenziger B, Jakob SM. Pulse-pressure variation and hemodynamic response in patients with elevated pulmonary artery pressure: a clinical study. Crit Care. 2010; 14(3):R111.

20. Jacques D, Bendjelid K, Duperret S, Colling J, Piriou V, Viale JP. Pulse pressure variation and stroke volume variation during increased intra-abdominal pressure: an experimental study. Crit Care. 2011;15(1):R33.

21. Audimoolam VK, McPhail MJ, Willars C, Bernal W, Wendon JA, Cecconi M, Auzinger G. Predicting fluid responsiveness in acute liver failure: a prospective study. Anesth Analg. 2017;124(2):480–6.

22. Magder S, Georgiadis G, Cheong T. Respiratory variations in right atrial pressure predict the response to fluid challenge. J Crit Care. 1992;1992(7):76–85.

23. Long E, Oakley E, Duke T, Babl FE. Paediatric research in emergency departments international C: does respiratory variation in inferior vena cava diameter predict fluid responsiveness: a systematic review and meta-analysis. Shock. 2017;47(5):550–9.

24. Das SK, Choupoo NS, Pradhan D, Saikia P, Monnet X. Diagnostic accuracy of inferior vena caval respiratory variation in detecting fluid unresponsiveness: a systematic review and meta-analysis. Eur J Anaesthesiol. 2018;35(11):831–9.

25. Vieillard-Baron A, Evrard B, Repesse X, Maizel J, Jacob C, Goudelin M, Charron C, Prat G, Slama M, Geri G et al. Limited value of end-expiratory inferior vena cava diameter to predict fluid responsiveness impact of intra-abdominal pressure. Intensive Care Med. 2018.

26. Vincent JL, Weil MH. Fluid challenge revisited. Crit Care Med. 2006;34(5):1333–7.

27. Muller L, Toumi M, Bousquet PJ, Riu-Poulenc B, Louart G, Candela D, Zoric L, Suehs C, de La Coussaye JE, Molinari N et al. An increase in aortic blood flow after an infusion of 100 ml colloid over 1 minute can predict fluid responsiveness: the mini-fluid challenge study. Anesthesiology. 2011; 115 (3):541–547.

28. Jozwiak M, Mercado P, Teboul JL, Benmalek A, Gimenez J, Depret F, Richard C, Monnet X: What is the lowest change in cardiac output that transthoracic echocardiography can detect? Crit Care. 2019 (In press).

29. Monnet X, Osman D, Ridel C, Lamia B, Richard C, Teboul JL. Predicting volume responsiveness by using the end-expiratory occlusion in mechanically ventilated intensive care unit patients. Crit Care Med. 2009;37(3):951–6.

30. Gavelli F, Shi R, Teboul JL, Azzolina D, Monnet X. The end-expiratory occlusion test for detecting preload responsiveness: a systematic review and meta-analysis. Ann Intensive Care. 2020;10(1):65.

31. Georges D, de Courson H, Lanchon R, Sesay M, Nouette-Gaulain K, Biais M. End-expiratory occlusion maneuver to predict fluid responsiveness in the intensive care unit: an echocardiographic study. Crit Care. 2018;22(1):32.

32. Biais M, Larghi M, Henriot J, de Courson H, Sesay M, Nouette-Gaulain K. End-expiratory occlusion test predicts fluid responsiveness in patients with protective ventilation in the operating room. Anesth Analg. 2017;125(6):1889–95.

33. Gavelli F, Teboul JL, Monnet X. The end-expiratory occlusion test: please, let me hold your breath! Crit Care. 2019; 23(1):274.

34. Jozwiak M, Monnet X, Teboul JL. Pressure waveform analysis. Anesth Analg. 2018;126(6):1930–3.

35. Jozwiak M, Depret F, Teboul JL, Alphonsine JE, Lai C, Richard C, Monnet X. Predicting fluid responsiveness in critically ill patients by using combined end-expiratory and end-inspiratory occlusions with echocardiography. Crit Care Med. 2017;45(11):e1131–8.

36. Silva S, Teboul JL. Defining the adequate arterial pressure target during septic shock: not a 'micro' issue but the microcirculation can help. Crit Care. 2011;15(6):1004.

37. Messina A, Montagnini C, Cammarota G, De Rosa S, Giuliani F, Muratore L, Della Corte F, Navalesi P, Cecconi M. Tidal volume challenge to predict fluid responsiveness in the operating room: an observational study. Eur J Anaesthesiol. 2019;36 (8):583–91.

38. Jabot J, Teboul JL, Richard C, Monnet X. Passive leg raising for predicting fluid responsiveness: importance of the postural change. Intensive Care Med. 2009;35(1):85–90.

39. Monnet X, Marik P, Teboul JL. Passive leg raising for predicting fluid responsiveness: a systematic review and meta-analysis. Intensive Care Med. 2016;42(12):1935–47.

40. Cherpanath TG, Hirsch A, Geerts BF, Lagrand WK, Leeflang MM, Schultz MJ, Groeneveld AB. Predicting fluid responsiveness by passive leg raising: a systematic review and meta-analysis of 23 clinical trials. Crit Care Med. 2016;44(5):981–91.

41. Rhodes A, Evans LE, Alhazzani W, Levy MM, Antonelli M, Ferrer R, Kumar A, Sevransky JE, Sprung CL, Nunnally ME, et al. Surviving sepsis campaign: international guidelines for management

of sepsis and septic shock: 2016. Intensive Care Med. 2017;43(3):304–77.

42. Cecconi M, De Backer D, Antonelli M, Beale R, Bakker J, Hofer C, Jaeschke R, Mebazaa A, Pinsky MR, Teboul JL et al. Consensus on circulatory shock and hemodynamic monitoring. Task force of the European society of intensive care medicine. Intensive Care Med. 2014; 40(12):1795–1815.

43. Monnet X, Teboul JL. Passive leg raising: five rules, not a drop of fluid! Crit Care. 2015; 19(1):18.

44. Monnet X, Rienzo M, Osman D, Anguel N, Richard C, Pinsky MR, Teboul JL. Passive leg raising predicts fluid responsiveness in the critically ill. Crit Care Med. 2006;34(5):1402–7.

45. Barjaktarevic I, Toppen WE, Hu S, Aquije Montoya E, Ong S, Buhr R, David IJ, Wang T, Rezayat T, Chang SY et al. Ultrasound assessment of the change in carotid corrected flow time in fluid responsiveness in undifferentiated shock. Crit Care Med. 2018; 46 (11):e1040–e1046.

46. Marik PE, Levitov A, Young A, Andrews L. The use of bioreactance and carotid Doppler to determine volume responsiveness and blood flow redistribution following passive leg raising in hemodynamically unstable patients. Chest. 2013;143(2):364–70.

47. Preau S, Saulnier F, Dewavrin F, Durocher A, Chagnon JL. Passive leg raising is predictive of fluid responsiveness in spontaneously breathing patients with severe sepsis or acute pancreatitis. Crit Care Med. 2010;38:989–90.

48. Girotto V, Teboul JL, Beurton A, Galarza L, Richard C, Monnet X. Can carotid and femoral Doppler assess the effects of passive leg raising? Ann Intensive Care. 2017; 7(suppl1).

49. Jalil B, Thompson P, Cavallazzi R, Marik P, Mann J, El-Kersh K, Guardiola J, Saad M. Comparing changes in carotid flow time and stroke volume induced by passive leg raising. Am J Med Sci. 2018; 355(2):168–173.

50. Chebl RB, Wuhantu J, Kiblawi S, Dagher GA, Zgheib H, Bachir R, Carnell J. Corrected carotid flow time and passive leg raise as a measure of volume status. Am J Emerg Med. 2019;37(8):1460–5.

51. Beurton A, Teboul JL, Girotto V, Galarza L, Anguel N, Richard C, Monnet X. Intra-abdominal hypertension is responsible for false negatives to the passive leg raising test. Crit Care Med. 2019;47(8): e639–47.

Systemic Venous Congestion

Korbin Haycock, Rory Spiegel,
and Philippe Rola

How to find what you're not looking for

Veera Hiranandani—American-Indian contemporary writer

Abstract

Systemic venous congestion is an underappreciated component of the hemodynamic system. The clinical significance of venous congestion has been demonstrated in multiple studies and has been shown to affect multiple organ systems, both in acute and chronic disease. A POCUS evaluation designated as the VExUS (Venous Excess with UltraSound) protocol was designed to assess venous congestion using the combination of hepatic, portal, and intrarenal venous Doppler in the setting of a plethoric IVC. The method of acquiring the various Doppler patterns and the VExUS scoring system is discussed.

K. Haycock
Emergency Medicine, Loma Linda University, Loma Linda, CA, USA

R. Spiegel
Attending Physician, Department of Emergency Medicine, University of Maryland, Baltimore, USA

P. Rola (✉)
Intensive Care Unit, Santa Cabrini Hospital CEMTL, Montreal, Canada
e-mail: philipperola@gmail.com

Keywords

Venous congestion · VExUS · Point-of-care ultrasound · Acute kidney injury · Fluid balance

Key Messages

- Systemic venous congestion is an often unappreciated but important hemodynamic entity and is associated with many adverse clinical outcomes.
- Systemic venous congestion is the result of volume overload, cardiac dysfunction, or a combination of both.
- Systemic venous Congestion can be quantified using the VExUS score, which utilizes hepatic, portal, and intrarenal venous Doppler to assess the degree of congestion and guide therapeutic progress.

Introduction

The most common approach to hemodynamic monitoring and resuscitation focuses on parameters such as blood pressure and cardiac output, therefore concentrating the clinician's efforts on the arterial side of the systemic circulation. The contribution of the venous side of the circulatory system is often largely ignored with little regard to right atrial pressures or the effect of venous congestion on tissue perfusion. It should be appreciated that the driving pressure of capillary refill is not the difference of the mean arterial pressure and central venous pressure, but rather the post-arteriolar resistors pressure minus the post-capillary venule pressure. Because of this, the importance of abnormally elevated venous pressure and the resulting congestion on tissue perfusion should always be considered in concert with the arterial blood pressure. In addition to the direct negative hemodynamic effects of venous congestion, the often coexistent and related interstitial tissue edema has negative effects on tissue perfusion. Increases in capillary hydrostatic pressure in combination with endothelial dysfunction and dysregulation, often the consequence of liberal fluid administration and/or inflammatory conditions, lead to the accumulation of interstitial fluid. This not only increases diffusional distances for gas and waste exchange, but in the setting of an encapsulated organ, perfusion pressures are further decreased as intracapsular pressures rise.

One hundred and fifty years ago, Ludwig demonstrated in animal hemodynamic studies that a central venous pressure exceeding 10 mmHg resulted in a decrease in urine output and Winton elegantly showed in 1931 that venous pressure rise actually impaired renal perfusion more so than an equivalent drop in arterial pressure [1].

The clinical significance of venous congestion has been well demonstrated. A positive fluid balance has repeatedly been shown to be associated with adverse outcomes in critically ill patients [2–10]. The kidney has been demonstrated to be highly susceptible to venous congestion. This has been shown in both the acutely ill and those with chronic congestive disease [11–20]. The portal system, being the venous drainage for most of the abdominal organs has been implicated in significant disease when portal hypertension is present due to venous congestion [21, 22]. Gut edema associated with

portal hypertension causes impaired absorption of nutrients and medications and the breakdown of the gut-blood barrier. This leads to malnutrition, systemic inflammation and the release of pro-inflammatory cytokines, bacterial translocation across the gut wall, and possibly the continuance of the sepsis syndrome [21–25]. Encephalopathy and ICU delirium correlates with portal vein pulsatility (a marker of venous congestion) [26] and cerebral perfusion is decreased in circumstances where venous drainage is impeded, or elevated central venous pressure is present [27–30].

The degree of venous pressure is an interplay of intravascular volume status, venous compliance, and right ventricular function. An upstream venous pressure that generates venous return to the heart is dependent on both the venous system's vascular tone and the volume filling the veins. Flow is opposed by the downstream right atrial pressure, which is determined by the efficiency of the right ventricle in its ability to pump the flow of venous return forward into the pulmonary arterial circuit [31]. Fluctuations in pressure at the right atrium associated with the cardiac cycle are always transmitted to the veins near to the heart. These pressure fluctuations are commonly described as the jugular venous pulse. In healthy individuals, with distance from the heart, these pulsations disappear, and venous flow becomes phasic in nature in the peripheral venous circulation. The reason for this phenomenon is that the venous system is quite compliant, and thus will dampen most variations in pressure as they are transmitted backward from the heart. However, when venous pressures rise to the point where the veins are stretched near to the limit of their compliance, venous pulsations are transmitted more peripherally, and these pressure oscillations can be observed as variations in flow using Doppler evaluation.

The VExUS (Venous Excess evaluation with UltraSound) protocol was developed to quantify the clinical significance of venous congestion (VExUS). When a plethoric IVC is present, the hepatic, portal, and intrarenal veins are interrogated using pulsed wave Doppler. Based on the Doppler findings, each of the three vessels'

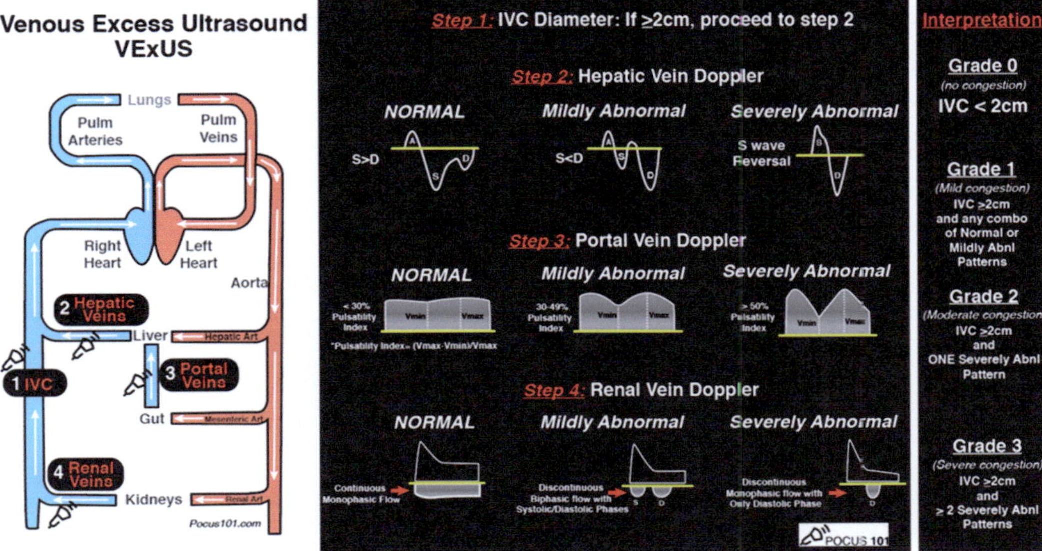

Fig. 1 VExUS scoring

characteristics are designated as either "normal", "mild congestion", or "severe congestion". In patients with normal or only mild congestion, the VExUS is assigned as "grade 1" congestion, with severe findings in one of the three veins evaluated, the VExUS is "grade 2", and if at least two of the three veins interrogated show severe congestion, the VExUS is "grade 3" (Fig. 1) [32]. The clinical significance of grade 3 congestion using the VExUS score has been demonstrated in multiple studies [32–34].

The Hepatic Vein

Due to its proximity to the right atria, Doppler signals of the hepatic vein mirror the pressure changes in the jugular venous pulse. With right atrial contraction some of the ejected blood, rather than filling the right ventricle, flows in a retrograde direction towards the hepatic veins. This is seen as an initial positive deflection above the baseline and is designated the "A" wave. With right ventricular contraction, blood flow normally reverses and then travels toward the right atria. This is due to right atrial relaxation, movement of the tricuspid annulus toward the

apex with right ventricular contraction, and ventricular ejection of their volumes, thus accommodating atrial filling within the limits of the non-compliant pericardium. The systolic flow is labeled the "S" wave. As forward flow slows at the end of systole, the Doppler signal becomes less negative and may cross the baseline. This is the "V" wave. Finally, during early diastole the tricuspid valve opens, and the atrium becomes a passive conduit for blood flow into the right ventricle. This final negative deflection is known as the "D" wave (Fig. 2).

Under normal circumstances, the A wave will have a small amplitude and duration and the S wave will have a more negative deflection than the D wave. With increasing venous congestion, the A wave will increase in both amplitude and duration and the S wave will progressively diminish, becoming smaller than the D wave. As congestion worsens, a more positive V wave is often noted. Eventually the S wave will reverse direction and often fuses with the A wave, giving the hepatic Doppler signal a biphasic appearance. With a normal hepatic Doppler pattern with the S wave greater than the D wave, the VExUS category is "grade 1". When the S wave becomes smaller than the D wave, VExUS classifies the

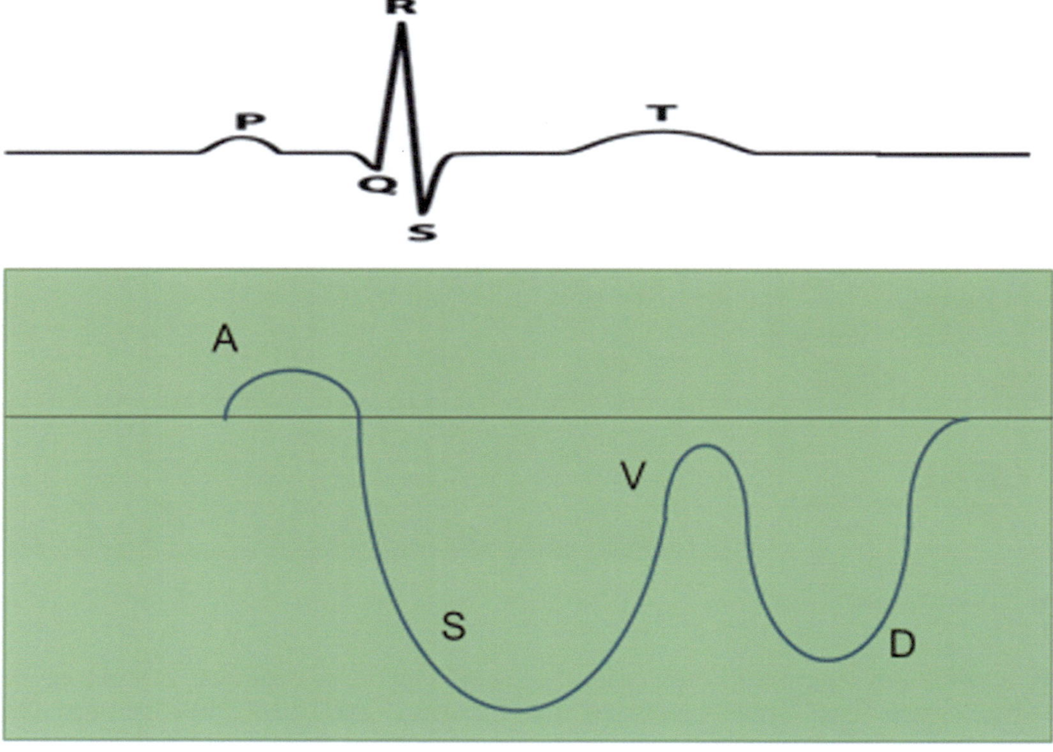

Fig. 2 Illustration of the temporal relationship between the EKG and the venous waveform

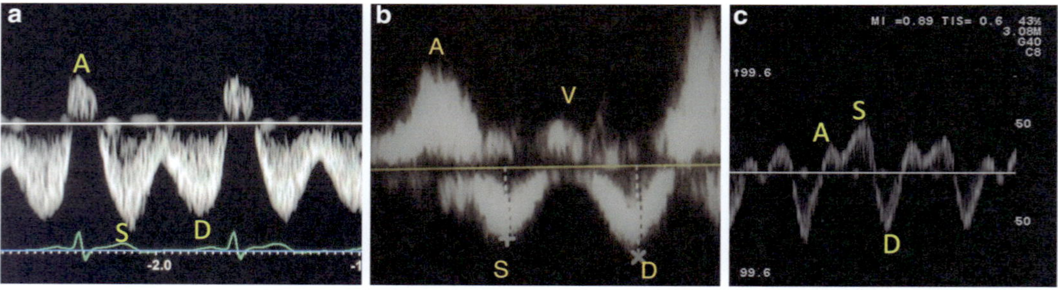

Fig. 3 Hepatic vein Doppler images showing the progression of congestion. (a) normal morphology, (b) grade 1 with S wave smaller than D wave, and (c) grade 2 with a retrograde S wave

Doppler findings as "grade 2" and with reversal of the S wave "grade 3" (Fig. 3). As stated above, these grades correspond to no significant congestion, mild congestion, and severe congestion respectively. Hepatic vein Doppler is limited in situations of severe tricuspid regurgitation, as S wave reversal may be present without significant venous congestion.

To Doppler the hepatic vein, from a subcostal echocardiography window, a pulsed wave Doppler gate is placed inside the hepatic vein about 1–2 cm within its junction with the inferior vena cava. If an adequate subcostal window is not obtainable, the right hepatic vein can often also be seen from a RUQ window at the anterior axillary or mid axillary line. It is always preferable to have a simultaneous ECG trace when interrogating the hepatic vein. This is because interpretation often becomes difficult and confusion can arise in multiple scenarios, such as when there is a prominent V wave that could be mistaken for an A wave or when there is fusion of various waves. The timing of the different deflections referenced to the ECG is thus of great assistance to interpretation of the hepatic Doppler pattern.

The Portal Vein

Most of the abdominal visceral organs' venous drainage is via the portal vein. The portal vein then branches multiple times and these branches drain into the hepatic sinusoids, which in turn will drain into the branches of the hepatic veins before finally emptying the blood into the inferior vena cava on the way to the heart. These sinusoids exhibit a significant dampening effect on hepatic vein pulsations, however once they become distended by venous congestion, the pressure waves of the hepatic vein can be transmitted up into the portal system. Normal portal blood travels at a velocity of about 20 cm/s on its way to the hepatic sinusoids. This flow is seen as an above the baseline monophasic undulating and continuous flow on Doppler.

When venous congestion is significant enough to overcome the dampening effect of the hepatic sinusoids, the portal vein will begin to exhibit a pulsatile nature, rather than the normal undulating appearance. Portal flow pulsatility is initially due to large amplitude A waves from the hepatic vein briefly slowing flow velocity as their pressures are transmitted across the sinusoids. When congestion is significant enough for S wave reversal, the pulsatile effect is amplified. The pulsatile effect can become significant enough to the point that portal flow can be interrupted or even reversed. The "pulsatility index" is used to describe the degree of portal venous congestion. The index can be calculated by taking the peak flow velocity and subtracting the minimum flow velocity, then dividing this by the peak flow velocity. A portal pulsatility index less than 0.3 is classified as "grade 1", 0.3–0.49 is "grade 2", and a pulsatility index greater than 0.5 is "grade 3" in the VExUS scheme (Fig. 4). In cases of fatty liver or cirrhosis the Doppler findings of congestion may be absent. Conversely, in young healthy thin individuals, a falsely positive pulsatile portal flow can often be seen [35, 36].

The portal vein can be imaged by placing a curvilinear or phased array probe with abdominal settings on the right upper quadrant in the anterior or mid-axillary line. The sonographer will most often need to use an intercostal window. The portal vein divides into left and right branches very near to the hilum of the liver, and the right branch usually offers near ideal Doppler angles from the above probe positioning. It may help to use the gallbladder as a reference to find the portal vein, but this is usually not required. The portal vein differs from the hepatic vein in that it is invested within the echogenic Glisson's capsule

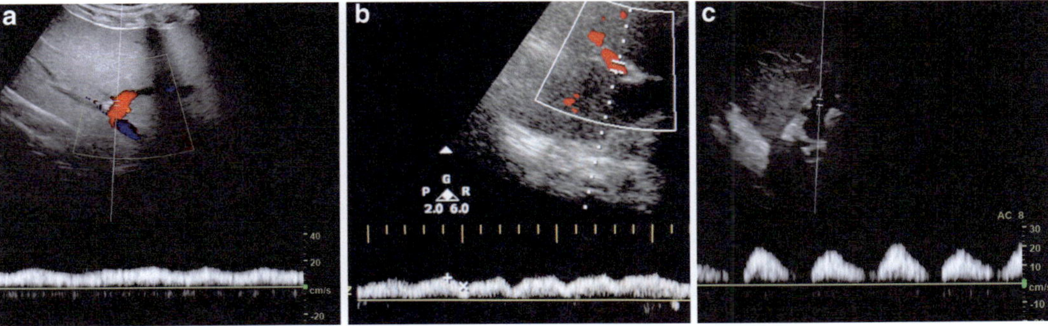

Fig. 4 Portal vein Doppler showing progression of congestion (a) normal with less than 30% pulsatility, (b) grade 1 with pulsatility between 30–50% and (c) greade 2 with pulsatility over 50%

and runs its course with the hepatic arteries and bile ducts. A pulsed wave Doppler gate is placed within the portal vein and then activated. Peak and trough velocities are measured and pulsatility index can then be calculated.

Intrarenal Venous Doppler

The renal veins enter the hilum of the kidney and travel in an antiparallel direction with the five intrarenal branches of the renal artery. Because of the proximity to the associated arteries and small size of the vessels, both the intrarenal arteries and veins are captured within the same pulsed wave Doppler gate. Therefore, when Doppler evaluation of the intrarenal vessels is performed, there will be an above the baseline pulsatile arterial trace with characteristics of a low resistance artery (with blood direction toward the probe) and a below the baseline venous trace (because blood flow is away from the probe). Flow irregularities of the intrarenal arteries manifest as a wide difference in the relative velocities of peak systolic and end-diastolic flow (calculated as a renal resistive index). In general, this difference in arterial velocities will increase with venous congestion [37], however the renal resistive index is multifactorial and generalizations about venous congestive status should not be made based on the arterial flow characteristics [38].

Normal intrarenal venous flow is similar in morphology to portal flow, being slowly undulating and non-pulsatile in nature. However, being more closely associated with the renal vein and its proximity to the inferior vena cava, the intrarenal venous Doppler characteristics share more in common with the hepatic flow patterns in the presence of venous congestion. Initially, flow does become pulsatile, just as in the portal vein, however the flow is always continuous, never crossing the baseline. As congestion worsens, the Doppler signal does cross the baseline and becomes discontinuous. When this happens, two distinct waveforms appear, one occurring during systole and one timed during diastole. These are analogous to the S and D waves of the hepatic vein and are also labeled as such. Indeed, the arterial trace that is above the baseline will demonstrate the timing of the S and D waves during the cardiac cycle. Just as the hepatic S wave diminishes in amplitude relative to the D wave and eventually reverses, the intrarenal S wave decreases in size until it disappears into the arterial trace above when it eventually reverses direction. This leaves a diastolic only interrupted waveform in severe congestion. The VExUS score of continuous and pulsatile uninterrupted flow is "grade 1", it is "grade 2" when there is interrupted flow with both S and D waves present, and "grade 3" when only the D wave is seen (Fig. 5).

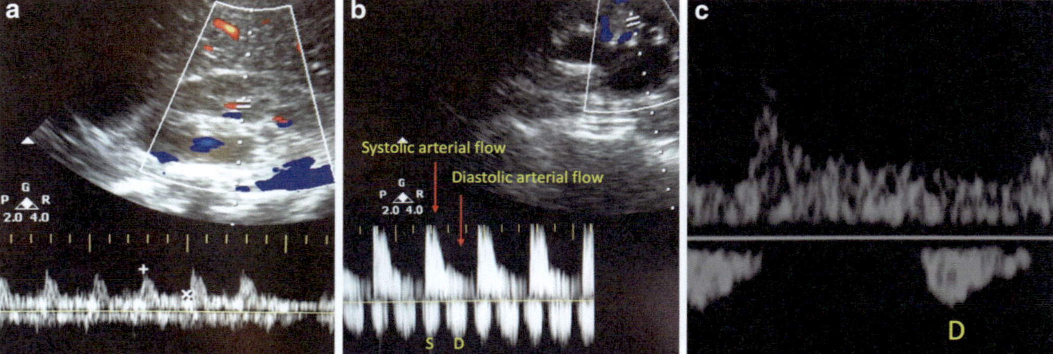

Fig. 5 Intrarenal venous Doppler showing progression of congestion (a) normal continuous venous flow (below baseline), (b) grade 1 discontinuous biphasic venous flow and (c) grade 2 discontinuous monophasic (only in diastole) venous flow

Intrarenal Doppler is the most challenging component of the VExUS exam due to the small size of the vessels. It is important that the sonographer uses Doppler on the intraparenchymal vessels, rather than the vessels closer to the hilum, as these more central vessels will often exhibit flow patterns closer to the hepatic vein profile even without venous congestion. The more peripheral interlobar branches are located in between the medullary pyramids and usually offer good Doppler angles for interrogation. To investigate these vessels, a color Doppler box is placed over the kidney and the gain increased to the point just before artifact is encountered. The color Doppler Nyquist limit should be set to between 20 cm/sec and 10 cm/s, with the lower limit often being required to locate where the pulsed wave Doppler gate will be placed. Once the interlobar vessel is located, the pulsed wave gate is placed, and the Doppler activated. Ideally, the pulsed wave Doppler scale is also adjusted to optimize visualization of the waveform.

Conclusion

Venous congestion is a significant (and often underappreciated) hemodynamic variable and when present is often associated with multiple important clinical outcomes. Indeed, common practice tends to either target higher CVP values than may be beneficial to organ function, or else have a very liberal approach to fluids, particularly in resuscitation as well as in the management of undifferentiated acute kidney injury, where a more physiologically tailored strategy would likely benefit patients. Quantification of venous congestion can be evaluated by the Doppler investigation of multiple organs. Each of these organs has its own inherent advantages, disadvantages, and limitations when assessing venous congestion. The VExUS scheme incorporates the evaluation of multiple organs to overcome some of these issues and give a global assessment of systemic venous congestion. In the

future, application of VExUS will likely have value in prognostication, hemodynamic monitoring, and guiding management in both the acute and outpatient clinical setting, as several clinical studies are currently underway.

References

1. Winton FR. The influence of venous pressure on the isolated mammalian kidney. J Physiol. 1931;72 (1):49–61.
2. Bouchard J, Mehta RL. Fluid accumulation and acute kidney injury: consequence or cause. Curr Opin Crit Care. 2009;15(6) 509–13.
3. Boyd JH, Forbes J, Nakada TA, Walley KR, Russell JA. Fluid resuscitation in septic shock: a positive fluid balance and elevated central venous pressure are associated with increased mortality. Crit Care Med. 2011;39(2):259–65.
4. Kasotakis G, Sideris A, Yang Y, de Moya M, Alam H, King DR, et al. Aggressive early crystalloid resuscitation adversely affects outcomes in adult blunt trauma patients: an analysis of the Glue Grant database. J Trauma Acute Care Surg. 2013;74 (5):1215–21; discussion 21–2.
5. Silva JM, Jr., de Oliveira AM, Nogueira FA, Vianna PM, Pereira Filho MC, Dias LF, et al. The effect of excess fluid balance on the mortality rate of surgical patients: a multicenter prospective study. Crit Care. 2013;17(6):R288.
6. Mitchell KH, Carlbom D, Caldwell E, Leary PJ, Himmelfarb J, Hough CL. Volume overload: prevalence, risk factors, and functional outcome in survivors of septic shock. Ann Am Thorac Soc. 2015;12(12):1837–44.
7. Zhang L, Chen Z, Diao Y, Yang Y, Fu P. Associations of fluid overload with mortality and kidney recovery in patients with acute kidney injury: A systematic review and meta-analysis. J Crit Care. 2015;30 (4):860 e7–13.
8. Danziger J, Chen K, Cavender S, Lee J, Feng M, Mark RG, et al. Admission peripheral edema, central venous pressure, and survival in critically Ill patients. Ann Am Thorac Soc. 2016;13(5):705–11.
9. Woodward CW, Lambert J, Ortiz-Soriano V, Li Y, Ruiz-Conejo M, Bissell BD, et al. Fluid overload associates with major adverse kidney events in critically Ill patients with acute kidney injury requiring continuous renal replacement therapy. Crit Care Med. 2019;47(9):e753–e60.
10. Hanberg JS, Tang WHW, Wilson FP, Coca SG, Ahmad T, Brisco MA, et al. An exploratory analysis of the competing effects of aggressive decongestion

and high-dose loop diuretic therapy in the DOSE trial. Int J Cardiol. 2017;241:277–82.

11. Iida N, Seo Y, Sai S, Machino-Ohtsuka T, Yamamoto M, Ishizu T, et al. Clinical implications of intrarenal hemodynamic evaluation by Doppler ultrasonography in heart Failure. JACC Heart Fail. 2016;4(8):674–82.

12. Damman K, Navis G, Smilde TD, Voors AA, van der Bij W, van Veldhuisen DJ, et al. Decreased cardiac output, venous congestion and the association with renal impairment in patients with cardiac dysfunction. Eur J Heart Fail. 2007;9(9):872–8.

13. Mullens W, Abrahams Z, Francis GS, Sokos G, Taylor DO, Starling RC, et al. Importance of venous congestion for worsening of renal function in advanced decompensated heart failure. J Am Coll Cardiol. 2009;53(7):589–96.

14. Williams JB, Peterson ED, Wojdyla D, Harskamp R, Southerland KW, Ferguson TB, et al. Central venous pressure after coronary artery bypass surgery: does it predict postoperative mortality or renal failure? J Crit Care. 2014;29(6):1006–10.

15. Chen KP, Cavender S, Lee J, Feng M, Mark RG, Celi LA, et al. Peripheral edema, central venous pressure, and risk of AKI in critical illness. Clin J Am Soc Nephrol. 2016;11(4):602–8.

16. Gambardella I, Gaudino M, Ronco C, Lau C, Ivascu N, Girardi LN. Congestive kidney failure in cardiac surgery: the relationship between central venous pressure and acute kidney injury. Interact Cardiovasc Thorac Surg. 2016;23(5):800–5.

17. Lankadeva YR, Kosaka J, Iguchi N, Evans RG, Booth LC, Bellomo R, et al. Effects of fluid bolus therapy on renal perfusion, oxygenation, and function in early experimental septic kidney injury. Crit Care Med. 2019;47(1):e36–43.

18. Maxwell MH, Breed ES, Schwartz IL. Renal venous pressure in chronic congestive heart failure. J Clin Invest. 1950;29(3):342–8.

19. Damman K, van Deursen VM, Navis G, Voors AA, van Veldhuisen DJ, Hillege HL. Increased central venous pressure is associated with impaired renal function and mortality in a broad spectrum of patients with cardiovascular disease. J Am Coll Cardiol. 2009;53(7):582–8.

20. Hanberg JS, Sury K, Wilson FP, Brisco MA, Ahmad T, Ter Maaten JM, et al. Reduced cardiac index is not the dominant driver of renal dysfunction in heart failure. J Am Coll Cardiol. 2016;67(19):2199–208.

21. Valentova M, von Haehling S, Bauditz J, Doehner W, Ebner N, Bekfani T, et al. Intestinal congestion and right ventricular dysfunction: a link with appetite loss, inflammation, and cachexia in chronic heart failure. Eur Heart J. 2016;37(21):1684–91.

22. Sandek A, Swidsinski A, Schroedl W, Watson A, Valentova M, Herrmann R, et al. Intestinal blood flow in patients with chronic heart failure: a link with bacterial growth, gastrointestinal symptoms, and cachexia. J Am Coll Cardiol. 2014;64(11):1092–102.

23. Byrne L, Obonyo NG, Diab SD, Dunster KR, Passmore MR, Boon AC, et al. Unintended consequences: fluid resuscitation worsens shock in an ovine model of endotoxemia. Am J Respir Crit Care Med. 2018;198(8):1043–54.

24. Niebauer J, Volk HD, Kemp M, Dominguez M, Schumann RR, Rauchhaus M, et al. Endotoxin and immune activation in chronic heart failure: a prospective cohort study. Lancet. 1999;353 (9167):1838–42.

25. Sundaram V, Fang JC. Gastrointestinal and liver issues in heart failure. Circulation. 2016;133 (17):1696–703.

26. Benkreira A, Beaubien-Souligny W, Mailhot T, Bouabdallaoui N, Robillard P, Desjardins G, et al. Portal hypertension is associated with congestive encephalopathy and delirium after cardiac surgery. Can J Cardiol. 2019;35(9):1134–41.

27. Dabrowski W, Kotlinska E, Rzecki Z, Czajkowski M, Stadnik A, Olszewski K. Raised jugular venous pressure intensifies release of brain injury biomarkers in patients undergoing cardiac surgery. J Cardiothorac Vasc Anesth. 2012;26(6):999–1006.

28. Lahiri S, Schlick KH, Padrick MM, Rinsky B, Gonzalez N, Jones H, et al. Cerebral pulsatility index is elevated in patients with elevated right atrial pressure. J Neuroimaging. 2018;28(1):95–8.

29. Nunez-Patino RA, Rubiano AM, Godoy DA. Impact of cervical collars on intracranial pressure values in traumatic brain injury: a systematic review and meta-analysis of prospective studies. Neurocrit Care. 2020;32(2):469–77.

30. Stone MB, Tubridy CM, Curran R. The effect of rigid cervical collars on internal jugular vein dimensions. Acad Emerg Med. 2010;17(1):100–2.

31. Guyton AC, Lindsey AW, Abernathy B, Richardson T. Venous return at various right atrial pressures and the normal venous return curve. Am J Physiol. 1957;189(3):609–15.

32. Beaubien-Souligny W, Rola P, Haycock K, Bouchard J, Lamarche Y, Spiegel R, et al. Quantifying systemic congestion with Point-Of-Care ultrasound: development of the venous excess ultrasound grading system. Ultrasound J. 2020;12(1):16.

33. Spiegel R, Teeter W, Sullivan S, Tupchong K, Mohammed N, Sutherland M, et al. The use of venous Doppler to predict adverse kidney events in a general ICU cohort. Crit Care. 2020;24(1):615.

34. Bhardwaj V, Vikneswaran G, Rola P, Raju S, Bhat RS, Jayakumar A, et al. Combination of inferior vena cava diameter, hepatic venous flow, and portal vein pulsatility index: venous excess ultrasound score (VEXUS score) in predicting acute kidney injury in patients with cardiorenal syndrome: a prospective cohort study. Indian J Crit Care Med. 2020;24 (9):783–9.

35. Wachsberg RH, Needleman L, Wilson DJ. Portal vein pulsatility in normal and cirrhotic adults without cardiac disease. J Clin Ultrasound. 1995;23(1):3–15.

36. Gallix BP, Taourel P, Dauzat M, Bruel JM, Lafortune M. Flow pulsatility in the portal venous system: a study of Doppler sonography in healthy adults. AJR Am J Roentgenol. 1997;169(1):141–4.

37. Song J, Wu W, He Y, Lin S, Zhu D, Zhong M. Value of the combination of renal resistance index and central venous pressure in the early prediction of sepsis-induced acute kidney injury. J Crit Care. 2018;45:204–8.

38. O'Neill WC. Renal resistive index: a case of mistaken identity. Hypertension. 2014;64(5):915–7.

POCUS in Monitoring: LV Diastolic Function and Filling Pressures

Matteo Cameli, Maria Concetta Pastore, and Marcelo Haertel Miglioranza

Don't tell me the moon is shining, show me the glint of light on a broken glass

Anton Chekov. Russian playwright and short-story writer (1860–1904 AD)

Abstract

In the last decade, the study of left ventricular (LV) relaxation properties to define diastolic dysfunction and the consequent increase in LV filling pressure has gained increasing importance for the assessment of heart failure, particularly the evaluation of the fluid status of the patient. Therefore, a thorough evaluation of diastolic function could be pivotal also in emergency and critical care settings for diagnosis, monitoring and guiding treatment. Noninvasive estimation of LV filling pressures and diastolic function by POCUS should be fully integrated into non-invasive bedside assessment of haemodynamics. This chapter describes the main grades of diastolic dysfunction and their evaluation with POCUS, highlighting their usefulness and limitations in daily clinical practice.

Keywords

Diastolic function · Filling pressures · Echocardiography · POCUS · Heart failure

Key Messages

- The study of left ventricular (LV) diastolic function and filling pressures is a pivotal element in acute clinical settings, for diagnostic, monitoring and therapeutic purposes
- The use of point-of-care ultrasound (POCUS) allows a bedside non-invasive and quick evaluation in emergency and critical care
- A simplified approach using trans-mitral filling pattern and tissue Doppler imaging in 4-apical chamber view provides a reliable assessment of LV diastolic function and filling pressure in most cases, and should be

M. Cameli (✉) · M. C. Pastore
Department of Medical Biotechnologies, Division of Cardiology, University of Siena, Viale Bracci N. 1, 53100 Siena, Italy
e-mail: matteo.cameli@yahoo.com

M. H. Miglioranza
Cardiology Institute of Rio Grande do Sul, Av. Princesa Isabel, 370, Porto Alegre/RS, Porto Alegre 90620-000, Brazil

integrated to POCUS assessment of haemodynamics

- Considering the technical limitations of these techniques, the evaluation should be tailored to every patient within the clinical and hemodynamic contexts.

Introduction

Left ventricular (LV) diastolic function is considered as the result of LV relaxation properties and, consequently, LV filling pressures. The assessment of diastolic function is a pivotal element in acute and chronic cardiac disease, especially when systolic function is preserved.

Thanks to the recent advances in technology and the increasing use of portable POCUS devices, the evaluation of diastolic function has become easier and feasible and has currently been fully integrated into clinical practice as part of every comprehensive echocardiographic examination. Particularly, in the emergency or critical care settings, the use of POCUS to determine LV diastolic dysfunction and filling pressures may help in assessing volume status, optimizing diuretic therapy in systo-diastolic heart failure (HF) and in differentiating between cardiogenic and non-cardiogenic respiratory failure [1]. In acute HF, hemodynamic congestion, determined as an elevation of LV filling pressures, precedes clinical manifestations by days to months [2, 3]. Moreover, some authors have shown that, at discharge, sometimes there is a persistence of hemodynamic congestion, with excess fluids in the intravascular and interstitial compartments, despite resolution of clinical manifestations, which is associated with symptoms recurrence [4].

The evaluation of LV diastolic function by POCUS relies on identifying structural heart changes which can be a cause (e.g., LV hypertrophy) or a consequence of diastolic dysfunction (LA enlargement) and on the estimation of markers of LV filling pressures and LV relaxation [5].

Diastolic Function and LV Filling Pressures

First of all, it is important to understand that the definition of diastolic function and LV filling pressures, although closely related and often regarded as interchangeable, are not the same concept. Diastolic function results from cardiac structural and functional characteristics and is more focused on LV compliance or stiffness. This could, on the one hand, influence LV filling pressures, with their growth over time in case of a "stiff" LV (which requires higher intracardiac pressures to reach a normal filling); on the other hand, LV filling pressures mainly depend on hemodynamic conditions, with an increase in LV filling pressures in case of volume overload, which could lead to LV diastolic dysfunction. Accordingly, even if often LV diastolic dysfunction and high LV filling pressures coexist, in clinical practice there are some cases in which LV filling pressures could be normal even in presence of LV diastolic dysfunction, or vice-versa (see paragraph 6). Therefore, it is important to assess and report separately both of these entities, particularly in the presence of discordant findings.

POCUS Parameters of Diastolic Function

According to the latest American Society of Echocardiography/European Association of Cardiovascular Imaging (ASE/EACVI) recommendations, to fully address the definition of diastolic function and LV filling pressures, a variety of echocardiographic parameters should be considered [6]. However, a meta-analysis showed that the application of these guidelines is subject to a high inter-operator variability (from 12 to 84%) for the diagnosis of diastolic dysfunction [7], as well as being time-consuming. This has led to an evidence-based expert consensus to not include diastolic dysfunction among the targets of the focus cardiac ultrasound (FoCUS) examination [1].

Of note, for POCUS purposes, a practical approach limited to one or two indices, acquired in apical 4-chamber view, is often sufficient to obtain information on the patient's volume status. The need for additional parameters could be reserved to doubtful cases, with requires more time for a thorough assessment (Fig. 1), or in case of missing parameters [8]. As compared to the invasive assessment of LV filling pressures by the pulmonary artery catheter (gold standard method), the 2016 guidelines have shown excellent interobserver accuracy and reproducibility, independent from the experience level of the operator [9]. In fact, it is important to make diastolic function analysis feasible for all clinicians—not only for cardiologists [10, 11].

The parameters included in assessing LV diastolic function and filling pressures are mitral inflow velocities, pulmonary venous flow, tissue Doppler imaging, and left atrial volume index. Of these, the preferred initial parameters are trans-mitral inflow and tissue Doppler imaging of the mitral annulus.

Pulsed-Wave Doppler (PWD)

The study of LV diastolic filling pattern by PWD allows to determine the trans-mitral flow velocity during the diastolic phases through the following parameters:

- Early diastolic filling, represented by the "E" wave, in which the LV relaxes and consequently it passively fills with blood after mitral valve opening.
- E-wave deceleration time (DT), which represents the duration of the early diastolic filling

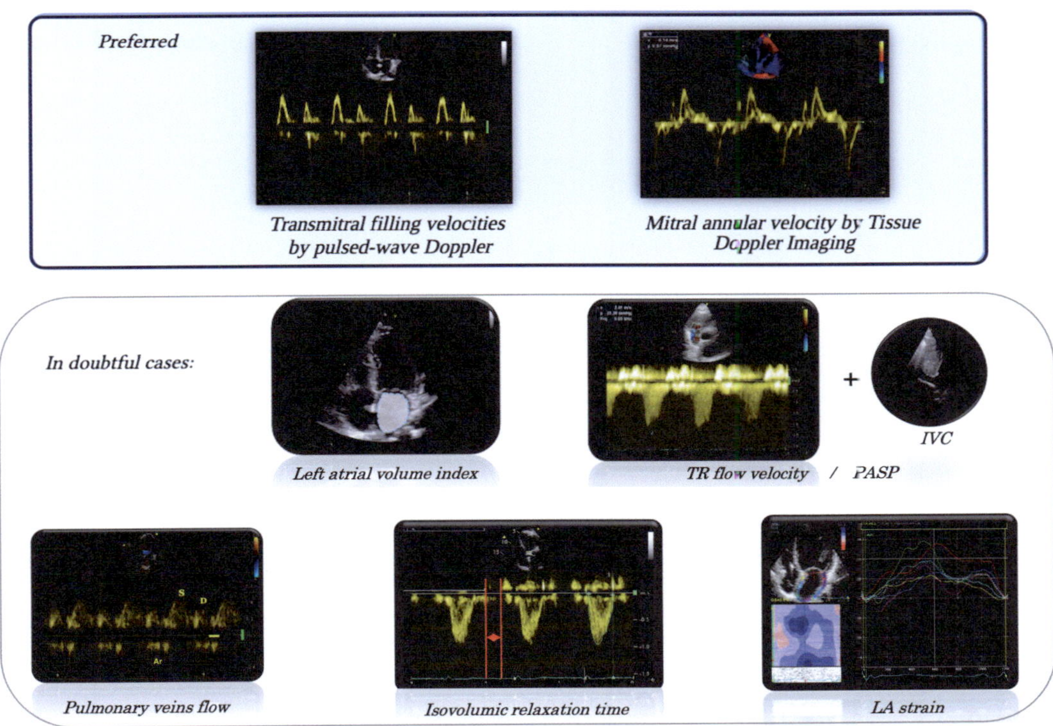

Fig. 1 Main parameters for noninvasive estimation of left ventricular diastolic function and filling pressures. IVC, inferior vena cava; LA, left atrial; LV, left ventricular; PASP, pulmomary artery systolic pressure; POCUS, point-of-care ultrasound

(= the time in which the E-wave returns to the baseline)

- Late diastolic filling, represented by the "A" wave, in which the left atrium (LA) actively contracts and consequently it pumps the remaining blood into the LV.

To obtain the flow tracing, the PWD function should be applied in the apical 4-chamber view by placing the sample volume between the tips of the opened mitral valve leaflets (Fig. 2). These parameters and their relationship are reliable indices of LA pressure. In young and healthy subjects, the highest part of the LV filling occurs in the "early diastolic filling" phase, therefore, the "E-wave" peak velocity is higher than the "A-wave" peak velocity (E/A ratio $\geq$ 0.8 m/s). Normal DT is 160–200 ms and a value <150 ms has been found to be predictive of a pulmonary capillary wedge pressure (PCWP) >15 mm Hg [12]. Conversely, in case of LV diastolic dysfunction and/or raised LA filling pressures, the trans-mitral flow velocity pattern gradually changes as follows:

(1) **Abnormal relaxation filling pattern**: with reduced LV compliance and relaxation properties, the early diastolic velocity reduces (E-wave < 0.5 m/s), therefore the LA should enhance its active contribution to LV filling in late diastole, generating a higher "A-wave" velocity -> E/A ratio < 0.8 m/s;

(2) **Pseudonormal filling pattern**: as diastolic dysfunction progresses and the LV becomes stiffer, LA pressures start to increase to compensate the higher LV diastolic pressures. Therefore, a significant amount of blood fills the LV during early diastole (E wave $\geq$ 0.5 m/s) due to high LA pressures (and not to LV relaxation, thus called "pseudonormal") -> E/A ratio $\geq$ 0.8 m/s;

(3) **Restrictive filling pattern**: due to worsening LV diastolic function, there is a considerable increase in LA pressures, which leads to a further increase in early diastolic filling velocity (large and narrow E wave), with less contribution from the LA (which is usually dilated due to chronic elevation in LV filling pressure at this phase) -> E/A ratio $\geq$ 2 m/s.

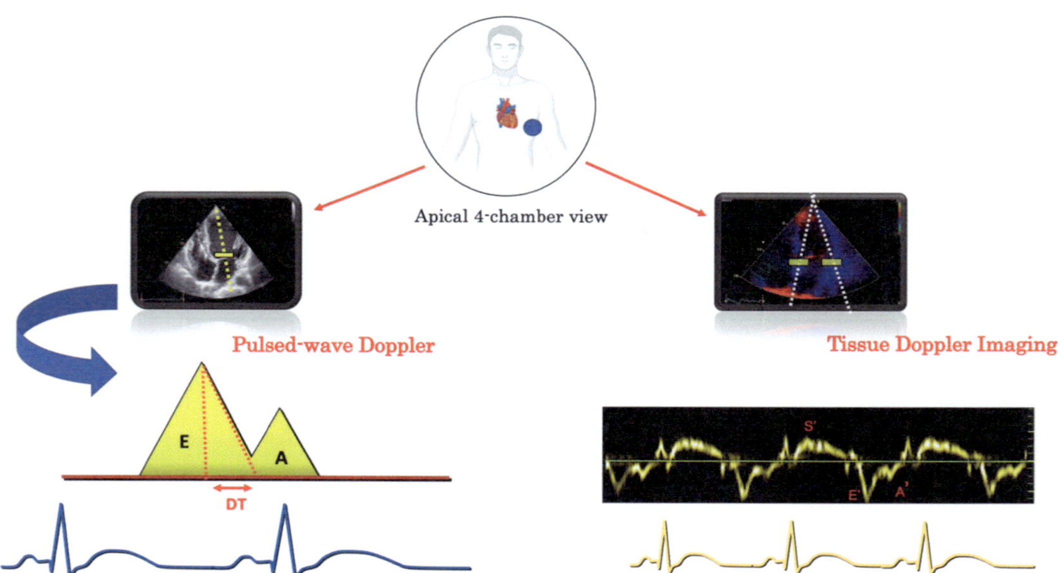

Fig. 2 Calculation of pulsed-wave Doppler and tissue Doppler imaging parameters for the assessment of left ventricular diastolic function. A = late diastolic wave by pulsed-wave Doppler; E, early diastolic wave by pulsed-wave Doppler; DT, deceleration time

According to the latest guidelines, in patients with reduced LV ejection fraction (EF), transmitral inflow pattern is usually sufficient to identify patients with increased LA pressures, which is directly correlated with diastolic dysfunction. It is feasible in the absence of atrial fibrillation (AF), significant mitral valve disease (at least moderate mitral annular calcification [MAC], any mitral stenosis or mitral regurgitation [MR] of more than moderate severity, mitral valve repair or prosthetic mitral valve), LV assist devices, left bundle branch block, and ventricular paced rhythm.

Moreover, DT of mitral E velocity is an important predictor of outcome [13] and it is influenced by LV relaxation, LV diastolic pressures after mitral valve opening, and LV stiffness. DT is also a high-feasibility and reproducibility measure and DT reduction in patients with reduced LV EF offers an accurate measure of increased LV end-diastolic pressure in patients with sinus rhythm and in AF. Moreover, it has also been suggested as a tool to monitor response to diuretic and vasodilator therapy in HF [14]. However, DT does not correlate to LV filling pressures in patients with normal LV EF, it should not be measured in case of E and A fusion (e.g., tachycardia) due to potential inaccuracy, and it commonly increases with age [6].

Tissue Doppler Imaging (TDI)

TDI represents a relatively recent method to assess LV relaxation and filling pressures. It allows for the study of the diastolic motion of the mitral annulus, which is influenced by the contraction of longitudinally oriented myocardial fibers. Therefore, this method indirectly assesses LV contraction and relaxation. In fact, three peak indices could be measured in the TDI wave in the two-point (septal and lateral wall) of mitral annulus (acquired in apical 4-chamber view, Fig. 2): a positive peak, called S' which reflects systolic function, two negative peaks: e', which corresponds to early diastole, and a', which corresponds to late diastole (atrial contraction). The mostly frequently used index is e', as the average value (e'avg) is a measure of the average of the velocities at early diastole in the two points of mitral annulus ($_{septal\ and\ lateral}$) and it is a good marker of diastolic function and LV filling pressures. This reflects LV relaxation and is independent of left atrial pressure (LAP) and acute changes in preload. Normal LV muscle relaxation will correspond to higher early diastolic velocity. Therefore, correcting E-wave velocity for LV relaxation with the E/e'avg ratio allows the accurate assessment of LAP or the mean PCWP [12]. The E/e'$_{avg}$ ratio demonstrated to follow directional changes in PCWP, which was found to be even better than brain natriuretic peptide (BNP) [15], and to be an independent predictor of mortality in patients with HF and reduced ejection fraction (HFrEF) [16]. PCWP can be estimated by the following equation: $PCWP = 1.24 * (E/e') + 1.9$ which has been proposed by Nagueh et al. in patients with reduced LV systolic function or structurally abnormal hearts.

E/e'avg ratio alone is useful in discriminating those patients having normal (E/e'avg < 8) or high (E/e'avg > 14) LVEDP. Particularly, a E/e' lateral ratio > 13 or a E/e' septal > 15 is considered indicative of elevated PCWP. In fact, individual cutoff values for individual e' (septal e' < 7 cm/s, lateral e' < 10 cm/s) are abnormal. However, in most patients with congestive HF, e' remains reduced even after diuretic therapy while E/e' ratio improves due to decrease in E-wave velocity [17]. Therefore, it is important to use E/e' ratio to guide decongestive therapy rather than isolated e'.

However, this technique is hampered by shortcomings related to the Doppler technology (angle misalignment, myocardial tissue movement) and by intrinsic characteristics of myocardial function (e.g. the presence of regional wall motion abnormalities). Moreover, E/e'avg ratio presents some limitations:

- It is less useful for classifying intermediate values [18];
- It is insensitive to preload changes in patients who have impaired relaxation but not in patients who have normal relaxation;

- It increases with age;
- It has limited accuracy in patients with mitral annular calcifications or prosthesis, left bundle branch block and pacemakers;
- It changes proportionally with afterload, so it is not a reliable index in patients with mitral regurgitation [19] and pericardial diseases [20] which influence loading conditions;
- It is limited by angle of incidence and tethering motion of the adjacent segment [21];
- It has a significant "grey zone" where it fails to predict filling pressures, in particular in case of severely depressed LVEF [22].

To optimize the acquisition in AF patients, cardiac cycles with controlled heart rate (<100 beats per minute) and similar preceding and pre-preceding RR intervals are required [23].

Classification of Diastolic Dysfunction

For POCUS application, a simplified approach including E/A ratio and E/e' ratio could be used to quickly classify diastolic dysfunction with sufficient accuracy [24]. It could be useful while performing POCUS at bedside not only for diagnosis (emergency settings) [25], but also for prognostication [26] and monitoring, especially in critical care, in order to guide therapy.

In patients with reduced LV EF and/or in patients with myocardial disease and normal LV EF, the diastolic dysfunction could be classified as follows:

Grade 0: Normal Mitral Inflow

- E/A $\geq$ 0.8
- e' septal $\geq$ 8 cm/s
- E/e' avg ratio < 8.

Grade 1 Diastolic Dysfunction: (impaired relaxation of the LV)

- **E/A < 0.8**
- **e' septal $\leq$ 8 cm/sec**

- **E/e'avg ratio $\leq$ 8** (since both the E and e' waves decreases, and the relative ratio is preserved).

As both in Grade 0 and Grade 1 Diastolic Dysfunction E/e' avg ratio is ≤ 8, the only difference is **E/A ratio**. Importantly, Grade 1 Diastolic Dysfunction can be a normal finding in the elderly (physiological aging).

Grade 2 Diastolic Dysfunction: (Pseudonormal)

- E/A $\geq$ 0.8 (pseudonormalization)
- **e' septal $\leq$ 8 cm/sec (due to moderately reduced LV relaxation)**
- **E/e'avg ratio: 8–15.**

The primary change highlighted by this diastolic pattern is worsening LV stiffness leading to increase in LV filling pressures and LAP (which is often accompanied by LA enlargement).

In this case, E/e' ratio is pivotal to identify the pseudonormal pattern and to differentiate Grade 0 from Grade 2.

Grade 3 Diastolic Dysfunction: (Restrictive)

- **E/A $\geq$ 2** (very high E wave)
- **e'septal << 8 cm/s** (significant decrease in LV compliance, with consequent severe increase in LAP)
- **E/e'avg ratio > 15.**

Usually, Grade 3 diastolic dysfunction is characterized by very high E wave, LA enlargement, and a small e' wave.

Of note, in subjects < 40 years of age, E/A ratios > 2 may be a normal finding, thus in this age group other signs of diastolic dysfunction should be sought. Importantly, normal subjects have normal annular E' velocity (e' > 8) which can be used to verify the presence of normal diastolic function.

In the previous guidelines, also **Grade 4** diastolic dysfunction was described. The only difference between Grade 3 and Grade 4 diastolic dysfunction is that Grade 3 was considered "reversible" and Grade 4 was considered "irreversible" after Valsalva maneuver → mitral inflow waveform changes from "restrictive" to "impaired relaxation" pattern.

Additional Parameters

According to the 2016 ASE/EACVI recommendations, in patients with preserved LV EF or with an E/A $\leq$ 0.8 and peak E velocity > 0.50 cm/sec, or an E/A ratio 0.8–2, additional parameters are required to classify diastolic function. Beyond TDI parameters, LA volume index (LAVi) and tricuspid regurgitant (TR) flow velocity and LA strain should be used [6], following the criteria described in Table 1. Then, in the latest EACVI consensus document for the use of multimodality imaging to evaluate HF with preserved ejection fraction (HFpEF), the use of LA strain is suggested in case of missing parameters with only 2 criteria available and 1 positive and 1 negative, with the cutoff value of LA reservoir strain < 18% to define elevated LV filling pressure [8].

Even if the formerly described simplified approach could offer a reliable assessment of diastolic function and LV filling pressures in most situations, there are some indeterminate conditions, e.g. E/A ratio $\leq$ 0.8 with E/e' ratio > 8 or E/A ratio = 0.8–2 and E/e' ratio $\leq$ 8, in which the integration of additional parameters becomes pivotal (Fig. 1).

For indeterminate diastolic function, the EACVI/ASE guidelines suggest the use of supplementary parameters such as pulmonary vein velocities, isovolumetric relaxation time, or methods, such as speckle-tracking echocardiography (STE) calculating LV global longitudinal strain in order to identify mild reductions in LV systolic function [6]. However, in the last years, LA strain by STE has proven a reliable index of LV filling pressures which could fill the gaps in the previous algorithm [27, 28], as recommended in the EACVI consensus document for the use of multimodality imaging in HFpEF [8]. Also, the use of diastolic stress test has been proposed as an additional method, however, it is not applicable for POCUS purposes, thus it falls outside the scope of this chapter (Table 2).

Table 1 Criteria to assess diastolic function in patients with reduced and preserved ejection fraction (EF) according to the American Society of Echocardiography/European Association of Cardiovascular Imaging 2016 recommendations [6], and according to a new unified algorithm recently proposed by Ho et al. [23]

Reduced EF	Preserved EF	All patients regardless of EF, except those with > moderate MAC, LBBB, PM, severe PH
E/e' ratio > 14	E/e' ratio > 14	E/e' > 15
	Septal e' < 7 cm/s or lateral e' < 10 cm/s	Septal e' < 7 cm/s
LAVi > 34 ml/m^2	LAVi > 34 ml/m^2	LAVi > 34 ml/m^2
TR velocity > 2.8 m/s	TR velocity > 2.8 m/s	TR velocity > 2.8 m/s
– Only 1/3 or none meet the cutoff value -> **grade I DD with normal LA pressure** – 2/3 or 3/3 meet the cutoff value -> **grade II DD with elevation of LA pressure** – Only 2 variables available and only 1/2 meet the cutoff value, **indeterminate diastolic function**	– 1/4 or none meet the cutoff value -> Normal diastolic function – 3/4 or 4/4 meet the cutoff value -> **DD** – 2/4 meet the cutoff value -> **Indeterminate diastolic function -> LA strain < 18% -> DD** [8]	– 1/4 or none meet the cutoff value -> **normal LV filling pressure with normal diastolic function or grade I DD** – 3/4 or all patients meet the cutoff value -> **increased LV filling pressure with grade 2 or 3 DD** – 2/4 meet the cutoff value -> **PV Doppler, IVRT, Valsalva, LA strain**

E, Early diastolic wave by pulsed-wave doppler; e', early diastolic velocity by tissue-doppler imaging; IVRT, isovolumic relaxation time; LA, left atrial; LAVi, left atrial volume index; PV, pulmonary veins; TR, tricuspid regurgitant

Table 2 Indications and pitfalls of noninvasive assessment of LV filling pressures and diastolic function in specific populations (according to ASE/EACVI recommendations [6])

Specific disease	Indications	Issues
Hypertrophic cardiomyopathy	*Recommended*: E/e' ratio (>14), LAVi (>34 mL/m^2), Pulmonary vein atrial reversal velocity (Ar-A duration $\geq$ 30 ms), Peak TR velocity > 2.8 m/sec (1) >50% of the variables meet the cutoff values $\rightarrow$ elevated LAP, **grade II DD** (2) <50% of the variables meet the cutoff values $\rightarrow$ LAP is normal, **grade I DD** (3) 50% discordance with 2 or 4 available variables $\rightarrow$ inconclusive (4) Restrictive filling pattern + abnormally reduced mitral annular e' velocity (e'septal < 7 cm/sec, e' lateral < 10 cm/sec) $\rightarrow$ **Grade III diastolic dysfunction**	Patients with > moderate MR: only Ar-A duration and peak TR velocity are still valid If only 1 parameter with a satisfactory signal $\rightarrow$ Estimation of LAP is **not** recommended
Restrictive cardiomyopathy	– *Early disease*: usually **grade I** DD that progresses to **grade II** as the severity of the disease advances – *Advanced disease*: **grade III DD:** mitral inflow E/A ratio > 2.5, DT < 150 ms, IVRT < 50 ms, decreased septal and lateral e' velocities (3–4 cm/sec) – *Constrictive pericarditis*: septal e' > lateral e'	E/E' not reliable in case of constrictive pericarditis
Mitral stenosis	– Consider IVRT, TE2e' and mitral inflow peak velocity at early and late diastole for estimation of mean LAP: – **Normal EF** -> time interval Ar-A and IVRT/TE2e' ratio may be applied for estimation for prediction of LV filling pressures if normal LVEF – **Depressed EF** -> E/e' ratio may be considered	
Heart transplantation	– After heart transplantation $\rightarrow$ restrictive filling pattern is common in patients with preserved EFs – **PASP** as surrogate of mean LAP (in the absence of pulmonary disease)	No single diastolic parameter appears reliable enough to predict graft rejection
Atrial fibrillation	– **Peak TR velocity > 2.8 m/sec** is suggestive of elevated LAP – Depressed EF $\rightarrow$ **DT** ($\leq$ 160 ms): increased LV diastolic pressures and adverse clinical outcomes – In patients with incomplete TR jet: peak acceleration rate of mitral E velocity $\geq$ 1,900 cm/sec, IVRT $\leq$ 65 ms, DT of pulmonary venous diastolic velocity $\leq$ 220 ms, E/Vp ratio $\geq$ 1.4, and E/e' ratio $\geq$ 11	Consider the variability of mitral inflow velocity with the RR cycle length, as patients with increased filling pressures have less beat-to-beat variation

(continued)

Table 2 (continued)

Specific disease	Indications	Issues
Atrioventricular block	– 1st degree AV block: common parameters if E and A velocities are not fused – If only mitral A velocity is present → use only **TR peak velocity > 2.8 m/sec**	Lower accuracy of mitral annular velocities and E/e′ ratio in the presence of LBBB, RV pacing, previous CRT

Ar-A, atrial reversal velocity—mitral late diastolic (A)-wave duration; AV, atrioventricular; CRT, cardiac resynchronization therapy; DD; diastolic dysfunction; DT, deceleration time; E Early diastolic wave by pulsed-wave doppler; E′, early diastolic velocity by tissue-doppler imaging; EF, ejection fraction; IVRT, isovolumic relaxation time; LAP, left atrial pressure; LAVi, left atrial volume index; LBBB, left bundle-branch block; MR, mitral regurgitation; PASP, pulmonary artery systolic pressure; TR, tricuspid regurgitant

Left Atrial Volume Index (LAVi)

LAVi could be calculated by manually tracing the LA endocardium in apical 4-chamber view in end-systole, obtaining LA maximum volume, and dividing this value for body surface area (BSA):

$$LAVi = LA\,maximum\,volume/BSA$$

Cardiac structural as well as functional information are of particular importance when assessing diastolic function in patients with preserved EF. An enlarged LA LA (LAVi > 34 ml/m^2) is strongly suggestive of chronically elevated LV filling pressure, after exclusion of anemia, atrial arrhythmias, bradycardia, heart transplantation, high cardiac output states, and >moderate mitral valve disease. Athletes may also have dilated atria without increased LV filling pressures [29]. However, a normal LAVi does not exclude the presence of diastolic dysfunction, in fact, LA is often not dilated in patients in the earliest stage of diastolic dysfunction and in situations with an acute increase in LV filling pressures, as LA volume reflects the chronic effects of increased LV filling pressures over time. Increased LA volume is an independent predictor of death, HF, AF, and ischemic stroke [30–33] and it is highly feasible and reproducible.

However, its measurement is limited by: suboptimal image quality, including LA fore-shortening; ascending and descending aortic aneurysms; large interatrial septal aneurysms.

Tricuspid Regurgitant (TR) Jet

TR jet peak velocity can be measured in apical 4 chamber view (or in parasternal RV inflow view) by continuous-wave (CW) Doppler, placing the sample volume on TR jet. A TR peak velocity >2.8 m/sec supports the presence of elevated LV filling pressures.

Moreover, the assessment of TR jet by CW Doppler offers a direct estimate of pulmonary artery systolic pressure when combined with right atrial pressure (which is indirectly assessed by inferior vena cava dimensions and collapsibility, from subcostal IVC view). In patients with systolic HF, it is uncommon to have coexisting primary pulmonary arterial disease, therefore, an elevated pulmonary artery systolic pressure (PASP) supports the presence of elevated LV filling pressures which reflected on the pulmonary circulation and the right heart [34]. However, in case of absent or minimum TR, these measures could be hardly obtained.

Pulmonary Veins Velocity

In patients in whom one of the three main criteria (E/e′, LAVi, TR velocity) is not available, the ratio of pulmonary vein peak systolic to peak diastolic velocity or systolic velocity time integral to diastolic velocity time integral (S/D) < 1 suggests the presence of elevated LV filling pressures. However, this should be taken cautiously in patients with preserved EF, since in healthy young people (<40 years of age), pulmonary venous S/D ratio is often < 1. In these cases, the normality of other parameters including mitral annular e' velocity and LAVi should discriminate between healthy and pathologic S/D < 1 [6].

IVRT

Isovolumetric relaxation time (IVRT) corresponds to the time interval between the aortic valve closure and the mitral valve opening, measured with PWD with the sample volume placed on the LV outflow tract in 5-chamber view, and is ≤ 70 ms in normal subjects. A prolongation of IVRT could be found in patients with impaired LV relaxation but normal LV filling pressures. Particularly, IVRT duration reduces in parallel to the increase in LA pressure, in fact it is inversely related to LV filling pressures in patients with cardiac disease. IVRT can be combined with other mitral inflow parameters as E/A ratio to estimate LV filling pressures in patients with HFrEF or other diseases [6].

LA Strain

LA strain has been described as a more sensitive parameter than LA volume for the early detection of LA structural and functional impairment. In fact, in the early phase of LV diastolic dysfunction, LA volume can still be normal, but, along with the progressive increase of LV volume and pressure, LA dilates, and its wall tension increases, presenting an initial improvement of its contractile function [28]. LA strain offers a quick analysis of LA deformation and has shown to be correlated to invasively assessed LV filling pressures [35] and to provide additive value for diastolic function classification [36, 37] and the HFpEF diagnosis [38, 39]. In fact, its use ad additional parameter to assess LV filling pressure in HFpEF has been indicated with a standardized cutoff value of LA reservoir strain < 18% [8].

However, the assessment of LA strain is commonly performed offline in dedicated workstation.

Some new echocardiographic machines allow to perform speckle tracking analysis in real-time. Hopefully in the future, since the application of this technique is still growing, the software implementation will lead to the wider application of STE on portable machines.

Clinical Applications of Diastolic Function by POCUS

The main question here is: why is it important to assess and classify diastolic function in the acute and critical care settings?

(1) **De-novo HF**: Due to the high influence of diastolic function on raised LV filling pressures, hence consequent congestion and possible HF symptoms, the evidence of diastolic dysfunction is considered an main parameter for the HF diagnosis, particularly for HFpEF. It is also considered an important prognostic marker. Moreover, serial assessment of ventricular filling pressures can be used to guide and titrate HF therapy [5].

(2) **Acute coronary syndromes**: The assessment of LA pressure has also been shown to be a useful parameter in evaluating patients with acute coronary syndromes, in order to recognize those with associated HF or those who are at risk of developing acute HF [40].

(3) **Chronic HF exacerbation**: In the acute phase of patients with known chronic HF, the assessment of diastolic function and LV filling pressures and their comparison with previous assessment would be useful to determine the severity of the current decompensation and the target for diuretic therapy. For example, if the patient had grade II diastolic dysfunction in stable conditions, this should represent the clinical focus to determine a possible worsening of LV filling pressures and for the therapeutic goal, rather than administering increasing amounts of diuretics as an attempt to reach grade I or normal diastolic function, which may potentially result in impaired forward flow and hypotension.

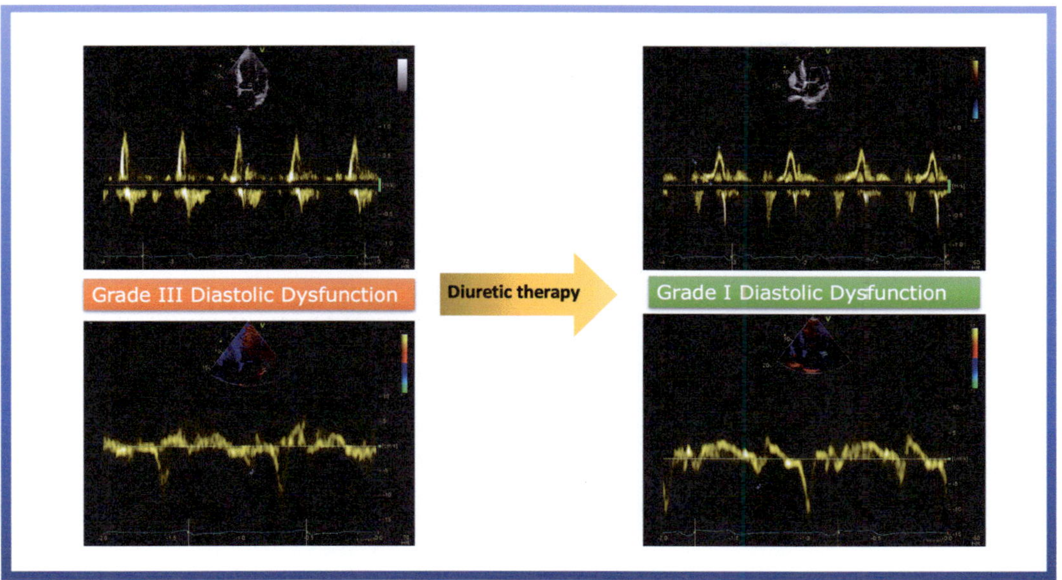

Fig. 3 Representative case of a patient with heart failure and grade III diastolic dysfunction with restrictive filling pattern and E/e' = 17, downgrading to grade I diastolic dysfunction and E/e' = 7 after being offloaded with diuretics

Moreover, trans-mitral filling pattern could be used to monitor diuretic response, as it would considerably change with the reduction of LV overload (Fig. 3).

(4) **Shock states**: Prior to intravenous fluids administration, the assessment of diastolic function could be useful, as a more liberal fluid approach could be used with normal LV diastolic function, while in the presence of diastolic dysfunction, fluid administration should be more cautious, with frequent reassessment of the patient's diastolic function, pulmonary congestion, and end-organ venous congestion (liver, gut, kidneys) [24].

(5) **Acute respiratory distress syndrome (ARDS)**: The diagnosis of ARDS implies that cardiogenic etiology of respiratory failure has been excluded (defined as pulmonary capillary wedge pressure <18 mmHg). Therefore, non-invasive assessment of left-sided intracardiac pressures with E/e' ratio as a surrogate of PCWP [41]. would be useful for differential diagnosis, aiding for the "rule out" of cardiogenic causes of lung congestion and diogenic causes of lung congestion and

hypoxia. Integration of lung ultrasound is vital while assessing LV filling pressures, as the presence of bilateral symmetrical B lines with thin pleural line is an indicator for increased extravascular lung water due to hydrostatic pulmonary oedema (See Chap. 12: Cardiogenic pulmonary oedema).

(6) **Caveat**: In the critically ill patients, LAP is not entirely related to the LV diastolic function: a patient with volume overload may have a very high LAP despite a normal LV diastolic function. Conversely, in the presence of hypovolaemia, there may be low LA pressure despite the presence of LV diastolic function [42].

Limitations

The assessment of LV diastolic function and filling pressures in the acute settings has some limitations that should be highlighted.

Some technical issues may be encountered in emergency or intensive care settings:

- The aforementioned parameters are strictly angle-dependent (except LA strain), therefore, if PWD or TDI parameters are measured off-axis (>20–$30°$) due to patient position, the values may be underestimated.
- In tachycardia, E and A waves may become fused, making it difficult to differentiate between them. Also, in AF with irregular heart rate there may be different waveform readings between each beat.
- Prosthetic mitral valve and MAC make TDI e' measurements unreliable.

Therefore, the echocardiographic indices of diastolic function should always be interpreted in a wider context that includes clinical status, they should be integrated with lung ultrasound and their use should be tailored to every single patient.

Conclusions

The study of diastolic function is of high additive value for bedside patient evaluation not only in the outpatient setting, but also emergency and critical care settings as it helps in the diagnosis, monitoring and guiding clinical decision-making. The ongoing technical advances and the use of quick and simplified approaches allows to rapidly obtain a noninvasive measurement of LV filling pressures and diastolic function, which is feasible for all advanced POCUS operators at the bedside. Therefore, integration of LV diastolic function and filling pressures in POCUS algorithms and targeted echocardiographic assessment if highly suggested. However, a comprehensive approach which integrates clinical, biochemical, and echocardiographic findings remains mandatory.

References

1. Neskovic AN, Skinner H, Price S, Via G, De Hert S, Stankovic I, Galderisi M, Donal E, Muraru D, Sloth E, Gargani L, Cardim N, Stefanidis A, Cameli M, Habib G, Cosyns B, Lancellotti P, Edvardsen T, Popescu BA. Reviewers: this document was reviewed by members of the 2016–2018 EACVI Scientific Documents Committee. Focus cardiac ultrasound core curriculum and core syllabus of the European Association of Cardiovascular Imaging. Eur Heart J Cardiovasc Imaging. 2018;19(5):475–481.

2. Gheorghiade M, Follath F, Ponikowski P, Barsuk JH, Blair JE, Cleland JG, et al. Assessing and grading congestion in acute heart failure: a scientific statement from the acute heart failure committee of the heart failure association of the European Society of Cardiology and endorsed by the European Society of Intensive Care Medicine. Eur J Heart Fail. 2010;12 (5):423–33.

3. Miller WL. Fluid volume overload and congestion in heart failure: time to reconsider pathophysiology and how volume is assessed. Circ Heart Fail. 2016;9(8): e002922.

4. Stevenson LW, Perloff JK. The limited reliability of physical signs for estimating hemodynamics in chronic heart failure. JAMA. 1989;261(6):884–8.

5. Litwin SE, Zile MR. Should we test for diastolic dysfunction? How and how often? JACC Cardiovasc Imaging. 2020;13(1 Pt 2):297–309.

6. Nagueh SF, Smiseth OA, Appleton CP, Byrd BF 3rd, Dokainish H, Edvardsen T, Flachskampf FA, Gillebert TC, Klein AL, Lancellotti P, Marino P, Oh JK, Popescu BA, Waggoner AD. Recommendations for the evaluation of left ventricular diastolic function by echocardiography: an update from the american society of echocardiography and the european association of cardiovascular imaging. J Am Soc Echocardiogr. 2016;29(4):277–314.

7. Nagueh SF, Abraham TP, Aurigemma GP, Bax JJ, Beladan C, Browning A, Chamsi-Pasha MA, Delgado V, Derumeaux G, Dolci G, Donal E, Edvardsen T, El Tallawi KC, Ernande L, Esposito R, Flachskampf FA, Galderisi M, Gentry J, Goldstein SA, Harb SC, Hubert A, Hung J, Klein AL, Lancellotti P, Mahmood RZ, Marino P, Popescu BA, Previato M, Sanghai SR, Smiseth OA, Xu J; for Diastolic Function Assessment Collaborators. Interobserver Variability in Applying American Society of Echocardiography/European Association of Cardiovascular Imaging 2016 Guidelines for Estimation of Left Ventricular Filling Pressure. Circ Cardiovasc Imaging. 2019;12(1):e008122.

8. Smiseth OA, Morris DA, Cardim N, Cikes M, Delgado V, Donal E, Flachskampf FA, Galderisi M, Gerber BL, Gimelli A, Klein AL, Knuuti J, Lancellotti P, Mascherbauer J, Milicic D, Seferovic P, Solomon S, Edvardsen T, Popescu BA. Reviewers: this document was reviewed by members of the 2018–2020 EACVI Scientific Documents Committee. Multimodality imaging in patients with heart failure and preserved ejection fraction: an expert consensus document of the European Association of Cardiovascular Imaging. Eur Heart J Cardiovasc Imaging. 2022 Jan 24;23(2):e34–e61. https://doi.org/10.1093/ehjci/jeab154. PMID: 34729586.

9. Selmeryd J, Henriksen E, Leppert J, Hedberg P. Interstudy heterogeneity of definitions of diastolic

dysfunction severely affects reported prevalence. Eur Heart J Cardiovasc Imaging. 2016;17:892–9.

10. Zawadka M, Marchel M, Andruszkiewicz P. Diastolic dysfunction of the left ventricle—a practical approach for an anaesthetist. Anaesthesiol Intensive Ther. 2020;52(3):237–44.

11. Ehrman RR, Russell FM, Ansari AH, Margeta B, Clary JM, Christian E, Cosby KS, Bailitz J. Can emergency physicians diagnose and correctly classify diastolic dysfunction using bedside echocardiography? Am J Emerg Med. 2015;33(9):1178–83.

12. Whalley GA, Doughty RN, Gamble GD, Wright SP, Walsh HJ, Muncaster SA, et al. Pseudonormal mitral filling pattern predicts hospital re-admission in patients with congestive heart failure. J Am Coll Cardiol. 2002;39(11):1787–95.

13. Logeart D, Saudubray C, Beyne P, Thabut G, Ennezat PV, Chavelas C, Zanker C, Bouvier E, Solal AC. Comparative value of Doppler echocardiography and B-type natriuretic peptide assay in the etiologic diagnosis of acute dyspnea. J Am Coll Cardiol. 2002;40:1794–800.

14. Nagueh SF, Middleton KJ, Kopelen HA, Zoghbi WA, Quiñones MA. Doppler tissue imaging: a noninvasive technique for evaluation of left ventricular relaxation and estimation of filling pressures. J Am Coll Cardiol 1997;15;30(6):1527–33.

15. Dokainish H, Zoghbi WA, Lakkis NM, Al-Bakshy F, Dhir M, Quinones MA, Nagueh SF. Optimal noninvasive assessment of left ventricular filling pressures: a comparison of tissue Doppler echocardiography and B-type natriuretic peptide in patients with pulmonary artery catheters. Circulation 2004;25;109 (20):2432–9.

16. Benfari G, Miller WL, Antoine C, Rossi A, Lin G, Oh JK, Roger VL, Thapa P, Enriquez-Sarano M. Diastolic determinants of excess mortality in heart failure with reduced ejection fraction JACC: Heart Failure 2019;1111. https://doi.org/10.1016/j.jchf.2019.04.024.

17. Little WC, Oh JK. Echocardiographic evaluation of diastolic function can be used to guide clinical care. Circulation. 2009;120(9):802–9.

18. Ommen SR, Nishimura RA, Appleton CP, Miller FA, Oh JK, Redfield MM, Tajik AJ. Clinical utility of Doppler echocardiography and tissue Doppler imaging in the estimation of left ventricular filling pressures: A comparative simultaneous Doppler-catheterization study. Circulation 2000;10;102(15):1788–94.

19. Olson JJ, Costa SP, Young CE, Palac RT. Early mitral filling/diastolic mitral annular velocity ratio is not a reliable predictor of left ventricular filling pressure in the setting of severe mitral regurgitation. J Am Soc Echocardiogr. 2006;19(1):83–7.

20. Park JH, Marwick TH. Use and limitations of E/e' to assess left ventricular filling pressure by echocardiography. J Cardiovasc Ultrasound. 2011;19:169–73.

21. Hillis GS, Møller JE, Pellikka PA, Gersh BJ, Wright RS, Ommen SR, Reeder GS, Oh JK. Noninvasive estimation of left ventricular filling pressure by E/e' is a powerful predictor of survival after acute myocardial infarction. J Am Coll Cardiol 2004;4;43 (3):360–7.

22. Pastore MC, Mandoli GE, Aboumarie HS, Santoro C, Bandera F, D'Andrea A, Benfari G, Esposito R, Evola V, Sorrentino R, Cameli P, Valente S, Mondillo S, Galderisi M, Cameli M; Working Group of Echocardiography of the Italian Society of Cardiology. Basic and advanced echocardiography in advanced heart failure: an overview. Heart Fail Rev. 2020;25(6):937–948.

23. Kotecha D, Mohamed M, Shantsila E, Popescu BA, Steeds RP. Is echocardiography valid and reproducible in patients with atrial fibrillation? A systematic review Europace. 2017;19:1427–38.

24. Lanspa MJ, Gutsche AR, Wilson EL, Olsen TD, Hirshberg EL, Knox DB, Brown SM, Grissom CK. Application of a simplified definition of diastolic function in severe sepsis and septic shock. Crit Care. 2016;20(1):243. https://doi.org/10.1186/s13054-016-1421-3. PMID:27487776;PMCID:PMC4973099.

25. Del Rios M, Colla J, Kotini-Shah P, Briller J, Gerber B, Prendergast H. Emergency physician use of tissue Doppler bedside echocardiography in detecting diastolic dysfunction: an exploratory study. Crit Ultrasound J. 2018;10(1):4.

26. Machino-Ohtsuka T, Seo Y, Ishizu T, Hamada-Harimura Y, Yamamoto M, Sato K, Sai S, Sugano A, Obara K, Yoshida I, Nishi I, Aonuma K, Ieda M. Clinical utility of the 2016 ASE/EACVI recommendations for the evaluation of left ventricular diastolic function in the stratification of post-discharge prognosis in patients with acute heart failure. Eur Heart J Cardiovasc Imaging. 2019;20(10):1129–37.

27. Oh JK, Miranda WR, Bird JG, Kane GC, Nagueh SF. The 2016 diastolic function guideline: is it already time to revisit or revise them? JACC Cardiovasc Imaging. 2020;13(1 Pt 2):327–35.

28. Mandoli GE, Sisti N, Mondillo S, Cameli M. Left atrial strain in left ventricular diastolic dysfunction: have we finally found the missing piece of the puzzle? Heart Fail Rev. 2020;25(3):409–17.

29. D'Ascenzi F, Anselmi F, Focardi M, Mondillo S. Atrial enlargement in the athlete's heart: assessment of atrial function may help distinguish adaptive from pathologic remodeling. J Am Soc Echocardiogr. 2018;31(2):148–57.

30. Njoku A, Kannabhiran M, Arora R, Reddy P, Gopinathannair R, Lakkireddy D, Dominic P. Left atrial volume predicts atrial fibrillation recurrence after radiofrequency ablation: a meta-analysis. Europace. 2018;20(1):33–42.

31. Katsiki N, Mikhailidis DP, Papanas N. Left atrial volume: An independent predictor of cardiovascular outcomes. Int J Cardiol. 2018;265:234–5.

32. Taniguchi N, Miyasaka Y, Suwa Y, Harada S, Nakai E, Kawazoe K, Shiojima I. Usefulness of left atrial volume as an independent predictor of development of heart failure in patients with atrial fibrillation. Am J Cardiol. 2019;124(9):1430–5.

33. Hashimoto N, Watanabe T, Tamura H, Tsuchiya H, Wanezaki M, Kato S, Nishiyama S, Arimoto T, Takahashi H, Shishido T, Watanabe M. Left atrial remodeling index is a feasible predictor of poor prognosis in patients with acute ischemic stroke. Heart Vessels. 2019;34(12):1936–43.

34. Cameli M, Pastore MC, Henein MY, Mondillo S. The left atrium and the right ventricle: two supporting chambers to the failing left ventricle. Heart Fail Rev. 2019;24(5):661–9.

35. Bytyçi I, Bajraktari G, Lindqvist P, Henein MY. Compromised left atrial function and increased size predict raised cavity pressure: a systematic review and meta-analysis. Clin Physiol Funct Imaging. 2019;39(5):297–307.

36. Potter EL, Ramkumar S, Kawakami H, Yang H, Wright L, Negishi T, Marwick TH. Association of asymptomatic diastolic dysfunction assessed by left atrial strain with incident heart failure. JACC Cardiovasc Imaging. 2020;13(11):2316–26.

37. Morris DA, Belyavskiy E, Aravind-Kumar R, Kropf M, Frydas A, Braunauer K, Marquez E, Krisper M, Lindhorst R, Osmanoglou E, Boldt LH, Blaschke F, Haverkamp W, Tschöpe C, Edelmann F, Pieske B, Pieske-Kraigher E. Potential usefulness and clinical relevance of adding left atrial strain to left atrial volume index in the detection of left ventricular diastolic dysfunction. JACC Cardiovasc Imaging. 2018;11(10):1405–15.

38. Dal Canto E, Remmelzwaal S, van Ballegooijen AJ, Handoko ML, Heymans S, van Empel V, Paulus WJ, Nijpels G, Elders P, Beulens JW. Diagnostic value of echocardiographic markers for diastolic dysfunction and heart failure with preserved ejection fraction. Heart Fail Rev. 2020. https://doi.org/10.1007/s10741-020-09985-1.

39. Reddy YNV, Obokata M, Egbe A, Yang JH, Pislaru S, Lin G, Carter R, Borlaug BA. Left atrial strain and compliance in the diagnostic evaluation of heart failure with preserved ejection fraction. Eur J Heart Fail. 2019;21(7):891–900.

40. Tachjian A, Sanghai SR, Stencel J, Parker MW, Kakouros N, Aurigemma GP. Estimation of mean left atrial pressure in patients with acute coronary syndromes: a doppler echocardiographic and cardiac catheterization study. J Am Soc Echocardiogr. 2019;32(3):365-374.e1.

41. Nagueh SF, Middleton KJ, Kopelen HA, Zoghbi WA, Quiñones MA. Doppler tissue imaging: a noninvasive technique for evaluation of left ventricular relaxation and estimation of filling pressures. J Am Coll Cardiol. 1997;30(6):1527–33.

42. Orde S, Slama M, Hilton A, Yastrebov K, McLean A. Pearls and pitfalls in comprehensive critical care echocardiography. Crit Care 2017;17;21(1):279.

POCUS in Monitoring: LV Systolic Function and Cardiac Output

Francisca Caetano and Hatem Soliman-Aboumarie

I would especially commend the physician who, in acute diseases, by which the bulk of mankind are cut off, conducts the treatment better than others

HIPPOCRATES. Greek physician and the father of modern medicine. (460 BC-370 BC)

Abstract

Echocardiography has been recognised as a haemodynamic monitoring device in the critically ill patients. Although transthoracic approach provides discontinuous haemodynamic monitoring, it can be readily repeated at the bedside. In this chapter, the authors will describe how to use POCUS to estimate cardiac output non-invasively which would be pivotal in the diagnosis and management of cardiogenic shock. Myocardial contractility is one of the determinants of cardiac output. Hence, its assessment is paramount. There are different echocardiographic tools to evaluate left ventricular myocardial contractility. The authors will describe different methodologies, their main strengths and limitations. Starting with two-dimensional echocardiography (e.g., Ejection Fraction), Doppler assessment (e.g., dP/dT) and M-mode techniques (e.g., MAPSE). Finally, a section dedicated to regional systolic function in which latest recommendations for segmentation of the LV and different aetiologies for regional wall motion abnormalities will be discussed.

Keywords

Cardiac output · Cardiogenic shock · Myocardial contractility · Doppler imaging · Regional systolic function

Key Messages

- Cardiac output is a measure of the amount of blood pumped by the heart every minute. There is no "normal" cardiac output value, instead, this depends on the specific conditions of the individual at the time of measurement.

F. Caetano
Department of Critical Care, Royal Papworth Hospital, Cambridge, UK
e-mail: ana.caetano@nhs.net

H. Soliman-Aboumarie (✉)
Department of Anaethetics and Critical Care, Harefield Hospital, Royal Brompton and Harefield Hospitals, London, UK
e-mail: hatem.soliman@gmail.com; h.solimanaboumarie@rbht.nhs.uk

School of Cardiovascular Medicine and Sciences, King's College London, London, UK

H. Soliman-Aboumarie et al. (eds.), *Cardiopulmonary Point of Care Ultrasound*,
https://doi.org/10.1007/978-3-031-29472-3_18

- The use of POCUS to estimate cardiac output has been extensively validated against pulmonary thermodilution in intensive care.
- Myocardial contractility can be defined as the quality of cardiac muscle that determines performance, independent of loading conditions.
- Ejection fraction is affected by preload and afterload. For example, the pathological decrease in afterload can cause a false impression of preserved left ventricular function even in the presence of serious myocardial compromise (e.g., mitral regurgitation).
- A combination of different echocardiographic tools to evaluate left ventricular myocardial contractility is likely to be the best approach in the critically ill patients.

Introduction

Early recognition of shock state is of paramount importance in order to reduce morbidity and mortality [1]. Prompt interventions aiming to restore normal haemodynamics and correcting the cause of shock may effectively change the clinical course of the disease [2].

In 2011, a consensus of experts in the field of haemodynamic monitoring has recognised echocardiography as a true haemodynamic monitoring device, although discontinuous [3]. Currently, echocardiography is used to help in the diagnosis of the source of the shock, to choose the correct therapy, and finally, to tailor the therapy at the bedside by reassessing the effects of the strategies adopted [4]. Thus, critical care echocardiography led to a paradigm shift towards a less invasive, qualitative, discontinuous and functional haemodynamic monitoring [5].

The use of POCUS to estimate the cardiac output and assess left ventricular systolic function is a cornerstone in the management of critically ill patients with haemodynamic compromise. 2D echocardiography, pulsed and continuous wave Doppler, M-mode, and tissue Doppler imaging are the main techniques used in POCUS for this purpose.

Diagnosis of Cardiogenic Shock with Echocardiography

Cardiogenic shock is often a form of low-cardiac output shock. It derives from ventricular failure caused by different pathological conditions (i.e., acute myocardial infarction, valvular heart disease, myocarditis, arrhythmias). In this type of shock, cardiac output is typically low, most of the times because of impaired ventricular contractility [6].

The cardiac output is a measure of the amount of blood pumped by the heart every minute. There is no "normal" cardiac output value; any cardiac output value can be inadequate or excessive depending on the specific conditions of the individual at the time of assessment [7].

Estimation of cardiac output can be performed with echocardiography. Using Doppler imaging, it is possible to measure the stroke distance. This refers to the distance travelled by a column of blood during a fixed time. Multiplying the stroke distance (velocity time integral: VTI) with the cross-sectional area (CSA) through which the column moves gives the stroke volume (SV).

Technique for Cardiac Output estimation from the LVOT:

This can be obtained at several sites, with the most common and accurate being the left ventricle outflow tract (LVOT) [8]. The PWD sample volume is placed at the aortic annulus and the flow through the LVOT should be laminar. The alignment of Doppler beam should be parallel to and through the center of the blood flow column in order to obtain the highest velocity. Note that the best view for Doppler estimation of LVOT VTI may not be necessarily the best 2D image. The LVOT VTI is obtained by tracing the modal velocity envelope (the chin and not the beard) which is the velocity at which most of the red blood cells are travelling at high intensity. Reducing the Doppler gain can help reducing non-modal velocities while improving the modal velocity.

Below is the equation to calculate the cardiac output (CO) with echocardiography [9]:

$$CO = SV \times HR$$
$$SV = CSA\,LVOT \times LVOT\,VTI$$
$$SV = 3.14 \times (LVOT/2)^2)] \times LVOT\,VTI$$

CO = cardiac output; CSA LVOT = cross sectional area of left ventricular outflow tract; HR = heart rate; SV = stroke volume; VTI = velocity time integral.

Cross sectional area is derived from the LVOT diameter measured from parasternal long axis view in mid-systole (Fig. 1). LVOT VTI is measured from apical 5-chamber view using pulsed wave (PW) Doppler (Fig. 2).

This method was extensively validated against pulmonary thermodilution in intensive care [9].

Because LVOT diameter is fixed, any change of SV can be tracked by the change in LVOT VTI. Therefore, LVOT VTI is considered a surrogate for SV. Normal values of the LVOT VTI are within the range of 18 to 22 cm with values of less than 15 cm suggestive of low cardiac output (Fig. 3). However, as mentioned earlier, LVOT VTI values should be always interpreted within the clinical context (e.g.:

LVOT VTI of 20 cm in a patient with profound vasoplegia and hyperdynamic state due to sepsis would indicate a combined cardiogenic and vasoplegic shock as pure vasoplegia would be expected to have higher values of LVOT VTI due to high cardiac output.) Moreover, an LVOT VTI of 14 cm can be enough to achieve adequate stroke volume in a patient with dilated LVOT.

By trans-oesophageal echocardiography, this can be calculated by obtaining the deep trans-gastric five-chamber view at 0° or the modified trans-gastric long-axis view at 120° as both provide fair alignment with the LVOT flow and the PWD beam (Table 1).

Pitfalls/Limitations:

– The cross-sectional area of the LVOT is calculated assuming a circular geometry, but in reality it is often elliptical [10].
– Small errors in diameter measurements become large errors in cross sectional area calculations, taking into account the square of the radius introduced in the recommended formula.
– Significant aortic regurgitation will lead to overestimation of the stroke volume and, consequently, the cardiac output. Assuming

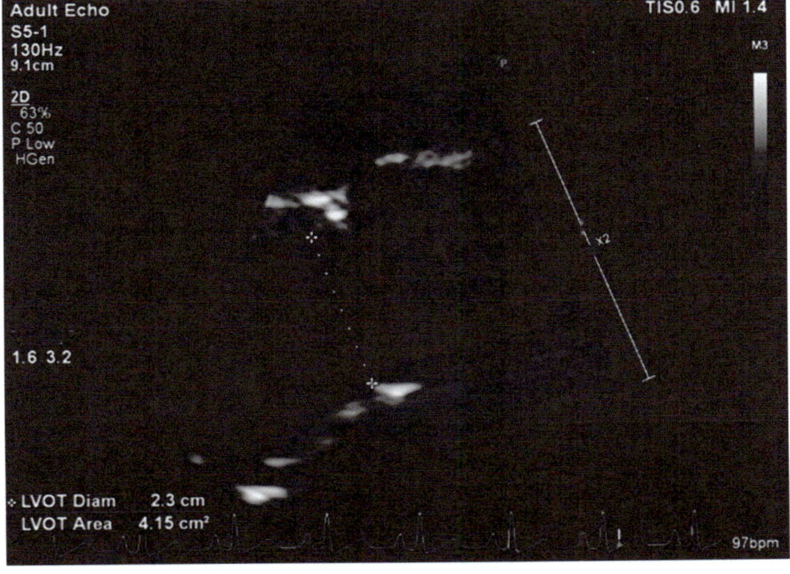

Fig. 1 LVOT diameter is measured from parasternal long axis view in mid-systole. In this case the LVOT diameter is 2.3 cm. Cross sectional area is 4.15 cm² $[\pi \times r^2 = 3.14 \times (2.3/2)^2]$

Fig. 2 LVOT VTI is measured from apical 5-chamber view using PWD. The estimated stroke volume is 87 mL [CSA LVOT x LVOT VTI = 4.15 × 20.9] and cardiac output 7.8L/min (SV x HR = 87 × 90)

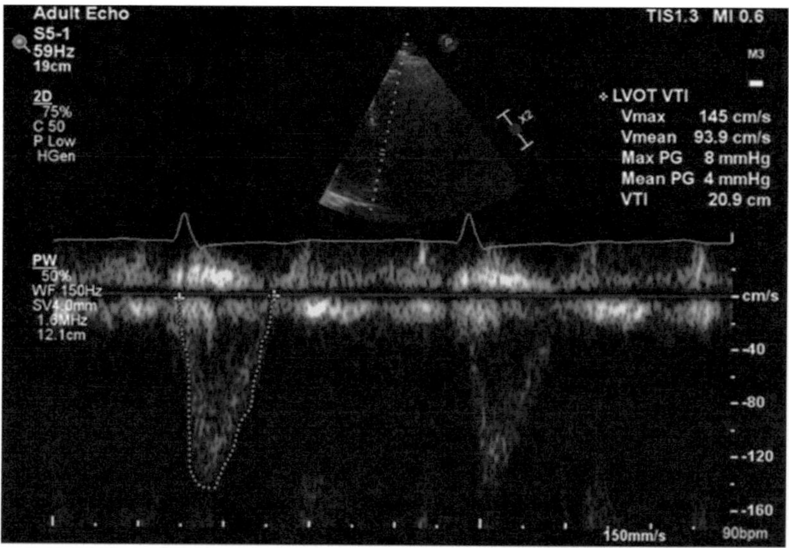

Fig. 3 In this case, the estimated stroke volume would be 31 mL and the cardiac output 2.8L/min (for the same CSA LVOT and heart rate)

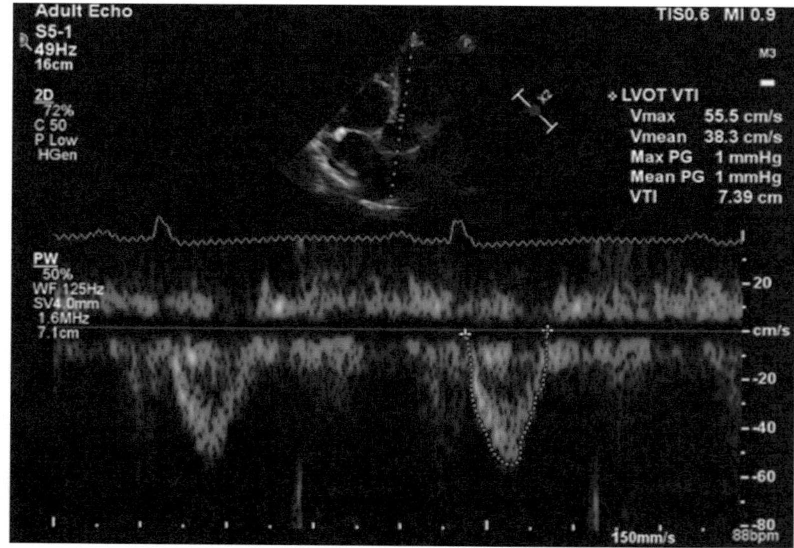

there is no pulmonic shunting and able to be visualised, the RV outflow tract can be used for assessment of stroke volume instead of the LVOT [11].

- In patients with atrial fibrillation. An average of 5–10 cardiac cycles estimation is recommended.

Tailored Management of Cardiogenic Shock with Echocardiography

Cardiac output is determined by four factors: heart rate, preload, afterload and myocardial contractility. Treatment of inadequate cardiac output therefore involves optimizing these four aspects.

Table 1 Parameters and pitfalls in LV systolic function and stroke volume assessment

Parameter	Pitfalls
• LVOT VTI/SV • MAPSE • TDI S′	• LVOT VTI: – Avoid plain foreshortening when measuring the LVOT diameter – Avoid SV under-estimation: 1. Optimize PWD settings to measure LVOT VTI 2. Put the PWD beam parallel to LVOT flow (use colour Doppler) – Shock -> check for dynamic LVOT obstruction ($\pm$ MV systolic anterior motion) [especially in case of hypovolemia, LV hypertrophy and hyperdynamic LV (e.g.: vasoplegia)] – Not applicable in aortic stenosis or subaortic obstruction – AF: average of 5 beats – AR: SV overestimation (the regurgitant diastolic flow is not considered) • MAPSE Mono-dimensional and regional parameter (only analyzes mitral annular LV portion) • TDI S′ Lower spatial resolution

Heart Rate

The optimal heart rate should be individualized for each patient. Echocardiography-guided heart rate optimization results in a significant increase in cardiac output. Total isovolumic time (t-IVT) has been shown to be the echocardiographic index with the highest sensitivity to determine the optimal hemodynamic profile [12].

Preload

Increasing preload can increase myocardial contractility by increasing myocardial fibre stretch, on the basis of the Frank-Starling relationship. To optimize fluid administration without causing fluid overload and its associated harmful effects, efforts should be taken to determine the patient's likely response to fluid administration (See Chap. 15 on volume responsiveness).

Afterload

Afterload represents the forces working to prevent ventricular emptying. In the normal heart, stroke volume is minimally affected by changes in afterload, whereas in the failing heart small changes in afterload can generate important changes in stroke volume [13]. Afterload can be decreased by using vasodilators.

Myocardial Contractility

Contractility is the force generated at any given end-diastolic volume. It may be defined as the quality of cardiac muscle that determines performance, independent of loading conditions [14]. However, its contribution to the haemodynamic process is difficult to study because no load-independent index of basal contractile state has been described yet [15].

There are different echocardiographic tools to evaluate left ventricle (LV) myocardial contractility.

a. **Ejection Fraction (EF)**

The most common quantitative approach of estimating LV systolic function is the ejection fraction (EF). It represents stroke volume as a percentage of end-diastolic volume. EF is a global index which expresses myocardial fibre shortening and requires the estimation of LV volumes [16]. Calculation of volume which is 3D from a 2D image requires mathematical calculations based on geometric models. The most frequently used technique for LV volume measurement is the biplane method of discs (modified Simpson's rule) [17]. This methodology is based on the principle of calculation of total LV volume as the summation of a series of elliptical discs of equal height, equally spaced along the long axis of the LV [18].

LV end-diastolic and end-systolic volumes (LVEDV and LVESV, respectively) are measured in two orthogonal planes (Apical 4-chamber, A4C; and Apical 2-chamber, A2C). LV ejection fraction is calculated as:

$$EF_{A4C} = (LVEDV_{A4C} - LVESV_{A4C})/$$
$$LVEDV_{A4C} \times 100 \,(Figure\ 4)$$
$$EF_{A2C} = (LVEDV_{A2C} - LVESV_{A2C})/$$
$$LVEDV_{A2C} \times 100 \,(Figure\ 5)$$

Mean ejection fraction is obtained as an average of A4C and A2C ejection fraction values. A normal ejection fraction is 53–73% [17] (Figs. 4 and 5).

3D echocardiographic methods of LV volume measurement are less geometry-dependent and give more accurate values of ejection fraction.

Pitfalls/Limitations:

- There are currently no validated reference values for EF in the haemodynamically unstable and critically ill patients and it is not in any of the definitions of shock.
- EF is affected by preload and afterload. Example: the pathological decrease in afterload (e.g., mitral regurgitation, or interventricular septal defect) can cause a false impression of preserved LV function even in the presence of serious myocardial compromise [19].
- Foreshortening of the ventricular apex causes overestimation of LVEF.
- When less than 80% of the endocardial border is adequately visualized, the use of contrast agents is highly recommended [20].
- Beat-to-beat variation of EF in the presence of arrhythmia, for example, atrial fibrillation, requires several measurements and averaging.

b. **Systolic index of contractility (dP/dT)**

The maximum rate of rise of LV pressure during the isovolumic contraction phase of LV systole is a good measure of LV contractility. Using continuous wave Doppler (CWD), dP/dT can be estimated, as long as the patient has mitral regurgitation (MR) [21]. If restricted to the early phases of systole, during isovolumic contraction, dP/dT is a relatively load-independent measure of ventricular contractility [22].

In the presence of global LV dysfunction, the LV pressure build-up will decrease, and the left atrium pressure will increase which will decrease the rate of rise of MR jet velocity. Time taken

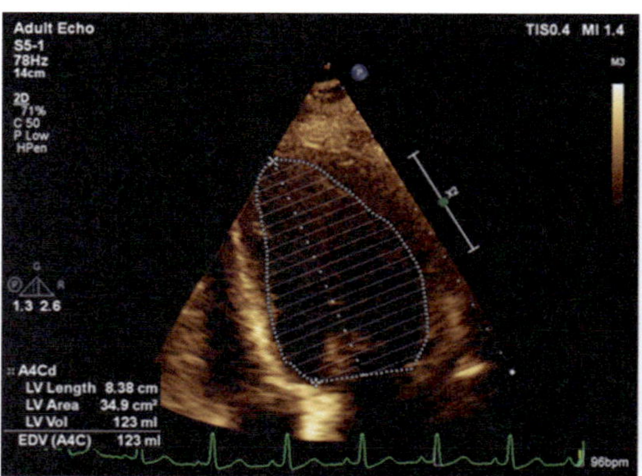

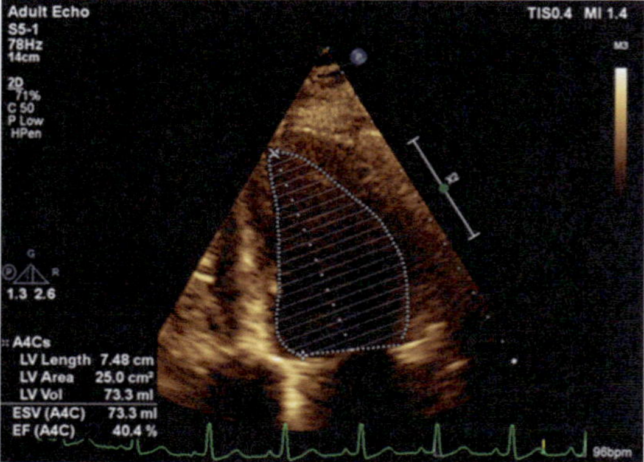

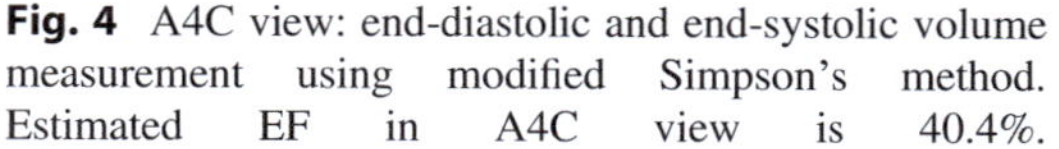

Fig. 4 A4C view: end-diastolic and end-systolic volume measurement using modified Simpson's method. Estimated EF in A4C view is 40.4%.

$$EF_{A4C} = (LVEDV_{A4C} - LVESV_{A4C})/LVEDV_{A4C} \times 100$$
$$EF_{A4C} = (123 - 73)/123 \times 100 = 40.4\%$$

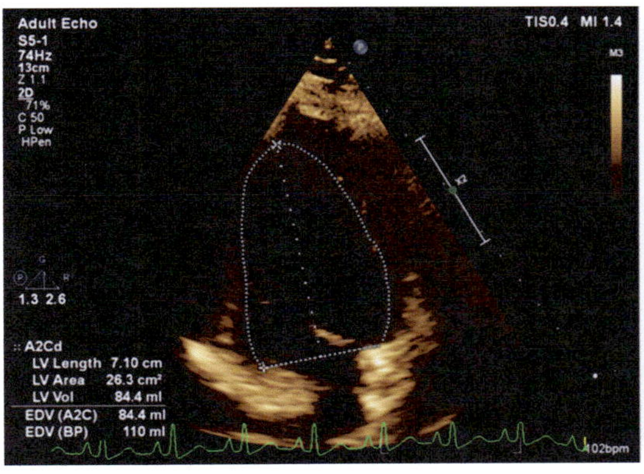
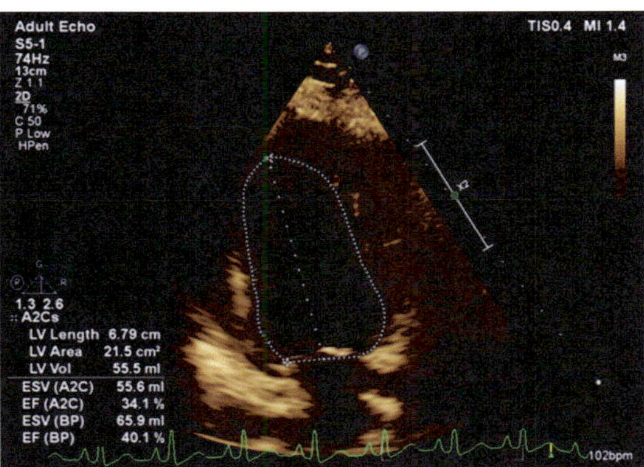

Fig. 5 A2C view: end-diastolic and end-systolic volume measurement using modified Simpson's method. Estimated EF in A2C view is 34.5%.

$$EF_{A2C} = (LVEDV_{A2C} - LVESV_{A2C})/LVEDV_{A2C} \times 100$$
$$EF_{A2C} = (84 - 55)/84 \times 100 = 34.5\%$$

(dT) for the velocity to rise from 1 m/s to 3 m/s (dP of 32 mmHg) is measured on the MR envelop (Fig. 6) [23]. Normal value is >1200 mmHg/s (dT $\leq$ 27 ms). Values <800 mmHg/s (dT $\geq$ 40 ms) are reduced. In situations of severe LV dysfunction, MR velocity might not reach 3 m/s. Any velocity can be selected, where a measurable time interval is possible, and can be used to calculate dP/dT [24].

In the presence of significant mechanical dyssynchrony, dP/dT may be reduced, as a consequence of contractile dyssynchrony in spite of preserved global systolic function.

Pitfalls/Limitations:

- A good MR signal is mandatory for estimation of dP/dT (which may not always be present)

Fig. 6 Systolic index of contractility (dP/dT) measurement. dP/dT = 32 mmHg/0.039 sec = 829 mmHg/sec

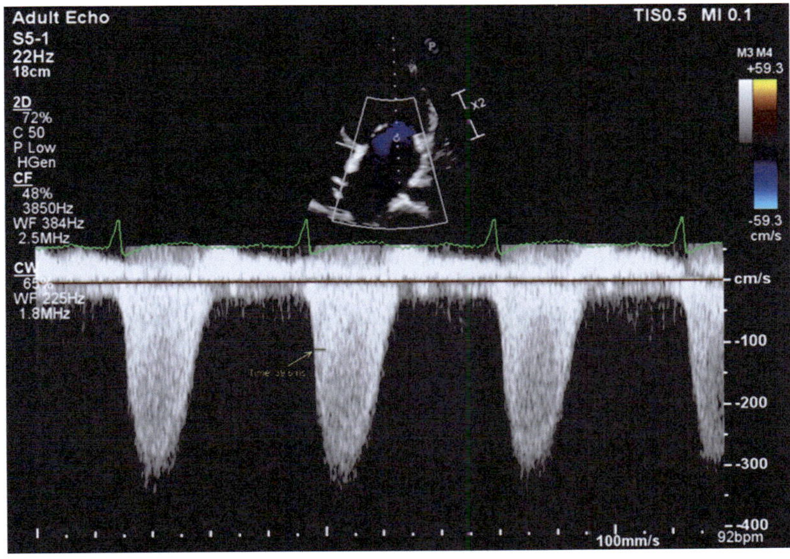

- A small error in the time interval will produce a large change in dP/dT value.
- This method is inappropriate in the presence of acute MR because of high left atrial pressures in acute MR.
- dP/dT is not an entirely load-independent index of LV function.

c. **Left ventricular outflow tract ejection acceleration**

In the absence of significant aortic valve disease, the time taken by the blood column to accelerate and reach the peak velocity through the LVOT is inversely related to the contractile function of the LV [24].

With PW Doppler sample volume positioned in the LVOT, the Doppler curve will give information regarding the LVOT peak velocity (Vmax) and LVOT acceleration time (ACT). LVOT ACT is the time from the beginning to the peak of the LOVT systolic flow and it provides information about global LV systolic function in the form of LVOT acceleration (LVOT ACC). LVOT ACC is calculated as follows:

$$\mathrm{LVOT\ ACC}\,(m/s^2) = V\mathrm{max}\ (m/s)/\mathrm{ACT}\,(s)$$

With impaired LV function, the ejection curve becomes flattened and round, instead of a sharp-angled triangle. This means decreased peak velocity and an increased ACT (Fig. 7).

LVOT ACC is not load-dependent. Normal range is 8–14 m/s^2.

Pitfalls/Limitations:

- This method is based on the measurement of a relatively short period of time that may be difficult and even misleading at times.
- It may be difficult to determine the peak velocity in a rounded velocity curve with no pronounced peak.

d. **Mitral annular plane systolic excursion (MAPSE)**

LV systolic function can also be assessed by mitral annular plane systolic excursion (MAPSE) measurement [25].

MAPSE should be measured using M-mode echocardiography with the M-mode cursor aligned parallel to the LV walls (Fig. 8). It corresponds to mitral annular displacement distance towards the apex and a reduced MAPSE thereby reflects impairment of the longitudinal LV contraction. The normal value of MAPSE ranges between 12 and 15 mm. A value <8 mm is

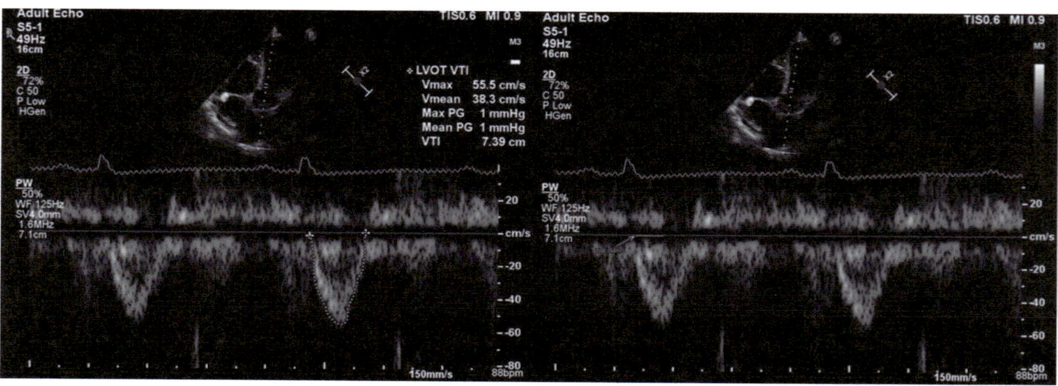

Fig. 7 Left ventricular outflow tract ejection acceleration measurement.
$\mathrm{LVOT\ ACC}\,(m/s^2) = V\mathrm{max}(m/sec)/\mathrm{ACT}\,(sec)$
$\mathrm{LVOT\ ACC} = 0.55\,m/sec/0.094\,sec = 5.8\,m/s^2$

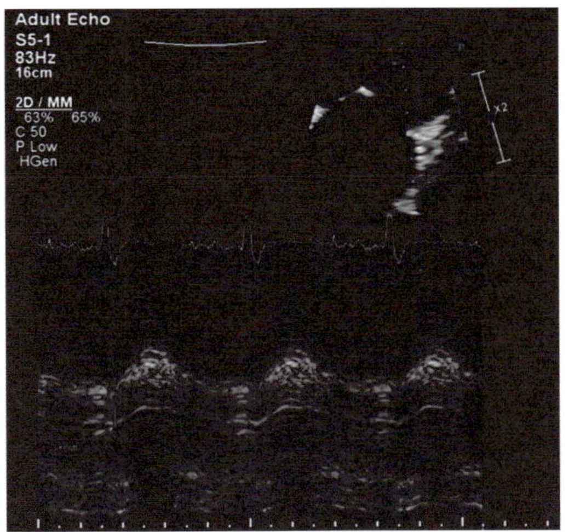

Fig. 8 MAPSE measurement using M-mode echocardiography. MAPSE is low (5.5 mm), reflecting impairment of the longitudinal LV contraction

associated with LV dysfunction (LVEF < 50%) [26].

MAPSE can be easily recorded even in patients with a poor acoustic window and for inexperienced POCUS operators.

e. Tissue Doppler Imaging (TDI)

Tissue Doppler imaging (TDI) measurements include both systolic and diastolic velocities.

TDI is acquired using PW Doppler from the apical views to acquire the mitral annular velocities [27]. Annular velocity in systole has

shown a good correlation with the LVEF. Usually, the systolic velocity of the mitral annulus is superior to 6 cm/s and has a strong correlation with normal EF [28]. Moreover, a decreased peak systolic velocity is a sensitive marker of mildly impaired LV systolic function, even in patients with normal LVEF (Fig. 9) [29]. However, TDI is not independent from preload [30].

Index of global myocardial performance

The index of global myocardial performance (MPI) or Tei index reflects global systolic and diastolic LV performance and is expressed by the formula:

$$MPI = ICT + IRT/ET$$

where *ICT* is the isovolumic contraction time, *IRT* is the isovolumic relaxation time, and *ET* the ejection time. Such time intervals can all be obtained using TD imaging. The normal value of the index is 0.4. Systolic dysfunction causes a prolonged ICT and a reduction of ET, while diastolic impairment prolongs the IRT. In patients with heart failure the Tei index is greater than 0.5.

Total isovolumic time (t-IVT) is the 'wasted' time of the cardiac cycle, during which the ventricle neither fill nor ejects, and it has been shown to be the echocardiographic index with the highest sensitivity to determine the optimal

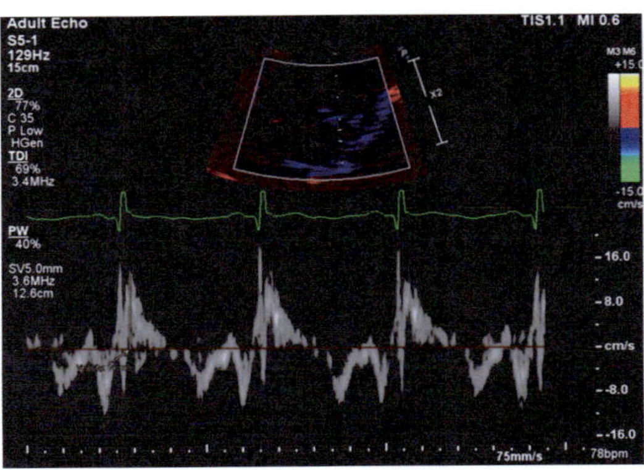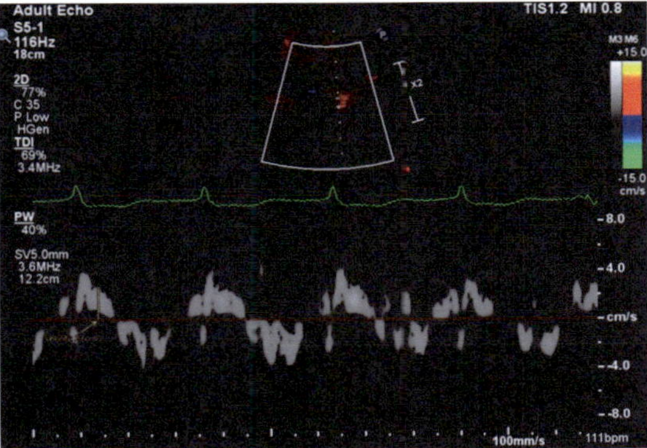

Fig. 9 TDI measurement of mitral annular velocity in systole. **a**—Normal peak systolic velocity (14 cm/s). **b**—Decreased peak systolic velocity (2.6 cm/s)

hemodynamic profile and it is a sensitive marker of LV electromechanical efficiency with a threshold value of >14 s/minute as an index for dyssynchrony and electromechanical inefficiency [12, 31].

$$t - IVT = ICT + IRT$$
$$= 60 - (t - FT + t - ET)$$

FT = filling time, ET = ejection time.
Longitudinal post systolic shortening (PSS).
Longitudinal post systolic shortening (PSS) is a typical finding if ventricular function is inhomogeneous (Fig. 10). It can be defined as shortening of the myocardium after aortic valve closure. Together with a reduced systolic function, PSS is a non-specific, but sensitive feature of regional ischaemia and scar [32].

f. **Left ventricle regional systolic function**

Segmentation of the Left Ventricle

Myocardial walls are divided according to the distribution of the coronary arteries. Although there is some degree of variability, there is a direct correlation between the LV segments and the coronary arteries. This allows the identification of which coronary artery is involved when a segmental wall motion abnormality is seen (Figs. 11 and 12) [17].

When using the 17-segment model to assess wall motion, the 17th segment (the apical cap) should not be included, because it doesn't move (Fig. 12) [33]. (See Chap 8: POCUS in acute myocardial ischaemia for more details).

Visual Assessment

Semi-quantitative wall motion score can be assigned to each segment to calculate the LV wall motion score index (sum score of all segments assessed/number of segments assessed) [34]. Each segment should be scored on the basis of its systolic motion and thickening. Results of the regional LV evaluation can be reported in a bull's eye graph (Fig. 12). The wall motion score index has been shown to be an important prognostic indicator in patients with coronary artery disease. (See Chap. 8: POCUS in acute myocardial ischaemia for more details).

Regional Abnormalities in the Absence of Coronary Artery Disease

Regional wall motion abnormalities (WMAs) may also occur in the absence of coronary artery disease (e.g., myocarditis, Takotsubo cardiomyopathy).

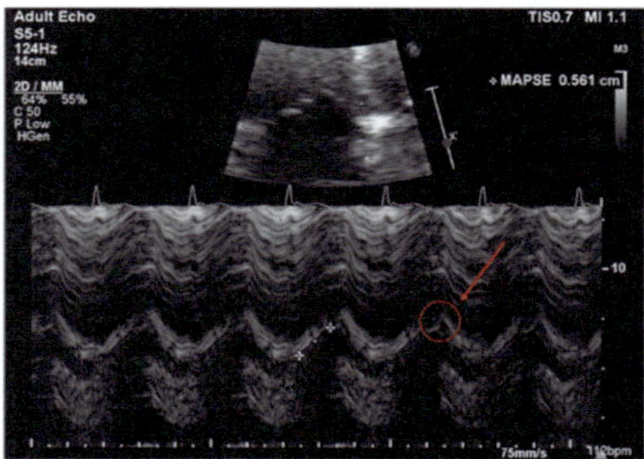
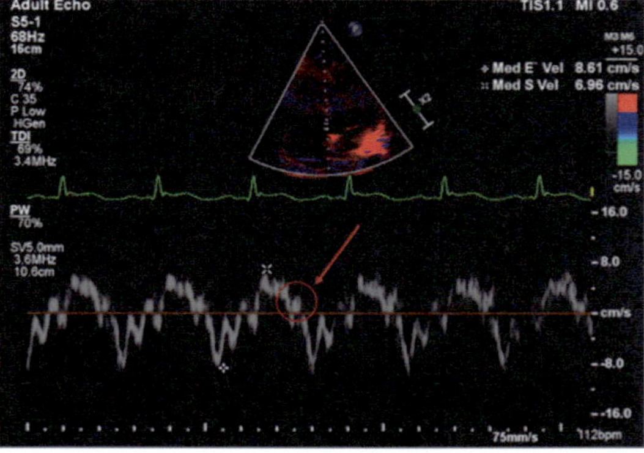

Fig. 10 Longitudinal post systolic shortening seen with M-mode and TDI

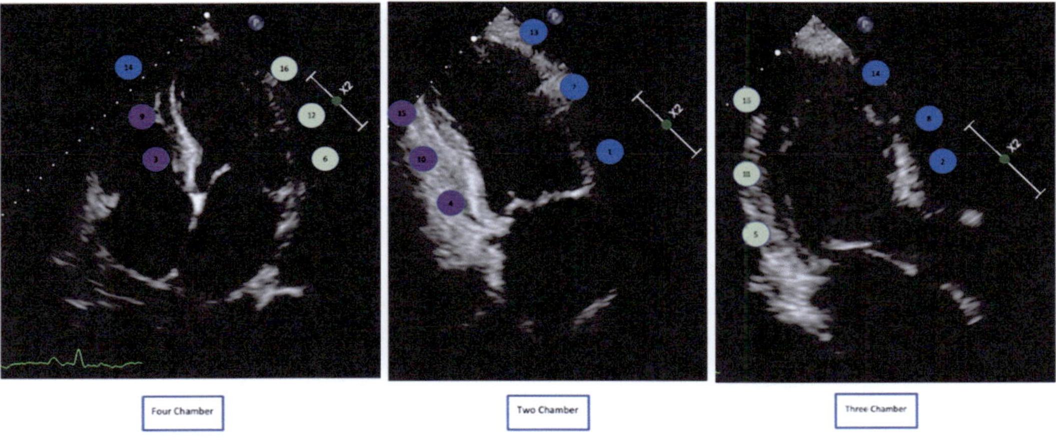

Fig. 11 Orientation of apical four-chamber, apical two-chamber, and apical three-chamber views in relation with the 17-segment model and corresponding coronary artery territories (Purple circles—right coronary artery; Green circles—left circumflex artery; Blue circles—left anterior descending artery) [17]

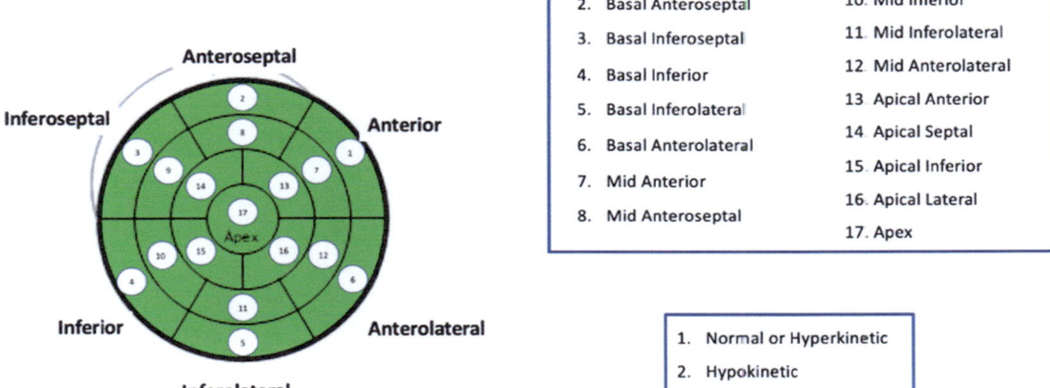

Fig. 12 Representation of each LV segment in the bull's eye graph (left side). 17-segment model (top right). Scoring system (bottom right)

The most common frequent non-ischaemic WMAs are as a consequence of conduction system abnormalities such as left bundle branch block and right ventricle pacing (Fig. 13a) [17]. The differential diagnosis of wall motion abnormalities caused by conduction system abnormalities or ischaemia might be challenging [35].

Another common form of non-ischaemic WMA is abnormal septal motion, observed after any form of cardiac surgery with pericardium opening and it results from the amplified anterior motion of the heart within the thorax due to loss of pericardial constraint [17].

Conditions involving pericardial constriction (Fig. 13b), or abnormal ventricular interaction caused by RV volume or pressure overload may be the origin of WMA of the interventricular septum (Fig. 13c). It is a consequence of exaggerated ventricular differential filling, often with respiratory variation, mainly as a consequence of volume overload or pericardial constriction [37].

Conclusion

POCUS should be a first line imaging method in the intensive care patients with haemodynamic compromise.

In patients with low cardiac output state, assessment of myocardial contractility is paramount. However, all the different techniques have inherent limitations, and the operator must

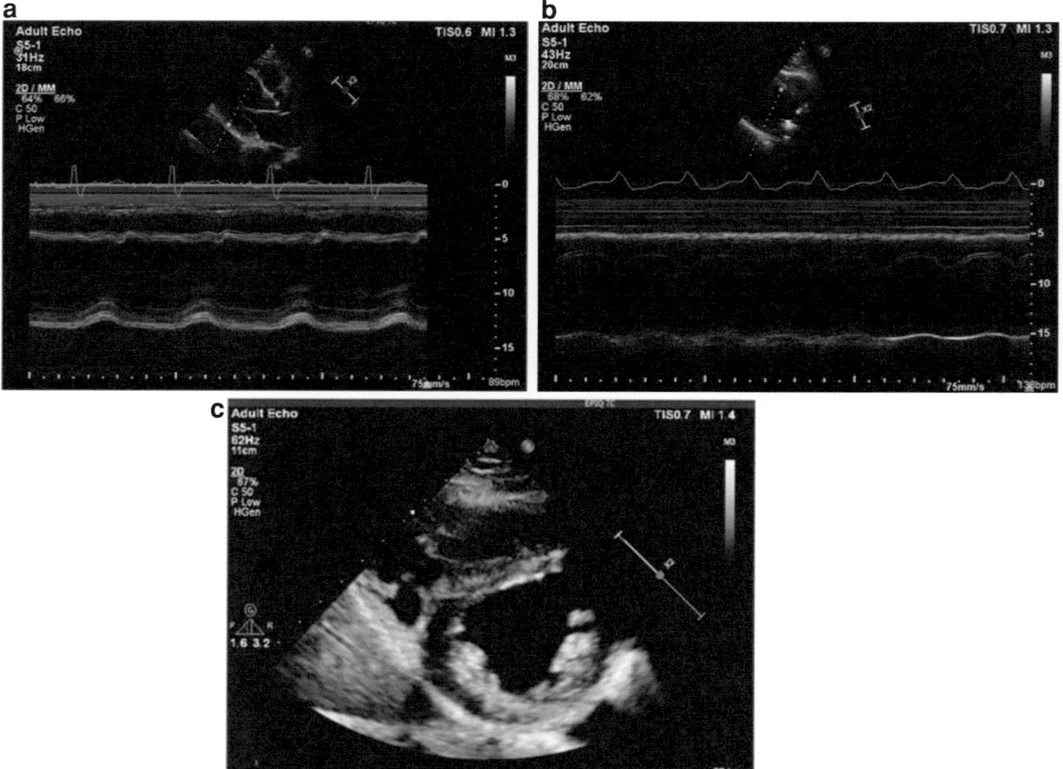

Fig. 13 **a–c** Regional abnormalities in the absence of coronary artery disease. **a** Patient with left bundle branch block. M-mode shows abnormal septal motion. **b** Patient with pericardial constriction. M-mode shows septal bounce. **c** Right ventricle volume overload causing abnormal septal motion/flattening in diastole

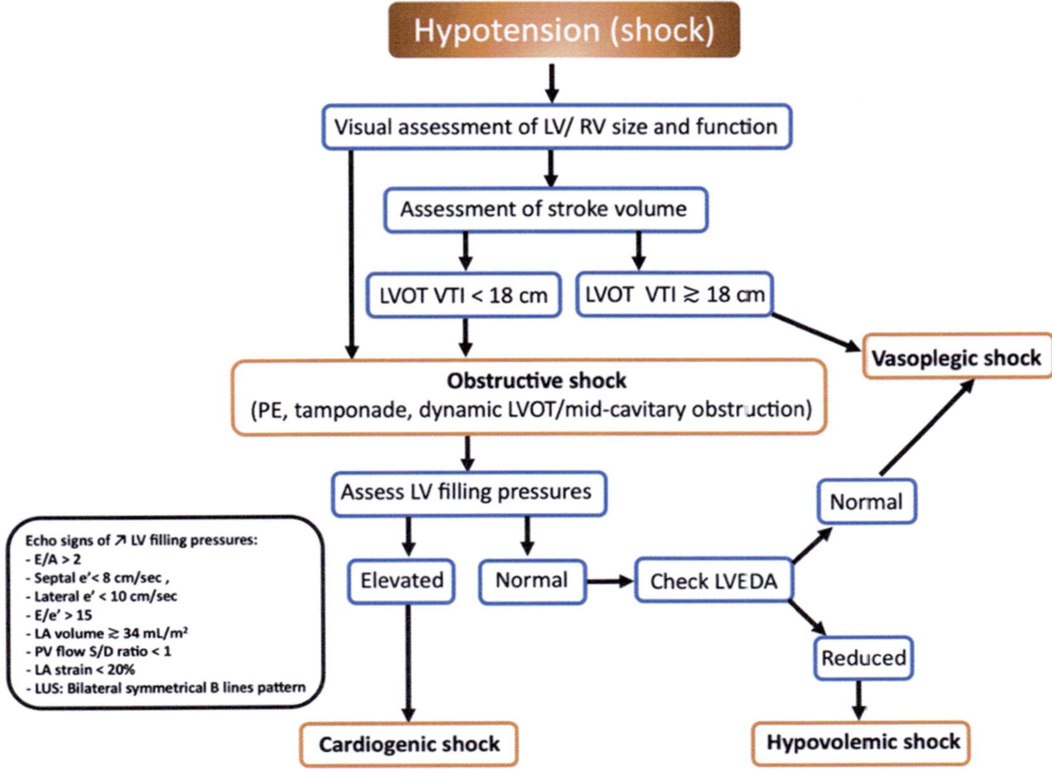

Fig. 14 Proposed algorithm showing POCUS-guided assessment of patients with hypotension/shock [36]

remain cautious and vigilant. An approach that combines the different POCUS modalities and techniques within the clinical context is likely to be the safest and the most successful.

References

1. Mervyn Singer CSD, Seymour CW, Shankar-Hari M, Annane D, Bauer M, Bellomo R, Bernard GR, Chiche J-D, Coopersmith CM, Hotchkiss RS, Levy MM, Marshall JC, Martin GS, Opal SM, Rubenfeld GD, van der Poll T, Vincent J-L, Angus DC. The third international consensus definitions for sepsis and septic shock (Sepsis-3). J Amer Med Assoc. 2016;315(8):801–10.

2. Maurizio Cecconi DDB, Antonelli M, Beale R, Bakker J, Hofer C, Jaeschke R, Mebazaa A, Pinsky MR, Teboul JL, Vincent JL, Rhodes A. Consensus on circulatory shock and hemodynamic monitoring. Task force of the European society of intensive care medicine. Intensive Care Med. 2014;40(12):1795–815.

3. Jean-Louis Vincent AR, Perel A, Martin GS, Rocca GD, Vallet B, Pinsky MR, Hofer CK, Teboul J-L, de Boode W-P, Scolletta S, Vieillard-Baron A, De Backer D, Walley KR, Maggiorini M, Singer M. Clinical review: Update on hemodynamic monitoring —a consensus of 16. Critical Care. 2011;15(4):229.

4. Philippe Vignon EB, Mari A, Silva S, Chimot L, Delour P, Vargas F, Filloux B, Vandroux D, Jabot J, François B, Pichon N, ClavelM, Levy B, Slama M, Riu-Poulenc B. Hemodynamic assessment of patients with septic shock using transpulmonary

thermodilution and critical care echocardiography: a comparative study. Chest. 2018;153(1):55–64.

5. Michael R, Pinsky DP. Functional hemodynamic monitoring. Crit Care. 2005;9(6):566–72.

6. Antonio Dell'Anna FT, Antonelli M. Shock: definition and recognition. In: Michael R Pinsky J-LT, Vincent J-L, editor. Hemodynamic Monitoring. Switzerland: Springer; 2019. p. 7–20.

7. Vincent J-L. Assessing the Adequacy of Cardiac Output. In: Vincent J-L, editor. Michael R Pinsky J-LT. Hemodynamic Monitoring. Switzerland: Springer; 2019. p. 21–6.

8. J F Lewis LCK, Nelson JG, Limacher MC, Quinones MA. Pulsed Doppler echocardiographic determination of stroke volume and cardiac output: clinical validation of two new methods using the apical window. Circulation. 1984;70:425–31.

9. Pablo Mercado JM, Beyls C, Titeca-Beauport D, Joris M, Kontar L, Riviere A, Bonef O, Soupison T, Tribouilloy C, de Cagny B, Slama M. Transthoracic echocardiography: an accurate and precise method for estimating cardiac output in the critically ill patient. Critical Care. 2017;21(1):136.

10. Alexander V Khaw RSvB, Strasser C, Mohr-Kahaly S, Blankenberg S, Espinola-Klein C, Münzel TF, Schnabel R. Direct measurement of left ventricular outflow tract by transthoracic real-time 3D-echocardiography increases accuracy in assessment of aortic valve stenosis. Int J Cardiol. 2009;136 (1):64–71.

11. James N, Kirkpatrick RML. Heart failure: hemodynamic assessment using echocardiography. Curr Cardiol Rep. 2008;10(3):240–6.

12. Guido Tavazzi AK, Guarracino F, Bergsland N, Martinez-Naharro A, Pepper J, Price S. Heart rate modification of cardiac output following cardiac surgery: the importance of cardiac time intervals. Critical Care Med. 2017;45(8):e782–e8.

13. Cohn JN. Vasodilator therapy for heart failure. The influence of impedance on left ventricular performance. Circulation. 1973;48(1):5–8.

14. Sheehan F. Ventricular shape and function. In: Otto C, editor. The Practice of Clinical Echocardiography. 3rd ed. Philadelphia: Saunders Elsevier; 2007. p. 212–36.

15. Alexandra Goncalves PA, Sogaard P, Zamorano JL. Assessment of systolic function. In: Galiuto L, editor. The EAE Textbook of Echocardiography. Glasgow: Oxford University Press; 2011. p. 117–34.

16. Jae Oh JS, Tajik J. Assessment of Systolic Function and Quantification of Cardiac Chambers. In: Oh J, editor. The Echo Manual. Third ed. Philadelphia: Lippincott Williams & Wilkins; 2006. p. 109–20.

17. Roberto M Lang LPB, Mor-Avi V, Afilalo J, Armstrong A, Ernande L, Flachskampf FA, Foster E, Goldstein SA, Kuznetsova T, Lancellotti P, Muraru D, Picard MH, Rietzschel ER, Rudski L, Spencer KT, Tsang W. Jens-Uwe Voigt Recommendations for cardiac chamber quantification by echocardiography in adults: an update from the American Society of echocardiography and the european association of cardiovascular imaging. J Amer Soc Echocardiogr. 2015;28(1):1–39

18. Harvey Feigenbaum WA, Ryan T, Evaluation of systolic and diastolic function of the left ventricle. Feigenbaum's Echocardiography. Sixth ed. Philadelphia: Lippincott Williams & Wilkins; 2005. p. 138–69.

19. H Goldfine GA, Zile M, Gaasch W. Left ventricular length-force-shortening relations before and after surgical correction of chronic mitral regurgitation. J Am Coll Cardiol. 1998;31(1):180–5.

20. T Nahar LC, Shapiro R, Fruchtman S, Diamond J, Henzlova M, Machac J, Buckley S, Goldman M. Comparison of four echocardiographic techniques for measuring left ventricular ejection fraction. Amer J Cardiol. 2000;86(12):1358–62.

21. G Bargiggia CB, Recusani F, Raisaro A, Servi S, Valdes-Cruz L, Sahn D, Tronconi L. A new method for estimating left ventricular dP/dt by continuous wave Doppler-echocardiography. Validation studies at cardiac catheterization. Circulation. 1989;80 (5):1287–92.

22. C Tei RN, Seward J, Tajik A. Noninvasive Doppler-derived myocardial performance index: correlation with simultaneous measurements of cardiac catheterization measurements. J Amer Soc Echocardiogr. 1997;10(2):169–78.

23. C Chen LR, Guerrero JL, Marshall S, Levine RA, Weyman AE, Thomas JD. Noninvasive estimation of the instantaneous first derivative of left ventricular pressure using continuous-wave Doppler echocardiography. Circulation. 1991;83(6):2101–10.

24. Chengode S. Left ventricular global systolic function assessment by echocardiography. Ann Card Anaesth. 2016;19:S26–34.

25. Lill Bergenzaun HO, Gudmundsson P, Willenheimer R, Chew MS. Mitral annular plane systolic excursion (MAPSE) in shock: a valuable echocardiographic parameter in intensive care patients. Cardiovascular Ultrasound. 2013;11:16.

26. Kai Hu DL, Herrmann S, Niemann M, Gaudron PD, Voelker W, Ertl G, Bijnens B, Weidemann F. Clinical implication of mitral annular plane systolic excursion for patients with cardiovascular disease. Europ Heart J Cardiovascular Imaging. 2013;14 (3):205–12.

27. A D Waggoner SMB. Tissue Doppler imaging: a useful echocardiographic method for the cardiac sonographer to assess systolic and diastolic ventricular function. J Amer Soc Echocardiogr. 2001;14 (12):1143–52.

28. V K Gulati WEK, Follansbee WP, J Gorcsan 3rd. Mitral annular descent velocity by tissue Doppler echocardiography as an index of global left ventricular function. Amer J Cardiol. 1996;77(11):979–84.

29. Sanderson JE. Heart failure with a normal ejection fraction. Heart. 2007;93(2):155–8.

30. Abdenasser Drighil JEM, Mathewson JW, El Mosalami H, El Badaoui N, Ramdani B, Bennis A.

Haemodialysis: effects of acute decrease in preload on tissue Doppler imaging indices of systolic and diastolic function of the left and right ventricles. Europ J Echocardiogr. 2008;9(4):530–5.

31. Duncan AM, Francis DP, Henein MY, Gibson DG. Limitation of car- diac output by total isovolumic time during pharmacologic stress in patients with dilated cardiomyopathy: activation-mediated effects of left bundle branch block and coronary artery disease. J Am Coll Cardiol. 2003;41:121–8.

32. Jens-Uwe Voigt GL, Exner B, Regenfus M, Werner D, Reulbach U, Nixdorff U, Flachskampf FA, Daniel WG. Incidence and characteristics of segmental postsystolic longitudinal shortening in normal, acutely ischemic, and scarred myocardium. J Amer Soc Echocardiogr. 2003;16(5):415–23.

33. Manuel D. Cerqueira NJW, Dilsizian V, Jacobs AK, Kaul S, Laskey WK, Pennell DJ, Rumberger JA, Ryan T, Verani MS. Standardized myocardial segmentation and nomenclature for tomographic imaging of the heart: a statement for healthcare professionals from the cardiac imaging committee of the council on clinical cardiology of the American heart association. Circulation. 2002;105:539–42.

34. G Kan CAV, Koclen JJ, Dunning AJ. Short and long term predictive value of admission wall motion score in acute myocardial infarction. A cross sectional echocardiographic study of 345 patients. British Heart J. 1986;56(5):422–7.

35. M L Geleijnse CV, Kasprzak JD, Rambaldi R, Salvatori MP, Elhendy A, Cornel JH, Fioretti PM, Roelandt JR. Usefulness and limitations of dobutamine-atropine stress echocardiography for the diagnosis of coronary artery disease in patients with left bundle branch block. A multicentre study. Europ Heart J. 2000;21(20):1666–73.

36. Soliman-Aboumarie H, Pastore MC, Galiatsou E, Gargani L, Pugliese NR, Mandoli GE, Valente S, Hurtado-Doce A, Lees N, Cameli M. Echocardiography in the intensive care unit: an essential tool for diagnosis, monitoring and guiding clinical decision-making. Physiol Int. 2021. https://doi.org/10.1556/1647.2021.00055. Epub ahead of print. PMID: 34825894.

37. I Kingma JVT, Smith ER. Effects of diastolic transseptal pressure gradient on ventricular septal position and motion. Circulation. 1983;68:1304–14.

POCUS in Monitoring: Right Ventricular Function and Pulmonary Hypertension

Arif Hussain, Rajkumar Rajendram, and Guido Tavazzi

... but there is no passage between these two cavities [right and left ventricles]; for the substance of the heart is solid in this region and has neither a visible passage, as was thought by some persons, nor an invisible one which could have permitted the transmission of blood, as was alleged by Galen. The pores of the heart there are closed, and its substance is thick.

And for the same reason, there exists perceptible passages (or pores, manafidh) between the two [blood vessels, namely pulmonary artery and pulmonary vein].

Ibn Al-Nafis, Medieval Arab Physician (1213–1288 AD). Commentary on Anatomy in Ibn Sina (Avicenna's) Canon of Medicine.

Supplementary Information The online version contains supplementary material available at https://doi.org/10.1007/978-3-031-29472-3_19.

A. Hussain (✉) · R. Rajendram
Departments of Cardiac Sciences and Medicine, King Abdulaziz International Medical Research Center, King Abdulaziz Medical City, Ministry of National Guard - Health Affairs, Riyadh, Saudi Arabia
e-mail: hussainar@ngha.med.sa

R. Rajendram
e-mail: rajkumarrajendram@doctors.org.uk

College of Medicine, King Saud Bin Abdulaziz, University of Health Sciences, Riyadh, Saudi Arabia

G. Tavazzi
Department of Clinical-Surgical, Diagnostic and Paediatric Sciences, Unit of Anaesthesia and Intensive Care, University of Pavia, Pavia, Italy
e-mail: guido.tavazzi@unipv.it

Anaesthesia and Intensive Care, Fondazione Instituto Di Ricovero E Cura a Carattere Scientifico Policlinico San Matteo Foundation, Pavia, Italy

Abstract

Increased understanding of heart–lung interactions in the critically ill patients has reignited intensivists' interest in the assessment of the right ventricle and pulmonary artery (PA) pressures. Recent studies have demonstrated the feasibility of using ultraportable ultrasound devices to perform advanced imaging studies at the beside of critically ill patients. In this context, we discuss several, clinically relevant techniques for the assessment of right ventricular anatomy and function, measurement of PA pressures and screening for pulmonary hypertension with point of care ultrasound. The use of bedside echocardiography may improve outcomes by guiding the application of emerging therapies including pulmonary vasodilators and extracorporeal life support.

Keywords

Point of care ultrasound · Echocardiography · Right ventricle · Cor pulmonale · Tricuspid annular plane systolic excursion · Pulmonary artery pressures · Pulmonary hypertension

Key Messages

- Assessment of the right ventricle (RV) requires an understanding of its peculiar anatomy and physiology.
- The physiology of the RV is very different from that of the left ventricle.
- Assessment of the RV and investigation of pulmonary hypertension requires the integration of data from all standard views and multiple modes of ultrasound.
- Several techniques for assessment of right ventricular function and pulmonary artery pressures have been described, some of which have been validated in critically ill patients.

Introduction

Increased understanding of heart–lung interactions coupled with the availability of novel pulmonary vasodilator medications and extracorporeal life support has reignited interest in the assessment of the function of the right ventricle (RV) and pulmonary artery (PA) pressures (PAP) in critical care. Whilst, relevant data can be obtained via a pulmonary artery catheter, right heart catheterization is invasive. Echocardiography is a widely available, relatively low-cost, non-invasive alternative. In addition, the feasibility of using ultraportable handheld ultrasound to perform advanced imaging studies at the beside of critically ill patients has been demonstrated [1]. In this chapter, we describe the techniques available for the assessment of the RV, PA pressures and pulmonary hypertension with point of care ultrasound (POCUS).

Assessment of the Right Ventricle

The anatomy and physiology of the RV is quite different from that of the left ventricle (LV). The pathophysiology of RV dysfunction results in characteristic changes to its anatomy and physiology that can be seen on bedside imaging. Echocardiographic assessment of the RV (Figs. 1 and 2) requires an understanding of these peculiarities.

Legend to Fig. 1. This figure shows the right ventricle in four standard echocardiographic views using Two-Dimensional (2D) imaging. A. Parasternal long axis. B. Parasternal short axis. C. Apical four chamber view. D Subcostal four chamber view. The right ventricle is outlined in blue in each view. This figure was provided by Dr Gabriele Via.

Legend to Fig. 2. This diagram illustrates the minimum data set which should be obtained for a basic but comprehensive assessment of the right ventricle. Abbreviations. FoCUS, focused cardiac ultrasound; LV, left ventricle, RV, right ventricle; TAPSE, tricuspid annular plane systolic excursion. This figure was provided by Dr Gabriele Via.

There are three main causes of RV dysfunction. These are: increased preload, decreased contractility and increased afterload (Fig. 3 and Videos 1A-C). Various dynamic combinations of these drivers of RV dysfunction may be present in critically ill patients. Thus, the application of a single modality of POCUS is not sufficient to obtain a full picture of RV function (Fig. 2). A comprehensive assessment exploiting different modes of ultrasound provides a much more clinically relevant analysis of the RV.

Legend to Fig. 3. These Two-Dimensional (2D) echocardiographic images show right ventricular (RV) dysfunction. A. Parasternal short axis view in diastole showing right ventricular volume overload. B. Parasternal short axis view in systole showing right ventricular volume overload. Note the leftward shift of septal motion during diastole (A). The septal curvature is

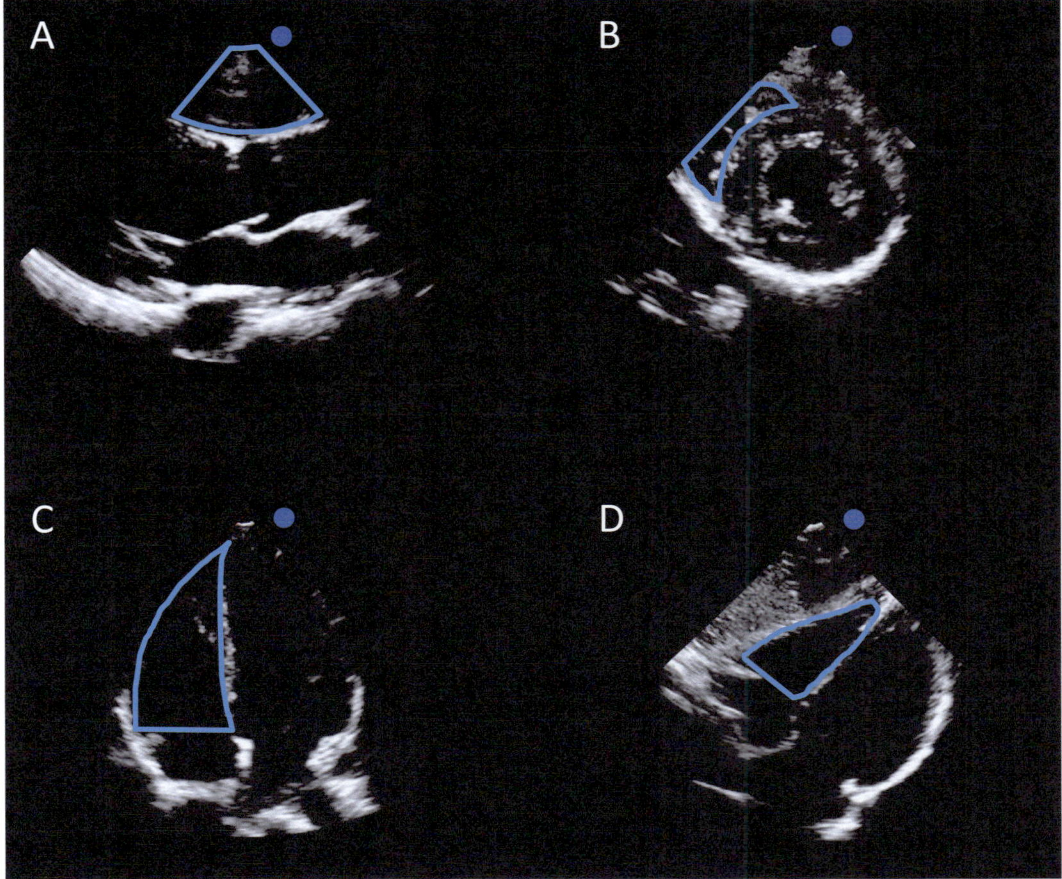

Fig. 1 Two-Dimensional echocardiographic imaging of the right ventricle

maximally reversed at mid-diastole but normalizes in systole (B). C. Parasternal short axis view in diastole showing a pressure overloaded right ventricle. D. Parasternal short axis view in systole showing a pressure overloaded right ventricle. Note the leftward shift of septal motion throughout the cardiac cycle. The septal curvature is maximally reversed at end-systole. E. Apical four chamber view in diastole showing systolic failure of the right ventricle. F. Apical four chamber view in systole showing systolic failure of the right ventricle. These still images were taken from videos 1A-C. The videos were provided by Dr Gabriele Via.

Video 1 A-C. Right ventricular dysfunction.

Legend to Videos 1A-C. These cine-loops of Two-Dimensional (2D) echocardiographic views show right ventricular dysfunction. A. Parasternal short axis view showing right ventricular volume overload. Note the leftward shift of septal motion during diastole. The septal curvature is maximally reversed at mid-diastole but normalizes in systole. B. Parasternal short axis view showing a pressure overloaded right ventricle. Note the leftward shift of septal motion throughout the cardiac cycle. The septal curvature is maximally reversed at end-systole. C. Apical four chamber view showing systolic

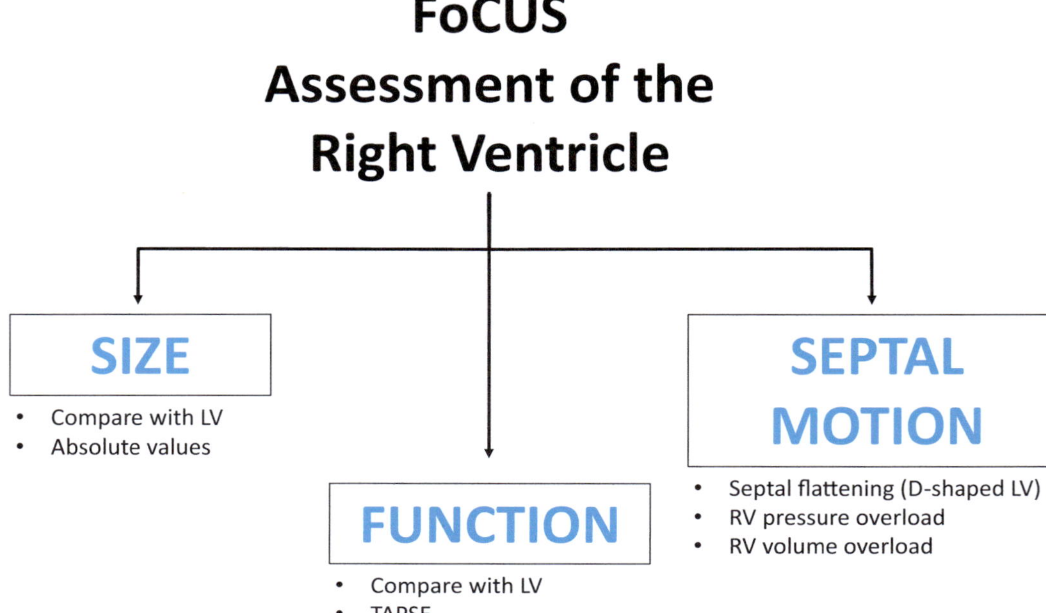

Fig. 2 Focused cardiac ultrasound assessment of the right ventricle

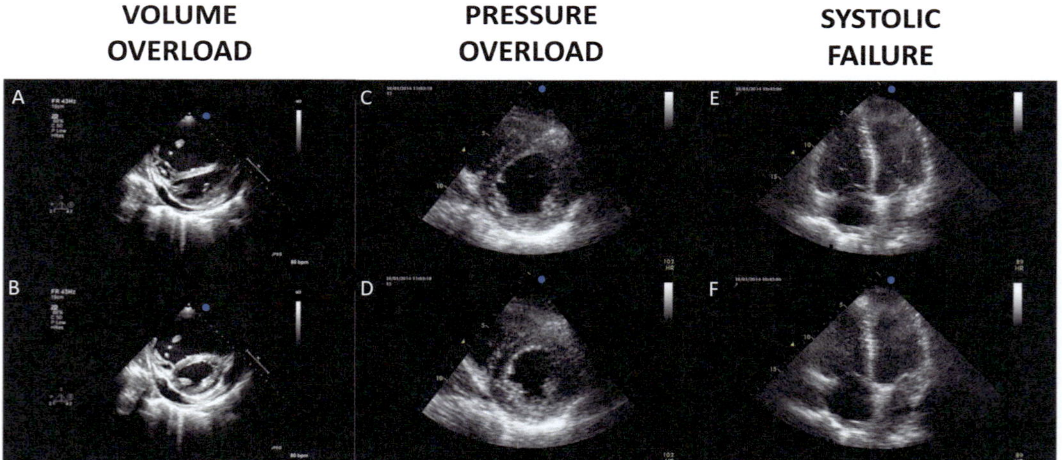

Fig. 3 Right ventricular dysfunction

failure of the right ventricle. Still images taken from these videos are shown in Fig. 3. The videos were provided by Dr Gabriele Via.

Anatomy

From the sonographic perspective, the RV has several peculiar features (Figs. 1 and 3). The RV lies anteriorly within the thorax, close to the chest wall. It is a triangular, crescent-shaped, sac-like structure that wraps around the LV somewhat like a hand grasping an ice cream cone. The tricuspid valve is situated at the inflow of the RV and the pulmonary valve is at the outflow. These valves may become regurgitant in response to ventricular dilation and increased afterload, respectively.

The presence and severity of valve regurgitation can readily be assessed with Doppler at the bedside, but functional assessment of the RV usually focuses on its free (i.e. lateral) wall. However, imaging the RV is hindered by the sternum. In ventilated patients, the heart is also obscured by inflation of the lungs, making the assessment of the free wall of the RV particularly difficult. These anatomical challenges significantly limit the utility of the parasternal and apical echocardiographic views for the assessment of the RV. However, a more comprehensive assessment of the RV can be achieved by integrating parasternal long/short axis and subcostal views. Hence, it is almost always possible to visualize the RV in most of the critically ill patients who are at risk of significant derangement of RV physiology.

Physiology and Pathophysiology

The pivotal role of the RV in cardiovascular physiology is often ignored. It is important to recognize that the RV is a cardiac chamber that tolerates volume to a greater extent than pressure overload (i.e. increased afterload due to pulmonary vascular resistance (PVR)). When discussing the use of POCUS for the assessment of RV function, preload must also be considered.

The severity of tricuspid valve regurgitation can be assessed from the resultant pulsed wave (PW) Doppler flow signals in the hepatic veins. Venous excess ultrasonography (VExUS) allows the recognition of elevated right atrial pressure (RAP) and venous congestion [2]. A detailed discussion of VExUS is presented in Chap. 16.

The size, shape and function of the RV are load-dependent. Myocardial ischemia can provoke rapid RV dilatation. This further exacerbates the ischemia, setting a vicious cycle in motion. Pathologies that increase afterload by raising the pulmonary arterial (PA) pressure, such as pulmonary vascular occlusion from thrombo-embolism, high airway pressures and the acute respiratory distress syndrome (ARDS) also cause the RV to dilate rapidly and impair its contractility. This is known as acute cor-pulmonale, the final stage of the RV compensatory mechanism. At this point, it is important to reduce the resistive load on the RV to avoid cardiogenic shock, and adverse outcomes [3].

Thus, clinical decisions may be supported by composite variables derived from integrated assessment of RV contractility, the load on the RV, RV dilatation and RAP (e.g. the load adaptation index) [4]. Whilst complex, such analyses can guide difficult decisions such as prognostication on the potential reversibility of RV dysfunction, when to implant a durable left ventricular assist device in the setting of congestive heart failure, and the timing of lung transplantation in the presence of pre-capillary pulmonary hypertension [4].

The influence of afterload on RV function is also evident in healthy individuals. Exercise tolerance is directly linked to the impact of exercise-induced changes in PA pressure on RV function. The age and sex-dependent measures of RV contractile reserve on stress echocardiography e.g. systolic PA pressure (sPAP), tricuspid annular plane systolic excursion (TAPSE), tissue Doppler systolic velocity (S') and (TAPSE/sPAP) correlate well with subjects' maximum exercise capacity [5]. These, in combination with other measures can provide a functional assessment of the RV.

Assessment of Right Ventricular Function

Understanding the anatomy and physiology of the RV described above greatly facilitates the bedside echocardiographic assessment of the RV.

Measurement of Right Ventricular Size and Wall Thickness

Unlike the LV, the RV is trabeculated and has a network of fibro-muscular strands. So, the wall of the RV is not as smooth as that of the LV. Quantifying the size of the RV is therefore challenging, particularly if the RV has hypertrophied (e.g. in response to chronic pressure overload from pulmonary hypertension). Furthermore, 2D evaluation of RV size underestimates the true dimensions as measured with 3D echocardiography or cardiac magnetic resonance imaging [6].

In the subcostal view, the RV wall thickness (excluding trabeculations and papillary muscles) is usually under 0.5 cm (Fig. 1d). This simple measurement allows a quick assessment for the presence of RV hypertrophy. However, it is important to be aware that RV hypertrophy may not be homogenous. The infundibulum is closest to the pulmonary valve and is therefore the first region of the RV to be exposed to any increase in afterload [7]. Thickening of the RV free wall usually occurs later [7]. Fig. 4 and Video 2 show a hypertrophied right ventricle.

Legend to Fig. 4. This still image of the Two-Dimensional (2D) subcostal four chamber view at end-diastole shows right ventricular hypertrophy. The thickness of the inferior wall of the right ventricle (arrowed) was approximately 1.2 cm. This still image was taken from video 2. The figure and the video were provided by Dr Gabriele Via.

Video 2. Right ventricular hypertrophy.

Legend to Video 2. This cine-loop of the Two-Dimensional (2D) subcostal four chamber view at end diastole shows right ventricular hypertrophy. The thickness of the inferior wall of the right ventricle was approximately 1.2 cm. A still image taken from this video is shown in Fig. 4. The video and the figure were provided by Dr Gabriele Via.

As the shape of the RV is unusual, quantification of its volume is difficult. Tedious calculations are required that are not practical for POCUS assessments. However, the normal and pathological size and shape of the RV can be more accurately determined with 3D echocardiography [8].

Fig. 4 Right ventricular hypertrophy

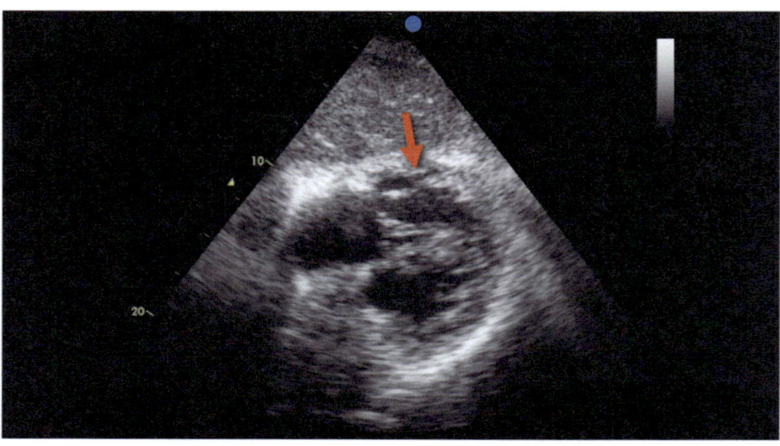

Measurement of the Shape and Area of the Right Ventricle

Indices for the quantification of the RV dimensions are available. Estimates obtained by 'eyeballing' compare well with the precise measurements detailed in guidelines. So, for expediency and quick reference, the detailed measures described by Lang et al., 2015 [9], are simplified in Table 1.

Figure 5 illustrates measurements of the diameter of the base of the right ventricle (Fig. 5a) and the right ventricular outflow tract (Fig. 5b). Figure 6 compares the end diastolic areas (EDA) of the left ventricle (LVEDA) and the right ventricle RVEDA of a normal RV (Fig. 6a) and a dilated RV (Fig. 6b). These Two-Dimensional (2D) echocardiographic images show the linear dimensions of the right ventricle. A. Apical four chamber view in diastole showing the basal diameter (RV B). B. Parasternal long axis view in diastole showing the diameter of the right ventricle outflow tract (RVOT P). Normal ranges for RV dimensions from Lang et al. [9]. The simplified reference ranges used in focused cardiac ultrasound (FoCUSFocused cardiac ultrasound (FoCUS)) facilitate bedside assessments. Abbreviations. cm, centimeter; mm, millimeter; SD,

Table 1 Reference ranges for POCUS quantification of the dimensions of the right ventricle

Parameter	Mean ± SD	Normal range
RV basal diameter (mm)	33 ± 4	25–41
RV mid diameter (mm)	27 ± 4	19–35
RV longitudinal diameter (mm)	71 ± 6	59–83
RVOT PLAX diameter (mm)	25 ± 2.5	20–30
RVOT proximal diameter (mm)	28 ± 3.5	21–35
RVOT distal diameter (mm)	22 ± 2.5	17–27
RV wall thickness (mm)	3 ± 1	1–5
RVOT EDA (cm^2)		
Men	17 ± 3.5	10–24
Women	14 ± 3	8–20
RV EDA indexed to BSA (cm^2/m^2)		
Men	8.8 ± 1.9	5–12.6
Women	8.0 ± 1.75	4.5–11.5
RV ESA (cm^2)		
Men	9 ± 3	3–15
Women	7 ± 2	3–11
RV ESA indexed to BSA (cm^2/m^2)		
Men	4.7 ± 1.35	2.0–7.4
Women	4.0 ± 1.2	1.6–6.4
RV EDV indexed to BSA (mL/m^2)		
Men	61 ± 13	35–87
Women	53 ± 10.5	32–74
RV ESV indexed to BSA (mL/m^2)		
Men	27 ± 8.5	10–44
Women	22 ± 7	8–36

Legend to Table 1. Abbreviations: EDA, end-diastolic area; ESA, end-systolic area; PLAX, parasternal long-axis view; RVOT, RV outflow tract. * RV wall thickness up to 10 mm is considered normal. Adapted from Lang et al., 2015 [9] with permission

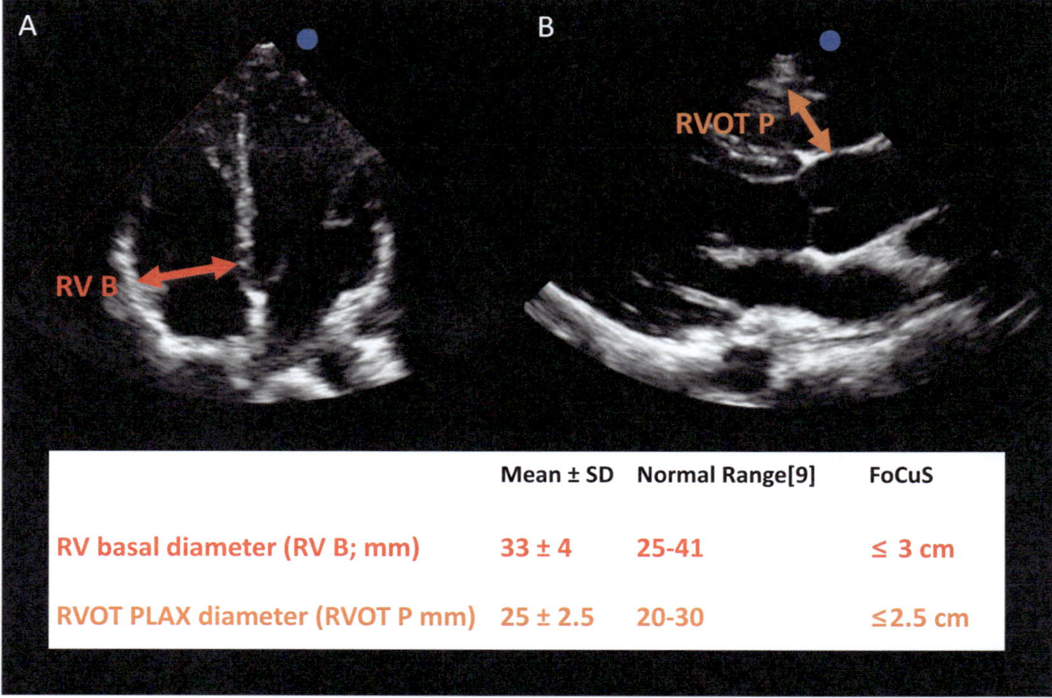

	Mean ± SD	Normal Range[9]	FoCuS
RV basal diameter (RV B; mm)	33 ± 4	25-41	≤ 3 cm
RVOT PLAX diameter (RVOT P mm)	25 ± 2.5	20-30	≤2.5 cm

Fig. 5 Linear dimensions of the right ventricle

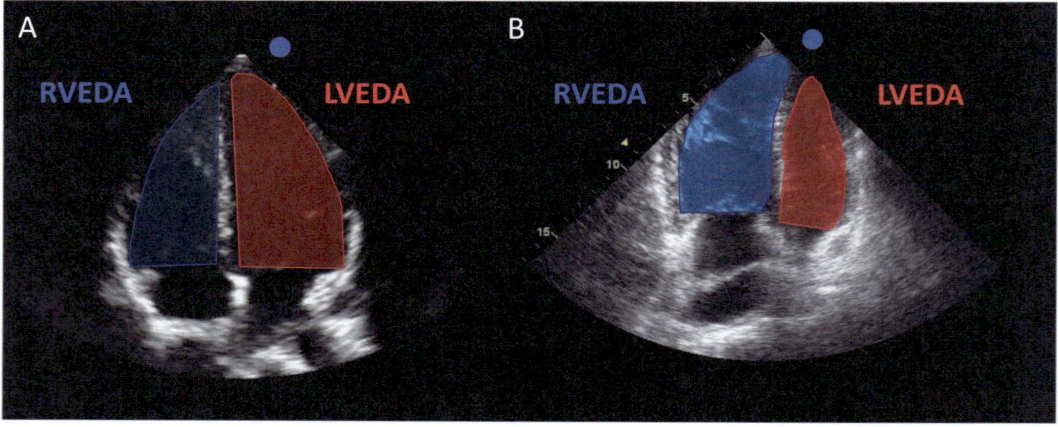

Fig. 6 Comparison of the areas of the left and right ventricles

standard deviation. The figure was provided by Dr Gabriele Via.

The cutoff values for RV maximum end diastolic dimension in the parasternal long axis view (PLAX) of 2.5 cm, RV diameter of 3 cm at the base of the RV and RV wall thickness of 0.5 cm in the subcostal four chamber view (SC4C) and RV to LV area ratio (i.e. RVEDA: LVEDA) 0.6:1 can be used as a reference for a quick assessment in focused cardiac ultrasound.

Legend to Fig. 6. These Two-Dimensional (2D) echocardiographic images compare the end diastolic areas (EDA) of the left ventricle (LVEDA) and the right ventricle (RVEDA). The RVEDA: LVEDA ratio is usually under 0.6: 1. Apical four chamber view in diastole showing normal left and right ventricular dimensions (RVEDA: LVEDA < 0.6: 1). B. Apical four chamber view in diastole showing a dilated right ventricle and a normal left ventricle (RVEDA: LVEDA > 0.6: 1). The figure was provided by Dr Gabriele Via.

Visual Assessment of Right Ventricular Contractile Function

Experienced echocardiographers can use visual assessments to rapidly gauge overall RV contractility, volume status and wall motion without the need for formal measurements. This is similar to the global assessment of the LV that is well recognized and commonly reported.

Right Ventricular Fractional Area Change

Albeit somewhat tedious to measure; the percentage fractional area change (RVFAC) is indicative of RV function (normal >35%). It is calculated by tracing the RV area at end-diastole (EDA) and end-systole (ESA) and using the formula [EDA-ESA/EDA] × 100. Excluding the trabeculations of the RV when delineating the endocardial borders is challenging. This measurement is particularly difficult in mechanically ventilated critically ill patients, in whom the RV may be obscured and the endocardial borders are poorly defined. However, when the RV is dilated, the endocardial borders are generally better defined.

Tricuspid Annular Plane Systolic Excursion by M-Mode

The use of TAPSE to assess RV contractility is strongly recommended [10]. To measure TAPSE, the longitudinal movement of a point on the lateral or medial aspect of the TV annulus is traced in M-mode (Fig. 7). The TAPSE reflects the movement of the longitudinal fibers of the RV which are the main determinant of RV function and it is less influenced by the circumferential and transverse fibers coming from the LV. Despite the complex anatomy, this simple, easily performed technique provides a reliable measure of the intrinsic RV systolic function. A TAPSE less than 17 mm suggests RV contractile dysfunction. With transesophageal (TEE) TAPSE is more difficult to track in M mode and may be less accurate. In the perioperative setting TEE speckle-tracking TAPSE may be used instead [10].

Legend to Fig. 7. The tricuspid annular plane systolic excursion (TAPSE) motion begins away

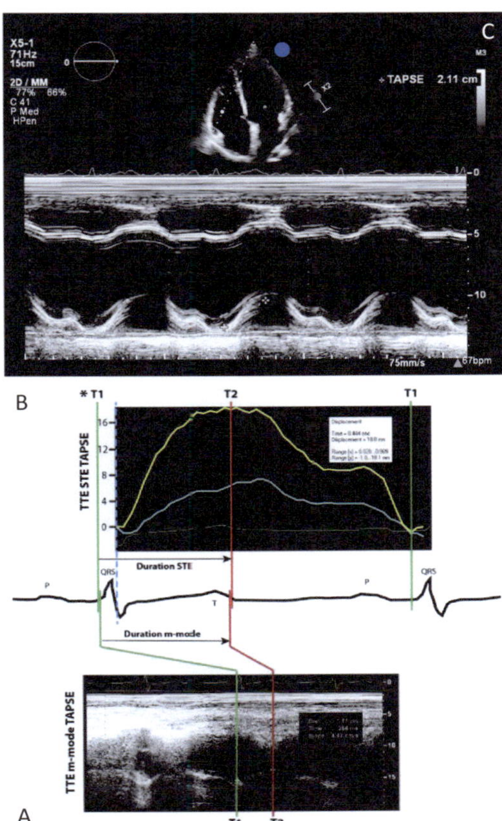

Fig. 7 Tricuspid annular plane systolic excursion assessed with M Mode and Speckle-tracking

from the apex on atrial contraction (before the QRS complex). Time point 1 (T1) is marked at the point farthest from the apex. It occurs before the QRS complex (i.e. before electrical ventricular contraction). Measurement of TAPSE ends at time point 2 (T2), the point closest to the apex. A. M-mode TAPSE. B. Speckle-tracked echocardiography (STE) tricuspid annular plane systolic excursion (TAPSE) on TTE. The tracked lateral tricuspid annular point is indicated by the yellow line. An asterisk indicates where T1 would be on the same electrical cycle as the M-mode measurement (A). The minimum point occurs at the end of the cycle selected by the TMAD option in CMQ. So, minimum and maximum displacement must be displayed to calculate STE TAPSE with TTE and transesophageal echocardiography (TEE). The starting point for STE and the arbitrary baseline (i.e. zero) from which positive and negative measurements are taken are shown by the dashed blue line. C. TTE apical 4 chamber view showing M-mode TAPSE. The M-mode cursor is aligned parallel to the motion of lateral TV annulus. Panels A and B reproduced with permission from Markin et al. [10].

Tissue Doppler S'

On tissue Doppler imaging (TDI), a trace can be obtained at the lateral and medial points of tricuspid annulus. The positive deflection S' depicts the tissue movement during systole (normal $\geq$ 10 cm/s; Fig. 8). This is analogous to the use of TDI at the mitral valve annulus where S' for LV systolic function and E/e' for assessment of LV diastolic function is more commonly used.

Legend to Fig. 8. The positive deflection S' depicts the tissue movement during systole (normal $\geq$ 10 cm/s). Abbreviations. a', tissue Doppler late diastolic velocity; e', tissue Doppler early diastolic velocity; ICT, isovolumic contraction time; IRT, isovolumic relaxation time; S ', tissue Doppler systolic velocity.

Right Ventricular Myocardial Performance Index

The RV Myocardial Performance Index (MPI), also known as the Tei Index (Fig. 9), is a useful measure of RV systolic and diastolic function. It

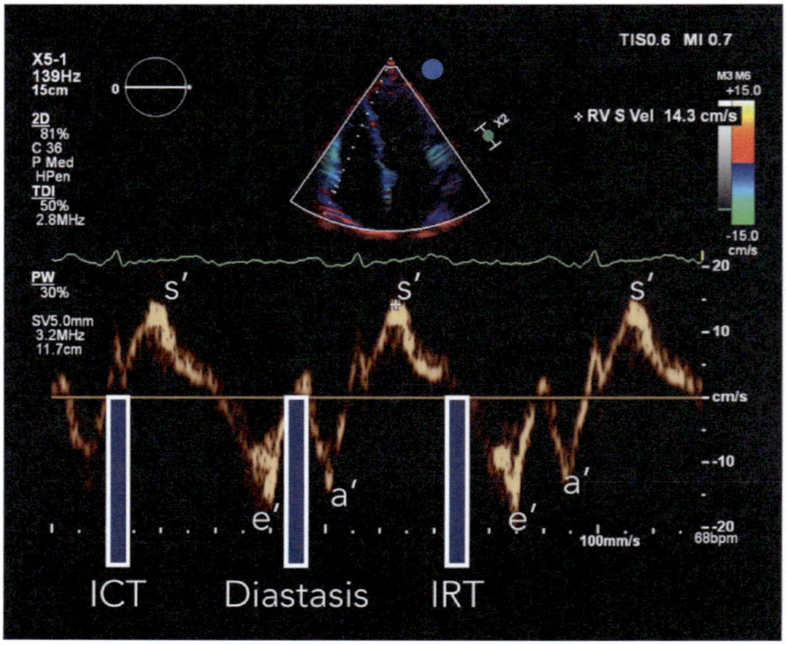

Fig. 8 Tissue Doppler tracing of the tricuspid annular plane for assessment of S' and the right ventricular myocardial performance index

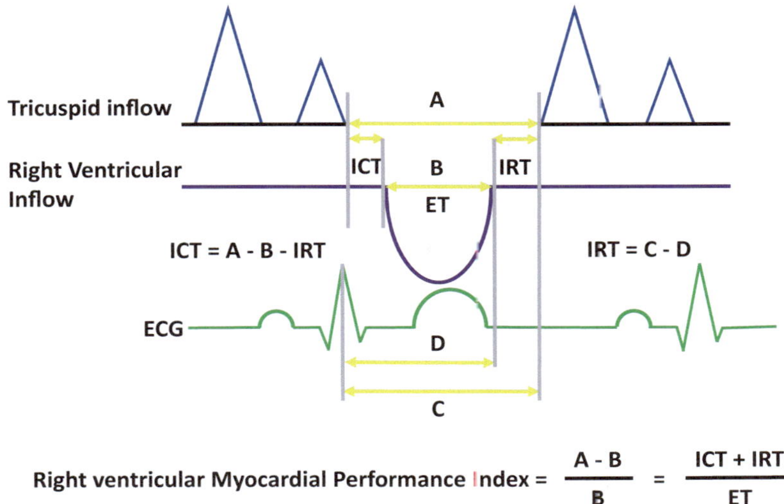

Fig. 9 Calculation of the right ventricular myocardial performance index using pulsed wave Doppler measurement of tricuspid inflow

$$\text{Right ventricular Myocardial Performance Index} = \frac{A - B}{B} = \frac{ICT + IRT}{ET}$$

takes into consideration the systolic and diastolic time intervals obtained from a single image with PW Doppler or TDI. Changes in the MPI (PW > 0.5 ms; TDI > 0.4 ms) reflect the severity and effects of pulmonary hypertension with many conditions. It also has prognostic implications.

Legend to Fig. 9. Abbreviations. A, Tricuspid Closure to Opening Time; B, RV Ejection Time; MPI, myocardial performance index; RV, right ventricular; ICT, Isovolumic Contraction Time; IRT, Isovolumic Relaxation Time; ET, RV Ejection Time.

Right Ventricular Strain

This relatively new technique, commonly referred to as speckle tracking, measures the percentage change in myocardial tissues during contraction and relaxation. This deformation, displayed as speckles on ultrasound, can be tracked in the long axis or the short axis. The composite measure generated from speckle tracking of individual regions of the myocardium provides a global, load independent assessment of RV function (Fig. 10 and Video 3). Whilst measurement of RV strain may be considered beyond the current scope of POCUS, it is possible with portable devices and is increasingly applicable in clinical practice. For example, using RV strain with TEE has recently provided an index that is particularly useful in the intra-operative and critical care settings [11].

Legend to Video 3. This cine-loop shows strain imaging of the right ventricle in the apical four chamber view. Abbreviations. RVFWSL, right ventricular free wall longitudinal strain; RV4CSL, right ventricular four chamber longitudinal strain. A still image taken from this video is shown in Fig. 10.

3D Assessment of Right Ventricular Volumes and Ejection Fraction

In some clinical situations, more accurate measurements of RV volumes and ejection fraction (EF) are required. For such cases 3D TTE and TEE assessment can be performed (Fig. 11 and Video 4). In recent years, the intra-operative application of these techniques has increased.

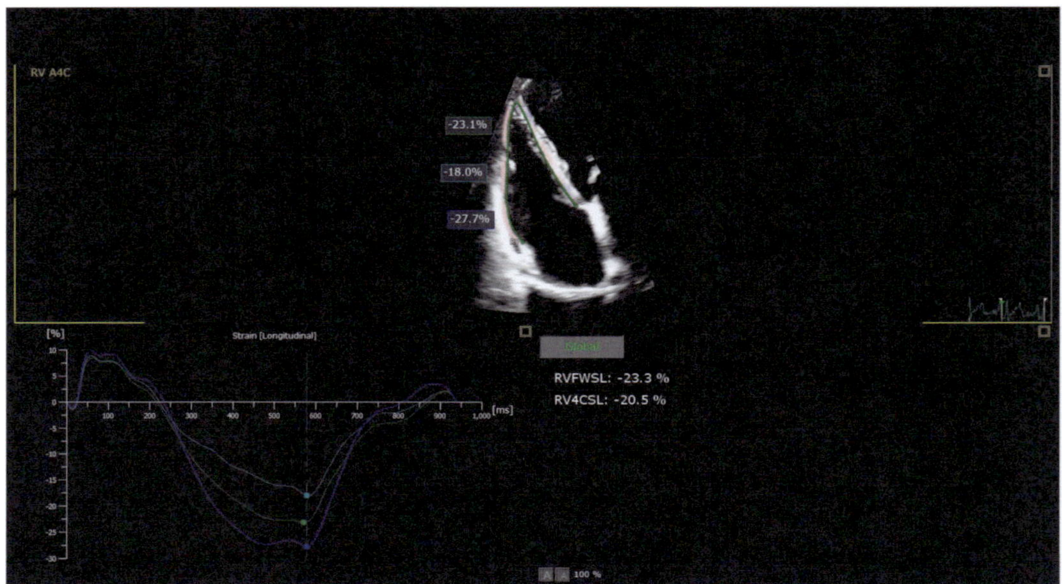

Fig. 10 Right ventricular strain with transthoracic echocardiography.
Legend to Fig. 10. This segment of a Two-Dimensional (2D) transthoracic apical four chamber view shows the right ventricle (RV). The RV free wall longitudinal strain (RV-fwLS) has been measured. The RV-fwLS was obtained by averaging the peak longitudinal strain of the 3 segments of the RV free wall. This frame is taken from Video 3

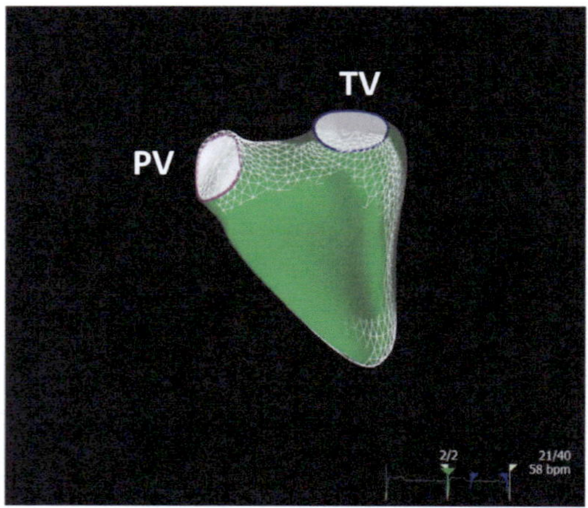

Fig. 11 Three-Dimensional (3D) transthoracic echocardiographic assessment of the right ventricle. Legend to Fig. 11. This frame is taken from Video 4. Abbreviations. PV, pulmonary valve; TV, tricuspid valve.▶ Video 4. Three-Dimensional (3D) echocardiographic reconstruction of the right ventricle. Legend to Video 4. This cineloop shows a Three-Dimensional (3D) reconstruction of the right ventricle generated from images obtained by transthoracic echocardiography. Abbreviations. PV, pulmonary valve; TV, tricuspid valve. A still image taken from this video is shown in Fig. 11

Estimation of Tricuspid Regurgitation, Right Ventricular Systolic Pressure and Pulmonary Artery Systolic Pressure

The TV can be viewed in multiple windows. Continuous wave Doppler measurement of the peak systolic velocity of TV regurgitation allows estimation of the pressure gradient (ΔP) between the RA and RV (Fig. 12). The use of this technique to estimate right ventricular systolic pressure (RVSP) or sPAP is discussed in more detail below.

Legend to Fig. 12. The upper part of the figure shows a thumbnail view of a Two-Dimensional (2D) transthoracic apical four chamber view with tricuspid valve regurgitation demonstrated by the overlying color Doppler. The continuous wave Doppler cursor has been aligned with the blood flow through the tricuspid valve.

The lower part of the figure shows the continuous wave Doppler trace of tricuspid

Fig. 12 Measurement of the tricuspid valve regurgitation maximum velocity with continuous wave Doppler

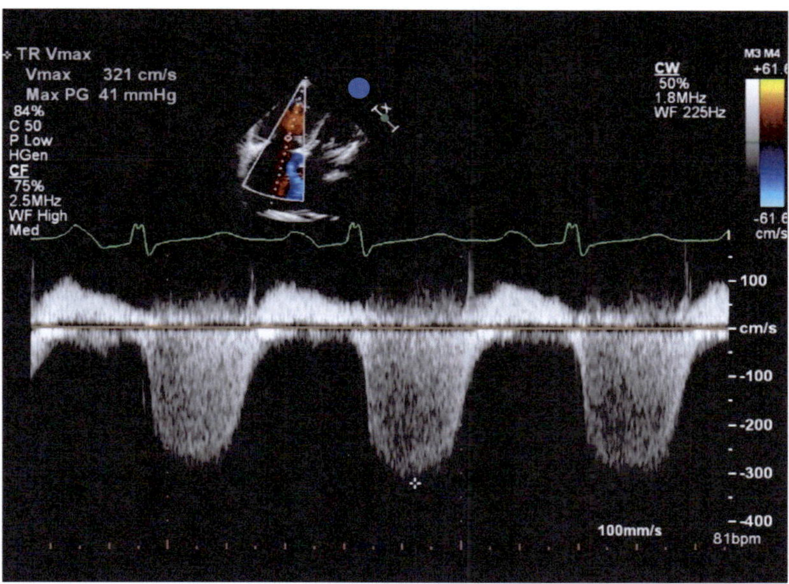

regurgitation. The color Doppler regurgitant signal can be used to guide the alignment of the cursor with the maximum velocity of the regurgitant flow. The modified Bernoulli equation can then be used to estimate the pressure gradient across the tricuspid valve. Adding the (measured or estimated) right atrial pressure (RAP) to the pressure gradient across the tricuspid valve allows estimation of the systolic pulmonary artery pressure.

Clinically relevant parameters which can be obtained by POCUS of the RV include measures of its dimensions, systolic and diastolic function, and the RVSP (Table 1 and Fig. 2). These tools are particularly useful for the beside assessment of acutely ill patients known or suspected to have pulmonary hypertension.

POCUS Assessment of Pulmonary Hypertension

Pulmonary hypertension is defined as mean PA pressure (mPAP) greater than 25 mmHg at rest in the 2015 European Society of Cardiology (ESC)/ European Respiratory Society (ERS) guidelines [12]. However, the most recent update from the World Symposium on pulmonary hypertension (2018) reduced the mPAP required for its diagnosis to mPAP > 20 mmHg [13]. The thresholds of pulmonary capillary wedge pressure (PCWP) and pulmonary vascular resistance (PVR) for the definition of pre-capillary pulmonary hypertension did not change (PCWP < 15 mmHg; PVR 3 Wood units). Reducing the mPAP threshold increases the sensitivity of the diagnostic criteria. However, this reduces their positive predictive value and increases the risk of false positives.

If pulmonary hypertension is suspected, echocardiography is the initial investigation of choice. To screen for pulmonary hypertension and its complications, measurements should be taken in several views using different modes of echocardiography. However, the decision to initiate treatment for pulmonary hypertension should not be based on echocardiography alone [12, 13]. Cardiac catheterization is required to confirm the diagnosis [12, 13]. Regardless, POCUS can be used to screen for pulmonary hypertension at the bedside.

M-Mode and Bidimensional Views

Hypertrophy (i.e. increased wall thickness) is the physiological compensatory response of the RV to chronically increased afterload. Hypertrophy of the RV begins at the infundibulum as this is closest to the pulmonary valve and is first subjected to the effects of any increase in impedance in the pulmonary vessels [6]. Dilatation of the RV occurs in response to acute pulmonary hypertension as well as at the advanced stages of chronic pulmonary hypertension.

Inter-ventricular interactions can be evaluated using the RV/LV ratio. This plays a key role in the hemodynamic assessment of the patient with pulmonary hypertension. A dilated, pressure-loaded RV compresses the LV (Fig. 3) and by distorting its geometry, impairs its filling, which consequently results in reduced cardiac output. The RV/LV ratio correlates with invasive measures of pulmonary hypertension. It takes into account the abnormal morphology and atypical movement of the interventricular septum, thereby incorporating characteristic features of RV failure, remodeling and hemodynamic dysfunction.

The ratio of the end systolic anterior–posterior diameters of the RV and LV is measured at the level of the papillary muscles of the LV in the 2D parasternal short-axis view (PSAX). The RV/ LV end diastolic area ratio can also be evaluated in the apical 4 chamber view (A4CV; Fig. 6). Severe RV enlargement (defined as RV/LV ratio > 0.9 1.0) is associated with increased mortality in patients with ARDS [14] and pulmonary embolism (PE) [15].

The PSAX also allows measurement of the eccentricity index in systole and diastole (Fig. 13). This ratio of two perpendicular minor axes of the LV is calculated by dividing the LV lateral dimension by the anterior–posterior dimension (Fig. 13). Whilst the eccentricity index is normally 1; flattening of the interventricular septum will increase the eccentricity index. This allows identification of LV compression by RV pressure overload (systolic inter-ventricular shift) or RV volume overload

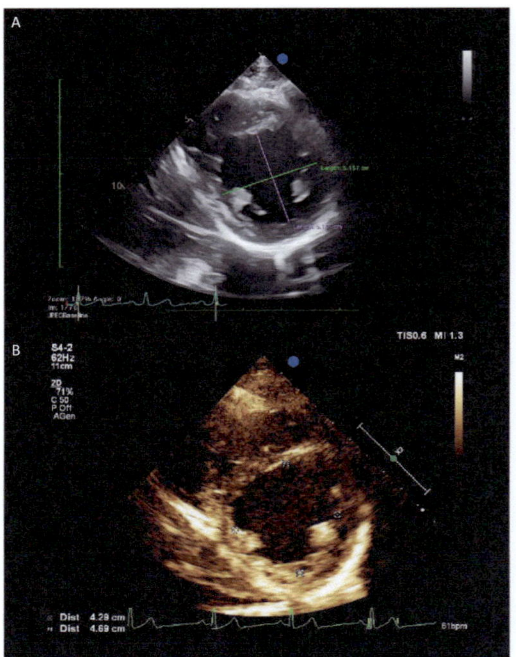

Fig. 13 The eccentricity index

(diastolic inter-ventricular shift). This index can also be measured using M-mode.

Legend to Fig. 13. The eccentricity index is calculated by dividing the lateral dimension of the left ventricle by its anterior–posterior dimension. A. Two-Dimensional (2D) parasternal short axis (PSAX) view showing a normal eccentricity index (5.17/5.14 ≈ 1.00). B. 2D PSAX view showing the eccentricity index (4.69/4.29 = 1.1) in a patient with increased right ventricular afterload.

Measurements of Pulmonary Artery Pressure

Systolic Pulmonary Artery Pressure

Although the definition of pulmonary hypertension is based on mPAP, the sPAP is the measurement of PA pressure most commonly estimated by echocardiography. The sPAP is calculated by addition of right atrial pressure

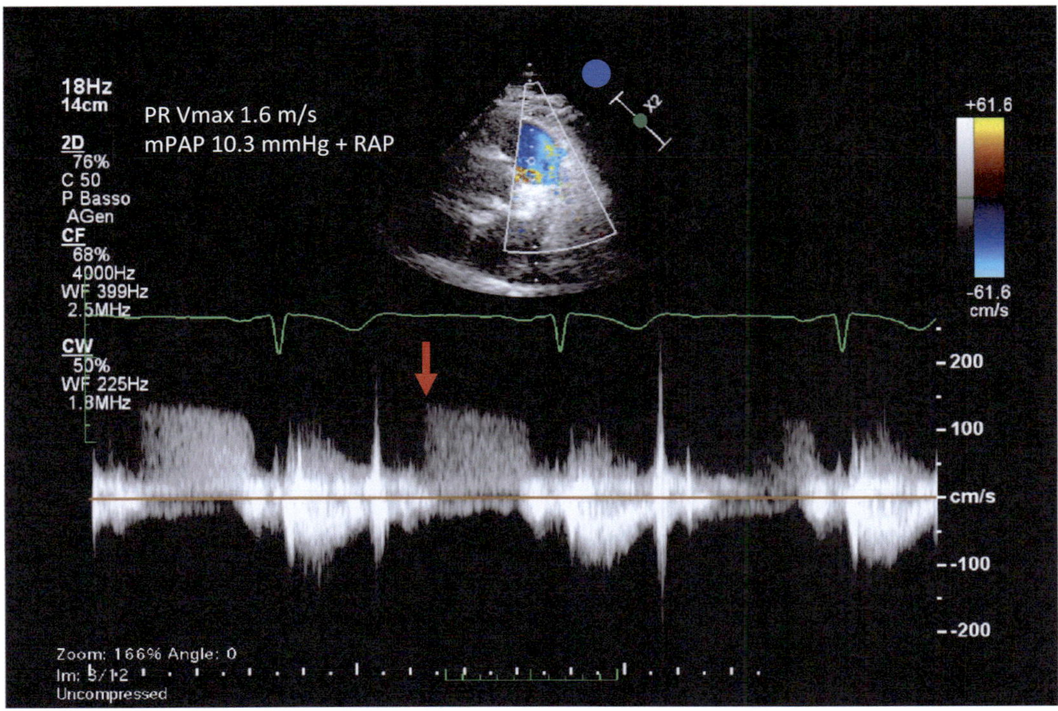

Fig. 14 Estimation of the mean pulmonary artery pressure from measurements of pulmonary valve regurgitation maximum velocity with continuous wave Doppler

(RAP) to the RVSP. The RVSP is estimated by the application of the modified Bernoulli equation to the tricuspid regurgitation maximum velocity (TRv) measured by continuous wave Doppler (Fig. 12) [16]:

$$sPAP = 4 * (TRv)^2 + RAP$$

$$sPAP = RVSP \text{ (if there is no pulmonary stenosis)}$$

$$sPAP = RVSP - \text{pulmonary stenosis gradient}$$

Normal resting values are usually defined as a peak TR gradient of >2.8 to 2.9 m/s (i.e. peak systolic pressure of 35 or 36 mmHg, assuming that RA pressure is 3–5 mmHg). This has been validated in several studies, some of which have included critically ill patients [17]. However, measurement of TRv may be inaccurate in some situations: a) incomplete TR Doppler signal; b) sub-optimal continuous wave Doppler cursor alignment; c) dagger-shaped TR due to severe/torrential TR; d) moderate to severe RV dysfunction [18–20]. It is important to be aware that the RA-RV gradient is also dependent on RV contractility. When significant impairment of RV systolic function occurs, the RA-RV gradient may be low. However, this reflects the loss of contractility. Therefore, the adjustment of TAPSE for sPAP (TAPSE/sPAP) can accurately identify patients with increased afterload and RV systolic dysfunction [10, 11].

Mean pulmonary artery pressure

The formula for calculation of mPAP from pressure measurements is:

$$mPAP = 2/3dPAP - 1/3sPAP$$

Using echocardiography, the mPAP is best estimated by application of the modified Bernoulli equation to pulmonary regurgitation (Fig. 14):

$$mPAP = 4 * (early\,PR\,velocity)^2 + RA$$

This measurement requires a well-defined continuous wave Doppler envelope of the pulmonary regurgitant jet in the PSAX view (Fig. 14).

Legend to Fig. 14. The upper part of the figure shows a thumbnail view of a Two-Dimensional (2D) parasternal short axis view with pulmonary valve regurgitation demonstrated by the overlying color Doppler. The continuous wave Doppler cursor is aligned with the regurgitant flow through the pulmonary valve. The lower part of the figure shows the continuous wave Doppler trace of pulmonary valve regurgitation. The modified Bernoulli equation can then be applied to the pulmonary regurgitation peak velocity (PR Vmax; red arrow) to estimate the pressure gradient across the pulmonary valve. Adding the (measured or estimated) right atrial pressure (RAP) to the pressure gradient across the pulmonary valve allows estimation of the mean pulmonary artery pressure.

A recently described alternative method to estimate mPAP adds estimated RA pressure to the velocity–time integral (VTI) of the TR jet [21].

$$MPAP = VTI_{TR} + RAP$$

However, this technique has not been validated in critically ill patients or those with RV dysfunction.

Pulmonary Flow

Assessment of the forward flow through the pulmonary valve provides important data about pulmonary hypertension. These include estimates of mPAP and PVR. The formula for calculation of PVR from cardiac catheterisation is:

$$PVR = (mPAP-PCWP)/cardiac\,output$$

where PCWP is the mean pulmonary capillary wedge pressure. However, as yet, no imaging technique has been validated for the measurement of PCWP in the critically ill.

The PVR can be estimated echocardiographically using the following formula:

$$PVR = 10$$
$$\times (TR\,peak\,systolic\,velocity/RVOT\,VTI) + 0.16$$

Flow through the pulmonary valve (Fig. 15a) is characterized by a 'rounded' Doppler curve with slower acceleration and a longer time from onset to the peak flow than the Doppler flow pattern of LV ejection. These differences reflect the lower vascular resistance of the pulmonary circulation.

Although, the presence of a mid-systolic wave notching (Fig. 15b) is highly suggestive of increased PA pressures and decreased vascular compliance, the absence of pulmonary notching does not demonstrate normal sPAP. The degree and timing of the arterial wave reflection is influenced by vascular resistance, the distance of the reflecting sites from the RVOT and the speed of the reflected wave (determined by the stiffness of medium and large vessels). If PVR is increased and the arterial compliance is low (e.g. due to pulmonary embolism and/or chronic vascular remodelling), the reflected waves have increased amplitude and propagate more rapidly creating an increased resistance which is propagated backward to the RVOT during systole which leads to the mid-systolic notching [20].

The PA acceleration time (PAAT; i.e. the time from the beginning of pulmonary flow to its peak velocity; Fig. 15) correlates with sPAP and PVR. The normal thresholds of the PAAT range from 136 to 153 ms [18, 22]. A finding of PAAT < 105 ms is highly suggestive of pulmonary hypertension and PAAT < 57 ms has a positive predictive value of 100% [18, 20, 22]. However, these parameters have not been specifically evaluated in critically ill patients.

Legend to Fig. 15. A. Modified Two-Dimensional (2D) parasternal long axis view with pulsed wave Doppler at the pulmonary valve demonstrating a normal systolic ejection wave and normal acceleration time (132 ms). B. 2D parasternal short axis view with pulsed wave

Fig. 15 Measurement of the pulmonary artery acceleration time

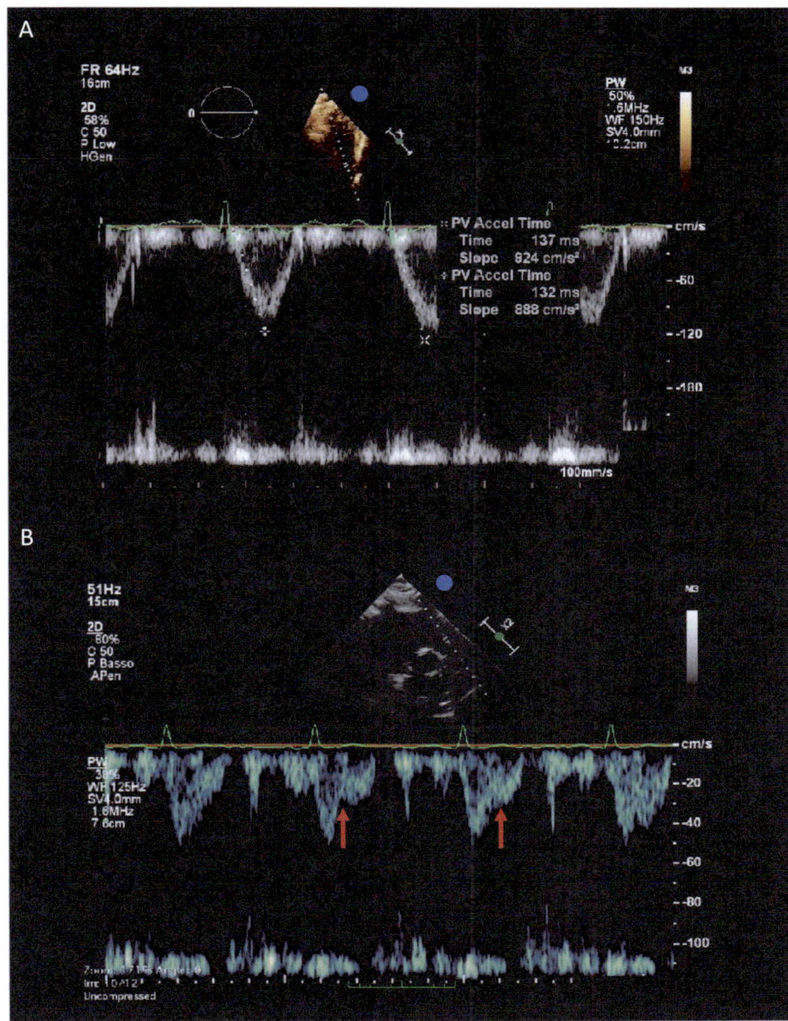

Doppler at the pulmonary valve showing mid-systolic notching (red arrow) of the ejection wave and reduced acceleration time (78 ms) in a patient with severe respiratory failure [23].

Conclusion

POCUS assessment of the RV and investigation of pulmonary hypertension requires integration of data from all standard views and multiple modes of ultrasound. Regardless, the assessment of the RV remains challenging in view of its complex morphology. Accurate echocardiographic estimation of PA pressures is equally difficult. Thus, as technology advances, the application of 3D echocardiography to POCUS for the RV and pulmonary hypertension are likely to increase. The bedside use of POCUS to assess the RV and pulmonary pressures is a milestone in the hemodynamic assessment of critically ill patients. Indeed, the use of POCUS to identify and monitor patients at risk of RV failure and pulmonary hypertension may improve outcomes by directing the application of game changing therapies such as pharmaceutical agents and mechanical cardiac support devices.

References

1. Rajendram R, Hussain A, Mahmood N, Kharal M. Feasibility of using a handheld ultrasound device to detect and characterize shunt and deep vein thrombosis in patients with COVID-19: an observational study. Ultrasound J. 2020;12:49. https://doi.org/10.1186/s13089-020-00197-0.PMID:33252722; PMCID:PMC7702202.

2. Beaubien-Souligny W, Rola P, Haycock K, Bouchard J, Lamarche Y, Spiegel R, Denault AY. Quantifying systemic congestion with Point-Of-Care ultrasound: development of the venous excess ultrasound grading system. Ultrasound J. 2020;9(12):16. https://doi.org/10.1186/s13089-020-00163-w.

3. Huisman MV, Barco S, Cannegieter SC, Le Gal G, Konstantinides SV, Reitsma PH, Rodger M, Vonk Noordegraaf A, Klok FA. Pulmonary embolism Nat Rev Dis Primers. 2018;4:18028. https://doi.org/10.1038/nrdp.2018.28.

4. Dandel M, Hetzer R. Echocardiographic assessment of the right ventricle: Impact of the distinctly load dependency of its size, geometry and performance. Int J Cardiol. 2016;221:1132–42. https://doi.org/10.1016/j.ijcard.2016.07.014.

5. D'Alto M, Pavelescu A, Argiento P, Romeo E, Correra A, Di Marco GM, D'Andrea A, Sarubbi B, Russo MG, Naeije R. Echocardiographic assessment of right ventricular contractile reserve in healthy subjects. Echocardiography. 2017;34:61–8. https://doi.org/10.1111/echo.13396.

6. Kawel-Boehm N, Maceira A, Valsangiacomo-Buechel ER, Vogel-Claussen J, Turkbey EB, Williams R, Plein S, Tee M, Eng J, Bluemke DA. Normal values for cardiovascular magnetic resonance in adults and children. J Cardiovasc Magn Reson. 2015;17:29. https://doi.org/10.1186/s12968-015-0111-7.

7. Simon MA, Deible C, Mathier MA, Lacomis J, Goitein O, Shroff SG, Pinsky MR. Phenotyping the right ventricle in patients with pulmonary hypertension. Clin Transl Sci. 2009;2:294–9. https://doi.org/10.1111/j.1752-8062.2009.00134.x.

8. Addetia K, Maffessanti F, Muraru D, Singh A, Surkova E, Mor-Avi V, Badano LP, Lang RM. Morphologic analysis of the normal right ventricle using three-dimensional echocardiography-derived curvature indices. J Am Soc Echocardiogr. 2018;31:614–23. https://doi.org/10.1016/j.echo.2017.12.009.

9. Lang RM, Badano LP, Mor-Avi V, Afilalo J, Armstrong A, Ernande L, Flachskampf FA, Foster E, Goldstein SA, Kuznetsova T, Lancellotti P, Muraru D, Picard MH, Rietzschel ER, Rudski L, Spencer KT, Tsang W, Voigt JU. Recommendations for cardiac chamber quantification by echocardiography in adults: an update from the American Society of Echocardiography and the European Association of Cardiovascular Imaging. J Am Soc Echocardiogr. 2015;28:1-39.e14. https://doi.org/10.1016/j.echo.2014.10.003.

10. Markin NW, Chamsi-Pasha M, Luo J, Thomas WR, Brakke TR, Porter TR, Shillcutt SK. Transesophageal speckle-tracking echocardiography improves right ventricular systolic function assessment in the perioperative setting. J Am Soc Echocardiogr. 2017;30:180–8. https://doi.org/10.1016/j.echo.2016.10.002.

11. Donauer M, Schneider J, Jander N, Beyersdorf F, Keyl C. Perioperative changes of right ventricular function in cardiac surgical patients assessed by myocardial deformation analysis and 3-dimensional echocardiography. J Cardiothorac Vasc Anesth. 2020;34:708–18. https://doi.org/10.1053/j.jvca.2019.08.026.

12. Galiè N, Humbert M, Vachiery JL, Gibbs S, Lang I, Torbicki A, Simonneau G, Peacock A, Vonk Noordegraaf A, Beghetti M, Ghofrani A, Gomez Sanchez MA, Hansmann G, Klepetko W, Lancellotti P, Matucci M, McDonagh T, Pierard LA, Trindade PT, Zompatori M, Hoeper M; ESC Scientific Document Group. 2015 ESC/ERS Guidelines for the diagnosis and treatment of pulmonary hypertension: The Joint Task Force for the Diagnosis and Treatment of Pulmonary Hypertension of the European Society of Cardiology (ESC) and the European Respiratory Society (ERS): Endorsed by: Association for European Paediatric and Congenital Cardiology (AEPC), International Society for Heart and Lung Transplantation (ISHLT). Eur Heart J. 2016 1;37:67–119. doi: https://doi.org/10.1093/eurheartj/ehv317.

13. Galiè N, McLaughlin VV, Rubin LJ, Simonneau G. An overview of the 6th world symposium on pulmonary hypertension. Eur Respir J. 2019;53:1802148. https://doi.org/10.1183/13993003.02148-2018.

14. Mekontso Dessap A, Boissier F, Charron C, Bégot E, Repessé X, Legras A, Brun-Buisson C, Vignon P, Vieillard-Baron A. Acute cor pulmonale during protective ventilation for acute respiratory distress syndrome: prevalence, predictors, and clinical impact. Intensive Care Med. 2016;42:862–70. https://doi.org/10.1007/s00134-015-4141-2.

15. Frémont B, Pacouret G, Jacobi D, Puglisi R, Charbonnier B, de Labriolle A. Prognostic value of echocardiographic right/left ventricular end-diastolic diameter ratio in patients with acute pulmonary embolism: results from a monocenter registry of 1,416 patients. Chest. 2008;133:358–62. https://doi.org/10.1378/chest.07-1231.

16. Rudski LG, Lai WW, Afilalo J, Hua L, Handschumacher MD, Chandrasekaran K, Solomon SD, Louie EK, Schiller NB. Guidelines for the echocardiographic assessment of the right heart in adults: a report from the American Society of Echocardiography endorsed by the European Association of Echocardiography, a registered branch of the European Society of Cardiology, and the Canadian Society of Echocardiography. J Am Soc

Echocardiogr. 2010;23:685–713. https://doi.org/10.1016/j.echo.2010.05.010.

17. Lafitte S, Pillois X, Reant P, Picard F, Arsac F, Dijos M, Coste P, Dos Santos P, Roudaut R. Estimation of pulmonary pressures and diagnosis of pulmonary hypertension by Doppler echocardiography: a retrospective comparison of routine echocardiography and invasive hemodynamics. J Am Soc Echocardiogr. 2013;26:457–63. https://doi.org/10.1016/j.echo.2013.02.002.

18. Fisher MR, Forfia PR, Chamera E, Housten-Harris T, Champion HC, Girgis RE, Corretti MC, Hassoun PM. Accuracy of Doppler echocardiography in the hemodynamic assessment of pulmonary hypertension. Am J Respir Crit Care Med. 2009;179:615–21. https://doi.org/10.1164/rccm.200811-1691OC.

19. Rich JD, Shah SJ, Swamy RS, Kamp A, Rich S. Inaccuracy of Doppler echocardiographic estimates of pulmonary artery pressures in patients with pulmonary hypertension: implications for clinical practice. Chest. 2011;139:988–93. https://doi.org/10.1378/chest.10-1269.

20. Mercado P, Maizel J, Beyls C, Kontar L, Orde S, Huang S, McLean A, Tribouilloy C, Slama M. Reassessment of the accuracy of cardiac doppler pulmonary artery pressure measurements in ventilated icu patients: a simultaneous doppler-catheterization study. Crit Care Med. 2019;47:41–8. https://doi.org/10.1097/CCM.0000000000003422.

21. Aduen JF, Castello R, Lozano MM, Hepler GN, Keller CA, Alvarez F, Safford RE, Crook JE, Heckman MG, Burger CD. An alternative echocardiographic method to estimate mean pulmonary artery pressure: diagnostic and clinical implications. J Am Soc Echocardiogr. 2009;22:814–9. https://doi.org/10.1016/j.echo.2009.04.007.

22. Tossavainen E, Söderberg S, Grönlund C, Gonzalez M, Henein MY, Lindqvist P. Pulmonary artery acceleration time in identifying pulmonary hypertension patients with raised pulmonary vascular resistance. Eur Heart J Cardiovasc Imaging. 2013;14:890–7. https://doi.org/10.1093/ehjci/jes309.

23. Arkles JS, Opotowsky AR, Ojeda J, Rogers F, Liu T, Prassana V, Marzec L, Palevsky HI, Ferrari VA, Forfia PR. Shape of the right ventricular Doppler envelope predicts hemodynamics and right heart function in pulmonary hypertension. Am J Respir Crit Care Med. 2011;183:268–76. https://doi.org/10.1164/rccm.201004-0601OC.

Assessment of Valves at the Point-of-Care

Shelley Rahman Haley

'The secret of science is to ask the right question'

—Sir Henry Tizard, English chemist, inventor and Rector of Imperial College (1885—1959)

Abstract

For over three decades following the recognition of echocardiography as the new cornerstone of cardiac imaging, it was accepted that accurate assessment of the heart valves was an often-complex challenge, which could only be met by formal "minimum standards" study acquisition in an echocardiography laboratory setting. However, over the past ten years, this view has changed, with the recognition that useful information about valve structure and function can be obtained at the bedside and may facilitate efficient clinical decision-making with minimal compromise in terms of the information quality. The key lies in understanding which pieces of information can be most reliably obtained in more challenging imaging conditions. As ever, "the secret of science is to ask the right question" *Sir Henry Tizard*

Keywords

Valvular heart disease · Mitral valve · Aortic valve · Tricuspid valve and pulmonary valve

Key messages

- POCUS assessment can include advanced assessment of valves in a targeted scan
- Point-of-care echocardiography is an excellent screening tool to pick up haemodynamically significant heart valve lesions and to allow assessment of the effects of these lesions on the function of the ventricles
- Echocardiographic assessment of valves should always be performed in the context of ventricular function.

Supplementary Information The online version contains supplementary material available at https://doi.org/10.1007/978-3-031-29472-3_20.

S. R. Haley (✉)
Royal Brompton and Harefield Hospitals, Uxbridge, England
e-mail: s.rahmanhaley@rbht.nhs.uk

S. R. Haley
Guys and St Thomas NHS Foundation Trust, London, UK

Introduction

For over three decades following the recognition of echocardiography as the new cornerstone of cardiac imaging, it was accepted that accurate assessment of the heart valves was an often-complex challenge, which could only be met by formal "minimum standards" study acquisition in an echocardiography laboratory setting. There is no doubt that full, detailed assessment and analysis of the structure and function of the heart valves can require a complex and time-consuming study. However, over the past ten years, technical advances, which have simplified the acquisition of quality images at the bedside have led to something of a "volte-face" in this opinion, with the result that it is now increasingly recognised that obtaining useful information about valve structure and function at the bedside can facilitate more efficient clinical decision-making and progress along the patient journey with minimal compromise in terms of the quality of the information. The trick lies in understanding which pieces of information can be most usefully and reliably acquired in more challenging imaging conditions. The converse of this is that the operator and interpreter (often the same person) must be aware of any limitations of the technique in this setting.

Overview

Point-of-care echocardiography is an excellent screening tool to pick up haemodynamically-significant heart valve lesions and to allow assessment of the effects of these lesions on the function of the ventricles [1]. Regardless of the setting in which the scan takes place, any finding of structural abnormality leading to impairment of valve function must be considered and interpreted in the context of ventricular function as a whole and indeed in the context of the patient's entire clinical presentation. For this reason, it is rarely, if ever, appropriate to do "nothing but" a valve assessment—this would risk other important abnormalities being overlooked.

Technical Tip

- *Always* connect an ECG, in whatever care setting the echo is being acquired—it takes just a few seconds and can be via stick-on electrodes or "internal" by slaving in the ECG of the patient monitor. The eye can play tricks on the brain when it comes to visually assessing points in the cardiac cycle, and events such as early valve closure can be very helpful pointers towards severity of lesions.

The Aortic Valve

2D Views, M-mode and Colour Flow Doppler

Technical tips:

- Perform 2D visual assessment ("eyeballing")
- M-mode or 2D measurements of LVOT/aortic root/Cardiac chambers
- Use colour flow Doppler across the valve
- Use the Zoom function to look more closely at the valve, which should look like a "Y" or "Mercedes-Benz sign" when closed
- The cusp adjacent to the interatrial septum is the non-coronary cusp
- Remember that the aortic "annulus" is a 3-dimensional crown shape, so make sure to tilt the probe in order to see the whole structure, not only one plane
- Colour Doppler—use colour M-mode to assess the width of the neck of any regurgitant jet as a proportion of the LVOT diameter
- The PSAX view with colour flow Doppler is good for spotting paraprosthetic leaks and complications of endocarditis e.g. abscess
- In the apical 4-chamber view, the aortic valve itself is *not* visible
- Be wary of overinterpreting colour Doppler from the apical 5-chamber view in aortic regurgitation—never base a grading decision on one colour flow view alone—look for corroborating CW/PW Doppler evidence
- Standalone Doppler remains a very useful skill, well-worth practising!

What are you looking out for?

- *Congenital abnormalities (bicuspid, quadricuspid valve)*—congenital aortic valve abnormalities are present in 4–5% of live births, bicuspid valve in 1–2% [2]
- *Aortic calcification/stenosis*—calcific AS is present in 2–4% of the European adult population aged > 70 y [3]
- *Aortic root dilatation*—suggests genetic aortopathy (Marfan's Loeys-Dietz, Ehlers-Danlos syndrome) or longstanding hypertension
- *Aortic valve prolapse*—may be isolated, or seen in association with dilated aortic root or as a complication of a previous valve-sparing root surgery
- *Aortic dissection*—caveat—reverberation artefact can mimic a dissection flap—look for movements of the suspected flap which are out of phase with the movements of the walls of the aorta
- Evidence of endocarditis—mobile masses, root abscess (unusual echo-free spaces or areas or high echogenicity), abnormal colour jets, leaflet destruction/perforation.
- When assessing the aortic valve and root in a patient who has had previous aortic surgery, it is useful to have full details of the previous surgery—ideally in the form of an operation note, or preferably a conversation with the surgeon!

In the PLAX view, the two visible cusps are the right coronary cusp (RCC) and the noncoronary cusp (NCC). Normally they should be thin and open virtually flush with the walls of the aortic root. A visual inspection will identify thickening and calcification—it is often difficult to be certain how much of any thickening seen is actually calcium (CT is the best imaging modality for this) but as the aortic valve tends to calcify with age, it is reasonable to conclude in the over 60s that thickening will represent calcium. Calcific aortic stenosis is present in 2–4% of the European adult population aged ≥ 70 years. (Video 1) Cusp motion and separation can be judged visually, but M-mode can be useful to measure cusp separation, which is the distance between the inner edges of the two visible cusps at mid-systole, when flow is greatest (at least 10 mm indicates adequate opening, and ≥ 12 mm is normal) (Fig. 1) and also to look for premature closure (seen in extremely severe mitral regurgitation, severe LV systolic dysfunction, hypertrophic cardiomyopathy and several other conditions) [4]. Thickening and calcification, along with reduced cusp mobility strongly suggest aortic stenosis. An assessment of the morphology and dimensions of the aortic root should be made—M-mode or 2D can be used to measure the dimensions of the LVOT/aortic annulus, sinus diameter, sinotubular junction and proximal ascending aorta (Fig. 2). The LVOT dimension is sometimes referred to as the "aortic annulus". It is the distance between the hinge points of the two visible cusps in the PLAX view. However, the aortic valve does not have a planar ring-shaped annulus, but a crown-shaped 3-dimensional one. It is therefore more correct to refer to this measurement as the LVOT diameter. Sometimes it is necessary to move the probe to a higher rib space in order to visualise the ascending aorta. All aortic measurements should be made at end-diastole *except* for the LVOT, which should be measured in mid-systole. This measurement is used in the continuity equation to calculate the effective valve orifice area (see Equations, below). In this calculation, the value for the LVOT diameter is squared and therefore, any error in measurement is also compounded. Poor operator reproducibility of the LVOT diameter measurement is one reason for criticism of the continuity equation as an objective quantitative measure of aortic stenosis. To reduce error and increase reproducibility, zoom in on the valve when taking this measurement.

The PSAX view is the best one for counting the number of cusps and for assessing whether one cusp is abnormally large or small, which can happen when the aortic root is asymmetrically dilated. If a bicuspid valve is suspected, a raphe may be identified between two fused cusps (Video 2). Although there is more than one accepted classification system for bicuspid aortic valves, the Sievers classification is simple and

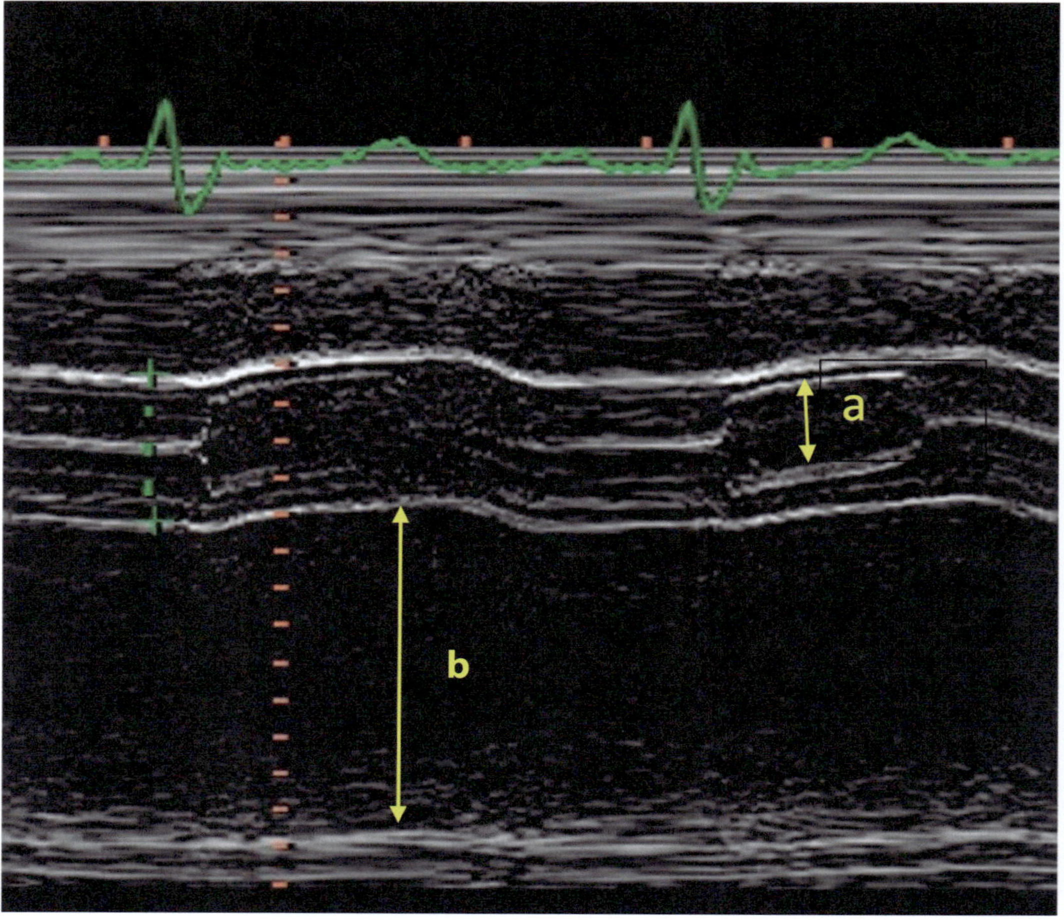

Fig. 1 M-mode evaluation of aortic valve. a: aortic cuspid separation during systole; b: left atrial diameter in measured in diastole

often used by cardiac surgeons and so is recommended here [5]. The annulus may be ovoid in the case of a true or "type 0" bicuspid valve—this is important to note if the patient is being considered for TAVR as the risk of paraprosthetic leakage is greater in the presence of an ovoid annulus. In aortic regurgitation, the PSAX view allows good appreciation of the width of the neck of the regurgitant jet (effectively the vena contracta)—a thin, central jet is likely to be mild—and also indicates where the leak is actually coming through the valve—central, or commissural.

The shape of the aortic root itself may be an important clue to the existence of pathology. Partial or complete effacement of the sino-tubular junction (STJ) is seen in patients with long-standing poorly-controlled hypertension and in patients with genetic aortopathy [6]. In a patient with known or suspected aortopathy presenting with chest pain, dilatation of the aortic root along with a change in morphology are causes for concern. Careful inspection should be made to look for a possible dissection flap, with the caveat that reverberation artefact can mimic this. To exclude artefact, look carefully for movements of the flap which do *not* follow the movements of the wall of the vessel. Often, multi-modality imaging is helpful if a diagnosis of acute ascending aortic dissection is suspected

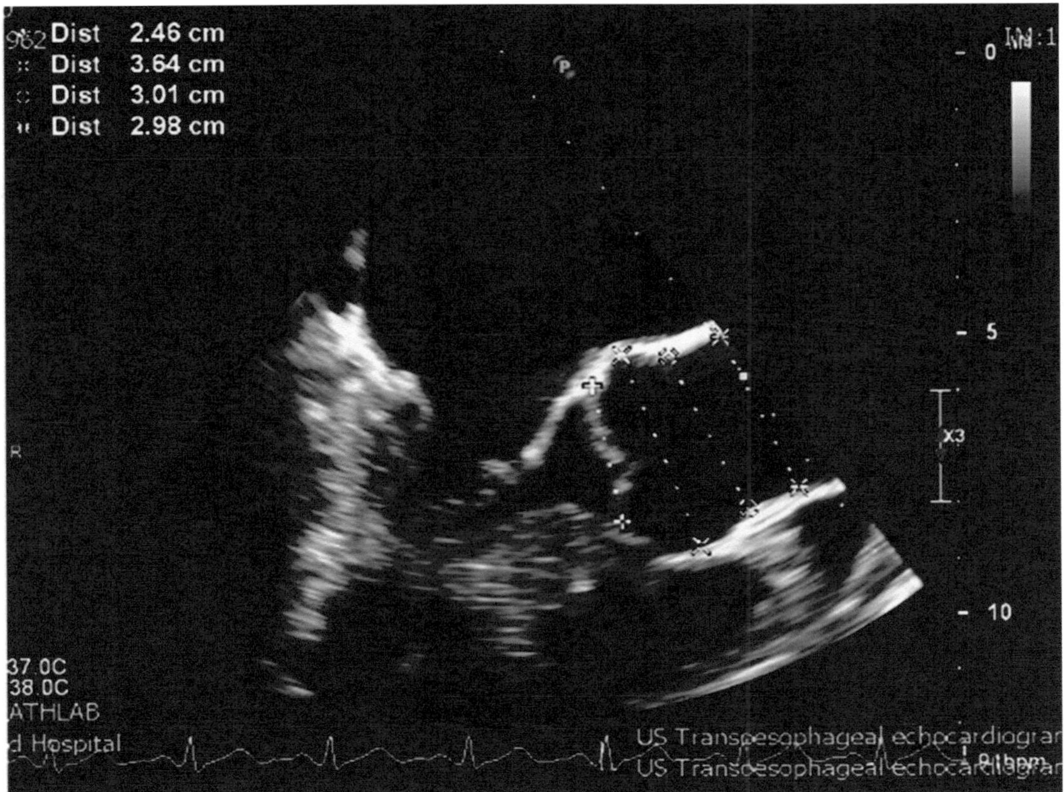

Fig. 2 Zoomed in mid-oesophageal long axis view (120 degrees) showing estimation of aortic valve, aortic root and ascending aorta diameters - note that if measuring in 2D, the internal diameter is taken - rather than the "leading edge-leading edge" measurement in M-mode

[7]. Transoesophageal echocardiography, whilst highly specific for AAD, should *not* be the first-line modality unless the patient is in the anaesthetic room or operating theatre, as the acute rise in blood pressure which may occur during intubation for TOE under light conscious sedation can precipitate disastrous extension of the dissection. A dilated aortic root may be associated with prolapse of one of the valve cusps, so this should be looked for. Finally, in the context of sepsis, infective endocarditis is a possibility and any signs of this—mobile masses, abscess cavities, fistulae, should be noted. Unusual high-velocity jets and aliasing on colour Doppler may indicate the presence of a fistula due to infection. It is common for a senile degenerative aortic valve to have small mobile masses (Lambl's excrescences) on the ventricular side of the cusps, and fibroelastomata are also seen, so a diagnosis of infective endocarditis can only be made in an appropriate clinical context.

Colour flow Doppler across the aortic valve allows the appreciation of turbulence in the LVOT, across the valve and in the aortic root. Turbulent flow in the LVOT may suggest LVOT obstruction and the operator should look carefully for asymmetric septal hypertrophy and systolic anterior motion of the mitral valve apparatus, both features of hypertrophic cardiomyopathy. Turbulent flow across the valve itself is often seen with age-related calcific degeneration as well as with haemodynamically-significant stenosis. Finally, aortic regurgitation is well-appreciated in this view using colour Doppler, which can be used to measure the width of the jet in the LVOT—a jet which

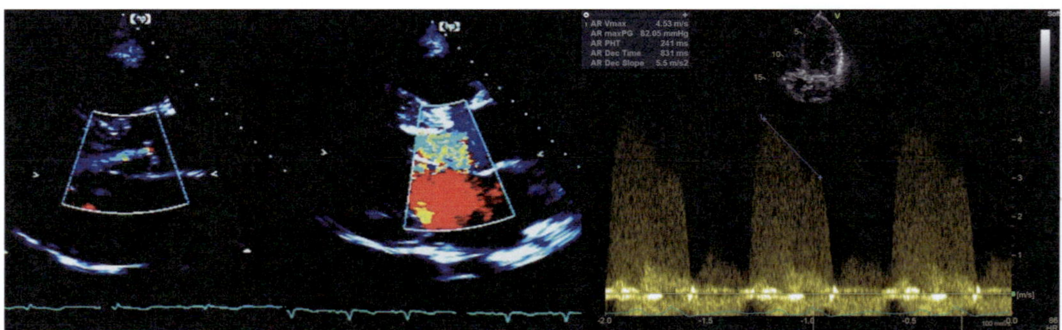

Fig. 3 Colour Doppler and continuous wave Doppler assessment of aortic regurgitation

occupies $\geq 50\%$ of the LVOT is likely to be severe, and one which occupies $\leq 30\%$ likely to be mild (Fig. 3). However, it must be remembered that echocardiography is a planar technique so the operator must look in other planes before drawing a firm conclusion regarding severity of a regurgitant lesion.

In the apical four chamber view, although the aortic valve itself is not visible, the effects of any valve lesion on the ventricles/atria can be appreciated. These include LV concentric or asymmetric hypertrophy and dilatation, reduced LVEF, hyperdynamic function in AR, regional abnormalities resulting from embolic events (in infection) or aortic dissection shearing off the RCA, and pericardial effusion (dissection, infective endocarditis). The left atrium is often dilated in longstanding aortic stenosis, due to raised LV filling pressure.

Using colour flow Doppler in the apical five chamber view, the extent of an aortic regurgitant jet into the ventricle can be well-seen, and this is also a good view to appreciate SAM of the mitral valve causing LVOTO. This the best view for measuring the velocities of blood flow across the aortic valve and in the LVOT in the majority of patients (see below).

The apical long axis or three chamber view is essentially identical to the PLAX view, except that it allows complete visualisation of the apex. It can be invaluable in patients with poor parasternal windows, such as those with COPD and occasionally provides just the right angle for

measuring the velocity across the aortic valve by CW Doppler.

The aortic valve is not visible in the apical two chamber view. The suprasternal window is used to visualise the aortic arch by 2D echocardiography. Colour flow across the aortic arch in this view gives a qualitative impression of the degree of aortic regurgitation, and colour M mode can show visually whether or not the reversal of flow is holo-diastolic, hence severe regurgitation.

CW, PW and standalone Doppler of the aortic valve

Doppler techniques are the cornerstone of assessment of aortic valve lesion severity. The continuous wave Doppler trace is used to measure the maximum and mean velocity of blood moving through the aortic valve in m/s. Using the modified Bernoulli equation, this can be converted into a peak and mean pressure drop, often called the peak and mean "gradient" across the valve. The shape of the CW trace itself indicates stenotic lesion severity—as the stenosis moves from "severe" to "critical", the shape of the trace becomes symmetrical or late-peaking as opposed to an asymmetrical trace with a more rapid upstroke. This symmetrical trace is sometimes referred to as "dagger-shaped" (Fig. 4). However, in a significant minority, either because of less-than-perfect image quality or, more likely, because of the angulation of the aortic root, the Doppler angle from the apex is

Fig. 4 The shape of continuous wave Doppler waveform in moderate versus severe aortic stenosis

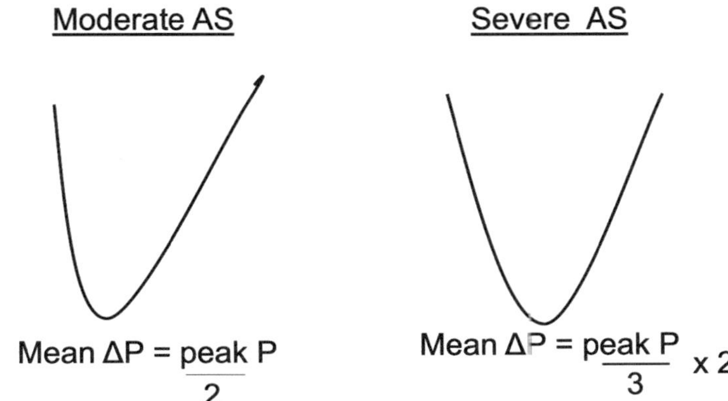

difficult and the trace is faint or incomplete. In these cases, it is *essential* that other views are used before a final assessment of lesion severity is made. The window from which the maximum stenotic gradient is measured should be recorded.

The effective regurgitant orifice of the aortic valve can be calculated using the continuity equation (below). This requires that the LVOT diameter be measured from the 2D image in mid-systole, and the velocity of blood in the LVOT 1cm below the valve using PW Doppler. Measurement of the LVOT diameter is prone to reproducibility error and in order to eliminate this, the dimensionless velocity index (DVI) can be used. This is a simple ratio of the maximum velocity of blood in the LVOT measured by PW Doppler to the maximum velocity of blood flowing across the valve measured by CW Doppler (Fig. 5). A dimensionless velocity index of 0.25 or less is consistent with severe AS.

When assessing aortic regurgitation, the density of the trace is itself proportional to the volume of blood in the regurgitant jet, and a regurgitant jet density that is similar to the density of the forward trace suggests severe AR. The key Doppler measurement in the evaluation of aortic regurgitation severity is the pressure half-time—the time taken for the velocity of blood in the regurgitation jet to fall to half its initial value. Accurate measurement depends on obtaining a trace with a clear edge, which in turn depends

upon the ability to line up the Doppler with the regurgitant jet. Pressure half-time may be arte-factually shortened if the LVEDP is raised. As with mitral regurgitation, the PISA method may be used to estimate EROA and regurgitant volume. The suprasternal window is perhaps the most useful single view when assessing the severity of AR. A PW Doppler trace from the descending limb of the aortic arch may be obtained and this will confirm whether the aortic regurgitation is holodiastolic and hence, severe. In addition, the end-diastolic velocity of the regurgitation has been shown to correlate with the regurgitant fraction: an EDV of 18 cm/s or greater suggests a regurgitant fraction of 40% or more [8]. Criteria for the assessment of severity of aortic regurgitation are shown below in Table 1.

Standalone Doppler is a very useful skill and one that is fast-disappearing from the regular armamentarium of many sonographers, especially those with a medical, as opposed to physiology background. The ability to precisely direct a single beam of Doppler ultrasound through a valve, which may be situated at an awkward angle is invaluable, and in particular, using standalone Doppler from the *right* parasternal window can add significantly to the measured velocity across a valve which is otherwise tricky to assess from the apical window.

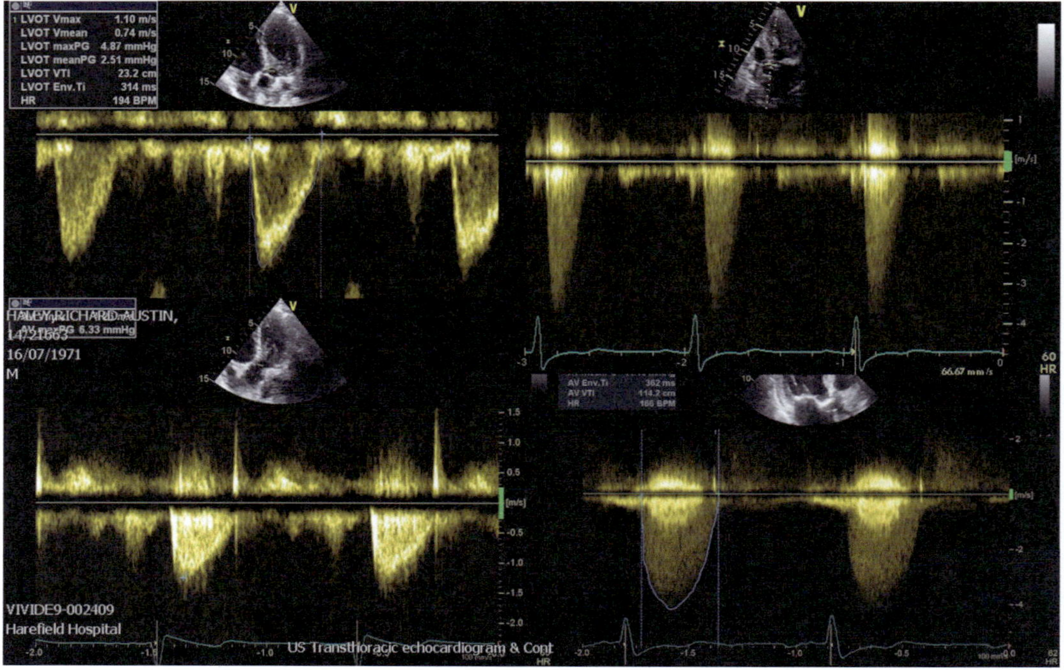

Fig. 5 Calculation of dimensionless index requires estimation of LVOT VTI using PW Doppler and aortic valve VTI using CW Doppler

The Continuity Equation and Dimensionless Velocity Index (DVI).

The assessment of aortic stenosis severity in patients with normal flow (≥ 200 ml/minute) is often made simply by measuring the Vmax across the valve and calculating the pressure gradient (PG) across the valve using the modified Bernouilli equation:

$$PG\,(mmHg) \;=\; 4V_m^2$$

In patients with reduced flow, whether due to reduced ejection fraction or small ventricular volumes, the gradient across the valve may be measurably lower despite a reduced orifice area. In such cases it is necessary to calculate the effective orifice area (EOAcm^2) using the continuity equation, which relies on the principle that

the flow rate through the LVOT and across the narrowed valve must be the same. The continuity equation is: A1 x V1 = A2 x V2.

A1: cross sectional area of the LVOT, V1: LVOT velocity time integral (VTI), A2: cross sectional area of the AV, V2: peak velocity of the AV VTI.

Current Assessment of Aortic Stenosis.

The most recent international guidelines for the assessment of aortic stenosis suggest that confirmation of the diagnosis depends on three parameters: mean pressure gradient (mmHg), peak transvalvular velocity (Vmax) and valve area (cm2). Taking into account conditions of flow, where low flow is defined by the stroke volume index ≤ 35 ml/min/m2, this allows differentiation of four categories of aortic stenosis, summarised in Table 2.

Table 1 Summary of qualitative and quantitative criteria for grading the severity of aortic regurgitation by Echocardiography

	Criterion	Mild	Moderate	Severe	**notes
Qualitative	Appearance of valve (morphology)	–	–	Obvious coaptation defect, flail leaflet, evidence of structural damage eg due to infection	
	Width of Colour M-mode jet as % of LVOT	<25	25–64	>65	For several of the parameters we use to assess AR severity, the moderate zone represents a "grey" area which may include any grade of AR!
	Regurgitant jet length	–	–	Extends to the LV apex	
	Regurgitant jet area	<5	5–59	>60	
	Regurgitant jet density	Faint or incomplete trace	Complete trace but not as dense as forward flow trace	Density similar to forward flow trace	
Semi-quantitative	Vena contracta width (mm)	≤ 3	**	≥ 6	
	Holodiastolic flow reversal in descending limb of the arch	Absent	Either absent or present but with a low end-diastolic velocity <18 cm/s	Present; End-diastolic velocity ≥ 13 cm/s	
	Pressure Half-time (ms)	>500	200–500**	<200	
Quantitative	EROA by PISA calculation (cm2)	<0.1	0.1–0.29	≥ 0.3	
	Regurgitant volume (ml)	<30	30–59	60	

The Mitral Valve

2D Views, M-mode and Colour flow Doppler

Technical Tips

- Ensure the image is "on-axis"
- Use "anatomical M mode" to make measurements if off-axis
- Do not rely on colour flow Doppler to assess severity of regurgitation

What are you looking out for?

- *Abnormalities of leaflet mobility/coaptation— tethering/prolapse*—a history of myocardial infarction would alert the sonographer to the possibility of tethering due to wall motion abnormality
- *Calcification—leaflets, annulus, chordae—* watch out for massive annular calcification [9]

Table 2 Summary of four categories of aortic stenosis assessed by Echocardiography*

	Criteria	Notes
High gradient Aortic Stenosis	Mean gradient $\geq$ 40 mmHg, Vmax $\geq$ 4 m/s, EOA $\leq$ 1cm^2 or indexed EOA $\leq$ 0.6 cm/m^2, LVEF normal OR reduced	This is severe AS, regardless of LVEF or flow (which does not need to be calculated, therefore!)
Low-flow, low-gradient Aortic Stenosis with reduced LVEF	Mean gradient < 40 mmHg, EOA $\leq$ 1cm^2, SVi < 35 ml/min, LVEF < 50%	Low-dose dobutamine stress echo may be used here to distinguish between true severe AS and pseudosevere AS, where the valve area increases to > 1cm2 when flow increases. This can also usefully identify contractile reserve in patients being considered for intervention
Low-flow, low-gradient Aortic Stenosis with preserved LVEF	Mean gradient < 40 mmHg, EOA < 1cm^2, LVEF $\geq$ 50% and SVi $\leq$ 35 ml/m^2	Typical patients are hypertensive women with small, hypertrophied ventricles, although other conditions which reduce forward flow such as severe MS/MR/TR can produce this pattern. After exclusion of measurement errors, further imaging by CT to assess the degree of valvar calcification can be helpful in distinguishing severe from moderate AS
Normal flow, low-gradient Aortic Stenosis with preserved LVEF	Mean gradient < 40 mmHg, EOA < 1cm^2, LVEF > 50% and SVi > 35 ml/m^2	These patients usually have moderate or even mild AS

*Based on ESC/EACTS 2021 Valve guidelines

- *Masses*—either associated with the valve itself or in the LA, causing obstruction to inflow
- *LA size*—in moderate-severe mitral valve lesions, it is almost certain that the LA will be dilated
- *LV size and function*—LV ejection fraction may not be a true guide to underlying intrinsic contractility in mitral regurgitation, so remember to interpret your findings in the context of the degree of MR and utilise strain measurements. Consider measuring forward ejection fraction [10].

General points

When assessing the mitral valve in any context, the most important thing to remember is that it is part of an intricate system consisting of the annulus, leaflets, chords, papillary muscles and left ventricle itself—the LV-mitral complex. Abnormalities of any one of these component parts may result in a valve that does not function normally and directing clinical management down the correct route depends on identifying the mechanism of the dysfunction and which components of the complex are involved. When mitral interventions are not successful, or are not durable, it is often the case (in the author's experience) that there has not been a full appreciation of the entire mechanism of the pathology, such that only one component has been addressed. An example of this is the early failure of mitral ring annuloplasty in the context of ischaemic heart disease—if the base of the inferolateral wall of the LV is fully-infarcted, then there is a significant risk that a ring annuloplasty will not give a durable repair, and replacement may be a better option for these patients [11].

2D and Colour flow Doppler

The parasternal long axis window is an excellent view for assessing leaflet thickening and

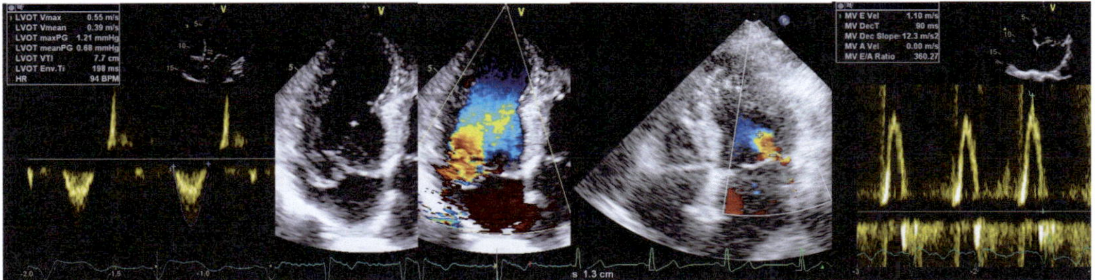

Fig. 6 Doppler assessment of mitral regurgitation (LVOT velocity time integral with PW Doppler, Proximal iso-velocity surface area with colour Doppler and trans-mitral flow using pulsed wave Doppler

mobility. Traditional M-mode through the valve is sometimes omitted nowadays but it remains a very useful high-temporal-resolution method of assessing leaflet motion. Thickened, calcified leaflets, in particular with an immobile posterior leaflet and "hockey-stick" (Video 3) movement of the anterior leaflet is virtually diagnostic of rheumatic mitral valve disease. Any associated thickening and calcification of the chords should be noted. Tethering or restriction of one or both leaflets into the LV can be well-appreciated and it is perhaps the best single view for demonstrating the classical appearance of ischaemic mitral regurgitation due to asymmetrical restriction of the posterior leaflet after and inferolateral myocardial infarction. The anteroseptal myocardium is also well-visualised and increased end-systolic dimensions causing separation of the papillary muscles with consequent tethering of the anterior leaflet by secondary chords may be noted. Tethering of both leaflets is seen in dilated cardiomyopathy (DCM) (Video 4). Asymmetric tethering predominantly affecting the posterior leaflet is typical of ischaemic regional LV dysfunction whereas symmetrical tethering of both leaflets is seen in global LV dilatation and dysfunction. Coaptation length and depth may be measured and tenting area as well as a posterior leaflet angle > 45° predict a higher failure rate after repair for ischaemic MR. A prolapsing leaflet or scallop may be visible but absence of an obvious prolapse in this view does not rule it out. Angling the probe inferiorly will bring in the relatively medial A3/P3 scallops and angling superiorly will bring in the lateral A1/P1 scallops

but these views are not always easy to obtain, especially in the sick or immobile patient. The vena contracta is the width of the mitral regurgitant jet as it emerges into the LA. It correlates well with MR volume but recent advances in technology have revealed that the VC measured from real time 3D TOE is more closely correlated with MR severity. Other important features to note with the colour Doppler include the presence of a zone of flow acceleration. If on the LV side of the mitral valve, its size correlates with the severity of MR and after adjusting the baseline, the radius can be used to measure effective regurgitant orifice area and regurgitant volume by the proximal isovelocity surface area (PISA) equation (Fig. 6). If a zone of flow acceleration is seen on the atrial side of the valve during diastole, this may indicate haemodynamically significant mitral stenosis (Video 5).

It is not always possible to obtain a high-quality in-plane PSAX image through the mitral valve, but it can be invaluable, especially in suspected mitral stenosis. This view shows the mitral orifice through the cardiac cycle and particular features to note include calcification (hyperechoic bright areas) and commissural fusion which reduces the wide, "smiling mouth shape" of the orifice to a restricted "fish-mouth" shape. Planimetry of the mitral valve from the 2D image remains an excellent and highly reproducible method of quantifying mitral stenosis. Congenital abnormalities of the mitral valve such as deep clefts may be spotted in this view, and any prolapse should be noted. Colour Doppler across the valve in the PSAX is particularly useful to precisely locate a regurgitant jet along the coaptation line in cases where a single scallop or commissure is prolapsing or restricted or alternatively to confirm that regurgitation is central or along the entire coaptation line in functional MR due to global LV dilatation resulting in increased papillary muscle separation.

The apical four chamber view gives the sonographer an appreciation of the entire mitral-LV complex, in particular the opportunity to "eyeball" the left ventricle and note global or regional dilatation and abnormalities of contraction. Left ventricular ejection fraction can be measured by biplane, triplane or 3D quantification. Dilatation of the left atrium can also be spotted easily, and the chamber area measured if deemed appropriate—surgeons sometimes ask about LA size if they are contemplating AF surgery at the same time as mitral surgery, but in general it is sufficient to describe the degree of dilatation qualitatively. Leaflet motion should be assessed, and any prolapse, or restriction noted. Wall motion abnormalities affecting the lateral wall (circumflex territory) are often seen along with restriction of the posterior leaflet. The degree of restriction should be noted because severe restriction secondary to ischaemic scarring of the LV myocardium is associated with poorer success rates after mitral annuloplasty. Accurate measurement of the leaflet angle should preferably be done by TOE [12].

The easiest way to screen for new or previously undiagnosed mitral lesions, particularly regurgitation, is by using colour flow Doppler across the valve in the apical four chamber view. The direction of the colour jet may give a clue as to the exact anatomical lesion: a general rule is that an anteriorly-directed jet results from posterior leaflet prolapse *or* anterior leaflet restriction, and a posteriorly-directed jet results from anterior leaflet prolapse *or* posterior leaflet restriction. A central jet suggests that both leaflets are involved equally, for example in the global dilatation that results from dilated cardiomyopathy (DCM) or that the annulus is dilated—or a combination of both. In reality, the mechanism of mitral regurgitation, especially when chronic, can be very complex and subtle, with the interplay between several abnormalities leading to multidirectional jets. As an example, in chronic myxomatous degenerative MR (Barlow's disease), there may be P2 prolapse, one of more ruptured chords, a dilated LA, annular dilatation and LV dilatation, with increased interpapillary muscle distance. These features would likely result in a combination of restricted/tethered and prolapsing scallops, with a regurgitant jet which has both central and anteriorly-directed components. While the subtleties of mechanism of mitral regurgitation are best appreciated by TOE and are invaluable to the cardiac surgeon when planning repair, I mention this here as a caution to the transthoracic sonographer—the mechanism of MR may be more complex than it appears! The *severity* of the MR, on the other hand, can be well-appreciated by transthoracic echocardiography using a combination of colour flow and other Doppler techniques. The caveat to this is that simply "eyeballing" the apparent size of the colour flow MR jet can be misleading and result in overestimation of the degree of MR severity—there should always be some objective CW or PW Doppler measurements to confirm that the physiology is consistent with the suspected lesion severity. In the apical two chamber view, the true anterior wall is shown (as opposed to the anteroseptal myocardium seen in the PLAX view) and also the inferior wall. It is a good view for identifying wall motion abnormalities which lead to ischaemic functional mitral regurgitation, in particular evidence of inferior or inferolateral myocardial infarction. This is virtually identical to the PLAX view and in some patients, particularly those with chronic lung disease, may be easier to obtain.

Colour jet size

Estimation of the area of the colour jet, either in absolute terms or indexed to the LA area is not a reliable method to estimate MR severity. The apparent area of the jet in the LA is highly variable depending on the exact mechanism of the MR and can be particularly misleading if the jet is eccentric. Nevertheless, if the structure of the valve and the LA size are normal (which is itself unusual in severe mitral valve lesions) then a jet are which takes up <10% of the LA area would be considered mild.

Vena Contracta Width

The width of the vena contracta should be measured – this is the smallest and most high-velocity point in the regurgitant jet and is situated at or just on the LA side of the regurgitant orifice. It is independent of flow-rate and dp/dt. A VC width of <3 mm indicates mild MR and >7 mm severe MR. Values from 4 to 6 mm may be measured in moderate or severe MR, hence other measurements must be taken before reaching a conclusion regarding MR severity.

Proximal isovelocity surface area (PISA) method

The PISA method allows the sonographer to calculate the effective regurgitant orifice are (EROA) and volume of mitral regurgitation. The four chamber view is also the most commonly-used view for measuring the proximal isovelocity surface area radius—in order to reduce error and increases reproducibility when measuring the PISA radius, this should be done by zooming in on the colour image showing the PISA shell. The baseline should be reduced until a clear hemi-sphere of yellow aliasing can be identified—usually at a baseline frequency of 38. Other measurements required for the calculation are the Vmax and VTI of the CW Doppler mitral regurgitant signal. Once obtained, measurements may be noted for an offline manual calculation, but most premium systems will perform the calculation automatically.

CW and PW Doppler of the mitral valve

Use of Doppler is essential to assess the severity of mitral lesions, whether qualitatively or semi-quantitatively. The density of the CW trace and whether or not it is holosystolic are reasonable indicators of the severity of MR, for the reason noted.

E wave velocity

In the awake patient (not under general anaes-thesia), the peak velocity of the E wave of the mitral inflow trace measured by PW Doppler at the tips of the mitral leaflets is consistent with severe MR if it is greater than 1.2 m/s. A dominant A wave is not consistent with severe MR.

Pulmonary vein flow reversal.

This is often assumed to be a failsafe method of confirming severe MR by demonstrating very high pressure in the LA during ventricular sys-tole but there are caveats. A complete pulmonary vein flow trace is relatively easy to acquire dur-ing TOE but can be trickier by TTE. Blunting of the systolic velocity or even systolic flow rever-sal may be seen in severe MR. However, any cause of raised LA pressure may lead to blunting of the systolic wave, and a false negative result may be seen if the jet is directed away from the pulmonary veins. Failure to demonstrate systolic blunting or reversal does not absolutely exclude severe MR. Finally, even a small MR jet, if directed right into a pulmonary vein, may blunt the systolic inflow trace, producing a false posi-tive result.

LV dp/dt

Although not a measure of mitral valve func-tion per se, LV dp/dt can be measured from the MR trace and gives additional information about underlying LV contractile function. It is estimated using the time interval during which the velocity of the MR signal rises from 1 to 3 m/s, i.e., the pressure rises from 4 to 36 mmHg—an increase of 32 mmHg. Normal values are ≥ 1200 mmHg/s, mild-moderate impairment 800-1200 mmHg/s, moderate-severe impairment <800 mmHg/s (Fig. 7). it can be seen that these are wide ranges, so the sonographer needs to synthesis all the relevant information before reaching a conclusion. (see also Chap. 18; POCUS assessment of LV systolic function).

Regurgitant index.

The ratio of the mitral inflow VTI: aortic VTI from the PW Doppler signal is a simple index for MR, if >1.4, this indicates severe MR. Another way to appreciate the same information is to calculate the so-called "forward" ejection frac-tion [10] (= Forward stroke volume / LV end-diastolic volume).

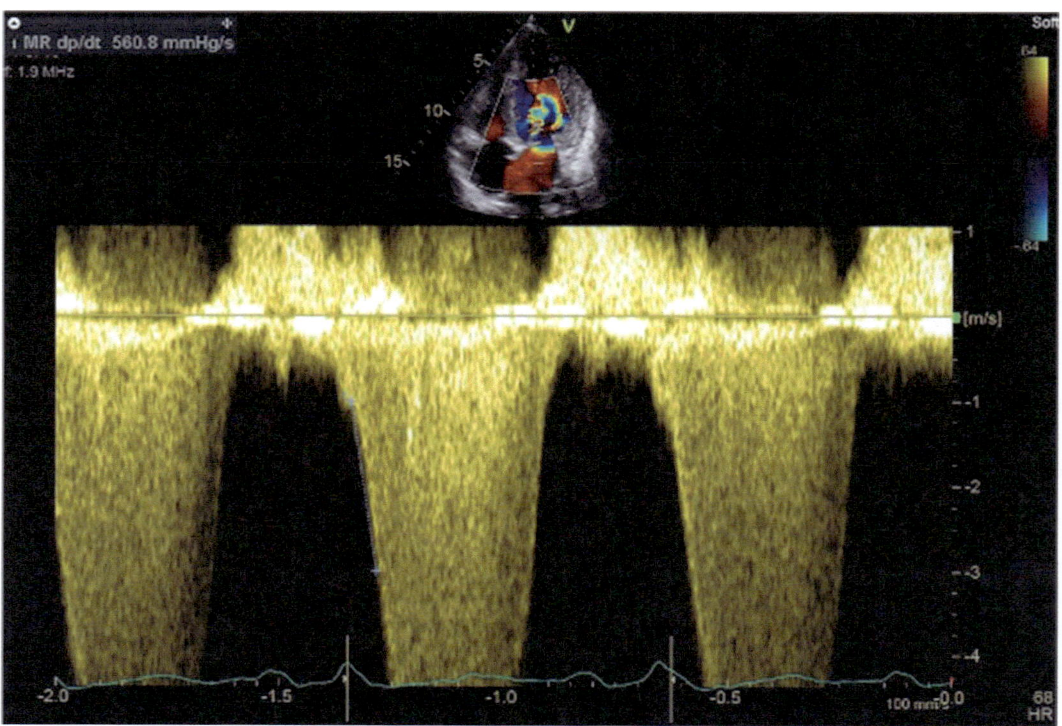

Fig. 7 Estimation of LV dP/dT using continuous wave Doppler envelope of mitral regurgitation as a measure of LV systolic function

Forward pressure gradient.

Peak and mean forward pressure gradients across the mitral valve are obtained by tracing the edge of the CW diastolic inflow trace with the CW cursor through the middle of the mitral valve leaflets. Mean gradient >10 mmHg indicates severe mitral stenosis, 5–10 moderate and <5 mmHg mild. However, as the gradient by echo is derived from *flow*, anything which increases forward flow across the valve such as significant mitral regurgitation, will give an apparently increased pressure gradient, even in the absence of severe MS.

Pressure half-time.

This is measured from the diastolic inflow CW signal and used to calculate the mitral orifice area using the formula MVA = 220/PHT. In certain contexts, pressure half-time may be less reliable.

These include: diastolic dysfunction, aortic regurgitation, after mitral valvuloplasty and in the case of severe mitral calcification. Figure 8 shows an extreme case of severe prosthetic mitral valve stenosis due to a thrombosed mechanical valve.

The Tricuspid valve

Technical Tips

- Use the modified parasternal long axis view to visualise the RV inflow
- Imaging the tricuspid valve in patients with electrodes in the right heart may be challenging because of artefacts
- In patients with a tricky parasternal acoustic window, the subcostal view can be particularly helpful when assessing tricuspid regurgitation

Fig. 8 An extreme case of severe prosthetic mitral valve stenosis due to a thrombosed mechanical valve (assessment using continuous wave Doppler) (Tables 3 and 4)

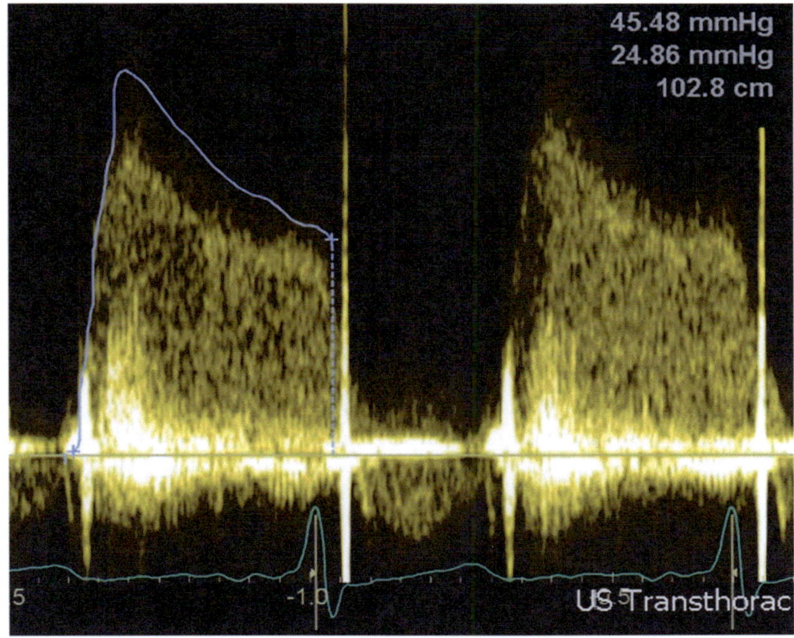

Table 3 Grading criteria for the severity of mitral regurgitation by echocardiography

	Criterion	Mild	Moderate	Severe
Qualitative	Visual assessment by 2D echo	May be no obvious abnormality seen	May or may not be abnormalities such as mild-moderate leaflet tenting, annular dilatation, leaflet degenerative changes	May be obvious flail leaflet or scallop, papillary muscle rupture, coaptation failure, perforation
Semi-quantitative	Vena contracta width (mm)	<3	4–6	≥7
	Jet area as a % of the LA area	<20	variable	> 40
	PISA radius (mm)			
Quantitative	EROA (cm^2)	0.20	0.2–0.39	≥ 0.40
	Regurgitant volume (ml)	<30	30–59	≥ 60
	Regurgitant fraction %	<30	30–49	≥ 50

Table 4 Grading criteria for severity of mitral stenosis by Doppler Echocardiography

	Mild	Moderate	Severe
Valve area (cm^2)	≥ 1.5	1.0–1.4	<1.0
Pressure half-time (ms)	<139	140–219	≥ 220
Mean pressure gradient (mmHg)	<5	6–9	≥ 10

What are you looking out for?

- Congenital abnormalities (Ebstein's anomaly, prolapse)

- Acquired leaflet abnormalities – masses, calcification, thickening, restriction, iatrogenic trauma

- Annular dilatation

- RA dilatation

- Abnormalities of RV size and function

General points.

It is relatively unlikely for emergent presentations in adult patients to result from tricuspid valve pathology, with the exception of *right-sided endocarditis*, which tends to present in intravenous drug-users or in patients with artificial material in the right side of the heart, such as implanted devices or long lines. In the latter case, associated immunosuppression may predispose to infection, particularly in oncology patients. Causes of tricuspid regurgitation, as with mitral regurgitation fall in to two broad categories—primary valve disease and secondary ventricular or atrial aetiology (the latter is often termed "functional" tricuspid regurgitation, as distinct from "degenerative" valve disease.

2D and Colour flow assessment.

As with any valve, the first question for the sonographer is whether the valve appears morphologically normal. Obvious congenital abnormalities of the leaflets should be noted, particularly the apical displacement of the septal leaflet seen in Ebstein's anomaly. Mobile masses may be identified in suspected endocarditis. Dilatation of the tricuspid annulus and RV suggest functional regurgitation due to lack of

coaptation, and this may also be caused by right atrial enlargement in chronic AF. Indeed, the presence of isolated TR in patients without concomitant left-sided heart disease or pulmonary hypertension is being increasingly recognised in the context of longstanding atrial fibrillation and it appears that this may have very significant adverse prognostic implications [11].

Colour flow Doppler

As with the mitral valve, "eyeball" assessment of the degree of TR from the colour flow jet alone may be misleading, although a very wide jet reaching the roof of the RA is more likely to be significant than a narrow jet. However, even semi-quantitative and quantitative criteria are less clear-cut on the right side than the left. Vena contracta width and PISA radius are the two quantitative measures most commonly used.

CW and PW Doppler assessment.

Echo criteria for grading the severity of TR have long been the subject of debate, with recent proposals that there should be a further category of "massive" or "torrential" TR in addition to the usual "mild, moderate and severe" which are the convention for all valves [12]. The rationale for this is increasing evidence that extremely severe TR has incrementally adverse prognostic implications over and above those for severe TR [10]. Identifying these individuals at greater risk may be important in the era of percutaneous valve interventions, when considering possible benefits of treatment. Severity criteria include the density and shape of the CW Doppler trace and the presence of hepatic vein systolic flow reversal or blunting (Table 5). Pulmonary artery systolic pressure (PASP) may be estimated by measuring the pressure drop across the tricuspid valve from the TR CW Doppler signal and adding this to the

Table 5 Grading criteria for severity of tricuspid regurgitation by echocardiography

Criterion	mild	moderate	severe	Torrential*
Qualitative				
Valve morphology by 2D	Normal/abnormal	Normal/abnormal	More often abnormal—coaptation failure, annular dilatation, flail leaflet	Abnormal
TR jet width by colour flow Doppler	Narrow, usually central	variable	Wide central or wall-hugging	Very wide
CW Doppler trace	Faint/incomplete, parabolic	Complete, intermediate density, parabolic	Dense, triangular, early peaking	Dense, triangular, early peaking, peak < 2 m/s
Semi-Quantitative				
Vena contracta width (mm)	Not defined	<7	<14	14–20
PISA radius** (mm)	≤ 5	6–9	≥ 10	–
EROA by PISA (mm^2)	<20	20–39	40–59	≥ 60
Regurgitant volume (ml)				≥ 60
Hepatic vein flow	Systolic dominant	Systolic blunting	Systolic flow reversal	Systolic flow reversal
Inflow Doppler trace	Normal	Normal	E wave dominant > 1 m/s	E wave dominant > 1 m/s
Quantitative**				

* It is now agreed that there should be a revised grading system to include extremely severe degrees of TR—referred to as "massive" and "torrential". The criteria for defining these has been suggested in the literature[15, 16] but is not formally agreed upon at the time of writing

RA pressure estimated from the IVC dimension and inspiratory collapsibility. However, in cases of severe chronic TR where the pressures in the RA and RV have virtually equalized, the TR signal is no longer a reliable method of estimating PASP. The presence of hepatic vein flow reversal has been shown to have a sensitivity of 80% for the presence of severe TR and E wave peak velocity of >1 m/s in the inflow signal is also consistent with severe TR, in the absence of previous annuloplasty surgery (Fig. 9).

Tricuspid Stenosis.

Tricuspid stenosis is relatively rare outside the context of congenital heart disease, but can occur in association with longstanding RV pacing where there have been electrodes in place across the valve for many years. Right-sided valve stenosis is also seen in association with neuroendocrine tumours (carcinoid syndrome), other masses (myxomata, hamartomata, thrombi) and rheumatic heart disease (Table 6). When considering whether significant TS is present, other findings should be taken into account to support the diagnosis. These include whether the RA inferior vena cava (IVC) are dilated.

The Pulmonary Valve

Technical Tips

- The pulmonary valve is the least well-seen by transthoracic echocardiography in the majority of patients with a normal cardiac anatomical arrangement

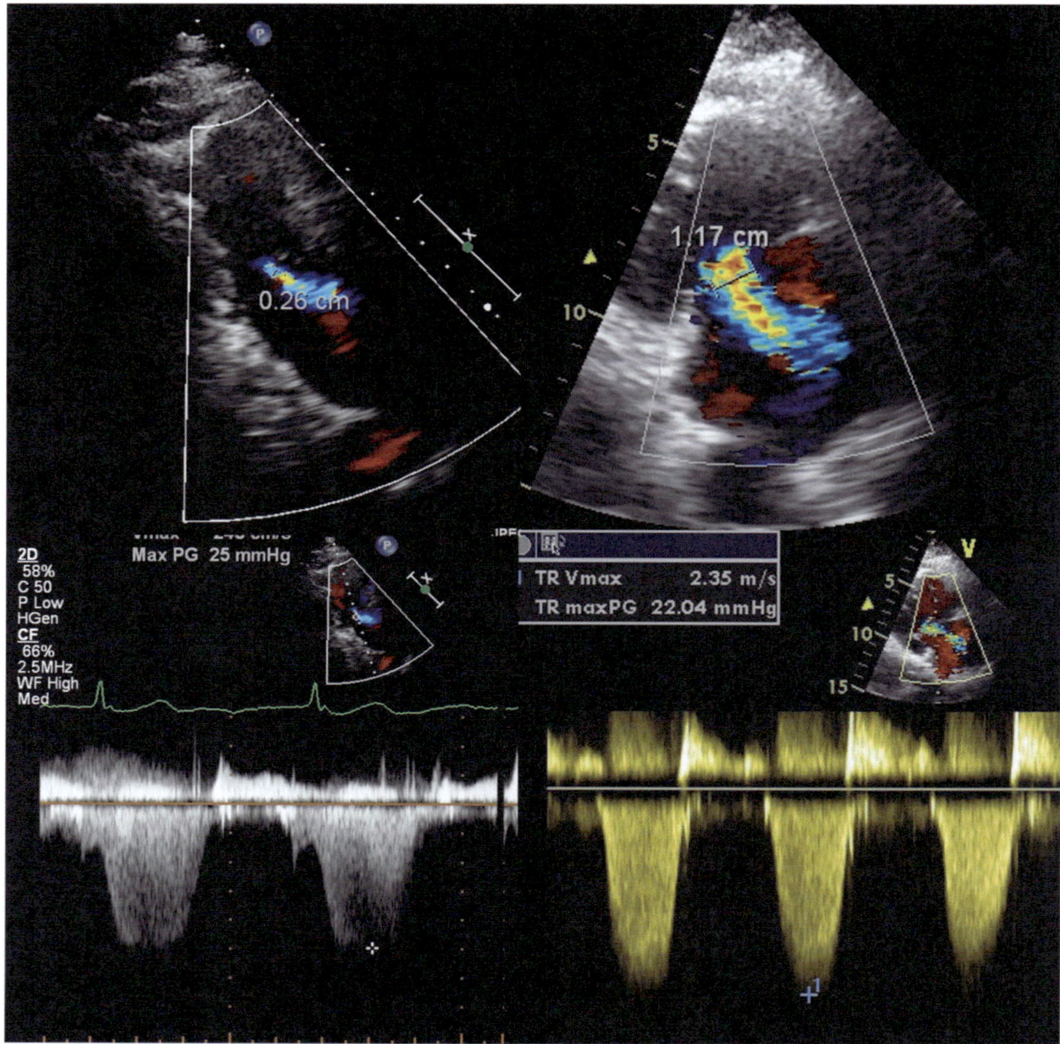

Fig. 9 Estimation of severity of tricuspid regurgitation using colour Doppler and continuous wave Doppler

Table 6 Criteria for diagnosing haemodynamically significant tricuspid stenosis by Echocardiography

Criterion	Threshold for haemodynamic significance*
Mean pressure gradient (mmHg)	≥ 5
Inflow VTI	≥ 60
Pressure half-time $t_{1/2}$ (ms)	≥ 190
Effective orifice area by continuity (cm^2)	≤ 1

* This could also be said to be "severe" tricuspid stenosis, and there are no specific criteria for mild and moderate narrowing

- The usual 2D views for the pulmonary valve are the parasternal RV outflow view (probe tail tilted caudad and rotated towards the left shoulder) and the left parasternal short axis view.
- If possible, ask the patient to turn as far onto their left side as possible –semi-prone—as this causes the pulmonary valve to drop forward close to the anterior chest wall.

What are you looking out for?

- Dilatation of the RVOT/MPA
- Thickening/immobility of the leaflets—if seen in conjunction with tricuspid leaflet thickening and fibrosis, consider carcinoid syndrome
- Masses—if the history is suggestive of infection or malignancy

General Points

The pulmonary valve is the least well-seen by transthoracic echocardiography. Nevertheless, it *can* be visualised to a greater or lesser extent, in the majority of patients. Features of the clinical context should alert the sonographer to the need to pay more attention to the pulmonary valve. These include likelihood of right-sided infective endocarditis (the gonococcus is said to have a predilection for the pulmonary valve, but the usual endocarditis-causing organisms will certainly also affect the pulmonary valve in susceptible individuals) and a history of congenital heart disease. A more unusual cause of pulmonary valve pathology is the presence of a hormone-secreting neuroendocrine tumour, leading to carcinoid syndrome, which causes fibrotic thickening of the leaflets of the right-sided valves. The pulmonary valve eventually becomes completely immobile with mixed stenosis and regurgitation. Patients typically give a clinical history of general malaise, weakness, fevers and weight loss, often accompanied by gastrointestinal symptoms.

Some patients may be noted to have an inappropriate affect, with a strangely elevated mood, despite their obvious ill-health.

2D and colour flow Doppler assessment.

The pulmonary valve has thin, delicate leaflets which are often difficult to visualise clearly. The normal valve is trivially-mildly regurgitant in up to 80% of subjects, whilst acquired moderate or severe PR is usually found in association with pulmonary hypertension and a dilated pulmonary artery. The lower pressure on the right side means that it can be particularly difficult to distinguish moderate from mild PR based on colour flow Doppler alone, but in general the width of the colour jet and the degree of aliasing are reasonable guides. It is generally accepted that if the colour flow Doppler appears normal by eye (i.e., laminar forward flow and trivial/mild regurgitation) then formal CW/PW Doppler assessment is not necessary unless the clinical context suggests a high likelihood of pulmonary pathology (see above).

CW and PW Doppler assessment.

RVOT VTI.

The RVOT VTI, measured by placing a PW Doppler sample volume just below the pulmonary annulus in the RVOT, can be useful to assess cardiac output/cardiac index in any patient but may be especially useful in those patients with a mechanically-supported left ventricle (e.g., left ventricular assist device).

Pulmonary acceleration time.

This is the time interval between the onset of pulmonary flow/pulmonary ejection and peak flow and should more accurately be referred to as RVOT acceleration time because it is measured by placing the PW cursor on the RVOT side of the pulmonary valve or just at the annulus in the parasternal short axis view through the aortic

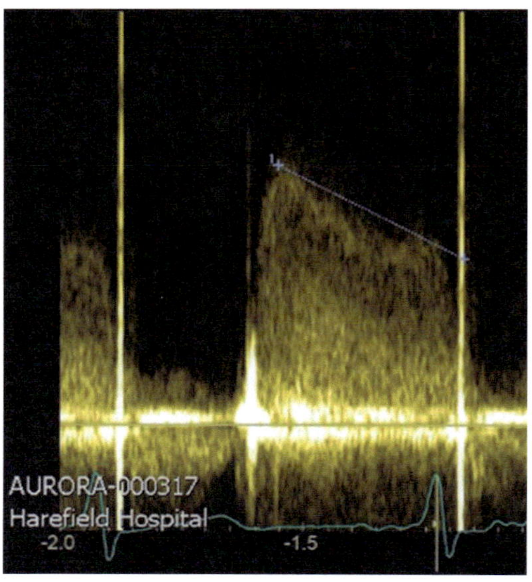

Fig. 10 Estimation of severity of pulmonary regurgitation using continuous wave Doppler

valve. A time of >140 ms is normal, and a time of <105 ms is suggestive (but by no means diagnostic of) pulmonary hypertension. It can be useful as a confirmatory finding. (see also Chap. 19: POCUS assessment of RV and pulmonary hypertension).

Pulmonary regurgitation trace

The regurgitant trace may be used to estimate pulmonary artery end-diastolic pressure, by applying the modified Bernoulli equation to the end-diastolic velocity of the regurgitant signal, whether normal (physiological) or pathological (Fig. 10 and Table 7).

Pulmonary stenosis

This is rarely diagnosed outside the context of congenital heart disease, but occasionally presents in patients with a neuroendocrine tumour. Grading criteria are shown in Table 8 below.

Table 7 Grading criteria for pulmonary regurgitation by echocardiography

	Criterion*	Mild	Moderate	Severe
Qualitative	Valve morphology	Normal	Variable	Abnormal (eg mass, prolapse, thickening)
	Width of PR jet on colour flow Doppler (mm)	<10–neck also narrow	Variable	≥ 11
	Qualities of Doppler trace	Faint or incomplete; slow deceleration	Variable but usually complete	Dense, steep, rapid deceleration

* Semi-quantitative and quantitative criteria such as EROA and vena contracta width are not fully defined for PR, however, increased pulmonary flow compared to aortic forward flow is a feature of significant pulmonary regurgitation and should be assessed

Table 8 Grading criteria for severity of pulmonary stenosis by echocardiography

	Mild	Moderate	Severe
Appearance*	Mild thickening and increased echogenicity of leaflets, possible doming or mild restriction of motion	Abnormal leaflet thickness, morphology and/or motion	Increased thickening or calcification, obviously restricted leaflet motion
Peak pressure gradient	<36 mmHg	36–63 mmHg	≥ 64 mmHg
Peak velocity (V_{max})	<3 m/s	3-4 m/s	>4 m/s
Valve area	–	–	$<1 cm^2$

* The pulmonary valve is not always easy to see by 2D echocardiography so the Doppler measurements are more reliable than the appearance

Recommended Reading

Vahanian A, Beyersdorf F, Praz F, Milojevic M, Baldus S, Bauersachs J et al. on behalf of the Task Force for the management of valvular heart disease of the European Society of Cardiology (ESC) and the European Association for Cardio-Thoracic Surgery (EACTS). 2021 ESC/EACST Guidelines for the management of Valvular Heart Disease Eur Heart J 2021; 00: 21–72.

References

1. Draper J, Subbiah S, Bailey R, Chambers JB. Murmur clinic: validation of a new model for detecting heart valve disease. Heart. 2019;105:56–9.
2. Huntington K, Hunter AGW, Chan K-L. A prospective study to assess the frequency of familial clustering of congenital bicuspid aortic valve. J Am Coll Cardiol. 1997;30(7):1809–12.
3. Zakkar M, Bryan AJ, Angelini GD. Aortic stenosis: diagnosis and management. BMJ. 2016;355:i5425.
4. Wong P, Cotter L, Gibson DG. Early systolic closure of the aortic valve. Br Heart J. 1980;44:386–9.
5. Sievers H-H, Schmidtke A. Classification system for he bicuspid aortic valve from 304 surgical specimens. J Thorac Cardiovasc Surg. 2007;133 (5):1226–33.
6. Paterick TE, Humphries JA, Afzal Ammar K, et al. Aortopathies: etiologies, genetics, differential diagnosis, prognosis and management. Am J Med. 2013;126(8):670–8.
7. Tolis G, Sundt TM. Contemporary insights into the management of type A aortic dissection. Expert Rev Cardiovasc Ther. 2016;14(10):1189–96.
8. Tribouilloy C, Avinee P, Shen WF, Rey JL, Slama M. Lesbre JP End diastolic flow velocityjust-beneath the aortic isthmus assessed by pulsed Doppler echocardiography: a new predictor of the aortic regurgitant fraction. Heart. 1991;65:37–40.
9. Caruso F, Ventura L, Viliani D, Della Sala SW. Massive mitral annula calcification mimicking intraardiac mass: multimodality approach to diagnosis. Radiol Case Rep. 2018;13(2):376–9
10. Dupuis M, Mahjoub H, Clavel M-A, et al. Forward left ventricular ejection fraction: a simple risk marker in patients with primary mitral regurgitation. J Am Heart Assoc. 2017;6:e006309.
11. Kongsaerepong V, Shiota M, Gillinov AM, et al. Evchocardiographic predictors of successful versus unsuccessful mitral valve repair in ischemic mitral regurgitation. Am J Cardiol. 2006;98(4):504–8.
12. Poelaert JI, Bouchez S. Perioperative echocardiographic assessment of mitral vale regurgitation: a comprehensive review. Eur J Cardiothor Surg. 2021;50(5):801–12.
13. Dietze MK, Goedemans L, Mai Vo N, Prihadi EA, Van der Bijl P, Gersh BJ. Prognostic Implications of significant tricuspid regurgitation in patients with atrial fibrillation without left-sided heart disease or pulmonary hypertension. Am J Cardiol. 2020;135:84–90
14. Go YY, Dulgheru R, Lancellotti P. The conundrum of tricuspid regurgitation grading. Front Cardiovasc Med. 2018;5:164
15. Kebed K, Addetia K, Henry M, Yamat M, Weinert L, Besser SA, et al Refining severe tricuspid regurgitation definition by echocardiography with a new outcomes based "Massive" grade. J Am Soc Echocardiogr. 2020;33(9):1087–94

POCUS in Monitoring: Echocardiography After Cardiac Surgery

Nicholas J. Lees and Ana I. Hurtado-Doce

Fundamental progress requires the reinterpretation of basic ideas.
Alfred North Whitehead. English Mathematician and Philosopher (1861–1947 AD)

Abstract

Patients after cardiac surgery require careful monitoring and both transthoracic (TTE) and transesophageal echocardiography (TOE) help during the daily assessment, guiding interventions, identifying complications and influencing decision-making at 'point of care'. Competence in echocardiography is an important skill for physicians involved in the care of these patients. Common complications as cardiac tamponade or ventricular failure are easily diagnosed and appropriate treatment can be promptly initiated, resulting in better outcome of our patients. This chapter will cover the use of echocardiography in the assessment and management of patients after cardiac surgery including those requiring mechanical circulatory support.

Keywords

Echocardiography · Cardiac surgery · Acute heart failure · Tamponade · Shock

Key Messages

- TTE and TOE are essential imaging modalities in postoperative cardiac surgical patients. Focused scans are often performed at point of care but performing comprehensive scans where possible with appropriate quantification is important.
- There are a variety of processes leading to haemodynamic instability in postoperative cardiac patients such as tamponade and acute heart failure in which Echocardiography can help in the diagnosis and management.
- Echocardiography is also an important monitoring device. cardiac output and other flow measurements can be estimated. This is particularly useful during dynamic assessments such as titrating inotropic drugs or weaning mechanical circulatory support.

N. J. Lees (✉) · A. I. Hurtado-Doce
Department of Anaesthetics and Intensive Care,
Harefield Hospital, London, UK
e-mail: n.lees@rbht.nhs.uk

A. I. Hurtado-Doce
e-mail: a.hurtadodoce@rbht.nhs.uk

N. J. Lees · A. I. Hurtado-Doce
Royal Brompton and Harefield Hospitals, London,
UK

© The Author(s), under exclusive license to Springer Nature Switzerland AG 2023
H. Soliman-Aboumarie et al. (eds.), *Cardiopulmonary Point of Care Ultrasound*,
https://doi.org/10.1007/978-3-031-29472-3_21

Introduction

Echocardiography is an essential part of a modern cardiac surgical patient's management and is utilised throughout the entire perioperative journey. Preoperatively it functions as an investigation to help diagnose heart disease, to quantify severity and to stratify risk. Intraoperatively, transoesophageal echocardiography (TOE) is used to guide the surgical repair, to help with haemodynamic management and as a dynamic tool in assessing response to interventions. This chapter will cover its use postoperatively, typically when the patient has arrived in the intensive care unit (ICU) or cardiac recovery unit.

TTE or TOE, indications and safety

The use of echocardiography is increasing rapidly in hospital medicine, in part due to improvement in machine technology, portability and improved accessibility—it is no longer limited to cardiology outpatients but now commonplace in emergency rooms, ICUs and operating theatres. Together with the advent of more training opportunities and accreditation in focused and critical care echocardiography it means that there are more appropriately trained staff available who can perform scans.

Transthoracic echocardiography (TTE) and transoesophageal echocardiography (TOE) are both used postoperatively in the care of the cardiac surgical patient. TTE is more convenient as it is minimally invasive and quick to perform. TTE is the first choice in most situations and usually useful images can be obtained despite limitations such as surgical dressings and drains, small pneumothoraces or artefacts due to mechanical ventilation. TOE is invasive and requires additional expertise in safe handling of the probe but overcomes these issues usually giving clearer images and has additional benefits in its closer proximity to the valves, atria and descending aorta. The potential for harm must be considered when inserting and operating the probe, particularly in anticoagulated or frail patients, during prolonged scans and with frequent probe insertions. Although generally safe, injury and bleeding related to the lips, oral cavity (hard and soft palate, teeth, tongue), oropharynx, laryngopharynx, oesophagus or stomach is easily caused. Morbidity related to TEE ranges from 0.2 to 1.2% and mortality (usually following oesophageal perforation) is often quoted as <0.01% [1].

Reasons for Performing Scans

Echocardiography is performed after surgery for several reasons. Firstly, as an imaging modality it allows rapid bedside diagnosis of a variety of pathophysiological conditions to which, once treatment has started, response to therapies can be assessed. The most common reason for performing a scan postoperatively is to assess haemodynamic instability, although it is also used to track progress and improvement, for example in patients recovering from cardiogenic shock or acute heart failure. Very often it is the images from the scans that provide the primary diagnosis, such as aortic dissections, mitral valve prolapse, pericardial collections and endocarditis; but more often echocardiography is used to complement clinical examination by providing additional information in the management of left and right ventricular failure for example. Echocardiography may be used as a monitoring device alongside vital signs measurements to provide information about cardiac function and various flow measurements and especially as a tool used during dynamic assessments such as fluid boluses, and inotrope or vasoactive drug titration. Echocardiography is used to ensure safe and accurate placement and positioning of invasive catheters and cannulas such as extracorporeal membrane oxygenation (ECMO) cannulas, intra-aortic balloon pumps and other mechanical circulatory support devices. Echocardiography is also used increasingly to scan the lungs and pleural spaces to demonstrate a number of pathologies which in conjunction with information from the heart scan can provide the clinician with important information which can guide management. Lung ultrasound is discussed in detail elsewhere.

Acute Heart failure After Cardiac Surgery

Acute heart failure (AHF) occurs perioperatively in more than 20% of cardiac surgical patients [2]. Severity varies from acute 'stunning' of the heart, which resolves in time with supportive care and inotropic support and is usually associated with good outcomes and seen in 45% of elective patients in one series [3], to cardiogenic shock which in the same study was seen in 67% of emergency patients. Risk factors for developing AHF perioperatively are unstable coronary syndromes, decompensated chronic HF, significant arrhythmias, valvular disease, cerebrovascular disease, diabetes mellitus, renal insufficiency and high-risk surgery. Echocardiography should be used to detect signs of cardiovascular dysfunction early and to understand the causes of AHF which can then guide appropriate management.

There are several processes leading to either haemodynamic compromise or deranged physiology commonly seen in postoperative cardiac surgery patients readily amenable to echocardiography evaluation which are summarised in Table 1, these will be covered in more detail below.

Table 1 Causes of haemodynamic instability and the echocardiography findings in postoperative cardiac surgical patients

Cause of instability	Echocardiography findings
Left ventricular failure/cardiogenic shock	Systolic impairment
	Regional wall motion abnormalities (RWMAs)
	Mitral regurgitation (MR)
	Diastolic impairment
Right ventricular failure	Systolic impairment
	Dilatation
	Tricuspid regurgitation
	Small 'underfilled' LV cavity, often good LV function
	Ventricular septal defect (as a cause)
Valves	Regurgitation/paravalvular leak/restriction related to surgical repair or injury
	Systolic anterior motion (SAM) of mitral valve
Aorta	Dissection
Pericardium: tamponade (obstructive shock)	Effusions/collections. POCUS features of tamponade. Dilated IVC
Lungs	Atelectasis, interstitial-alveolar oedema, pneumonia
Pleural space	Effusions/collections, pneumothorax
Hypovolaemic/haemorrhagic shock	Small RV
	Hyperkinetic LV, small end systolic area
	Small/collapsible inferior vena cava (IVC)
Distributive shock (sepsis/vasoplegia)	Hyperkinetic LV (usually, although septic cardiomyopathy may be present)
	Small collapsible IVC
Pulmonary embolism (obstructive shock)	RV dilatation and impairment, pulmonary hypertension, presence of thrombus
Cardiac arrest	To confirm asystole/pulseless electrical activity
	To diagnose potentially reversible causes i.e., tamponade, hypovolaemia, pulmonary embolism

Focused Versus Comprehensive Echocardiography in Postoperative Patients

Many of the causes of haemodynamic instability are suitable to 'point of care' or 'focused' scanning techniques and protocols. The emergency setting may be such that a comprehensive scan is too time consuming and in fact unnecessary when what is needed under time-pressure is a binary (yes/no) answer, such as presence or absence of collection, normal or poor ventricular function without detailed quantification. The term 'FoCUS' has been used to define this method of cardiac ultrasound scan, performed according to standardised but restricted scanning protocols to add information to the clinical assessment, by an operator not necessarily fully trained in echocardiography but appropriately trained in FoCUS, who is at the same time usually responsible for immediate decision-making based on the findings [4]. There are a variety of different FoCUS techniques promoted by different organisations, some of which offer accreditation, but most follow similar protocols. The main concerns relate to inadequate training and not performing a comprehensive echocardiography examination, i.e., potentially missing pathology or making decisions based on misdiagnosis and inaccurate assumptions. Caution also applies to the experienced sonographer when performing a focused and limited scan, as to not miss other potential pathology (e.g., pleural collections, aortic dissection) which may not be immediately apparent. The scope of POCUS expands beyond focused basic scanning to focused advanced assessment to allow answering questions at the bedside in a short time.

Common Conditions in Postoperative Cardiac Surgical Patients Readily Evaluated by Echocardiography

Tamponade

Pericardial collections after cardiac surgery are common. Pericardial, mediastinal and pleural drains are placed at the time of surgery to prevent collections of blood. In the absence of a functioning drain, blood may accumulate in the intrapericardial space. Without intervention, this can give rise to the clinical condition of cardiac tamponade. A rapid increase of only a relatively small volume of fluid in the pericardial space may lead to this condition, whereas slow (subacute or chronic) accumulation of effusions as seen in patients with chronic heart failure may not cause instability because over time the pericardium stretches and becomes more compliant. Whether or not an accumulation of intrapericardial fluid becomes haemodynamically significant depends on the pressure–volume relationships between the pericardium and the cardiac chambers. With increasing volumes of fluid, the increased intrapericardial pressures eventually exceed the end-diastolic pressures within the cardiac chambers and reduce diastolic filling. This will reduce stroke volume and therefore cardiac output [5]. The clinical signs described are tachycardia, hypotension, muffled heart sounds, pulsus paradoxus, a rising right atrial (central venous) pressure and oliguria. Electrocardiogram (ECG) may show reduced voltages on ECG. CXR may show an enlarged cardiac silhouette, or a new opacity round the heart. Often a worsening base deficit or rising serum lactate is seen on blood gas analysis. Patients are often bleeding so emergency surgery, anticoagulation/coagulopathy and complex operations are risk factors. Very often not all these features are present, so performing a TTE or TOE examination is essential. TTE is a Class 1, Level C recommendation for all patients suspected of having a pericardial effusion [6].

The presence of a circumferential pericardial effusion is usually easily confirmed with TTE or TOE. Loculated effusions may be less obvious, and TOE is usually more diagnostic. Isolated left and right atrial tamponade following cardiac surgery is well-recognised and this may be caused by only small collections of blood. In the case of postoperative bleeding, the collection may be mixture of liquid blood and organised clot, which may be recognised by seeing heterogenous and irregular echo-dense areas around the heart. By

Table 2 Classical echocardiography findings in cardiac tamponade

2D findings

- Early diastolic collapse of the right ventricular free wall
- Late diastolic compression or collapse of the right atrium
- Swinging of the heart in the pericardial sac (with large circumferential collections)
- Dilated inferior vena cava with minimal or no collapse with inspiration
- Septal bounce into the left ventricle during inspiration

Doppler findings

- 40% relative inspiratory augmentation of blood flow across the tricuspid valve
- 25% relative decrease in inspiratory flow across the mitral valve
- Inspiratory decrease and expiratory increase in pulmonary vein diastolic forward flow
- Respiratory variation in aortic outflow velocity (echocardiographic pulsus paradoxus)

measuring the effusion in two dimensions (2D), size may be semi-quantitively assessed as being mild (<10 mm), moderate (10–20 mm) or large (>20 mm). Tamponade remains a clinical diagnosis, but echocardiographic confirmation comes down to demonstrating evidence of impaired chamber filling and certain changes with respiration, in the presence of a collection. Respiratory variation in transmitral flow is pronounced during standard positive pressure mechanical ventilation, decreases in the presence of pericardial effusion, and becomes almost non-existent when cardiac tamponade is present [7]. The 'classic' echocardiography features of tamponade are listed below in Table 2. It is very important however to appreciate that many of these signs are not seen, or only seen with large volume effusions and a pericardial collection may still be haemodynamically significant and affect the patient in an adverse way, even if it does not meet these 'tamponade criteria'. In one series, TTE failed to identify any pericardial collection in 60% of patients presenting in the first 72 h following surgery and moreover, the classical POCUS features of tamponade were absent in 79%. At re-exploration, the volumes found in patients presenting within 72 h were <200 ml in 85% of cases [8]. It is the author's recommendation to strongly consider reopening a patient with a pericardial collection and haemodynamic compromise, even if these classical echo findings are not present.

Left Ventricular Assessment and Dysfunction

Left ventricular (LV) function analysis is a common reason for performing an echocardiographic study postoperatively. An assessment of LV systolic function gives a visual indication of myocardial performance. This is often performed semi-quantitatively without measurements ('eye-balling') which in experienced users usually correlates well with formal quantitative measurements. A systematic approach will start with measurements of LV size in end-diastole and end-systole, then assessments of LV global function, regional function and diastolic function. Lang et al. [9] global function measurements include ejection fraction, fractional area change and fractional shortening. Ejection fraction (EF), which refers to the relative change in LV volume in systole and diastole, is the most commonly quoted measurement in clinical practice and this should be taken in accordance with recommended guidelines i.e., using Simpson's biplane method, although modern machines with 3D or speckle tracking can calculate this automatically.

Speckle tracking technology allows measurement of strain of the myocardial fibres and Global longitudinal strain (GLS) is a validated assessment of systolic function [10]. The normal value is $-20 \pm 2\%$ with more negative values indicative of better systolic function. EF has been shown to suffer from significant intra- and interobserver variability and GLS has been shown to be a more reproducible method of evaluating LV function regardless of level of echocardiography training [11]. Furthermore it has been shown that patients may have a normal EF but reduced LV systolic function as demonstrated by reduced GLS, as GLS detects subtle longitudinal abnormalities that do not affect EF globally. EF tends to remain normal in a small LV with a thick wall, yet these ventricles will often show reductions in both longitudinal and circumferential shortening when strain analysis is performed. Other patients in whom a normal EF may be seen but with reduced GLS are those with diastolic dysfunction, coronary artery disease, diabetes mellitus, hypertensive heart disease, hypertrophic obstructive cardiomyopathy and electrical disease, which reduces the usefulness of EF as a reliable measurement of systolic function in these groups and support the use of strain as an alternative [12]. However, the evaluation of GLS remains limited in everyday POCUS practice as it is not yet available on most handheld and portable machines.

It is important to recognise the limitations of EF and other methods of LV function assessment, in particular the presence of regional wall motion abnormalities (RWMAs), measurement error due to lack of clarity of the blood/ myocardial border or foreshortening. EF can be normal in the presence of impaired LV systolic function, since it does not reflect intrinsic myocardial contractility. In addition, EF is highly load-dependent such that LV function may be overestimated in the presence of mitral regurgitation or ventricular septal defect. In these situations where the LV is unloaded, LV function should be assessed using additional methods such as dP/dT and caution applied when deciding that function is adequate. Another situation to bear in mind is the effect of inotropic drugs. An EF >55% may be indicative of 'good' function but if the patient is receiving high doses of inotropic agents to achieve this then this is clearly a different situation to a patient with the same EF but not needing support and this should be noted in the POCUS report.

Regional function is important to look at next. The standard 17-segment model should be used [13] and the relative thickening of each segment assessed. This is done using 2D echocardiography and examining the three-standard apical TTE views (or mid-oesophageal four chamber, two chamber and long-axis views in the case of TOE) of the LV where all 17 segments will be visualised. Longitudinal strain is another way of identifying RWMAs and may make it easier to discern them. New RWMAs may be indicative of regional ischaemia which may result from obstructed coronary artery bypass grafts (mechanical kinking, air, debris or acute thrombosis) or disruption/ obstruction of a native coronary artery (e.g., during aortic valve or root surgery). It is very common to see paradoxical septal wall movement (systolic movement toward the right ventricle despite normal thickening) after even uncomplicated cardiac surgery. The aetiology is likely to be multifactorial and theories include altered mobility of the heart after incision of the pericardium, damage to the interventricular septum during surgery and ischaemia. It is most likely to be associated with valve surgery rather than coronary artery bypass surgery and the use of cardiopulmonary bypass (CPB), especially prolonged [14].

Other causes of RWMAs are left bundle branch block, epicardial pacing and dilatation of the RV due to volume or pressure overload causing a bowing of the interventricular septum (Table 3).

Diastolic Dysfunction

Diastolic dysfunction (DD) leads to increased filling pressures (left atrial and left ventricular end diastolic pressures), reduced cardiac output and pulmonary venous congestion and may be a cause of heart failure or pulmonary oedema. It is commonly seen in cardiac surgical patients (>40%) and is an important cause of poor outcomes. Patients with more severe DD have been shown to have more difficulties separating from CPB, higher creatinine levels and rates of prolonged

Table 3 Evaluation of the left ventricle

Assessment	Notes	Normal values
1: Systolic function assessment		
Global 'Eyeballing'	Qualitative, risks interobserver variability	EF Normal ♂ >52% ♀ >54%
Ejection fraction	Change in volume EF = EDV-ESV / EDV × 100% Avoid foreshortening. May be hard to see endocardial borders accurately	Mildly impaired 41–51%♂/53♀% Moderately impaired 30–40% Severely impaired <30%
Fractional area change	Change in area *in just one plane* FAC = EDA-ESA / EDA × 100% Not recommended in guidelines preload and afterload-dependent Caution with RWMAs	>35%
Fractional shortening	Change in length *in just one plane* FS = EDD-ESD / EDD × 100% caution with RWMAs preload and afterload dependent	28–44%
Global longitudinal strain	Angle independent, technology-dependent (speckle-tracking)	Peak of −20%
dP/dT	Not so affected by preload/afterload Need good MR Doppler trace	>1200 mmHg/s
Regional	Use 16 or 17 (16 plus apical cap) segment models. Visual assessment most commonly used. Can also use speckle tracking and tissue Doppler	Report: normal/hyperdynamic, hypokinetic, akinetic, dyskinetic
2: Diastolic function assessment		
Transmitral	E, A waves (Pulse wave Doppler)	Diastolic dysfunction present if:
Pulmonary veins	S, D, A waves (Pulse wave Doppler)	
Tissue Doppler	E' (Tissue Doppler) Inaccurate in presence of RWMA/mitral surgery/pericardial disease	Septal E' <7 Lateral E' <10 Average E/E' >14
LA volume		LA volume index >34 ml/m2
Tricuspid regurgitation velocity		TR velocity >2.8 m/s
3: Combined systolic and diastolic function assessment		
Myocardial performance (Tei) index	IVCT + IVRT/ET	Normal < 0.39–0.44

EDV end-diastolic volume, ESV end-systolic volume, EDA end diastolic area, ESA end-systolic area, EDD end-diastolic dimension, ESD end-systolic dimension, IVCT isovolumic contraction time, IVRT isovolumic relaxation time, ET ejection time mechanical ventilation post-operatively, longer hospital length of stay, and higher rates of in hospital mortality independent of systolic function [15]. The new development or worsening of DD after CPB is likely a consequence of the ischaemia–reperfusion injury. New or worsened DD was found to be a significant predictor of postoperative atrial fibrillation [16].

The recommended echocardiographic assessment of LV diastolic function includes Doppler measurements of mitral flow velocities, pulmonary vein velocities, mitral annular e' velocity, E/e' ratio, the peak velocity of the tricuspid regurgitation (TR) jet; and the size/volume of the left atrium [17].

Cardiac Output Assessment

Cardiac output can be estimated by echocardiography using Doppler techniques. Using the principle of the continuity equation and measuring the velocity time integral (VTI) of the LV outflow tract (LVOT) and the dimensions of the LVOT, stroke volume is established (Fig. 1). This often correlates with measurements from the pulmonary artery catheter (PAC), but echocardiography is not interchangeable with this and is better used for tracking trends [18]. It is common to use the VTI alone as a surrogate of cardiac output. Indeed, this may be a more accurate technique as it negates the need to incorporate the area of the LVOT, which is prone to measurement error due to its elliptic shape and then potentially increasing the error by squaring of the radius.

It is especially useful to measure the VTI during dynamic changes, such as initiation of inotropic agents or fluid boluses. LVOT (or aortic) VTI is often incorporated as part of the echo assessment when weaning patients from mechanical circulatory support such as venoarterial (VA) ECMO, typically with a value of 10 cm or greater associated with more success [19] (Fig. 2).

Right Ventricular Failure

Right ventricular (RV) failure is an important cause of morbidity and mortality for haemodynamic instability postoperatively particularly after complex surgery, valvular surgery, congenital surgery, heart transplantation and left ventricular assist device surgery. The presence of RV failure after CPB is associated with a mortality rate ranging from 44 to 86% [20]. Causes can be divided into factors affecting preload (e.g., excess volume), contractility (e.g., ischaemia/reperfusion injury, intra-coronary air and post-surgical stunning) and afterload (increases in pulmonary vascular resistance) [21] (Fig. 3).

Methods of Assessment

Assessment with echocardiography can help identify RV failure and sometimes give the aetiology (e.g., presence of large interatrial or interventricular shunts, anomalous pulmonary veins or thrombus causing pulmonary embolism). The development of tricuspid regurgitation is usually a consequence rather than a cause of RV impairment, developing as the failing RV dilates and leads to annular dilatation. Current guidelines for RV function analysis involves assessment of size and function using a variety of methods (Table 4), also see [22].

Stroke Volume (SV)=LVOT VTI × Cross sectional area of the LVOT

Cardiac output=SV x heart rate

Cardiac index= CO/ body surface area (normal >2.2L/min/m^2)

Fig. 1 Estimating cardiac output with echocardiography

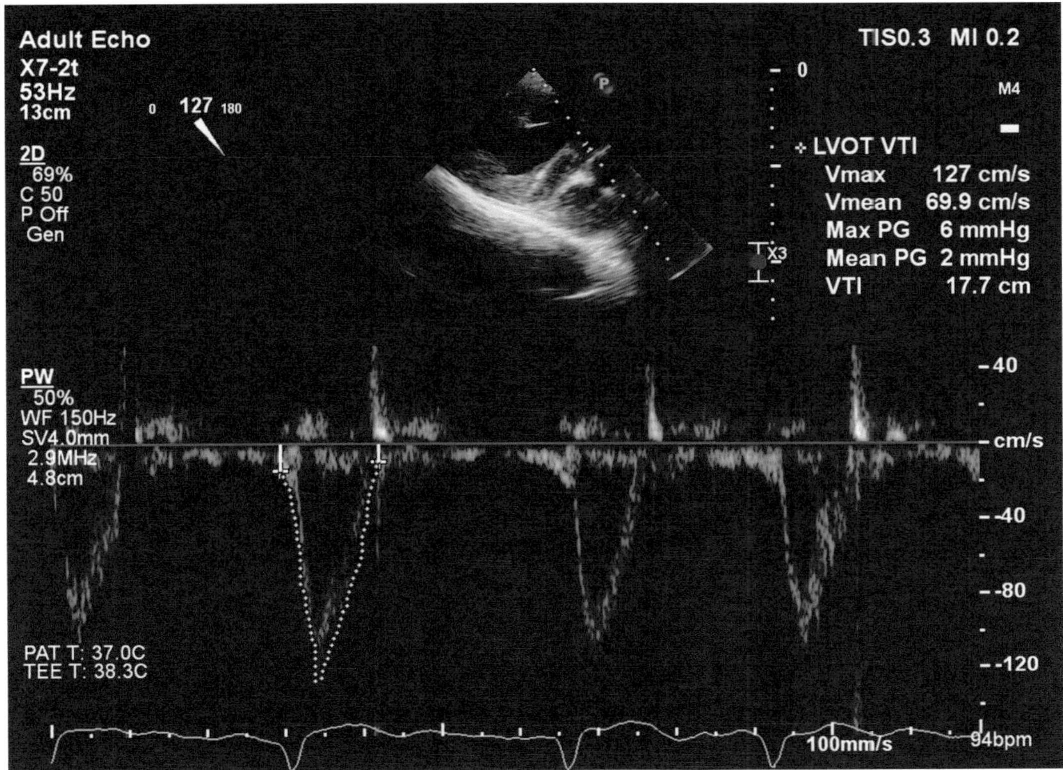

Fig. 2 LVOT VTI measured from TOE in a patient weaning from VA ECMO. The extracorporeal blood flow has been reduced from 4 to 2 L/min, demonstrating a favourable VTI of 17.7 cm. This equates to a stroke volume of 56 ml, cardiac output of 5 L/min and cardiac index of 2.5 (assuming LVOT diameter of 2 cm, heart rate of 90 and body surface area of 2 m^2)

The usual approach to POCUS assessment of the RV starts with 'eyeballing'. Signs of RV failure will be dilatation and reduced systolic motion or contractility. Fractional area change is a method of assessing RV function (the difference between the traced area of the RV in diastole and systole, divided by diastolic area, expressed as a percentage). Owing to its irregular shape, the RV is harder to quantify than the LV using methods where the endocardial borders are traced, but newer 3D methods are better able to track the complex geometry and entire surface of the RV over a number of cardiac cycles, therefore overcoming these limitations and allowing evaluation of the volume, function and provide an accurate EF. Good correlation has been shown with cardiac magnetic resonance imaging (cMRI) [22].

In the normal RV, longitudinal contraction contributes more to overall RV function than transverse shortening with longitudinal shortening accounting for almost 80% of overall RV function [23]. Tricuspid annular plane systolic evaluation (TAPSE) is easy to measure and reproducible and is a useful index of RV systolic function, although it is only a measure of longitudinal function. After cardiac surgery and in particular pericardiotomy and cardiopulmonary bypass (CPB), the RV changes its contractility pattern with a decrease in longitudinal shortening and an increase in transverse shortening which weakens the correlation between TAPSE and RV function [24]. A reduced TAPSE has been shown to persist some months after cardiac surgery despite no clinical signs of RV impairment so this should be appreciated when comparing

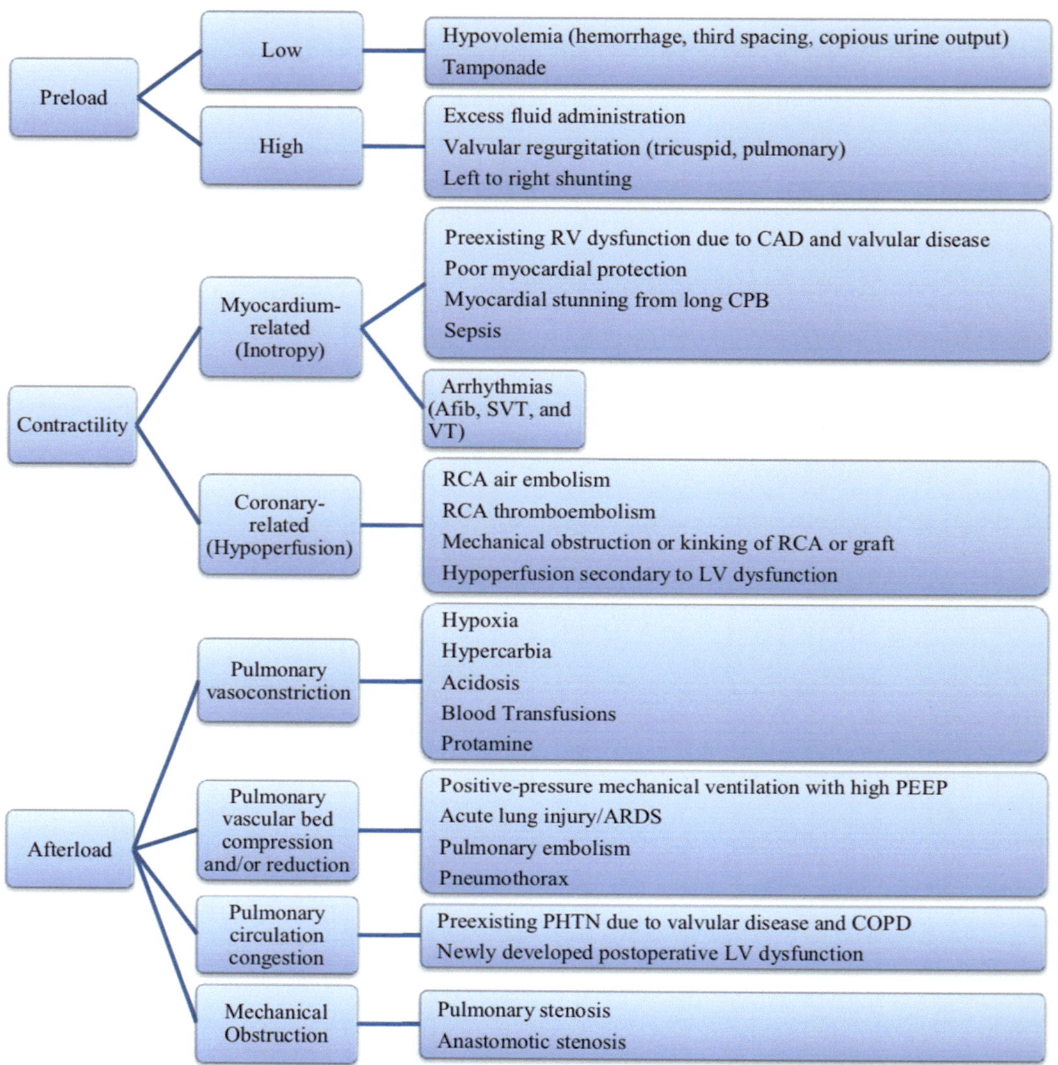

Fig. 3 Aetiology of RV failure. Reprinted from Seminars in Thoracic and Cardiovascular Surgery Vol 24/edition 3, Shinobu Itagaki, Leila Hosseinian, Robin Varghese, Right Ventricular Failure After Cardiac Surgery: Management Strategies, 188–194, Copyright (2012), with permission from Elsevier

values with non-surgical patients [25]. TAPSE should be assessed routinely in every assessment of RV function. It is important that the correct angle is obtained when measuring this. The apical four chamber view (TTE) usually allows good alignment; however, it is often harder to achieve good alignment in TOE studies. In this situation one should obtain multiple different views of the tricuspid annulus (e.g., mid-oesophageal four chamber, inflow-outflow, deep transgastric) in order to achieve the clearest view of the lateral annulus. M mode should only be used if the cursor is parallel to the motion.

Tissue Doppler imaging is another simple and reproducible way of measuring longitudinal (rather than global) RV function. Similar to TAPSE, the motion of the myocardium at the level of the tricuspid annulus in systole gives rise to the S prime (S') when measured with pulse wave tissue Doppler imaging. Like TAPSE it is

Table 4 Assessment of the RV

Variable	Notes	Normal values
RA size	Measure size/area/volume	Minor axis
RV size	Measure dimensions at base, midpoint, RV outflow tract proximally and distally	Base 25–41 mm Midpoint 19–35 mm Length 59–83 mm RVOT prox 21–35 mm RVOT distal 17–27 mm
TAPSE	Readily obtainable Established prognostic variable Angle and load dependent	>17 mm
S'	Readily obtainable Established prognostic variable Angle and load dependent	>9.5 cm/s
FAC	Need good endocardial definition, without foreshortening, high inter/intraobserver variability. Load dependent	>35%
EF	Unreliable with 2D, promising with 3D (use restricted to availability)	>45%
Myocardial performance (Tei) index	Less load dependent	>0.43 (measured with PWD) >0.54 (measured with TDI)
Diastolic function	E/A, E/e' (infrequently used)	E/A 0.8–2.0 e'>7.8 E/e'<6
Strain (GLS)	Promising, machine/software dependent Angle independent Prognostic validation	>20
Tricuspid regurgitation	Quantify severity	
RV load measurements using Doppler	RV (PA) peak systolic pressure RV end diastolic pressure Pulmonary artery acceleration time	>37 mmHg >90 ms

fairly easy to measure, and it has been shown to correlate well with other measures of global RV systolic function. It is unreliable after thoracotomy, pulmonary thromboendarterectomy and heart transplantation [22].

Pulmonary Hypertension

Load on the RV should be assessed by means of Doppler. Pulmonary hypertension (PHT) after cardiac surgery may be associated with RV failure. Causes of post-operative PHT include left-sided cardiac pathology, through dysfunction within the pulmonary vasculature caused by reperfusion; by cytokine release and the inflammatory response as a result of surgery or cardiopulmonary bypass; by blood transfusions, drugs (e.g., protamine); by the effects of mechanical ventilation and intrathoracic pressures or impaired gas exchange causing hypoxia or hypercarbia; and by thromboembolism [26]. In cardiac surgery, it is typically 'post-capillary' (World Health Organisation Group 2), of cardiac origin. The most common cause is LV systolic or diastolic impairment causing a rise in the LVEDP and LA pressure; or valvular pathology (e.g., after mitral valve surgery).

If the pulmonary vascular resistance (PVR) is high, afterload on the RV increases which can lead to RV failure and a drop in cardiac output. If this is the case then characteristic 2D echo signs are the triad of RV dilatation, RV systolic impairment and interventricular septal bowing towards the LV.

PA systolic pressure (PASP) is estimated by applying the principle of the simplified Bernoulli equation (PASP = $4 \times V^2$ + RAP) of the peak velocity of a tricuspid regurgitation jet (ensuring good parallel alignment between the jet direction and continuous wave Doppler cursor and optimising the view so as to obtain the highest velocity). Assuming no pulmonary stenosis, the RV systolic pressure is the same as the PA pressure. Diastolic PA pressures can also be estimated (diastolic PAP = $4 \times$ V2 PR + RAP), although this is dependent on the presence of pulmonary regurgitation, which is less likely to be present and harder to interrogate than tricuspid regurgitation.

PA acceleration time is another measure associated with a raised PVR or PA pressure and an acceleration time of 90 ms was associated with elevated pulmonary artery pressure and pulmonary vascular resistance [27]. This is easy to measure by using pulsed wave Doppler in the main PA. In addition, a normal flow pattern in the RV outflow tract has a smooth envelope on spectral Doppler whereas if elevated PVR is present, a systolic notching can be seen (see Chap. "POCUS in Monitoring: Right Ventricular Function and Pulmonary Hypertension": POCUS assessment of RV and pulmonary hypertension).

Acute pulmonary embolism (PE) is an uncommon occurrence acutely after cardiac surgery but remains an important cause of haemodynamic instability from 'obstructive shock' and mortality during a patient's stay in critical care. A sudden increase in PVR from an acute PE which may exceed the systolic capabilities of the RV so causing RV failure and cardiogenic shock.

2DE will demonstrate an impaired and dilated RV, so the methods used to assess systolic function (TAPSE etc.) will be abnormal. McConnell's sign is commonly seen, with basal to mid RV impairment and 'buckling' hinge point seen around the apex, however, it is not specific for PE. Thrombus is rarely seen unless in severe cases in which case this may be intracardiac.

Valvular Heart Disease

Valvular heart pathology seen in postoperative cardiac patients may be related to the complications of valve surgery (such as a paravalvular leak or dehiscence), from ischaemic tethering, or from worsening cardiac function and 'functional' regurgitation due to ventricular distension. The use of intraoperative TOE is now routine for valvular surgery, with benefit seen particularly in valve repair and mitral replacement surgeries and with low complication rates [28], so valvular pathologies seen postoperatively are more likely to be of new onset.

Systolic anterior motion (SAM) of the mitral valve occurs after around 4% of mitral valve surgeries [29] but is also seen in cases of hypertrophic obstructive cardiomyopathy (HOCM) and flail mitral leaflet. The anterior mitral valve leaflet and/or supporting chordae moves anteriorly towards the interventricular septum during systole, causing LVOT obstruction and MR. The effects may be severe, with hypotension, severe MR and low cardiac output. As management is specific (volume loading, reducing or stopping inotropic agents, giving vasoconstrictor drugs, slowing heart rate) and the condition is dynamic, echocardiography is essential for diagnosis so as to ensure correct management. Predisposing factors which increase the likelihood of SAM include a small LV cavity size in diastole, a tall posterior leaflet, narrow aorto-mitral angle and enlarged basal septum [30] and preoperative LV EF >60% [29].

Volume Status Assessment and Hypovolaemic Shock

Echocardiography is a useful tool in the assessment of volume status in postoperative cardiac surgical patients. These are often incorporated during dynamic assessments such as passive leg raising or exogenous fluid challenges. In hypovolaemic shock two-dimensional echocardiography may demonstrate small hyperdynamic LV with 'kissing' papillary muscles. The RV will also be small. Note in cases of RV failure, the LV will also appear small and 'underfilled', with a dilated RV; and excess fluid would not be appropriate in this case. The inferior vena cava (IVC) size is assessed routinely with echo, just below the junction of the RA (normal size 17–29 mm) and in a healthy, euvolaemic individual, the IVC will collapse by up to 50% in quiet inspiration. When the IVC is distended, its compliance reduces, so a large IVC that doesn't vary with respiration suggests that the patient is not on the steep (volume responsive) portion of the Starling curve [31]. In mechanically ventilated patients, the opposite is seen, with positive inspiratory intrathoracic pressure increasing its size. Ventilator settings and lung pathology significantly affect the size and collapsibility, with increasing intrathoracic pressures such as PEEP affecting it. Therefore, static absolute measurements of IVC size are unreliable guides to ascertain volume status. It is more useful to look at changes of size during the respiratory (mechanically ventilated) cycle. Septic patients who respond to fluid by increasing their cardiac output have been shown to have changes in IVC diameter of >12% [32], >18% [33] or >21% [34] during respiration. The Superior vena cava can also be measured in this way with TOE, and it may outperform the IVC method; with a value of >29% seen in responders [34]. Fluctuational swings (variability) in aortic blood flow during controlled mechanically ventilation as measured by TOE have also been studied, with a value of >15% indicating fluid-responders [35]. Methods of assessing preload responsiveness during mechanical ventilation are inaccurate if the patient has LV or RV dysfunction, ARDS [36] or an open chest. (See Chap. "POCUS in Monitoring: Volume Responsiveness": POCUS for volume responsiveness).

Distributive Shock and Vasoplegic Syndrome

Distributive shock is commonly caused by sepsis or systemic inflammatory response syndrome. It is characterised by a relative hypovolaemia due to redistribution of the intravascular volume due to vasodilatation and endothelial dysfunction. The vasoplegic syndrome is well-known in cardiac surgical patients occurring in 5–50% of patients post-operatively [37] and is characterised by a normal or raised cardiac output and low systemic vascular resistance (SVR); but a shock state, with hypotension and organ hypoperfusion. Proinflammatory cytokines are released as a consequence of CPB, leading to release of nitric oxide, dysregulation of adrenoreceptors and vasodilatation. Risk factors for the vasoplegic syndrome are preoperative low EF, use of angiotensin converting enzyme (ACE) inhibitor drugs, preoperative need for vasopressors and the CPB technique. POCUS will show a hyperkinetic LV or mildly reduced LV function and evidence of high cardiac output (raised aortic VTI). The low SVR may mask LV impairment however, which becomes apparent when vasoconstrictors are started.

Septic cardiomyopathy occurs in around 40% of patients with septic shock, with reduced LVEF seen in 50% and impaired RV function (up to 80%) [38]. Diastolic function may also be impaired. Echocardiography will therefore be useful in guiding therapies, i.e., introduction of inotropic agents rather than increasing vasopressor drugs. A study of 360 mechanically ventilated septic patients showed that patients fell into five different categories of TOE findings, highlighting the heterogenous cardiovascular behaviour seen between patients in sepsis and the importance of echocardiography: Group 1: '*well-resuscitated*' / normal function (no ventricular impairment and no fluid responsiveness as measured by SVC variability), Group 2: *LV systolic impairment*, Group 3: *hyperkinetic* LV function without fluid responsiveness, Group 4: *RV impairment* with normal LV and not fluid responsive, Group 5: normal LV function but *fluid responsive* [39].

Cardiac Arrest

During cardiac arrest, POCUS has a potential role in helping diagnose potential reversible causes as mentioned above, or to assess response to therapies. The 2020 ALS guidelines concluded that if echocardiography can be performed without interfering with the resuscitation protocols and chest compressions, it may be considered as an additional diagnostic tool to identify potentially reversible causes (weak recommendation, very low-quality evidence) [40]. POCUS is incorporated into some algorithms during the pulse-check phase, in order to differentiate pulseless electrical activity (lack of organised motion or contractility), from severe LV impairment. A prognostic benefit has not been shown from its use in this setting, however. There is caution against overinterpreting the finding of RV dilation in isolation as a diagnostic indicator of massive PE, as RV dilation has been shown to occur shortly after the onset of cardiac arrest due to causes other than PE, as blood moves from the systemic circulation to the right heart along a pressure gradient.

References

1. Hilberath JN. Safety of transesophageal echocardiography. J Am Soc Echocardiogr. 2010;23(11):1115–27.
2. Mebazaa AP. Clinical review: practical recommendations on the management of perioperative heart failure in cardiac surgery. Crit Care. 2010;14(101):1–14.
3. Rudiger A, Businger F, Streit M, Schmid E, Maggiorini M, Follath F. Presentation and outcome of critically ill medical and cardiac-surgery patients with acute heart failure. Swiss Med Wkly. 2009;139 (7–8):110–6.
4. Neskovic AN, Edvardsen T, Galderisi M, Garbi M, Gullace G, Jurcut R, Dalen H, Hagendorff A, Lancellotti P, European Association of Cardiovascular Imaging Document Reviewers:, Popescu BA. Focus cardiac ultrasound: the European Association of Cardiovascular Imaging viewpoint. Eur Heart J Cardiovasc Imaging. 2014; 15(9):956–60.
5. Hoit B. Pericardial effusion and cardiac tamponade in the new millenium. Curr Cardiol Rep. 2017;19(7):57.
6. Adler Y, Charron P, Imazio M, Badano L, Barón-Esquivias G, Bogaert J. 2015 ESC guidelines for the diagnosis and management of pericardial diseases: the task force for the diagnosis and management of pericardial diseases of the european society of cardiology (ESC). Eur Heart J. 2015; 36(42):2921–64.
7. Faehnrich JA. Effects of positive-pressure ventilation, pericardial effusion, and cardiac tamponade on respiratory variation in transmitral flow velocities. J Cardiothorac Vasc Anesth. 2003;17(1):45–50.
8. Price S, Prout J, Jaggar SI, Gibson DG, Pepper JR. 'Tamponade' following cardiac surgery: terminology and echocardiography may both mislead. Eur J Cardiothorac Surg. 2004; 26:1156–60.
9. Lang RM, Badano LP, Mor-Avi V, Afilalo J, Armstrong A, Ernande L, Flachskampf FA, Foster E, Goldstein SA, Kuznetsova T, Lancellotti P. Recommendations for cardiac chamber quantification by echocardiography in adults: An update from the American Society of Echocardiography and the European Association of Cardiovascular Imaging. Eur Heart J Cardiovasc Imaging. 2015; 16:233–71.
10. Abou R. Global longitudinal strain: clinical use and prognostic implications in contemporary practice. Heart. 2020;106:1438–44.
11. Karlsen SD. Global longitudinal strain is a more reproducible measure of left ventricular function than ejection fraction regardless of echocardiographic training. Cardiovasc Ultrasound. 2019; 17(18).
12. Stokke TM, Hasselberg NE, Smedsrud MK, Sarvari SI, Haugaa KH, Smiseth OA, Edvardsen T, Remme EW. Geometry as a confounder when assessing ventricular systolic function. J Am Coll Cardiol. 2017; 70(8):942–54.
13. Cerqueira MD, Weissman NJ, Dilsizian V, Jacobs AK, Kaul S, Laskey WK, Pennell DJ, Rumberger JA, Ryan T, Verani MS. Standardized myocardial segmentation and nomenclature for tomographic imaging of the heart. A statement for healthcare professionals from the cardiac imaging committee of the council on clinical cardiology of the american heart association. Circulation. 2002; 105:539–42
14. Reynolds HR, Tunick PA, Grossi EA, Dilmanian H, Colvin SB, Kronzon I. Paradoxical Septal Motion After Cardiac Surgery: A Review of 3,292 Cases. Clin Cardiol. 2007; 30(12):621–3.
15. Metkus TS, Suarez-Pierre A, Crawford TC, Lawton JS, Goeddel L, Dodd-o J, Mukherjee M, Abraham TP, Whitman GJ. Diastolic dysfunction is common and predicts outcome after cardiac surgery. J Cardiothorac Surg. 2018; 13(67).
16. Ashes CM, Yu M, Meineri M, Katznelson R, Carroll J, Rao V, Djaiani G. Diastolic dysfunction,

cardiopulmonary bypass, and atrial fibrillation after coronary artery bypass graft surgery. Br J Anaesth. 2014; 113(5):815–21.

17. Nagueh SFSO. Eur Heart J Cardiovasc Imaging. 2016; 17(12):1321–60.

18. Wetterslev M, Møller-Sørensen H, Johansen RR, Perner A. Systematic review of cardiac output measurements by echocardiography vs. thermodilution: the techniques are not interchangeable. Intensive Care Med. 2016; 42(8):1223–33.

19. Aissaoui N, Luyt CE, Leprince P, Trouillet JL, Léger P, Pavie A. Predictors of successful extracorporeal membrane oxygenation (ECMO) weaning after assistance for refractory cardiogenic shock. Intensive Care Med. 2011; 37(11):1738–45.

20. Dávila-Román VG, Waggoner AD, Hopkins WE, Barzilai B. Right ventricular dysfunction in low output syndrome after cardiac operations: assessment by transesophageal echocardiography. Ann Thorac Surg. 1995; 60(4):1081–6.

21. Itagaki S, Hosseinian L, Varghese R. Right ventricular failure after cardiac surgery: management strategies. Semin Thorac Cardiovasc Surg. 2012; 24 (3):188–94.

22. Lang RM, Badano LP, Tsang W, Adams DH, Agricola E, Buck T, Faletra FF, Franke A, Hung J, de Isla LP, Kamp O. EAE/ASE recommendations for image acquisition and display using three-dimensional echocardiography. Eur Heart J Cardiovasc Imaging. 2012; 13(1):1–46

23. Brown SB, Raina A, Katz D, Szerlip M, Wiegers SE, Forfia PR. Longitudinal shortening accounts for the majority of right ventricular contraction and improves after pulmonary vasodilator therapy in normal subjects and patients with pulmonary arterial hypertension. Chest. 2011; 140:27–33.

24. Raina A, Vaidya A, Gertz ZM, Chambers S, Forfia PR. Marked changes in right ventricular contractile pattern after cardiothoracic surgery: Implications for post-surgical assessment of right ventricular function. J Heart Lung Transplant. 2013; 32(8).

25. Grønlykke L, Ravn HB, Gustafsson F, Hassager C, Kjaergaard J, Nilsson JC. Right ventricular dysfunction after cardiac surgery–diagnostic options. Scand Cardiovasc J. 2016; 51(2):114–21

26. Denault A, Deschamps A, Tardif JC, Lambert J, Perrault L. Pulmonary hypertension in cardiac surgery. Curr Cardiol Rev. 2010; 6(1):1–14.

27. Tousignant C, Van Orman JR. Pulmonary artery acceleration time in cardiac surgical patients. J Cardiothorac Vasc Anesth. 2015; 29(6):1517–23.

28. Michelena HI, Abel MD, Suri RM, Freeman WK, Click RL, Sundt TM, Schaff HV, Enriquez-Sarano M. Intraoperative echocardiography in valvular heart disease: an evidence-based appraisal. Mayo Clin Proc. 2010; 85(7):646–5.

29. Loulmet DF, Yaffee DW, Ursomanno PA, Rabinovich AE, Applebaum RM, Galloway AC, Grossi EA. Systolic anterior motion of the mitral valve: a 30-year perspective. J Thorac Cardiovasc Surg. 148(6):2787–93.

30. Varghese R, Itagaki S, Anyanwu AC, Trigo P, Fischer G, Adams DH. Predicting systolic anterior motion after mitral valve reconstruction: using intra-operative transoesophageal echocardiography to identify those at greatest risk. Eur J Cardiothorac Surg. 2014; 45(1), 132–7.

31. Boyd JS. Echocardiography as a guide for fluid management. Crit Care. 2016; 20(274).

32. Feissel M, Michard F, Faller JP, Teboul JL. The respiratory variation in inferior vena cava diameter as a guide to fluid therapy. Intensive Care Med. 30 (9):1834–7.

33. Barbier C, Loubières Y, Schmit C, Hayon J, Ricôme JL, Jardin F, Vieillard-Baron A. Respiratory changes in inferior vena cava diameter are helpful in predicting fluid responsiveness in ventilated septic patients. Intensive Care Med. 2004; 30(9):1740–6.

34. Charbonneau H, Riu B, Faron M, Mari A, Kurrek MM, Ruiz J, Geeraerts T, Fourcade O, Genestal M, Silva S. Predicting preload responsiveness using simultaneous recordings of inferior and superior vena cavae diameters. Crit Care 2014; 18(5):473.

35. Feissel M, Mangin I, Ruyer O Faller JP, Michard F, Teboul JL. Respiratory changes in aortic blood velocity as an indicator of fluid responsiveness in ventilated patients with septic shock. Chest. 2001; 119(3):867–73.

36. Liu Y, Wei LQ, Li GQ, Yu X, Li GF, Li YM. Pulse pressure variation adjusted by respiratory changes in pleural pressure, rather than by tidal volume, reliably predicts fluid responsiveness in patients with acute respiratory distress syndrome. Crit Care Med. 2016; 44(2):342–51.

37. Busse LW, Barker N, Petersen C. Vasoplegic syndrome following cardiothoracic surgery-review of pathophysiology and update of treatment options. Crit Care. 2020; 24(1):36.

38. Ehrman RR. Pathophysiology, echocardiographic evaluation, biomarker findings, and prognostic implications of septic cardiomyopathy: a review of the literature. Crit Care. 2018;22(1):112.

39. Geri G, Vignon P, Aubry A, Fedou AL, Charron C, Silva S, Repessé X, Vieillard-Baron A. Cardiovascular clusters in septic shock combining clinical and echocardiographic parameters: a post hoc analysis. Intensive Care Med. 2019; 45(5):657–67.

40. Soar JE. Adult advanced life support: 2020 International consensus on cardiopulmonary resuscitation and emergency cardiovascular care science with treatment recommendations. Resuscitation. 2020;156:A80–119.

Echocardiography in Mechanical Circulatory Support

Susanna Price and Guido Tavazzi

The real benefit to the patient [of echocardiography] is not the technical skill, but rather the application of intellectual input.... Information, communication and teamwork are essential.
Jos Roelandt, a Dutch cardiologist and a POCUS Pioneer (1993)

Keywords

ECMO · Mechanical circulatory support · Echocardiography · FoCUS

Key Messages

- Echocardiography in MCS is the domain of the echocardiography expert
- The intelligent application of FoCUS with expert interpretation can be potentially lifesaving where no other practitioner is directly and immediately available
- Specialized training is required to perform and interpret echocardiography in MCS
- Multidisciplinary teamwork is crucial for managing patients with MCS.

S. Price (✉)
Adult Intensive Care Unit, Royal Brompton Hospital, London, UK
e-mail: s.price@rbht.nhs.uk

National Heart and Lung Institute, Imperial College London, London, UK

G. Tavazzi
Fondazione IRCCS Policlinico S. Matteo, Pavia, Italy
e-mail: guido.tavazzi@unipv.it

Background

Echocardiography in mechanical circulatory support (MCS) is a highly specialist imaging area in its own right, and the relevance of focused cardiac ultrasound may seem counter-intuitive or questionable. Nonetheless, application of focused imaging in the context of cardiogenic shock (CS) by an expert in echocardiography may be appropriate in certain circumstances, in particular where the patient is peri-arrest, and a comprehensive study is precluded by the timeframe allowed. Further, although echocardiography in MCS is the domain of the echocardiography expert, intelligent application of FoCUS with expert interpretation can be potentially lifesaving where no other practitioner is directly and immediately available. Here, the images acquired by an appropriately trained FoCUS practitioner can be used to 'understand underlying pathophysiology, narrow the differential diagnosis, initiate therapy and/or to trigger further diagnostic work-up' when interpreted by an expert in the field. Additionally, a basic evaluation using trans-oesophageal echocardiography, with appropriate training is achieved, may be helpful in specific situations (e.g., cardiac arrest) or to address specific questions (e.g., thrombosis, tamponade, offloading, etc.).

© The Author(s), under exclusive license to Springer Nature Switzerland AG 2023
H. Soliman-Aboumarie et al. (eds.), *Cardiopulmonary Point of Care Ultrasound,*
https://doi.org/10.1007/978-3-031-29472-3_22

In this chapter we will describe where focused imaging undertaken by an expert might be used in the application of MCS in the emergency setting, including identification of the patient potentially needing MCS, exclusion of contra-indications, confirmation of appropriate cannulation and identification of complications. The final stage of MCS, weaning, is complex, requires high-end imaging knowledge and techniques and as FoCUS is not applicable in this setting, weaning from MCS is not covered in this chapter.

Cardiogenic Shock and Acute Mechanical Circulatory Support

Cardiogenic shock (CS) is a syndrome of circulatory failure due to low cardiac output from left and/or right heart failure, where the cardiac output is insufficient to meet the demands of the body. International guidelines for the diagnosis and treatment of acute and chronic heart failure recommend short-term MCS to support patients with acute left or biventricular failure (INTERMACS I) until cardiac and other organ systems have recovered. In addition, recommendations are that MCS systems, particularly extracorporeal membrane oxygenation (ECMO) can be used as a 'bridge to decision' in patients with acute and rapidly deteriorating heart failure/CS to stabilise haemodynamics, recover end-organ function and allow for a full clinical evaluation for the possibility of either heart transplant or a more durable MCS device.

Although none of the definitions of CS include echocardiography, current guidelines do recommend the use of echocardiography in the presence of CS in order to determine the underlying cause, and resuscitation guidelines recommend the use of FoCUS to diagnose/exclude potentially reversible causes of cardiac arrest where an appropriately trained practitioner is present. In CS, where the clinical status of the patient precludes a comprehensive study (i.e., profound instability and rapid deterioration), a FoCUS may demonstrate severe left and/or right ventricular dysfunction and/or dilatation, indicate the presence/absence of pre-existing cardiac disease and/or gross acute valvular abnormalities that may be useful to guide immediate interventions up to and including MCS. If time allows, progression to comprehensive echocardiography should be undertaken however, this is not always possible. Where no expert is immediately available, remote review of by an expert of emergently acquired FoCUS imaging can be sufficient to guide decision-making, in particular in patients with CS of severity SCAI D or E and when further delay might lead to significant compromise in delivery life-saving interventions.

Types of MCS

A range of acute MCS devices are available which will support the left and/or right ventricles, with/without additional oxygenation. The main devices currently used include IABP (left heart), Impella (left heart), Impella RP/Protek Duo (right heart) or VA-ECMO (both ventricles + oxygenation). The different configurations for devices are shown in Fig. 1. Any imaging practitioner involved in decision-making in acute MCS should be fully aware of the potential MCS configurations, their indications, contra-indications, the effects on the heart & circulation, cannula positioning, complications and echocardiographic features of optimal MCS and weaning.

Key Information Required for Emergency Decision-Making

If focused imaging is used, either TTE or TOE, all images must be obtained or reviewed by an expert in the specialty. There are certain factors that are key for decision-making in the very acute setting that can be identified, even using FoCUS, and where imaging is undertaken by a non-expert for emergency remote review, the imager must take care to ensure that images are adequate to inform expert decision-making. Key questions to answer include:

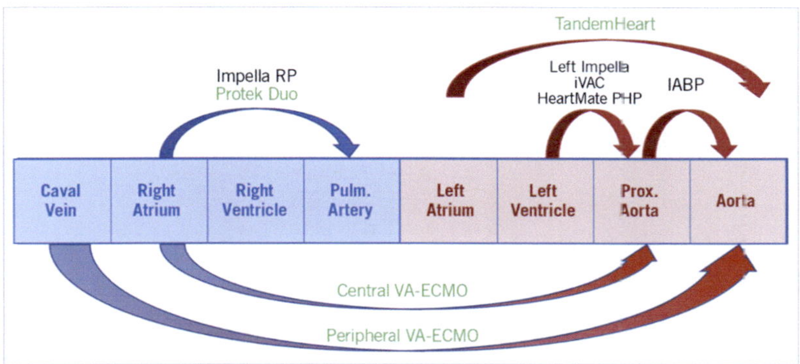

Fig. 1 Different options for acute MCS. Arrows indicate which part of the circulation is supported by the modality used. Devices in green can add blood oxygenation in addition to mechanical support. IABP: intra-aortic balloon pump, VA-ECMO veno-arterial extracorporeal membrane oxygenation (from EACVI/ACVC position paper on pMCS 2021)

1. Is this acute or acute-on-chronic cardiac disease (pre-existing cardiac disease)?
2. Is there involvement of one or other side of the heart (or both)?
3. What is the potential cause(s) of cardiogenic shock?
4. Are there any contraindications to MCS (relative and absolute)?

The main role of the practitioner in this setting is to obtain as high-quality images as possible in order to allow the expert MDT to make a decision as to the best MCS support for the individual patient based on the information available and in the clinical context. An expert echocardiographer trained in MCS imaging will be able to do this intuitively, however this is not routine echocardiographic practice, and specific training is required. The presence/absence of pulmonary oedema can be demonstrated using LUS, but the decision to include a device that can oxygenate the blood is not made based in this finding, but rather the arterial blood gas analysis, ventilatory settings and inspired oxygen content.

Exclusion of Contraindications

Echocardiography is widely used to exclude/diagnose relative contraindications to acute MCS. A focused study may be sufficient to rule in/out some of these, but, as with all imaging in the very acute setting, where suboptimal the sensitivity may be insufficient to rule in/out with absolute certainty. Some of the echocardiographic features that are *relative* contraindications to acute MCS are shown in Table 1. Clearly, they cannot all be identified using focused imaging with 100% sensitivity and specificity, and echocardiographic techniques beyond those used in FoCUS are required. Nonetheless, where one of these features is identified or cannot be excluded, the finding should be noted, and a more comprehensive assessment undertaken.

Cannulation and Institution of Support for VA-ECMO: The Role of FoCUS

Cannulation may be undertaken at the bedside in an emergency (VA-ECMO) or in the catheter laboratory. If the patient is transferred to the catheter lab for the procedure, expert echocardiography should be undertaken in conjunction with TTE (and/or TOE), and all echo modalities, in conjunction with fluoroscopy should be used as required.

In the event that an emergent decision is made for bedside cannulation it is possible to use focused imaging to guide the procedure,

Table 1 Relative contra-indications to acute MCS identifiable on echo

VA-ECMO	pLVAD	pRVAD
• Unrepaired aortic dissection • Severe aortic regurgitation • Unrepaired coarctation of the aorta • Severe aortic atheroma • Abdominal/thoracic aneurysm with intraluminal thrombus	• Unrepaired aortic dissection • Severe aortic stenosis • Mechanical aortic valve replacement • Left ventricular thrombus Unrepaired coarctation of the aorta • Severe aortic atheroma • Abdominal/thoracic aneurysm with intraluminal thrombus	• Reconstruction of the right heart • Right-sided valvular stenosis

VA-ECMO; veno-arterial extracorporeal membrane oxygenation, pLVAD; percutaneous left ventricular assist device, Impella, pRVAD; percutaneous right ventricular assist device, Protek Duo or Impella RP

provided it is undertaken by a practitioner expert in applying the technique in this setting. US-related imaging used for the procedure includes the following steps:

1. Real-time US-guided vascular access
2. US-confirmation (transhepatic shoot-through view) that the wires in IVC and aorta
3. Continued demonstration that wires have not migrated during cannula exchange
4. Confirmation that the venous wire has not crossed into the RV and is extending to the SVC
5. Confirmation of venous cannula placement towards the SVC
6. Confirmation of arterial cannulation in the aorta
7. Exclusion of immediate complications (i.e. pericardial collection, aortic dissection, incorrect cannula placement).

It cannot be overemphasized that that this is not basic echo, but rather focused, protocolized, precise, procedure-guiding imaging, performed by an expert and intended to facilitate an immediate life-saving intervention. It is not intended to substitute for a comprehensive echo for evaluation of the heart, which is preferred at every stage before and after cannulation. If possible and if time allows, a combination of US, TTE and TOE is preferred, with a comprehensive TOE undertaken following/during cannulation, in particular to confirm positioning of the venous cannula and diagnosis/exclusion of any unsuspected cardiac pathology not diagnosed on TTE.

Immediate Effects of VA-ECMO Seen on FoCUS

Immediate effects seen should be gradual decrease in ventricular size. Where left ventricular function is poor, there may be only intermittent (or even no) aortic valve opening, and on occasion the ventricle will not reduce in size and appear to be filled with spontaneous echo contrast (Fig. 2). These findings should be communicated clearly to the practitioner in charge of the MCS procedure as additional strategies will likely be needed to decompress the left ventricle. This is not an emergency, and comprehensive echocardiographic evaluation of the heart on MCS should be undertaken in order to confirm the diagnosis and pathology, evaluate filling pressures and determine the optimal unloading strategy (Fig. 3).

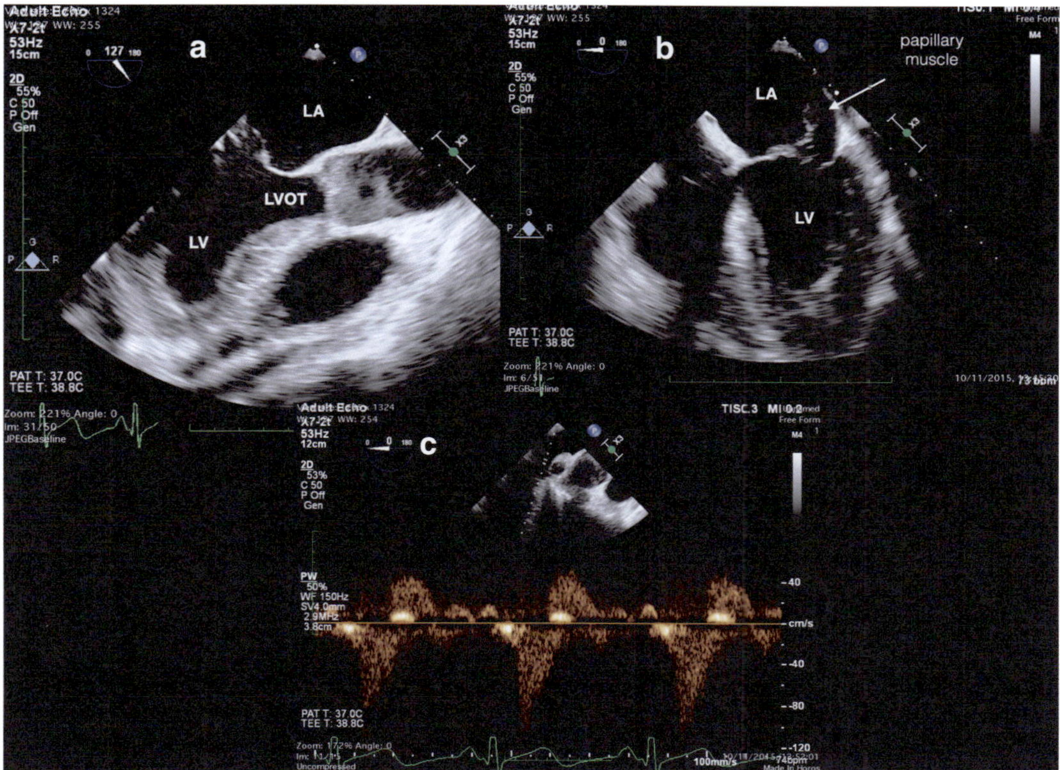

Fig. 2 Transesophageal echocardiography of patient on VA ECMO due to papillary muscle rupture as consequence to acute myocardial infarction. The 2D evaluation of cardiac chambers allows both the visualization of mitral valve flail with papillary muscle attached to the sub-valvular apparatus bouncing in left atrium during systole and the closure of the aortic valve with blood stasis on the aortic side. Pulmonary vein pulse wave Doppler demonstrating reverse systolic flow as sign of high left atrial pressure related to LV ineffective offloading

Troubleshooting and Complications

Every patient receiving acute MCS should have a daily echocardiogram. In the event an acute haemodynamic deterioration is seen, and/or the circuit is not functioning normally, the critical care team may request a focused study as a rapid rule in/rule out of specific complications. Findings may include:

- Pericardial collection: this can be relatively large and with no haemodynamic effects, or small with significant effects where cardiac drainage is impeded (Fig. 4)
- Cannula displacement or migration (with/without cannula obstruction)
- Cannula-related thrombus (with/without cannula obstruction) (Fig. 5)
- Excessive ventricular offloading
- Valve/cardiac thrombosis (Figs. 2 and 6)
- Worsening valvular regurgitation (volume and/or duration)
- Inadequate left ventricular offloading and associated features (LV contrast, biphasic retrograde transmitral flow, retrograde pulmonary systolic flow) (Figs. 2 and 3)
- Post-ejection shortening on TAPSE/MAPSE (Fig. 7).

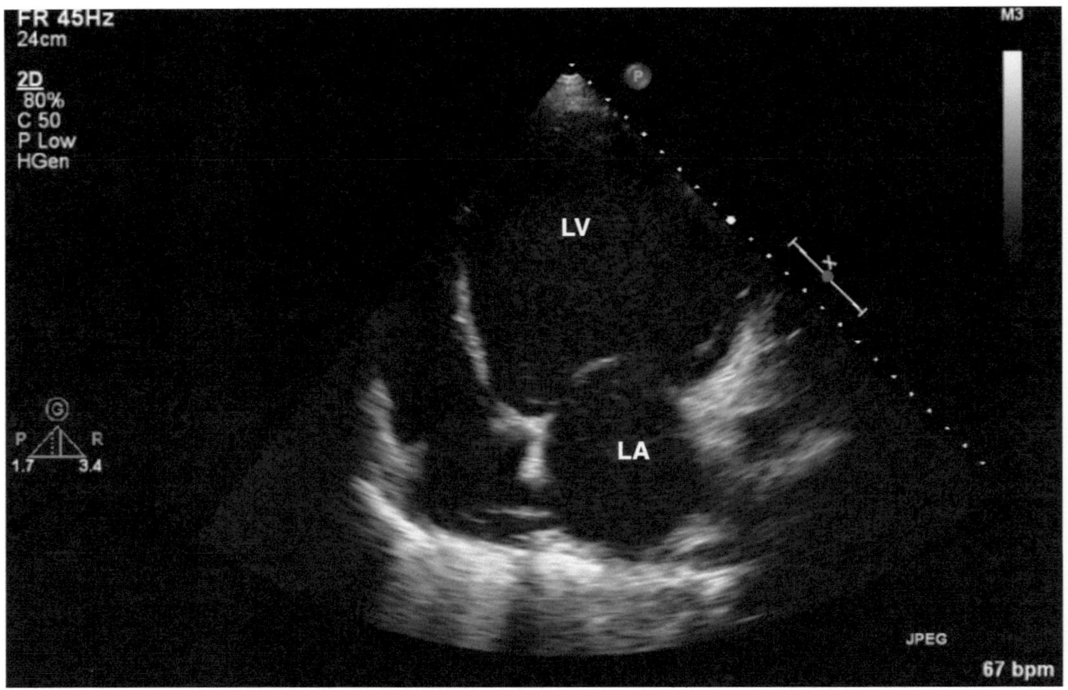

Fig. 3 Transthoracic echocardiography apical four chambers view with an overdistended left ventricle due to ineffective offloading after placement of veno-arterial ECMO. The grainy aspect inside the left side cardiac chambers is the smoke effect related to blood stasis

Clearly all these cannot be diagnosed/ excluded using FoCUS protocols, but a focused study, undertaken by an experienced practitioner should readily be able to demonstrate/exclude all these findings where present. As with all critical care echo examinations, findings must be evaluated in the clinical context and discussed with the responsible clinician by the bedside and where TTE images are inadequate, unless contraindicated, TOE undertaken. Of note, the use of left-sided contrast to improve image interpretation in patients receiving MCS should only be undertaken by those experienced in its use, as with certain MCS devices, detection of the bubbles will result in instant cessation of the MCS circuit. Once an intervention has been undertaken to reverse the problem (i.e., increase/reduction in MCS flows, cannula repositioning) the effects on the heart and circulation should be re-evaluated in real time.

In the event that univentricular support is used, in addition to the standard potential

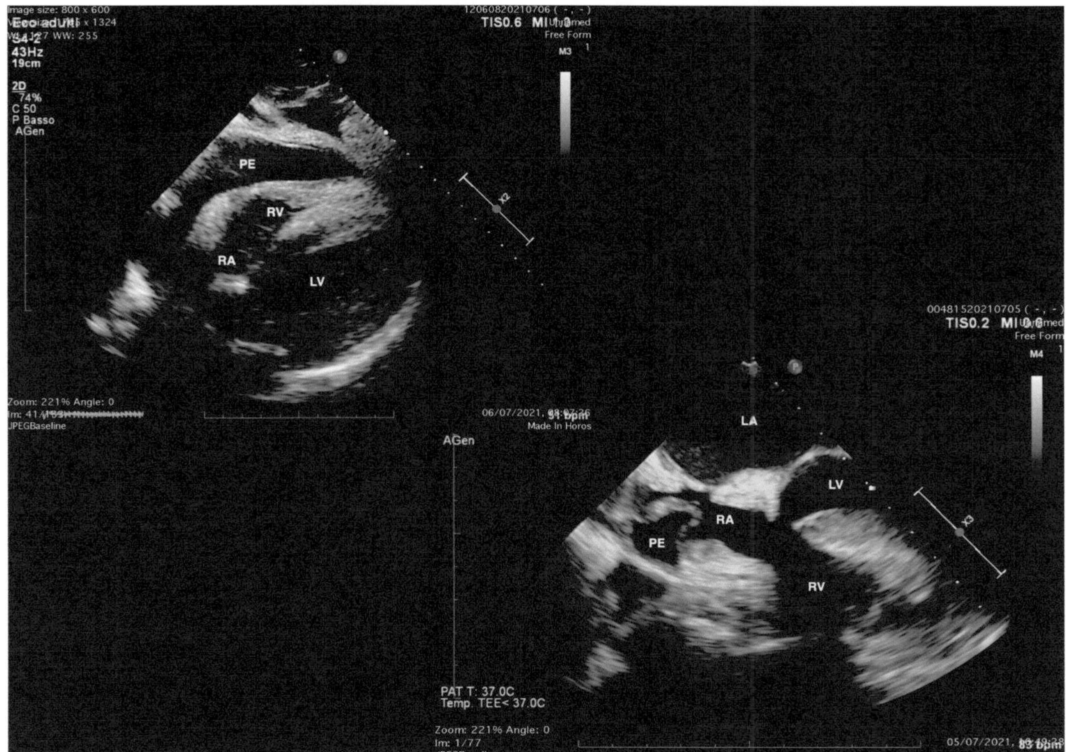

Fig. 4 Sub-costal view of a patients on VA ECMO with significant pericardial effusion (PE) encompassing the right-sided chambers. Focus transesophageal echocardiography 4 chambers view (0°) of the same patient demonstrating the right atrium collapse due to PE

complications identified using imaging described above, the effects on the contralateral ventricle must be evaluated, together with any shift in the interventricular septum. This is highly specialized echocardiography, requires in-depth understanding of cardiac physiology, MCS, and potentially the use of advanced techniques including global longitudinal strain, this is not the domain of FoCUS.

Assessment of Offloading and Weaning

A number of protocols exist for weaning from VA-ECMO and percutaneous left-sided support. These are complex, usually paired with invasive haemodynamic monitoring and individualised to the patient's clinical status. This is beyond the

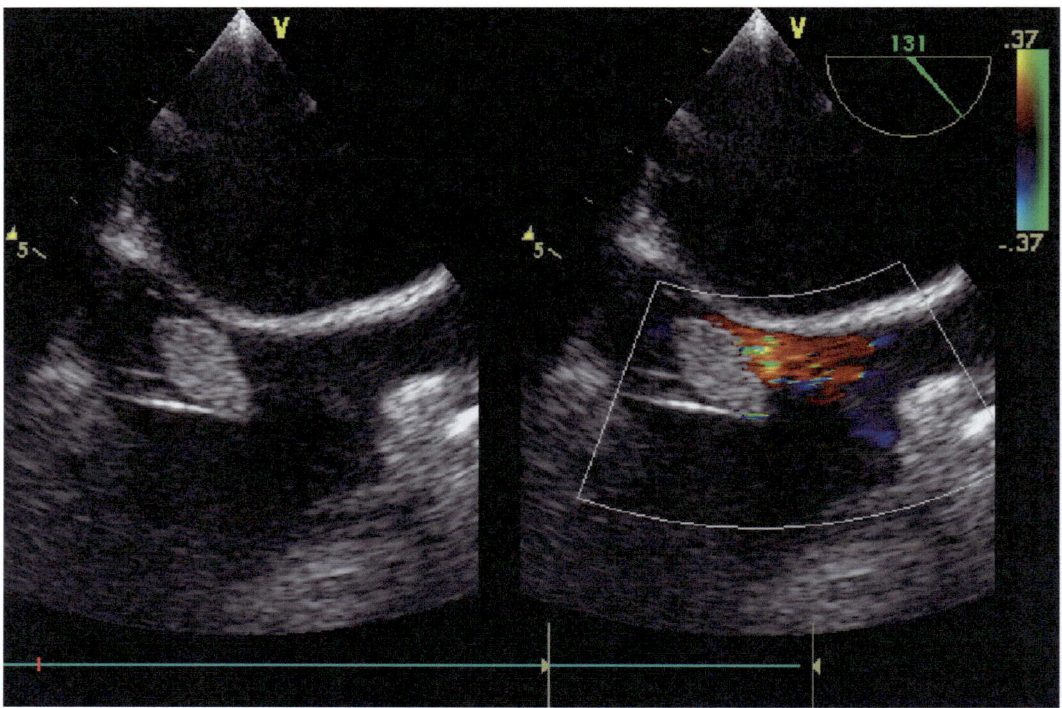

Fig. 5 Focus transesophageal echocardiography demonstrating drainage cannula in the middle of the right atrium (RA) with a thrombus on the cannula tip causing partial obstruction

scope of any focused imaging protocols, demands the full spectrum of advanced echo techniques to be available to the imager. It is likely, however, that in the future these will become more standardized, and as our knowledge of weaning from acute MCS increases, the role of imaging, and focused studies may well increase.

Summary and Conclusions

Accurate imaging and interpretation are key to guide expert decision-making in all critical care echocardiography including the field of acute MCS. Here the stakes are high, and there is no

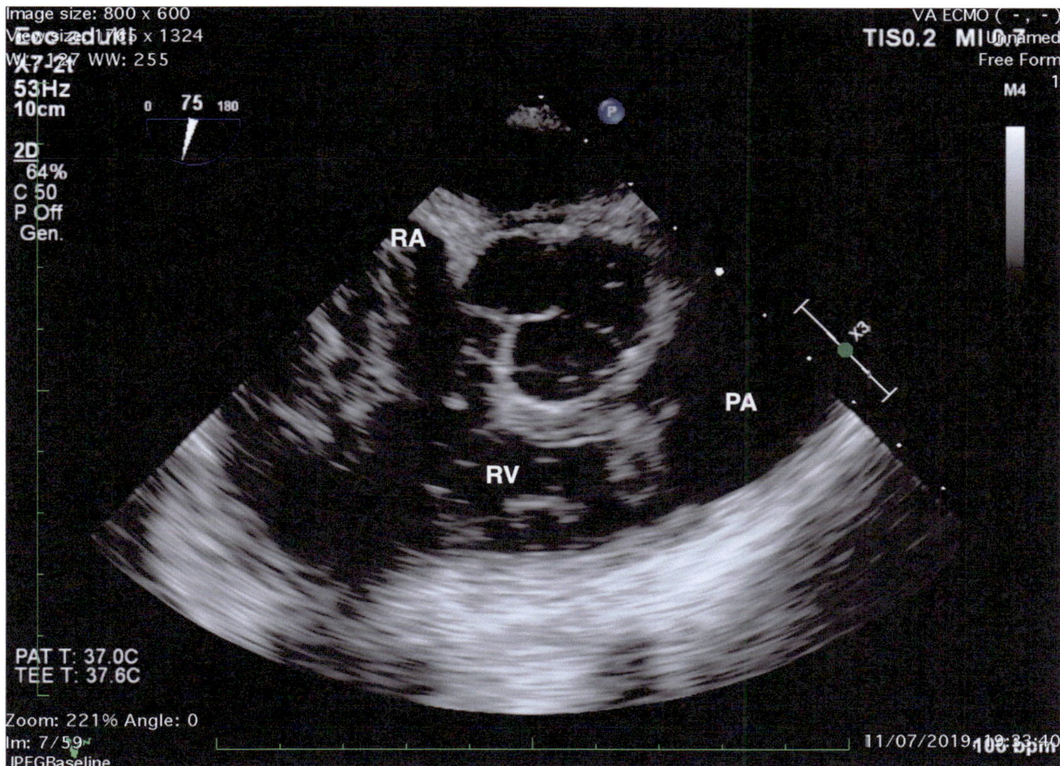

Fig. 6 Focus transesophageal echocardiography of a patient on cardiac arrest being evaluated for potential extra-corporeal cardiac resuscitation. Right ventricular inflow-outflow view demonstrating diffuse thrombosis of all the right side chambers and pulmonary valve

place for over-confidence on the part of any practitioner, no matter how experienced, as major decisions which may prove lifesaving will be made on the basis of this imaging. On occasion, time constraints will mean that focused imaging alone is available. Specific training is required, not only to understand the appropriate application of focused imaging and echocardiography in

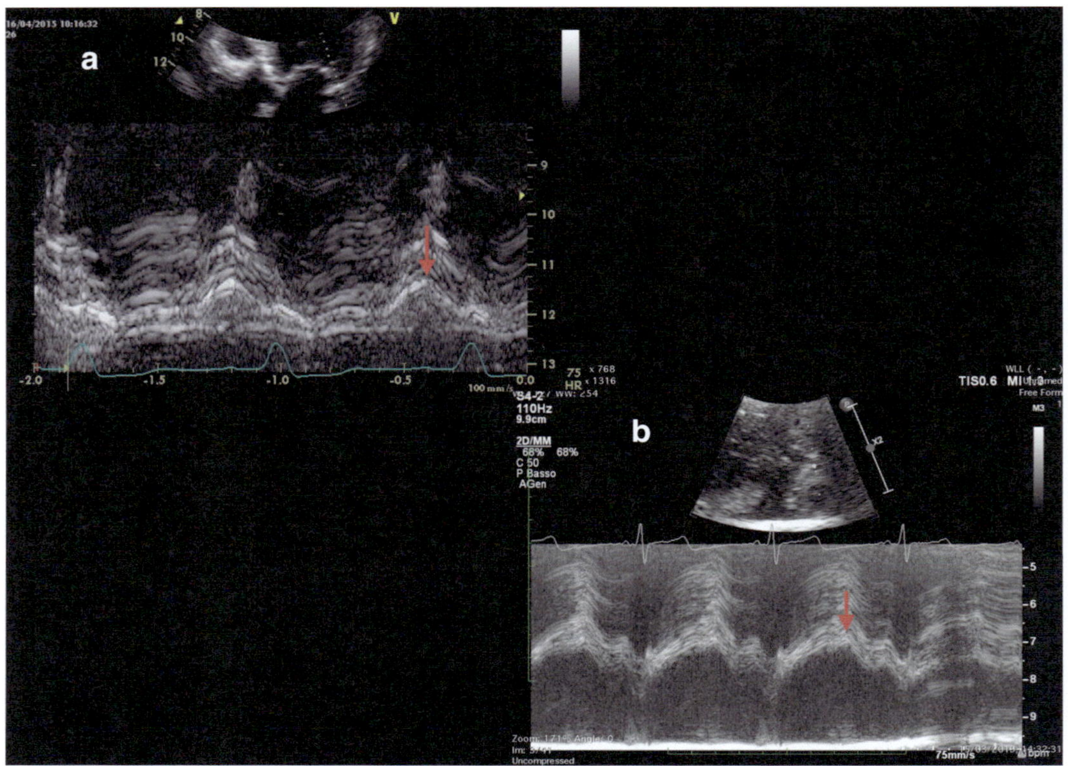

Fig. 7 Post-ejection shortening at MAPSE (**a**) and TAPSE (**b**) of respectively a patients with ongoing myocardial ischemia and a patient with hypoxemia, hypercarbia and increased right ventricular afterload (in absence of acute cor pulmonale) due to severe respiratory failure. The peak contraction (red arrow) occurs after the T wave at ECG entailing electro-mechanical dyssynchrony and reduction of effective diastolic filling time

this context, but also the scope of acute MCS, its potential complications, and the ability of comprehensive echocardiography to direct assessment and management of these highly complex patients.

Point of Care Ultrasound in Chest Trauma

Serena Rovida, Salman Naeem, and Andrew Kirckpatrick

To study the phenomena of disease without books is to sail an uncharted sea, while to study books without patients is not to go to sea at all.

Sir William Osler—Canadian physician and pioneer (1849–1919 AD)

Abstract

Point of care ultrasound (POCUS) allows immediate recognition of life-threatening disorders, leading to prompt clinical decisions in trauma settings. When compared to plain chest radiography it has higher accuracy in diagnosing injuries of chest wall, lung parenchyma and heart. The advent of portable handheld devices has allowed POCUS to be adopted in the pre-hospital environment as well as in retrieval medicine, mainly for diagnosis of pneumothorax with good results. Besides its diagnostic power, US can assist or guide chest drain insertion and regional anaesthesia making the physician more comfortable during the invasive procedure. This chapter will explain the uses of POCUS in chest trauma.

Keywords

Trauma · Lung ultrasound · Chest ultrasound · Pneumothorax · Lung contusion · POCUS

Supplementary Information The online version contains supplementary material available at https://doi.org/10.1007/978-3-031-29472-3_23.

S. Rovida (✉)
General Intensive Care Unit, St Georges Hospital, London, UK
e-mail: sererovida@gmail.com

S. Naeem
Department of Emergency Medicine, Barts Health NHS Trust, London, UK

A. Kirckpatrick
Acute Care, Trauma, and General Surgery and Critical Care Medicine, University of Calgary, Calgary, Canada
e-mail: andrew.kirkpatrick@albertahealthservices.ca

Key Messages

- POCUS of chest can easily rule out massive pneumothorax and pericardial effusion in trauma.
- It does not pose any risk to the patient and can be repeated allowing the opportunity to perform enhanced examination at the bedside
- It can also be used to monitor lung parenchymal changes and allow guidance during procedures.

Ultrasound for the Chest Wall

Rib & sternal fractures: Compared to standard chest radiography, ultrasound has higher diagnostic sensitivity even in case of minimal discontinuities of the cortical bone [1]. Direct evidence of a cortical step or indirect evidence of a local hematoma are the two diagnostic criteria for rib fractures [1] (Fig. 1). Detection of rib and sternal fractures correlate to a relatively high-energy trauma, suggesting the clinician to perform a meticulous examination looking for further parenchymal or great vessel injuries.

Subcutaneous emphysema: This condition refers to the presence of gas in the subcutaneous tissues that usually dissects into the deeper soft tissues and musculature along fascial planes. Its presence indicates possible serious injuries in the setting of a chest trauma of an otherwise healthy patient and is indicative of pneumothorax and/or rupture of the upper airways [2] that do require urgent management. Air collection between the skin and the chest wall prevents visualisation of the pleural line, impairing the 'bat sign' view. In this circumstance, chest US cannot be used to draw any diagnostic conclusions regarding underlying pleura and lung conditions.

Ultrasound for the Pleura

Pneumothorax(Fig. 2)

Pneumothorax (PTX) is a common complication of trauma to the chest. The pathophysiology and technique for scanning for PTX is explained in previous chapters **(see Chap. 11 for more details)**. Scanning technique of chest in a trauma patient differs from the standard scan as majority of patients are lying supine. Air rises to the least dependent area of the chest which corresponds to anterior region at approximately 2nd to 4th intercostal space in mid-clavicular line while it's in the apico-lateral location in an upright patient [3]. Therefore, in trauma patients, anterior location will identify majority of significant pneumothoraces [4].

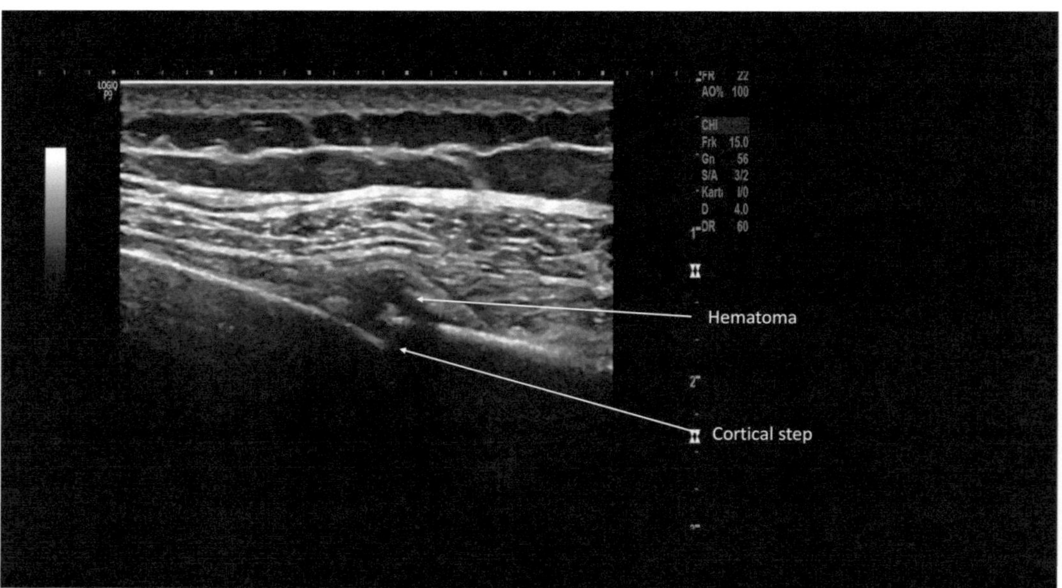

Fig. 1 Rib fracture. Chest wall structures above and a hyperechoic line in the middle with post-acoustic shadowing representing the cortex of the rib. There is a break in the cortex (arrow) surrounded by anechoic shadow representing the hematoma (arrow)

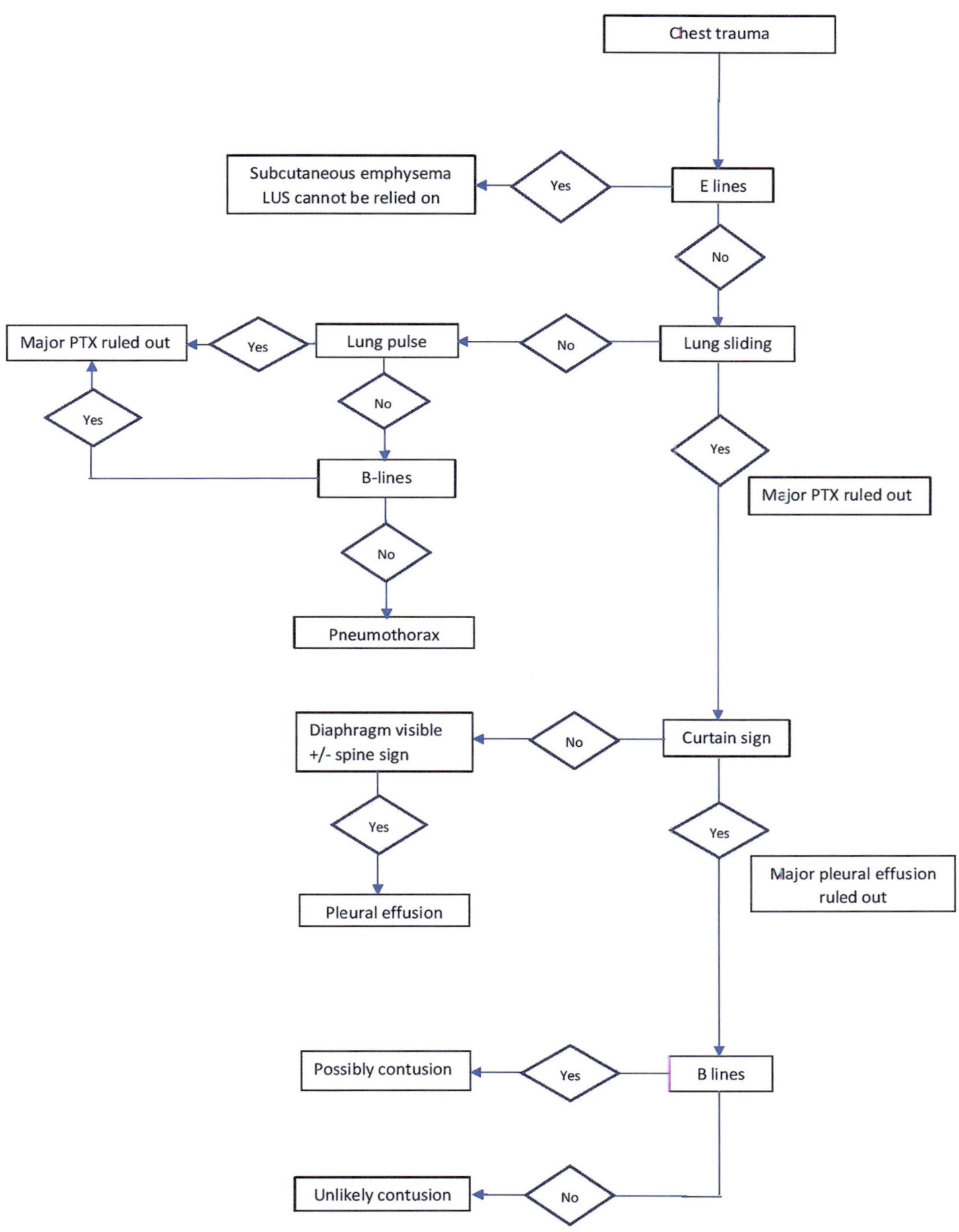

Fig. 2 Proposed algorithm for POCUS in chest trauma, "E" stands for emphysema (subcutaneous). E lines are vertical lines visualized when there is gas trapped in the subcutaneous space. These lines do not arise from the pleural line, but from the subcutaneous tissue; as the gas does not move, they are not synchronous with respiratory movements.

Specific sonographic signs of PTX

Lung Point: In a patient with partially collapsed lung due to PTX, part of the visceral and parietal pleura slide against each other producing normal lung sliding and a part of the pleural cavity is filled with air, hence absence of lung sliding. At this transition point, both distinct sonographic signs (normal pleural sliding & loss of pleural sliding due to PTX) are visible and this is called lung point [5] which oscillates with each respiratory cycle. It is 100% specific for PTX, however, its sensitivity is only about 65% [6]. Lung point can used to quantify the pneumothorax as well as guide chest drain insertions. In certain patients with underlying lung parenchymal pathologies i.e. blebs, bullae or restrictive lung disease, it can be falsely positive.

Hydro point: In cases where there are both fluid and air in the pleural space, it creates a specific sonographic pattern at the interface which is called 'hydro-point'. Air in the pleural space is depicted by the absence of lung sliding and A-lines, while pleural effusion is demonstrated by anechoic fluid collection [7].

Heart point: Usually, heart is visualised in systole and diastole due to absence of free air in the thorax and pre-cardiac space. In the presence of pneumothorax, as the heart contracts in systole air can fill the space between heart and the anterior chest wall, preventing the conduction of ultrasound waves, hence the heart disappears from the view. This is called the 'heart point' and this might be one of first signs of pneumothorax [8].

Estimation of size of pneumothorax

Lung point can be used to estimate the size of pneumothorax. With the patient in supine position, using sternum as the reference, if the lung point is visualised before the anterior axillary line (AAL), lung collapse is less than 10% which is classified as small PTX. If the lung point is between the AAL and mid-axillary line (MAL), it is classified as medium PTX with approximately 10% to 15% lung collapse. When lung point visualisation is beyond MAL the collapse is greater than 15% and is classified as large PTX

[9]. This estimation can help guide conservative versus invasive management approach for pneumothoraces.

Key message:

POCUS of the chest can reliably detect PTX in trauma patients when lung sliding, lung pulse and B-lines are absent, while lung point and A-lines are present. Other specific signs such as hydro point and heart point can aid in the diagnosis of PTX.

Haemothorax: Fluid is an excellent medium for transmission of US waves, hence it appears as an anechoic space in between the two pleural layers, collecting in the baso-lateral area of the thorax in a supine patient. It allows the visualisation of thoracic structures which would not be normally visible i.e. thoracic spine which is called the 'thoracic spine sign' [1]. The collapsed lung can be seen floating in the pleural fluid, the tip of the lower lobe which appears like a tongue can be seen moving with each respiratory cycle and is called the 'tongue sign' (Fig. 3) (Video 1). Depending upon the consistency of the pleural fluid some debris can be seen floating in the thoracic cavity which is called the 'plankton sign' [10] (Fig. 4). The presence of 'curtain sign', defined as sonographic image of normal lung pattern overlapping the diaphragm and abdominal organs intermittently and synchronously with respiration can rule out pleural effusion [11, 12] (see Chap. 6 for more details).

Estimation of pleural effusion:

It can be helpful to estimate the size of pleural effusion in a trauma patient as it can guide further management and investigations. Moderate sized pleural effusion can be estimated using the following formula:

Volume of pleural fluid (millilitres) = 16 × distance between visceral and parietal pleurae (mm).

With interpleural distance measured in the sagittal plane at mid-scapular line between base of lung and mid-diaphragm. Alternatively, if pleural effusion is spanning more than three intercostal spaces in a sitting patient then it is

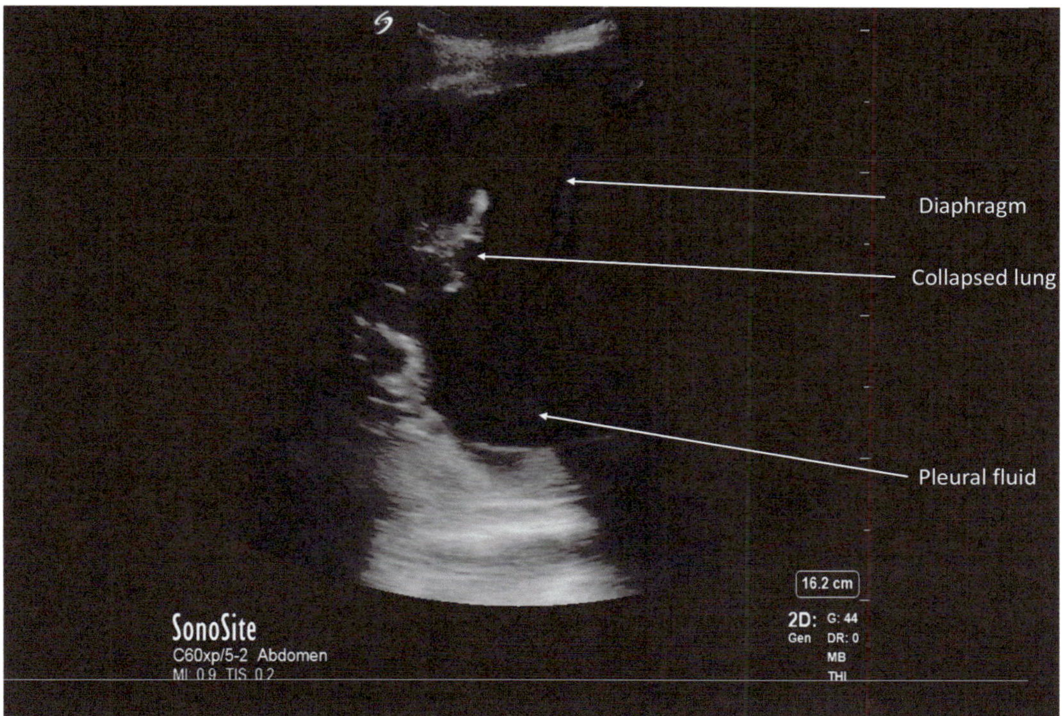

Fig. 3 Tongue sign. Anechoic fluid in the right hemithorax compressing the right lower lobe of the lung which appears like a tongue (arrow)

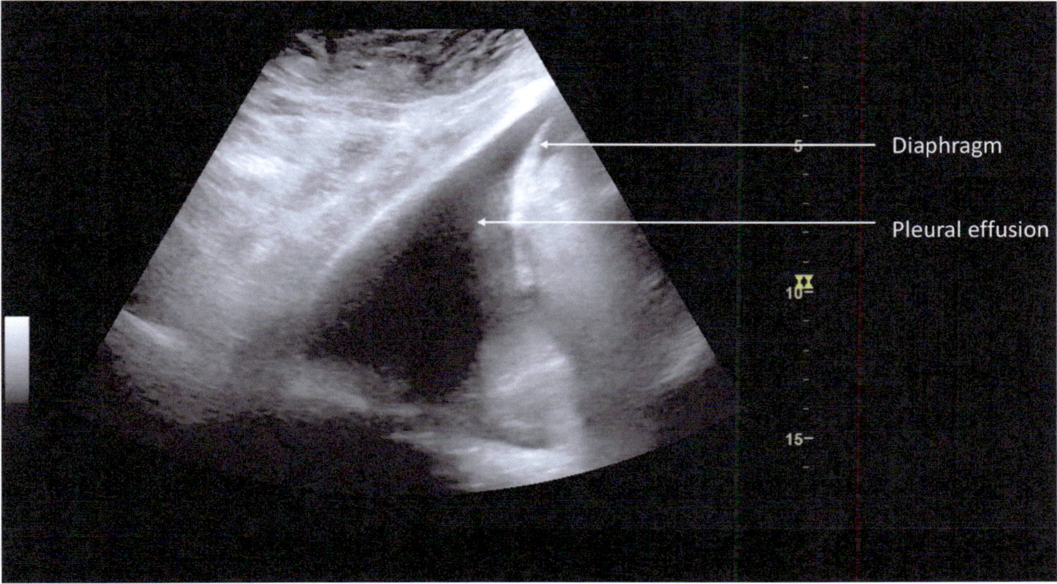

Fig. 4 Haemothorax. Anechoic fluid (arrow) in the left hemithorax above the hyperechoic band like diaphragm (arrow)

estimated to be more than 1 L. (see Chaps. 6 and 27 for more details).

Key message:

Chest US has very high accuracy to diagnose pleural fluid and can be used to quickly quantify amount of fluid in the hemithorax which can aid in decision making.

Ultrasound for Lung Parenchyma

Lung contusion: Lung contusion results from trauma to lung parenchyma by either direct trauma to the lung tissue (in penetrating injuries) or through indirect transmission of forces through the chest wall (blunt trauma) [13]. The injured parenchyma begins to accumulate fluid/blood due to the initial insult and then resulting in inflammation [14]. Conventionally chest radiography has been used to assess lung contusion, which often appears as increased opacity of lung tissue. However, it is not very sensitive as it can take several hours for the changes to appear on a chest radiograph. On POCUS, the first sign of reduced aeration appears as B-lines 'interstitial pattern' often associated with irregularity of pleural line. This can then progress to sub pleural consolidations (Fig. 5) (Video 3) and then complete loss of aeration and hepatisation of the lung (Fig. 6) (Video 4) where air content is fully replaced by inflamed, oedematous tissue. Although the sensitivity of POCUS is high in detecting increased fluid content of lung (extravascular lung water), however, it is not very specific for diagnosing lung contusion and the physician should be aware that similar changes are detected in other conditions for example, pneumonia and non-cardiogenic pulmonary oedema [15]. However, the presence of these

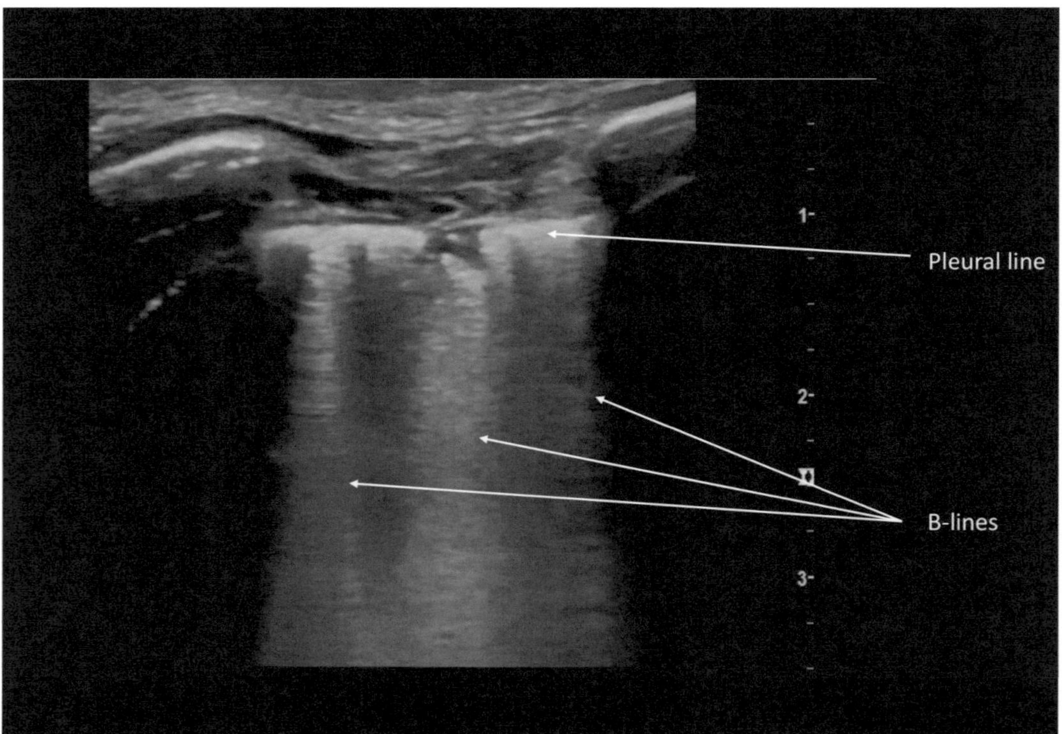

Fig. 5 B-lines & sub-pleural consolidation. Hyperechoic thickened pleura (arrow) with multiple (b-lines) hyperechoic reverberation artefacts originating from the pleura and going to the end of screen (arrows). There is a paucity of the pleural line in the middle replaced by hypoechoic lung tissue which represents sub-pleural consolidation

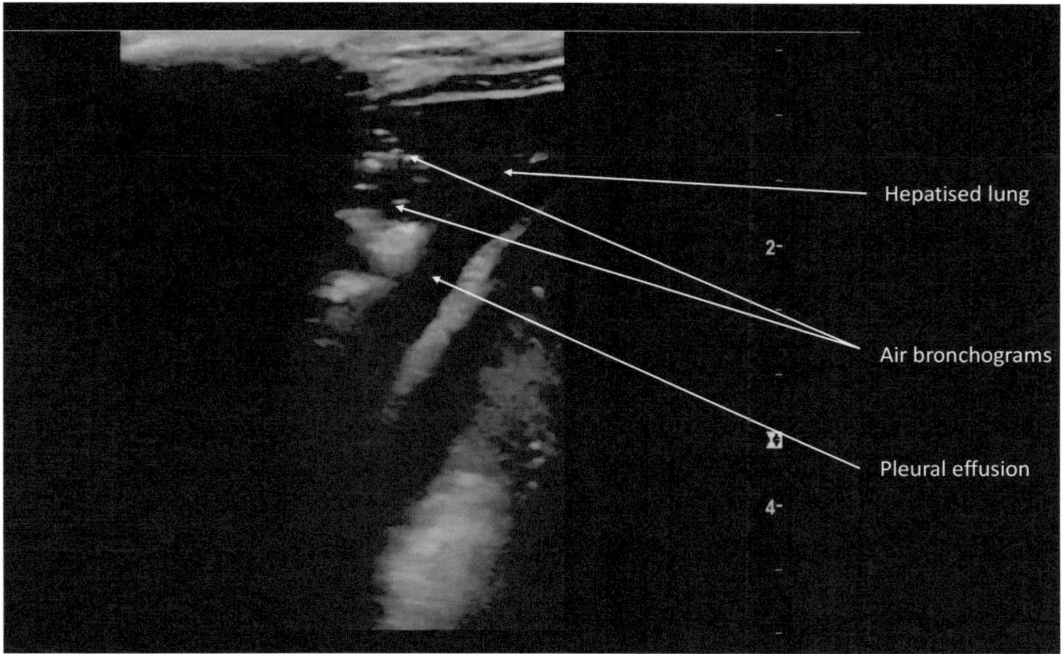

Fig. 6 Lung hepatisation: Consolidated right lower lobe of lung (arrow) appearing as isoechoic structure above the diaphragm resembling liver. Multiple hyperechoic shadows (arrows) within the hepatised lung known as dynamic air bronchograms along with pleural effusion (arrow)

findings, in the context of trauma, raises suspicion of lung contusion.

Key Message

POCUS is more sensitive than plain chest radiography in diagnosing lung contusion in the context of trauma and it can be safely repeated to monitor the progression of the contusion without additional radiation.

Ultrasound of the Heart

Pericardial effusion (see Chap. 26 for further details):

Accumulation of blood in the pericardial sac can occur after trauma leading to sudden increase in pressure in the pericardial sac and collapse of right atrial and then right ventricle free wall [16, 17]. Diagnosis of pericardial tamponade is challenging as signs and symptoms are not very specific [17]. ATLS protocol suggests POCUS to diagnose pericardial effusion as bedside ultrasonography can reliably diagnose pericardial effusion with a greater than 95% accuracy [18, 19]. Subcostal 4 chamber view is the most common window utilised to assess pericardial effusion in trauma. Fluid appears as anechoic rim between the parietal pericardium and right ventricle free wall as this is most dependent part of pericardium. Although cardiac tamponade is a clinical diagnosis, echocardiographic features of tamponade appear before clinical deterioration, specifically, right atrial free wall collapse during right ventricular systole, right ventricular free wall collapse during ventricular diastole along with a dilated non-collapsing IVC are diagnostic of cardiac tamponade (Video 4). Of note, the presence a collapsing IVC has a high negative predictive value for cardiac tamponade. In haemorrhagic pericardial effusion, a hyperechoic fibrinous band can be seen attached to the right ventricular free wall which is due to clotted blood.

POCUS for Procedural Guidance in Chest Trauma

US guided chest drain:

Blunt trauma to the chest can cause pneumothorax, haemothorax or a combination of both. POCUS can be used to guide placement of a small bore 12–18 French chest drain using a modified-Seldinger technique for isolated pneumothorax as a large bore catheter is recommended for haemothorax. Identifying lung point and then inserting the chest tube anterior to it can improve the safety of the procedure.

US guided serratus anterior block:

Rib fractures are very painful and can limit ventilatory effort. This can lead to development of lower respiratory tract infection after a few days if pain is not controlled adequately. Regional anaesthetic administration has now become a preferred method for analgesia in such patients. US-guided serratus anterior [21] and errector spinae plane [22] blocks are most commonly used.

Pearls and highlights

Despite the feasibility and accuracy of POCUS in detecting PTX, there are several complex situations, which the POCUS practitioner should be aware of, to avoid misdiagnosis:

(a) *Pleural adhesions*: can be due to previous surgical pleurodesis or due to lung contusion in a trauma setting. Adherence of pleural layers in some specific areas, prevents air from moving freely inside the pleural cavity [4, 7, 23] and results in the loss of respiratory movement (absence of lung sliding). In contrast to normal physiology, air may also collect in the lower chest area. In a stable patient with known pleural adhesions, the absence of lung sliding alone should not be considered as a direct sign to make the diagnosis of PTX and the entire chest surface should be properly scanned. A more detailed chest computed tomography may be required.

(b) A very small (loculated) pneumothorax: may show the '*double lung point sig'n*. This phenomenon consists of two lung points moving with respirations intermittently appearing at the two opposite sides of the scan. It does not have clinical relevance unless in ventilated patients and in those requiring helicopter transport. In these two specific situations, even the smallest PTX need to be monitored or may warrant prophylactic drainage [7].

(c) Absence of lung sliding: is not a pathognomonic sign of PTX. Lung disorders such as atelectasis, ARDS, selective right mainstem intubation, pneumonectomy, apnea, cardiorespiratory arrest, pleurodesis and bullae abolish the physiological pleural layers movement. Therefore, in the absence of lung sliding, in a stable patient, it is necessary to look for other basic sonographic signs to make a diagnosis.

(d) In hemodynamically unstable/cardiac arrest patients, a fast-track technique is applied to diagnose pneumothorax, consisting of checking for lung sliding, B lines and lung pulse in the least dependent areas of the chest bilaterally, known as 'hot zones'. Absence of these three signs is an indication for immediate drainage whereas in a stable patient, the technique should be extended to the lateral chest looking for the lung point.

(e) Surgical emphysema: The presence of subcutaneous emphysema and loculated pneumothorax can lead to errors when POCUS is used to diagnose pneumothorax in trauma patients. Air in the subcutaneous space prevents the visualisation of the standard normal view of the pleura layers between the two-ribs shadow, known as 'bat sign'.

(f) Lung contusions: cause immediate increase in the density of the peripheral area of the injured lung parenchyma with loss of alveolar air and haemorrhagic infarction, and progression to oedema and infiltrates. This phenomenon can be visualized and monitored accurately over time through the analysis of B lines and consolidations. One of the limitations is that only the consolidation reaching the pleura can be visualised with ultrasound.

Limitations:

1. Trauma patients benefit from rapid POCUS-guided evaluation at the bedside due to ease of use, low cost, no risk of ionizing radiation and reproducibility. In blunt chest trauma, LUS has demonstrated accuracy and safety superior to conventional radiography for conditions such as pneumothorax, lung contusion or haemothorax at the early stage.

2. Given that, POCUS remains strictly 'operator dependent', the use of inappropriate probes, inadequate optimization of the images, lack of knowledge of the possible differential diagnoses are some of the common mistakes reported in literature. To overcome these limitations, the use of standardized guidelines, clinical integration with ultrasound findings are mandatory steps to avoid unnecessary invasive treatment in trauma patients.

References

1. Volpicelli G, Boero E, Sverzellati N, et al. Semi-quantification of pneumothorax volume by lung ultrasound. Intensive Care Med. 2014;40(10):1460–7. https://doi.org/10.1007/s00134-014-3402-9.

2. Steenvoorden TS, Hilderink B, Elbers PWG, et al. Lung point in the absence of pneumothorax. Intensive Care Med. 2018;44(8):1329–30. https://doi.org/10.1007/s00134-018-5112-1.

3. Groote-Bidlingmaier F, Koegelenberg C. A practical guide to transthoracic ultrasound. Breathe. 2012;9:132–42. https://doi.org/10.1183/20734735.024112.

4. Rovida S, Orso D, Naeem S, et al. Lung ultrasound in blunt chest trauma: a clinical review. Ultrasound. 2021. https://doi.org/10.1177/1742271X21994604.

5. Husain L, Hagopian L, Wayman D, et al. Sonographic diagnosis of pneumothorax. J Emerg, Trauma, Shock 2012;5:76–81. https://doi.org/10.4103/0974-2700.93116

6. Lichtenstein D, Mezière G, Biderman P, et al. The "lung point": an ultrasound sign specific to pneumothorax. Intensive Care Med. 2000;26(10):1434–40. https://doi.org/10.1007/s001340000627

7. Volpicelli G, Boero E, Stefanone V, et al. Unusual new signs of pneumothorax at lung ultrasound. Crit Ultrasound J. 2013;5:10. https://doi.org/10.1186/2036-7902-5-10

8. Agricola E, Bove T, Oppizzi M, et al. "Ultrasound comet-tail images": a marker of pulmonary edema: a comparative study with wedge pressure and extravascular lung water. Chest. 2005;127(5):1690–5. https://doi.org/10.1378/chest.127.5.1690

9. Francisco MJ Neto, Rahal A Junior, Vieira FA, et al. Advances in lung ultrasound. Einstein (Sao Paulo, Brazil). 2016;14(3):443–8. https://doi.org/10.1590/s1679-45082016md3557

10. Dickman E, Terentiev V, Likourezos A, et al. Extension of the thoracic spine sign: a new sonographic marker of pleural effusion. J Ultrasound Med. 2015;34(9):1555–61. https://doi.org/10.7863/ultra.15.14.06013.

11. De Luca C, Valentino M, Rimondi MR, et al. Use of chest sonography in acute-care radiology. J Ultrasound. 2008;11(4):125–34. https://doi.org/10.1016/j.jus.2008.09.006.

12. Lee FCY. The curtain sign in lung ultrasound. J Med Ultrasound. 2017;25(2):101–4. https://doi.org/10.1016/j.jmu.2017.04.005.

13. Staub LJ, Biscaro RRM, Kaszubowski E, Maurici R. Chest ultrasonography for the emergency diagnosis of traumatic pneumothorax and haemothorax: a systematic review and meta-analysis. Injury. 2018;49(3):457–66. https://doi.org/10.1016/j.injury.2018.01.033.

14. Soldati G, Sher S, Copetti R. If you see the contusion, there is no pneumothorax. Am J Emerg Med. 2010;28(1):106–7; author reply 107–8. https://doi.org/10.1016/j.ajem.2009.09.003.

15. Helmy S, Beshay B, Hady MA, et al. Role of chest ultrasonography in the diagnosis of lung contusion. Egypt J Chest Dis Tuberc. 2015;64(2), 469–475. https://doi.org/10.1016/j.ejcdt.2014.11.021.

16. Volpicelli G, Mussa A, Garofalo G, et al. Bedside lung ultrasound in the assessment of alveolar-interstitial syndrome. Am J Emerg Med. 2006;24(6):689–96. https://doi.org/10.1016/j.ajem.2006.02.013.

17. Longmore JM; Murray L Wilkinson I, et al. Oxford handbook of clinical medicine (6th ed.). Oxford [Oxfordshire] (2004): Oxford University Press. ISBN 978-0-19-352558-5.

18. Tsang TS, Oh JK, Seward JB. Diagnosis and management of cardiac tamponade in the era of echocardiography. Clin Cardiol. 1999;22(7):446–52. https://doi.org/10.1002/clc.4960220703.

19. Mandavia DP, Hoffner RJ, Mahaney K, et al. Bedside echocardiography by emergency physicians. Ann Emerg Med. 2001;38(4):377–82. https://doi.org/10.1067/mem.2001.118224.

20. Vignon P, Chastagner C, François B, et al. Diagnostic ability of hand-held echocardiography in ventilated critically ill patients. Crit Care. 2003;7(5):R84–91. https://doi.org/10.1186/cc2360.

21. Kunhabdulla NP, Agarwal A, Gaur A, Gautam SK, Gupta R, Agarwal A. Serratus anterior plane block for multiple rib fractures. Pain Physician. 2014;17(4): E553–5.

22. Luftig J, Mantuani D, Herring AA, et al. Successful emergency pain control for posterior rib fractures with ultrasound-guided erector spinae plane block. Am J Emerg Med. 2018;36(8):1391–1396. https://doi.org/10.1016/j.ajem.2017.12.060.

23. Blanco P, Volpicelli G. Common pitfalls in point-of-care ultrasound: a practical guide for emergency and critical care physicians. Crit Ultrasound J. 2016. https://doi.org/10.1186/s13089-016-0052-x.

POCUS in Monitoring: How Monitor Pulmonary Aeration/Deaeration?

Aileen Tan, Antonio Rubino, Sundeep Kaul, and Hatem Soliman-Aboumarie

'It is strange that only extraordinary men make the discoveries, which later appear so easy and simple.'

Georg C. Lichtenberg, German Physicist (1742–1799 AD)

Abstract

Quantitative computerised tomography (CT) looks at lung tissue density and is currently the gold standard in assessing lung aeration in patients with acute respiratory distress syndrome [1]. Lung ultrasound (LUS) is now being proposed as a practical alternative tool for the bedside evaluation and assessment of lung abnormalities [2]. LUS artifacts such as A-lines and B-lines are directly determined by lung density on CT [3]. The relationship between the number of B-lines and lung density in mechanically ventilated patients has been reported in a previous study [4]. In this chapter, we look at how LUS can be used to assess lung aeration and its clinical significance.

Supplementary Information The online version contains supplementary material available at https://doi.org/10.1007/978-3-031-29472-3_24.

A. Tan · A. Rubino
Department of Cardiothoracic Anaesthesia and Intensive Care, Royal Papworth Hospital NHS Foundation Trust, Cambridge, UK
e-mail: aileen.tan@nhs.net

A. Rubino
e-mail: a.rubino@nhs.net

S. Kaul
Departments of Respiratory Medicine and Intensive Care, Harefield Hospital, Lonon, UK
e-mail: s.kaul@rbht.nhs.uk

H. Soliman-Aboumarie (✉)
Department of Anaesthetics and Intensive Care, Harefield Hospital, London, UK
e-mail: hatem.soliman@gmail.com;
h.solimanaboumarie@rbht.nhs.uk

Keywords

Acute respiratory distress syndrome · Lung ultrasound · Lung aeration score · B-lines · Consolidation

Key Messages

- Lung ultrasound can be used to assess lung aeration by calculating a global lung aeration score.
- A re-aeration score can be used to monitor changes in lung aeration over time.
- This scoring system has been widely used in patients with acute respiratory distress syndrome.
- Modifications of this scoring system has been used to monitor lung aeration in other clinical scenarios.
- There is a good correlation between lung aeration score and the degree of aeration in lung tissue on CT scan.

How to assess lung aeration with LUS?

Lung aeration can be assessed directly on lung ultrasound (LUS) in acute lung conditions such as acute respiratory distress syndrome (ARDS), acute cardiogenic pulmonary oedema, community-acquired and ventilator-associated pneumonia, and alveolar proteinosis (post whole lung lavage). POCUS findings should include assessment of A-lines, B-lines and lung consolidation. B-lines are a direct marker of lung aeration which correspond to lung density [2, 5].

Lung aeration in different lung regions and current scoring system:

Lung aeration can be assessed using a scoring system based on a simplified LUS pattern developed by Bouhemad et al. [6]. Using the anterior and posterior axillary lines to divide each hemithorax into three lung regions, each of these lung regions can be further divided into superior and inferior halves to identify twelve regions of interest. A lung aeration score for each region of interest is allocated based on the worst LUS appearance detected (Table 1). A global lung aeration score can be calculated by summating the lung aeration score for all twelve lung regions.

An alternative scoring system has recently been developed by Mongodi et al. to overcome the spatial limitation of LUS scans and take into account non-homogeneous lung pathologies with focal disease. It includes transverse scans and takes into account the percentage of pleural involvement in each region of interest. It also takes into account sonographic changes such as subpleural consolidation and the number of B-lines [7] (Table 2).

Lung reaeration and clinical relevance:

Re-aeration can be assessed by tracking the changes in sonographic findings over an observational period. A lung re-aeration score can be

Table 1 Lung ultrasound patterns corresponding to lung aeration

Degree of lung aeration	Points	Description	Lung ultrasound pattern
Normal lung aeration (N)	0	Normal pulmonary aeration	Visualization of pleural line, horizontal A-line artefacts, presence of lung sliding
Moderate loss of lung aeration (B1)	1	Interstitial oedema resulting from fluid within the interstitial space or thickening of interlobular septa	Presence of multiple and regularly spaced (non-coalescent) vertical B-lines arising from the pleural line
Severe loss of lung aeration (B2)	2	Alveolar-interstitial edema resulting from fluid within the alveolar space, or confluent bronchopneumonia	Presence of coalescent B-lines arising from the pleural line
Complete loss of lung aeration (C)	3	Lung consolidation due to aeration of distal bronchioles and fluid-filled alveoli	Tissue-like structure Lack of variation in lung movement during respiration Hyperechoic punctiform images corresponding to distal air bronchograms

Table 2 Modified lung ultrasound aeration score

Degree of lung aeration	Traditional score	Modified score
Normal lung aeration (N)	0	A-lines
Moderate loss of lung aeration (B1)	1	Artefacts occupying $\leq 50\%$ of the pleura
Severe loss of lung aeration (B2)	2	Artefacts occupying >50% of the pleura
Complete loss of lung aeration (C)	3	Tissue-like structure

Table 3 Lung re-aeration score

1 point	3 points	5 points	−5 points	−3 points	−1 point
B1 → N	B2 → N	C → N	N → C	N → B2	N → B1
B2 → B1	C → B1			B1 → C	B1 → B2
C → B2					B2 → C

calculated based on the LUS pattern change observed over a defined period. A score is given for each region of interest based on Table 1 and 3. This can be summated to obtain a global lung re-aeration score [6].

Assessment of lung re-aeration has been reported in various clinical contexts described below:

– *Daily monitoring of lung aeration*:

LUS gives significant information about the baseline severity of lung aeration and allows for the monitoring over the disease course and eventual lung recovery. This is useful in patients with ARDS, in whom chest x-ray (CXR) has low accuracy and computerised tomography (CT) scan is potentially harmful both due to the higher levels of radiation and risks associated with patient transfer [8]. This becomes even more significant in patients on veno-venous extracorporeal membrane oxygenation (VV-ECMO). A progressive reduction in lung aeration score corresponding to an improvement in lung aeration is seen in patients successfully weaned off VV-ECMO [9, 10].

– *PEEP titration and lung recruitment*:

LUS can be used to titrate positive end-expiratory pressure (PEEP) levels in patients receiving invasive mechanical ventilation in order to optimise lung recruitment in patients with ARDS. There is a significant correlation between lung recruitment as measured by a pressure–volume curve method and the lung re-aeration score resulting in an increase in PaO_2 levels [18].

LUS has enabled us to gain a better understanding of lung aeration and re-aeration patterns in patients with ARDS. Loss of lung aeration was predominantly present in the dependent (lower parts of the posterior lung) regions of the lungs. PEEP-induced lung re-aeration can be confirmed on LUS as the disappearance of B-lines in the anterior and lateral lung regions. Consolidation occurring largely in the lower parts of the lungs were only marginally modified.

Lung recruitment is dependent on the type of lung pathology. Patients with diffuse loss of lung aeration have multiple B-lines or consolidation in all lung regions. Lung re-aeration can be seen in the anterior and lateral lung regions. Patients with focal loss of lung aeration tend to have multiple B-lines or consolidation in the dependent lung regions. Lung re-aeration can be seen in the lower parts of the anterior and lateral lung regions and the upper parts of the posterior lung regions [11].

– *Prone positioning*:

LUS provides constant monitoring of regional lung aeration changes to prone positioning (PP) in patients with ARDS. At one hour after PP, patients with focal ARDS had higher re-aeration changes on LUS in the posterior lung regions and greater aeration loss in the anterior lung regions. Patients with non-focal ARDS had greater re-aeration of the anterior lung regions one hour after returning to the supine position [12].

LUS also allows clinicians to predict which group of patients responded to PP. At baseline, aeration of the lower part of the anterior lung regions on LUS was associated with >20 mmHg improvement in the PaO_2/FiO_2 ratio up to 2 h after returning to supine [13]. Improvement in lung aeration scores 3 h after PP was seen in patients with a PaO_2/FiO_2 ratio <300 mmHg after 7 days and survival at 28 days [14].

– Weaning failure after a spontaneous breathing trial:

LUS aeration changes after a 1 h spontaneous breathing trial (SBT) accurately predicts post-extubation distress in patients who have been mechanically ventilated for >48 h. Loss of lung aeration and a higher lung aeration score at the end of the SBT is greater in patients who fail a SBT. In patients who passed the SBT, a lung aeration score ≤ 12 at the end of the SBT is predictive of post-extubation success whereas a score ≥ 17 is predictive of post-extubation failure [15].

– Antibiotic treatment of ventilator-associated pneumonia:

A lung aeration score, that was adapted to detect the presence of pneumonia, was predictive of the response to a 7 day course of antimicrobial therapy in patients with ventilator-associated pneumonia. A re-aeration score >5 on day 7 was predictive of success whereas a score <−10 was predictive of antimicrobial therapy failure [16].

– Paediatric patients:

A neonatal-adapted lung aeration score with fewer scanning zones in neonates with signs of respiratory distress was shown to predict the need for surfactant administration. LUS was performed in the first few hours of life under continuous positive airway pressure. The lung aeration score correlated with all indices of oxygenation based on transcutaneous blood gas measurements. Furthermore, it predicted the need for surfactant in preterm babies with a gestational age of less than 34 weeks with good reliability [17].

– Lung aeration and CXR:

Using a dedicated software to digitally process CXR, Wallet et al. showed good correlation between changes in lung density and lung recruitment, as measured by a pressure–volume curve method, at different levels of PEEP [18]. At present, this method is not routinely used in clinical practice.

Various studies have reported low accuracy of bedside CXR in detecting alveolar interstitial syndrome and alveolar consolidation [19, 20]. CXR has been known to have limited diagnostic accuracy in patients with ARDS [19] due to its potential to miss early ARDS changes [21]. Furthermore, portable anteroposterior CXRs [22] have technical limitations that may reduce the quality of the CXR images [19]. Similarly, Bouhemad et al. found that CXR was inaccurate in predicting lung re-aeration in patients undergoing antimicrobial therapy for ventilator-associated pneumonia [16].

– Lung aeration and CT scan as gold standard:

CT quantitative analysis is the gold standard in computing lung aeration. It allows an accurate assessment of the volumes of both gas and lung tissue [1]. However, it requires a dedicated software and manual delineation of lung parenchyma in each image which is a time-consuming and cumbersome process [23, 24]. The high ionizing radiation also limits repeatability of the procedure [25]. Furthermore, it requires transportation of the patient to the radiology department, which is a risky procedure that necessitates the presence of trained physicians and specific cardiorespiratory monitoring [26].

Both global and regional lung aeration scores have been shown to correlate with lung tissue aeration on CT quantitative analysis at different levels of PEEP. However, lung aeration scores do not correlate with PEEP-induced lung recruitment when assessed on CT. This is possibly due to the definition of lung recruitment being a decrease in non-aerated lung tissue on CT. This does not take into consideration patients with incomplete loss of tissue aeration

(B1 and B2) who respond to PEEP with a decrease in lung aeration score [27].

When lung aeration was defined as the additional volume of gas present in the lungs on CT, a significant correlation was found with the lung re-aeration score in patients with ventilator-associated pneumonia after one week of antimicrobial therapy [16].

References

1. Rouby JJ, Puybasset L, Nieszkowska A, Lu Q. Acute respiratory distress syndrome: lessons from computed tomography of the whole lung. Crit Care Med. 2003;31(4 Suppl):S285–95. https://doi.org/10.1097/01.CCM.0000057905.74813.BC.

2. Volpicelli G, Elbarbary M, Blaivas M, et al. International evidence-based recommendations for point-of-care lung ultrasound. Intensive Care Med. 2012;38(4):577–91. https://doi.org/10.1007/s00134-012-2513-4.

3. Soldati G, Inchingolo R, Smargiassi A, et al. Ex vivo lung sonography: morphologic-ultrasound relationship. Ultrasound Med Biol. 2012;38(7):1169–79. https://doi.org/10.1016/j.ultrasmedbio.2012.03.001.

4. Baldi G, Gargani L, Abramo A, et al. Lung water assessment by lung ultrasonography in intensive care: a pilot study. Intensive Care Med. 2013;39(1):74–84. https://doi.org/10.1007/s00134-012-2694-x.

5. Via G, Lichtenstein D, Mojoli F, et al. Whole lung lavage: a unique model for ultrasound assessment of lung aeration changes. Intensive Care Med. 2010;36(6):999–1007. https://doi.org/10.1007/s00134-010-1834-4.

6. Bouhemad B, Mongodi S, Via G, Rouquette I. Ultrasound for "lung monitoring" of ventilated patients. Anesthesiology. 2015;122(2):437–47. https://doi.org/10.1097/ALN.0000000000000558.

7. Mongodi S, Bouhemad B, Orlando A, et al. Modified lung ultrasound score for assessing and monitoring pulmonary aeration. Ultraschall Med. 2017;38(5):530–7. https://doi.org/10.1055/s-0042-120260.

8. Mongodi S, Bonaiti S, Stella A, et al. Lung ultrasound for daily monitoring and management of ARDS patients. Clin Pulm Med. 2019;26(3):92–7.

9. Mongodi S, Pozzi M, Orlando A, et al. Lung ultrasound for daily monitoring of ARDS patients on extracorporeal membrane oxygenation: preliminary experience. Intensive Care Med. 2018;44(1):123–4. https://doi.org/10.1007/s00134-017-4941-7.

10. Lu X, Arbelot C, Schreiber A, Langeron O, Monsel A, Lu Q. Ultrasound assessment of lung aeration in subjects supported by venovenous extracorporeal membrane oxygenation. Respir Care. 2019;64(12):1478–87. https://doi.org/10.4187/respcare.06907.

11. Bouhemad B, Brisson H, Le-Guen M, Arbelot C, Lu Q, Rouby JJ. Bedside ultrasound assessment of positive end-expiratory pressure-induced lung recruitment. Am J Respir Crit Care Med. 2011;183(3):341–7. https://doi.org/10.1164/rccm.201003-0369OC

12. Haddam M, Zieleskiewicz L, Perbet S, et al. Lung ultrasonography for assessment of oxygenation response to prone position ventilation in ARDS. Intensive Care Med. 2016;42(10):1546–56. https://doi.org/10.1007/s00134-016-4411-7.

13. Prat G, Guinard S, Bizien N, et al. Can lung ultrasonography predict prone positioning response in acute respiratory distress syndrome patients? J Crit Care. 2016;32:36–41. https://doi.org/10.1016/j.jcrc.2015.12.015.

14. Wang XT, Ding X, Zhang HM, et al. Lung ultrasound can be used to predict the potential of prone positioning and assess prognosis in patients with acute respiratory distress syndrome. Crit Care. 2016;20(1):385. https://doi.org/10.1186/s13054-016-1558-0.

15. Soummer A, Perbet S, Brisson H, et al. Ultrasound assessment of lung aeration loss during a successful weaning trial predicts postextubation distress*. Crit Care Med. 2012;40(7):2064–72. https://doi.org/10.1097/CCM.0b013e31824e68ae.

16. Bouhemad B, Liu ZH, Arbelot C, et al. Ultrasound assessment of antibiotic-induced pulmonary reaeration in ventilator-associated pneumonia. Crit Care Med. 2010;38(1):84–92. https://doi.org/10.1097/CCM.0b013e3181b08cdb.

17. Brat R, Yousef N, Klifa R, Reynaud S, Shankar Aguilera S, De Luca D. Lung ultrasonography score to evaluate oxygenation and surfactant need in neonates treated with continuous positive airway pressure. JAMA Pediatr. 2015;169(8): e151797. https://doi.org/10.1001/jamapediatrics.2015.1797.

18. Wallet F, Delannoy B, Haquin A, et al. Evaluation of recruited lung volume at inspiratory plateau pressure with PEEP using bedside digital chest X-ray in patients with acute lung injury/ARDS. Respir Care. 2013;58(3):416–23. https://doi.org/10.4187/respcare.01893.

19. Lichtenstein D, Goldstein I, Mourgeon E, Cluzel P, Grenier P, Rouby JJ. Comparative diagnostic performances of auscultation, chest radiography, and lung ultrasonography in acute respiratory distress syndrome. Anesthesiology. 2004;100(1):9–15. https://doi.org/10.1097/00000542-200401000-00006.

20. Xirouchaki N, Magkanas E, Vaporidi K, et al. Lung ultrasound in critically ill patients: comparison with bedside chest radiography. Intensive Care Med. 2011;37(9):1488–93. https://doi.org/10.1007/s00134-011-2317-y.

21. See KC, Ong V, Tan YL, Sahagun J, Taculod J. Chest radiography versus lung ultrasound for identification of acute respiratory distress syndrome: a retrospective observational study. Crit Care. 2018;22(1):203. https://doi.org/10.1186/s13054-018-2105-y.

22. Rubinowitz AN, Siegel MD, Tocino I. Thoracic imaging in the ICU. Crit Care Clin. 2007;23(3):539–73. https://doi.org/10.1016/j.ccc.2007.06.001.

23. Chiumello D, Marino A, Brioni M, et al. Visual anatomical lung CT scan assessment of lung recruitability. Intensive Care Med. 2013;39(1):66–73. https://doi.org/10.1007/s00134-012-2707-9.

24. Arbelot C, Ferrari F, Bouhemad B, Rouby JJ. Lung ultrasound in acute respiratory distress syndrome and acute lung injury. Curr Opin Crit Care. 2008;14(1):70–4. https://doi.org/10.1097/MCC.0b013e3282f43d05.

25. Mayo JR, Aldrich J, Muller NL, Society F. Radiation exposure at chest CT: a statement of the Fleischner Society. Radiology. 2003;228(1):15–21. https://doi.org/10.1148/radiol.2281020874.

26. Beckmann U, Gillies DM, Berenholtz SM, Wu AW, Pronovost P. Incidents relating to the intra-hospital transfer of critically ill patients. An analysis of the reports submitted to the Australian Incident Monitoring Study in Intensive Care. Intensive Care Med. 2004;30(8):1579–85. https://doi.org/10.1007/s00134-004-2177-9.

27. Chiumello D, Mongodi S, Algieri I, et al. Assessment of lung aeration and recruitment by CT scan and ultrasound in acute respiratory distress syndrome patients. Crit Care Med. 2018;46(11):1761–8. https://doi.org/10.1097/CCM.0000000000003340.

POCUS in Cardiac Arrest

Liana Shirley and Christopher Shirley

Even the right tool if used in the wrong way can lead to failure rather than success

The authors

Abstract

The use of focussed ultrasound in cardiac arrest continues to develop as an effective source of identifying and excluding the reversible causes. In this chapter we will explore the value of this point of care diagnostic tool; and what information this gives us to guide treatment with certainty and expedience during time critical resuscitation. This chapter will also examine the pitfalls of incorporating focused ultrasound into a cardiac arrest setting and explore the human factors that can enhance or impede the delivery of care. The effective integration of POCUS into established cardiac arrest algorithms without detriment to the evidence-based treatment such as CPR and defibrillation, is essential. Non-technical aspects such as planning, communication, leadership and team membership are all critical to success. These skills must be honed by specific training in rapid focussed image acquisition and scenario-based simulations to co-ordinate the team. It is only when all of these technical and non-technical skills are effectively applied together, that the success of diagnostic ultrasound during cardiac arrest resuscitation completely emerges.

Supplementary Information The online version contains supplementary material available at https://doi.org/10.1007/978-3-031-29472-3_25.

L. Shirley (✉)
Advanced Imaging Specialist Cardiology, MSc Advanced Clinical Practice & PwSI in Cardiology, Betsi Cadwaladr University Health Board, Wales, UK
e-mail: liana.shirley@wales.nhs.uk

C. Shirley
Professional Development Lead: Resuscitation Services, Betsi Cadwaladr University Health Board, Wales, UK
e-mail: christopher.shirley@wales.nhs.uk

Keywords

Cardiac arrest · POCUS · Point of care ultrasound · Tamponade · Resuscitation

Key messages

- POCUS during cardiac arrest has the potential of identifying reversible causes of cardiac arrest and guiding further management.
- The effective integration of POCUS into established cardiac arrest algorithms without detriment to the evidence-based treatment such as CPR and defibrillation, is essential.
- Understanding the role of human factors which can enhance or impede the delivery of care during CPR is crucial for effective resuscitation.
- It is important to understand that if both the technical and non-technical skills required are considered and employed; POCUS can be safely and effectively embedded into cardiac arrest management.

Introduction

Cardiac arrest is the most extreme end point of acute emergency care and is the leading cause of disability and death Worldwide [1]. Many causes of cardiac arrest are reversible therefore Identifying and treating this cause is crucial in an attempt to improve the patient outcome.

POCUS is increasingly recognised as having a valuable role in timely and effective decision making during this critical phase of acute care by identifying or excluding these reversible causes and guiding further management. This diagnostic tool is only successful when its application does not hinder evidence-based treatments. There have been numerous papers, chapters and studies written on the use of POCUS in cardiac arrest and its use is not novel practice, however, there are still reservations and reluctance of its standard use with topics mainly comprising of training limitations, interruption to CPR and disruption of teamwork. Part I of this chapter will

initially provide a brief overview of the technical aspects of the use of POCUS in cardiac arrest, in terms of identifying and excluding the reversal causes, and Part II of the chapter will proceed to examine in more detail the non-technical 'human factors' that can in many respects lead its use being underutilised.

Part I: What Information Can Point of Care Ultrasound (POCUS) Give Us?

Since the origins of clinical echocardiography credited to Carl Helmuth Hertz and Inge Edler back in the 1950s [2], substantial advancements have been made, they are, regrettably, too many to include in this chapter. However, with the developments of image quality and transportability of handheld diagnostic ultrasound machines it is unsurprising that the use of ultrasound has magnified in clinical practice, but its use in cardiac arrest still appears to be underutilised.

It is important to recognise that if applied appropriately POCUS will provide additional diagnostic information that can, and has, led to changes in cardiac arrest management [3, 4]. When a non-electrical cause of cardiac arrest is identified (PEA) the focus is to identify and treat the underlying cause of the cardiac arrest, without this intervention the outcome is poor. Reversible causes of cardiac arrest are often defined as the 'Hs and Ts' some of these can be diagnosed at the bedside (Hypoxia, Hypothermia and Hypo/hyperkalaemia. Hypovolemia) may be obvious in the case of a severe trauma or bleed but equally it may not be.

The remaining reversible causes rely on subjective clinical assessment 'best guess' decisions (Tamponade, coronary and pulmonary embolism, tension pneumothorax) or laboratory investigations with Toxins. However, with the introduction of focussed ultrasound appropriately applied and interpreted, we can identify / exclude all but one by the bedside with certainty.

Tamponade

A rapid accumulation even of a small amount of pericardial fluid resulting in tamponade can, if not treated, lead to cardiac arrest, unless this was an identified diagnosis prior to the collapse, this would be a challenging judgement. During a cardiac arrest the traditional clinical features of tamponade, known as the Beck's triad of hypotension, jugular venous distention and muffled heart sounds are not available [5]. In the situation of a cardiac arrest, the use of POCUS changes this degree of uncertainty to assurance including the opportunity for guided intervention (POCUS-guided pericardiocentesis) (see Chap. 27 for further details).

Figure 1 shows left parasternal long axis view and Fig. 2 shows an apical four chamber image of a clear pericardial effusion, noted by the echo-free space surrounding most of the heart as indicated by the arrows. Note this is an obvious abnormality which can be detected even by novice sonographers. Further details on POCUS features of cardiac tamponade are discussed in detail in Chap. 27.

Pulmonary Embolism

A pulmonary embolism that results in cardiac arrest is likely to be massive/submassive and mortality rates from this are generally dismal with records as high as 95% [6]. Their presentation can be fairly non-specific, and this can cause difficulty identifying a definitive diagnosis. POCUS findings of right ventricular dilatation without an underlying cause (pulmonary disease, valve disease etc.) would indicate a high probability of pulmonary embolism, potentially facilitating a more timely management and treatment. Figure 3 shows an apical four chamber view, and highlights a significantly dilated right ventricle, as indicated by the arrow, note again this right ventricle will be noticeably larger than the left ventricle.

Coronary Embolism

Whilst a dilated right ventricle in the presence of a large pulmonary embolism will be obvious using POCUS even by the relatively inexperienced sonographers, in the case of a coronary

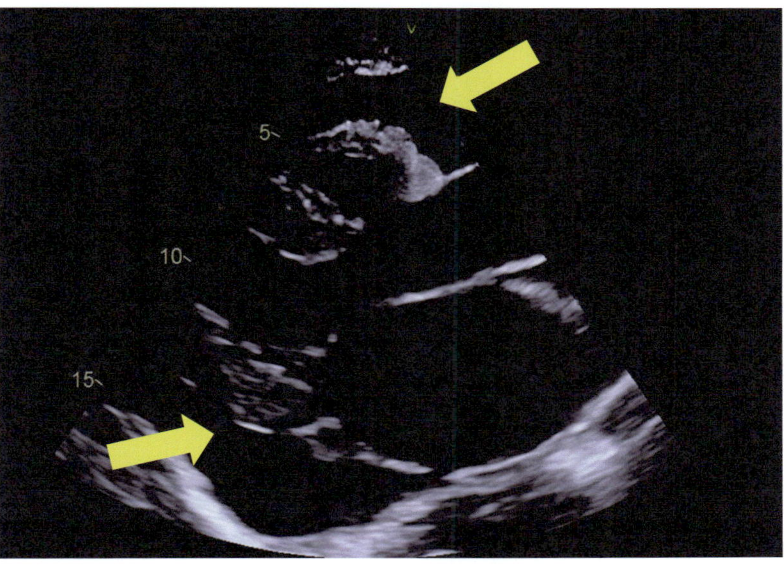

Fig. 1 Left parasternal view showing a collection of pericardial fluid (indicated by yellow arrows) around the heart

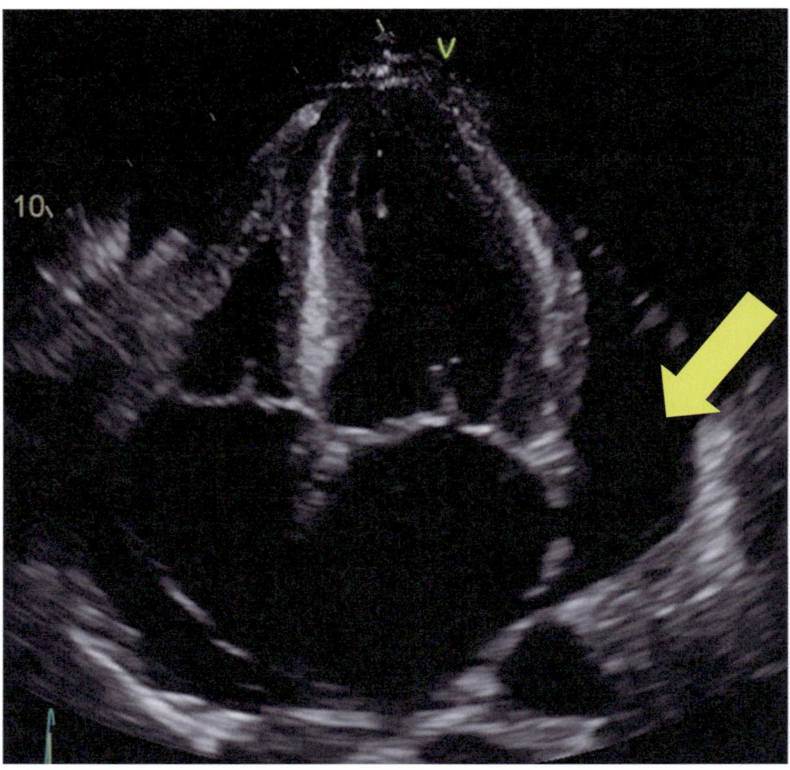

Fig. 2 Apical four chamber view with pericardial fluid (indicated by the yellow arrow)

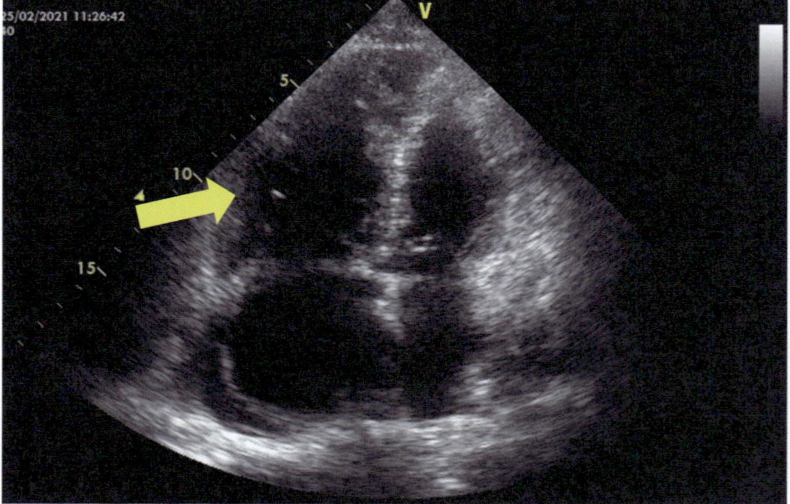

Fig. 3 Apical four chamber view showing a dilated right ventricle (indicated by the yellow arrow)

embolism, unless a thrombus is directly observed the diagnosis may be more challenging. During cardiac arrest where there is ongoing activity, the more experienced sonographer would be able to identify regional wall motion abnormalities which would indicate a previous myocardial infarction or new ischaemia. If this is noted in a cardiac arrest setting, coupled with the clinical presentation, it may indicate a change to the therapeutic intervention.

Hypovolaemia–Hypercontractile 'Kissing' Ventricle

Although hypovolaemic causes of cardiac arrest may be externally obvious such as haemorrhage or diarrhoea and vomiting, equally they may be hidden for example in sepsis or internal bleeding. A number of Echocardiographic features have been shown to correlate with severe hypovolaemia, these include the presence of a hyperkinetic small left ventricle with an end systolic cavity obliteration (kissing ventricle), and a small inferior vena cava in the context of normal RV size and function. In the collapsed patient where clinical findings and POCUS findings suggest severe hypovolaemia, volume resuscitation can be instigated guided by POCUS. Figure 4 shows a left parasternal long axis view of a left ventricle in diastole, and Fig. 5 shows the same ventricle with near cavity obliteration in systole. In a cardiac arrest with a normal right ventricle this would suggest a significantly underfilled heart.

Tension Pneumothorax

The use of POCUS to detect tension pneumothorax in a cardiac arrest has gained increasing validity and there are many articles declaring its usefulness. However, the optimal transducer for this would be a linear array or micro convex probe for scanning the pleura rather than the cardiac phased array probe which is used for identifying the other reversible causes of cardiac arrest.

Diagnosing tension pneumothorax using POCUS focuses on four key features:

Absence of lung sliding, absence of B lines, presence of lung point and absence of lung pulse.

However, in a clinical emergency with features suggestive of a tension pneumothorax, the treatment by needle de-compression must not be delayed in order to gain POCUS confirmation [7].

On reflection, there is no doubt that POCUS has the potential to detect and exclude reversible causes of cardiac arrest and there have been studies to suggest a significant change in the clinical management following a POCUS scan

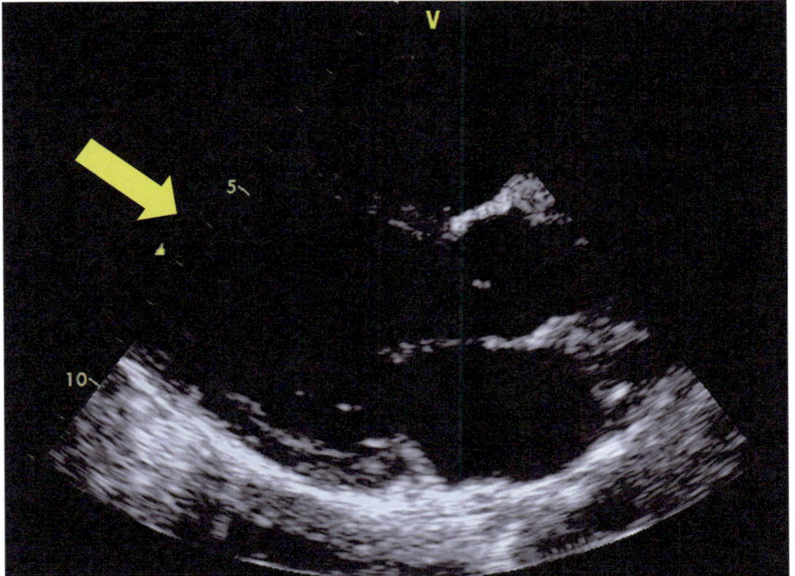

Fig. 4 Parasternal long axis view showing the left ventricle in diastole

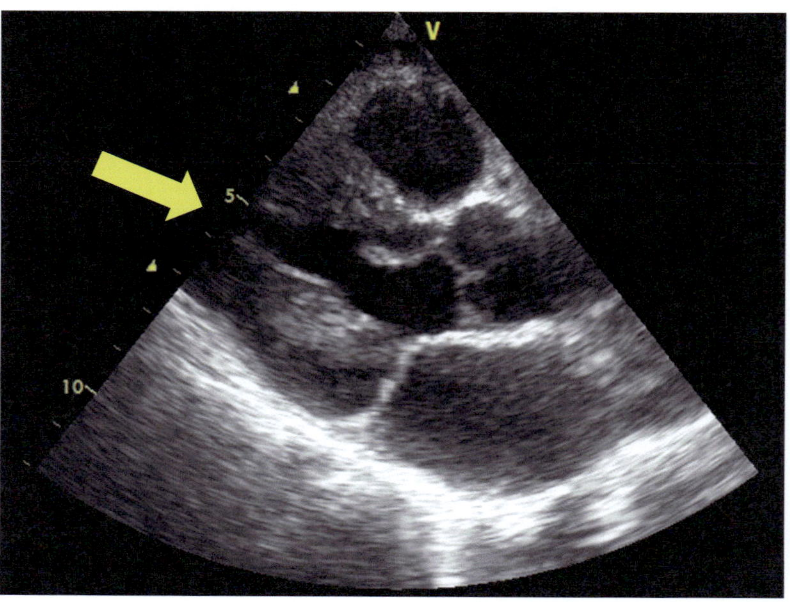

Fig. 5 The same scan this time in systole showing hyper contractile left ventricle and near obliteration of the cavity

[3] so why is this modality not a standard practice yet?

In the beginning of this chapter, we referred to training limitations, interruption to CPR and disruption of teamwork so let us explore that further!

Part II: The 'Right Tool', Used in the 'Right Way'…

Even the right tool if used in the wrong way can lead to failure rather than success. As a keen walker in my local mountains, a very simplified example of the right tool for me could be my walking boots. However even wearing the right boots could lead to me having to abandon the trip through pain and discomfort, if I put them on the wrong feet as shown in Fig. 6. An example of using the right tool, but in the wrong way leading to failure.

In the context of this chapter, the use of the 'right tool in the wrong way' is to employ POCUS in cardiac arrest management, without considering how it will affect the behaviours of the other members of the resuscitation team. Resuscitation teams can be analogous to complex mechanisms with individual components having to behave and perform in specific and consistent ways. When placed in concert with one another, these individual components work together to produce the overall effect, much like the cogs in a clock or watch. If we introduce a new 'cog' it will undoubtedly affect the behaviour of the others and this must therefore be taken into account for the new component to fit into the overall process. In cardiac arrest management, the introduction of a new component into a known algorithm (especially with new equipment); without clear communication, planning, and training to create familiarity, creates an environment with an increased likelihood of confusion and distraction which can quickly lead to loss of situational awareness by the team. Such breakdowns in the teamwork are often attributed to 'Human Factors' and can be deleterious to the patient outcomes.

The concept of employing POCUS as part of cardiac arrest management is not new, and if you go back over a decade and read journals in the subjects of resuscitation, critical care, and sonography; you will see that the conversation of the merits/demerits of the use of POCUS in cardiac arrest was certainly active as far back as 2010 and beyond [3, 8–10]. Given the benefits of POCUS in cardiac arrest already discussed in this

Fig. 6 When applied incorrectly (in this case the boots have been put on the wrong feet), even using the right boots will result in failure

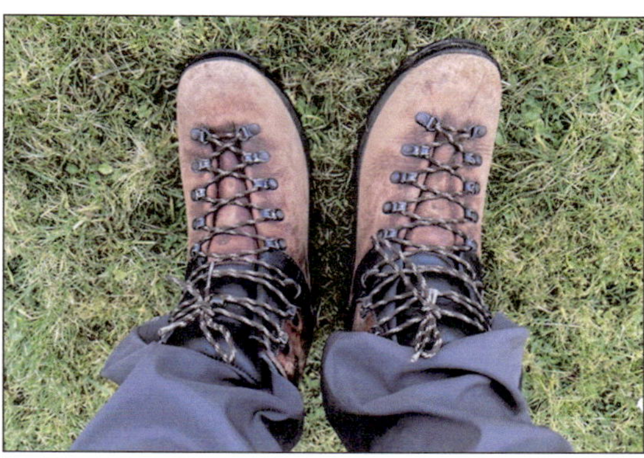

chapter, it is apt to consider that while its use is growing, over a decade later it has not yet become standard routine practice to see ultrasound being used in cardiac arrest management.

The most common demerit would be the position that the inclusion of POCUS may lead to delays in other therapies or extend the 'hands off' periods during CPR [11, 12]. Clearly such delays may be highly detrimental to the patient and should be avoided. On the 'other side of the coin' there are papers showing that with the right training, interpretable images can be reliably obtained within the 10s limit of a pulse check, even by those not already familiar with sonography; and that if POCUS is applied appropriately the scan findings can positively alter decision making and resuscitation management [3]. It is these factors; the training and subsequent 'drilling' of the technical skills already discussed, and non-technical skills/'human factors' that together are the key elements to the success or failure of implementing POCUS into cardiac arrest management.

The Window of Opportunity

Resuscitation in cardiac arrest is a time critical process. It is vital that POCUS imaging does not impede treatments such as defibrillation or increase the 'hands-off' time in CPR. Consensus from bodies such as the Resuscitation Council UK (RCUK), European Resuscitation Council (ERC), and American Heart Association is that the placement of POCUS within their existing algorithms should be during the 10s pulse check on the 'non-shockable' side of the algorithm. Figure 7 shows the algorithms for the ERC and RCUK and illustrates that the POCUS scan would take place during the pulse check on the 'non shockable side' of the algorithm as indicated by the arrow and dashed red rectangle.

It may be helpful to refer to this as our 'window of opportunity', and 10s is a very short time when you consider all the simultaneous actions that need to take place including: the identification of the underlying rhythm; a pulse check; and the acquisition, optimisation, and recording of interpretable POCUS images. However, this is achievable within the window of opportunity if the following factors are employed in a structured and meaningful way:

- Training
- Planning & Preparation
- Communication
- Teamwork

Training: *Train, Train, & Train Again...*

Train: For first time learners, sonography is a completely new discipline and is an unfamiliar skillset requiring visualisation skills, and a high degree of hand–eye coordination. For more experienced sonographers, POCUS is a different

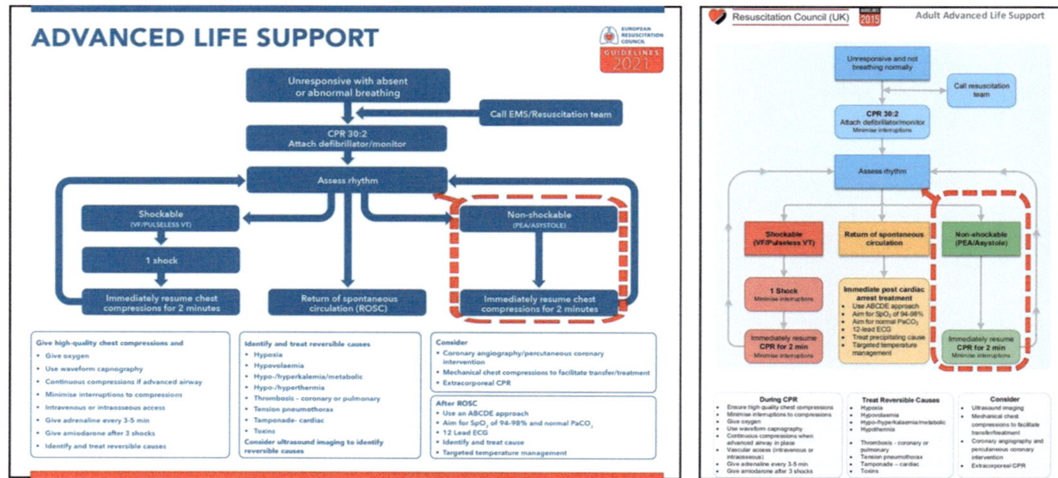

Fig. 7 Algorithms reproduced with the kind permission of RCUK, and ERC 2021

mindset than their day to day 'elective' practice; with different challenges including limitations to what views are obtained, extreme time constraints, and sub optimal environments and patient positioning. For these reasons, specific training is essential to develop the technical skills required for new learners, and to equip more experienced scanners with the mindset to strip away all but the basics and answer only very specific questions and nothing more. There are several courses designed for POCUS in critical care / emergency care settings and while primarily designed to develop the technical skills, they also touch on an awareness of the human factors concepts.

Train: The courses designed to introduce and develop these skills, are really just the start of a journey of competence. Attending a one-day course does not immediately lead to a competent POCUS sonographer who is able to perform interpretable scans under challenging and stressful conditions. The technical skills require development and 'honing' and many of the courses require a portfolio of scans to be completed over a time period under the mentorship of experienced sonographers before certified status is awarded.

Train again: The final training aspect is the drilling of both the technical and non-technical skills in resuscitation-based simulations, ideally using the members of the cardiac arrest teams. This leads to familiarity to the process for all of the team. It enables the human factors to be practiced in a safe environment and the team can explore where their strengths and weaknesses are and jointly come up with solutions that support one another. As the team practice and become more familiar with the new process, a POCUS scan can mesh seamlessly into the resuscitation without distraction or impairment to any other treatments or actions.

Planning and Preparation

Before the emergency… The planning in terms of POCUS in cardiac arrest begins far in advance of the emergency event itself. POCUS is growing in popularity for a number of uses in different settings and purposes. As a result, ultrasound machines are increasingly found in many different critical care settings, and it is important to find and become familiar with the different machines around the hospital. Knowing where the nearest machine is, and how to turn on,

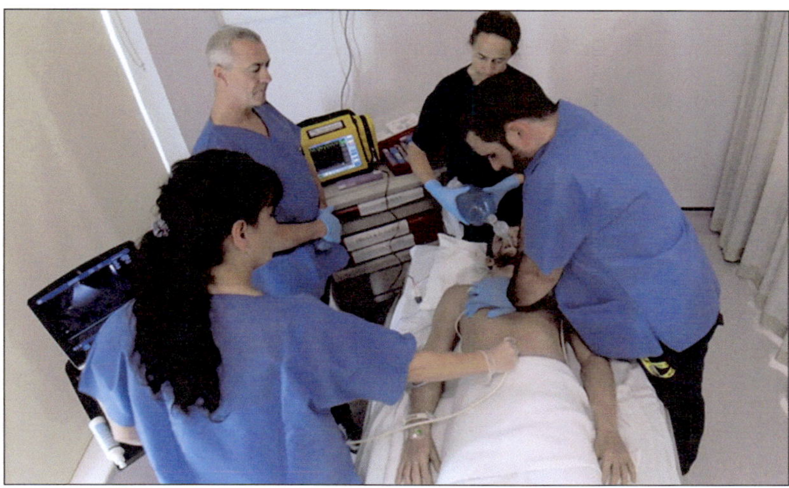

Fig. 8 Effective positioning of team members means the sonographer can be in position ready to scan without interrupting CPR

optimise, and record an image before an emergency saves valuable time during an actual resuscitation. Additionally, handheld devices are increasingly capable and popular for POCUS and compared to the larger models are relatively inexpensive. While they often have less features than larger machines, the images these handheld devices produce are certainly of sufficient quality for use in this setting.

During the emergency… Planning is important during a resuscitation and it is too late to ask for a POCUS scan just before a pulse check. Time is required to obtain, power up, and prepare a machine to be ready to perform a scan in the next window of opportunity. Resuscitation team leaders need to have this in mind and the key here is…Ask early!!!

Pulse checks occur at predictable intervals and do not arrive suddenly and without warning. This gives the team leader the ability to plan ahead and discuss the actions that will be required during the next pulse check with the team and assign those actions to individual team members. Remember multiple actions have to occur simultaneously during the pulse check and getting everyone into position and ready before CPR is halted means that no time is wasted. A well-positioned team means that everyone can carry out their tasks without impeding anybody else. Team members with direct roles should have enough space to carry out their tasks effectively.

For the sonographer, positioning the probe for a subcostal view is often optimal as it can easily be ready before CPR is paused and without getting in the way of chest compressions. Overcrowding at cardiac arrests is not uncommon, and team leaders should not be afraid to limit and control the number of people in the patient's direct vicinity.

In Fig. 8 you can see that effective positioning of the team enables the ultrasound probe to be positioned for a subcostal view; ready to obtain an image prior to the pause in CPR at the next pulse check. You can also see that the ultrasound machine is powered on and has been optimised ready to scan.

Communication

For resuscitation to be effective, and for the team to function as a coherent unit, communication is paramount. Team leaders can only put into practice the planning discussed in the above paragraph, if there is effective two-way communication between the team leader and team members. When planning the actions in the next window of opportunity, team leaders need to allocate tasks to individuals rather than to the room as a whole. Each team member should know what is expected of them during the rhythm check, and what others will be doing at

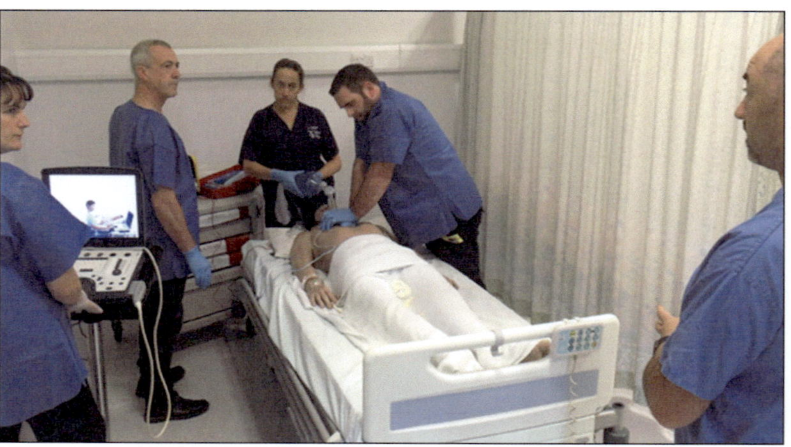

Fig. 9 Clear planning and communication is essential to identify each team members roles before CPR is paused

the same time. In respect of the POCUS scan, the sonographer can be instructed to prepare the machine and optimise settings, then place the probe prior to stopping CPR; ready to scan as soon as CPR stops. Contingencies for whether to complete or abandon the scan should be in place before CPR is paused. Once the team leader is happy that everyone has their allocated tasks and understands their actions, then the rhythm check should be 'counted in' and the tasks are carried out simultaneously. Figure 9 gives an example of a team leader communicating with the whole team in this manner prior to the pause in CPR.

Teamwork

Obtaining the images… Here in Fig. 10, you can see that chest compressions have now stopped, and in this brief period the following actions are being carried out simultaneously: the POCUS image is recorded; the underlying cardiac rhythm is assessed; and the presence of a palpable pulse is confirmed/excluded.

For the sonographer especially, situational awareness is an important factor. Several things could happen that will affect their required actions:

- If a shockable rhythm is identified they must immediately abandon the scan in order to enable the rapid and safe delivery of a defibrillation shock.

- If an image cannot be obtained in the first few seconds, then the sonographer should declare this to the team leader, and the scan should be abandoned. Additional time spent 'hunting' for an image risks delaying the pause in CPR beyond the 10 s window which is detrimental to the overall resuscitation. A plan for the next rhythm check can be made based on the nature of the issue identified. It may be that different depth settings may be required, or that the acoustic window was poor in that particular view, and an alternative view such as parasternal long axis might be more useful. Requests for "just a few more seconds" are indicative of a loss of situational awareness, and that the 10 s window is at risk of breach. Remember there will be another opportunity to scan again in a few minutes and it is better to abandon and make a new plan, than to extend the break in CPR.

- If the sonographer can rapidly acquire an interpretable image, then the rest of the time should be spent recording the scan and continuing to optimise the image on screen. The sonographer should not attempt to interpret the scan during acquisition, as this can lead quickly to a loss of situational awareness and again risks prolonging the 'hands off' time for CPR. Instead, an 'acquire and withdraw' approach can be adopted. This enables the time during the scan to be spent optimising the recorded image to obtain the best possible quality for review. As soon as the 10 s are finished the

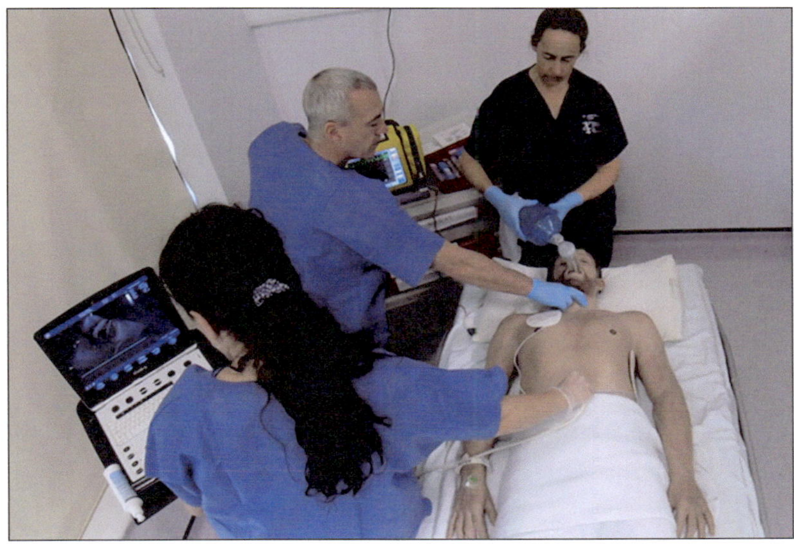

Fig. 10 During the ten second pause in CPR for a rhythm check, an effective team with identified roles completes their tasks quickly with no distractions from the POCUS scan

sonographer can withdraw away from the resuscitation to review and report on the best quality recorded image they could obtain.

Reviewing & Reporting… Once an optimised image has been obtained at the patient's side it may be beneficial to withdraw away from the resuscitation area to review the images and form a focussed report. This has two possible advantages:

- It enables the resuscitation to continue without distraction and also reduces the personnel and equipment in the immediate resuscitation area.
- It enables the sonographer to analyse the images away from the potentially stressful resuscitation environment and under better lighting conditions.

When reviewing the images, it is important to only look to answer the questions relating to identifying the potentially reversible causes of cardiac arrest as discussed earlier in the chapter. To avoid a human factors term known as 'anchoring bias' in which increased emphasis is given to just a part of the available information, limiting decision making options; it is important to ensure that all possible questions (evidence of each of the reversible causes) are answered in turn, rather than just reporting on one 'piece of the puzzle'. Formalising the report may be a useful way to ensure that all possible questions are answered. Additionally, as the sonographer it is useful to report on what they can see and also what they cannot see or confirm. Stating that something cannot be seen or confirmed is not the same as stating that particular cause can be excluded and is often equally useful to the team leader. It may be helpful to report using terms such as:

- There is evidence of…'x'
- There is no evidence of…'y'
- 'z'… could not be confirmed or excluded due to the limitations of the image obtained.

The sonographer should report their findings back to the team leader at the earliest opportunity.

Video 1 showing the implementation of POCUS into cardiac arrest simulation.

Conclusion

Decision-making is a human factor trait that can become impaired under stress, and in time critical situations where information may be limited [13]. If we think of decision making as choosing a course of action, using sound judgement, based on the available information; then when employed within the setting of cardiac arrest resuscitation, POCUS can be a useful decision-making tool. It improves both the availability and quality of the information upon which our decisions can be made. When such information is available, actions can be chosen rapidly and based on evidence rather than on a 'best guess' basis; and the effective use of POCUS can positively influence patient management in many resuscitation events [3].

It is also important to understand that if both the technical and non-technical skills required are considered and employed; POCUS can be safely and effectively embedded into cardiac arrest management.

References

1. Hussein L, Rehman M, Sajid R, Annajjar F, Al-Janabi T (2019) Bedside ultrasound in cardiac standstill: a clinical review. The Ultrasound Journal. https://doi.org/10.1186/s13089-019-0150-7
2. Maleki M, Esmaeilzadeh M. The Evolutionary Development of Echocardiography. Iranian Journal of Medical Sciences. 2012;37:222–32.
3. Price S, Uddin S, Quinn T. Echocardiography in cardiac arrest. Curr Opin Crit Care. 2010;16:211–5.
4. El Sayed M, Zaghrini E. Prehospital Emergency Ultrasound: A Review of Current Clinical Applications, Challenges, and Future Implications. Emergency Medicine International. 2013;2013:1–6.
5. Jensen JK, Poulsen SH, Mølgaard H. Cardiac tamponade: a clinical challenge. Кардиология: от науки к практике. 2017(4):107–13.
6. Laher A, Richards G. Cardiac arrest due to pulmonary embolism. Indian Heart J. 2018;70:731–5.
7. Price S, Uddin S, Pitcher D, Lockey A, Mitchell S, Harris S, Jaggar S, Hampshire S (2013) Focused Echocardiography in Emergency Life Support, 2nd ed. 33
8. Hayhurst C, Lebus C, Atkinson P, Kendall R, Madan R, Talbot J, Ross P, Lewis D (2010) An evaluation of echo in life support (ELS): is it feasible? What does it add? Emerg Med J 28:119-121.
9. Labovitz A, Noble V, Bierig M, Goldstein S, Jones R, Kort S, Porter T, Spencer K, Tayal V, Wei K (2010) Focused cardiac ultrasound in the emergent setting: a consensus statement of the American society of echocardiography and American college of emergency physicians. J Am Soc Echocardiogr. 23:1225–30.
10. Jan M. Shoenberger S (2021) The Use of Bedside Ultrasound in Cardiac Arrest. In: PubMed Central (PMC). https://www.ncbi.nlm.nih.gov/pmc/articles/PMC2860421/. Accessed 29 Mar 2021
11. Moskowitz A, Berg K (2017) First do no harm: Echocardiography during cardiac arrest may increase pulse check duration. Resuscitation 119:A2–3.
12. Huis in 't Veld M, Allison M, Bostick D, Fisher K, Goloubeva O, Witting M, Winters M,. Ultrasound use during cardiopulmonary resuscitation is associated with delays in chest compressions. Resuscitation. 2017;119:95–8.
13. Groombridge C, Kim Y, Maini A, Smit D, Fitzgerald M. Stress and decision-making in resuscitation: A systematic review. Resuscitation. 2019;144:115–22.

POCUS in Pericardial Effusion and Cardiac Tamponade

Eftychia Galiatsou and Clara Hernandez Caballero

The envelope becomes filled in hydrops of the heart; the walls of the heart are compressed by the fluid settling everywhere so that the heart cannot dilate sufficiently to receive the blood; then the pulse becomes exceedingly small, until finally it becomes utterly suppressed by the great inundation of fluid whence succeed syncope and death itself.

Dr. Richard Lower, English physician and pioneer, (1631–1691 AD)

Abstract

In the acute settings, echocardiography, which is widely available, rapid, repeatable, and non-invasive, is the modality of choice for the diagnosis of pericardial disease and especially pericardial effusion (PEF) and cardiac tamponade. A PEF will appear as an anechoic (echo-free) space separating the visceral from the parietal pericardium and can be circumferential or loculated. Two important questions for the POCUS practitioner are: how to estimate of the size of the effusion? and how to assess its haemodynamic impact? The haemodynamics of a PEF depend not only on the volume of the pericardial fluid but more importantly on the rate of accumulation. Acute cardiac tamponade is a form of obstructive shock that is lethal if left untreated. Clinical suspicion of tamponade in the setting of undifferentiated shock should prompt immediate bedside echocardiographic examination. However, tamponade is a predominantly clinical diagnosis: any interpretation of echocardiographic findings should be made within the clinical context and any decision making will be firstly guided by the patient's clinical condition. Emergency pericardiocentesis is a life-saving procedure with no absolute contraindications in the case of life-threatening tamponade and should be performed under echocardiography or fluoroscopic guidance.

Supplementary Information The online version contains supplementary material available at https://doi.org/10.1007/978-3-031-29472-3_26.

E. Galiatsou (✉) · C. H. Caballero
Department of Anaesthetics and Intensive Care, Harefield Hospital, Royal Brompton and Harefield Hospitals, London, UK
e-mail: e.galiatsou@rbht.nhs.uk

C. H. Caballero
e-mail: c.hernandezcaballero@rbht.nhs.uk

Key Messages

- In the acute settings, echocardiography is the modality of choice for the diagnosis of pericardial disease and especially pericardial effusion (PEF) and cardiac tamponade.
- The haemodynamics of a PEF depend not only on the volume of the pericardial fluid but more importantly on the rate of accumulation.
- Acute cardiac tamponade is a clinical diagnosis and is a form of obstructive shock that is lethal if left untreated.
- Emergency pericardiocentesis is a life-saving procedure with no absolute contraindications in the case of life-threatening tamponade and should be performed under echocardiography or fluoroscopic guidance.

Introduction

Pericardial disease represents a whole spectrum of clinical syndromes with acute pericarditis on one end and pericardial tamponade or pericardial constriction on the other end. The haemodynamics of pericardial tamponade or constriction delineate a fascinating model of cardiovascular physiology, intersecting heart- lung interactions, ventricular interdependence, and atrio-ventricular coupling. Diagnosis can be challenging and involves history, physical examination, imaging, and invasive monitoring. Patients with pericardial disease can present in various settings. A non-exhaustive list of such scenarios would be, in an emergency department post trauma, chest pain and pericardial rub following viral illness, post-myocardial infarction, post-cardiac surgery or percutaneous cardiac procedures, oncology patient post chest radiotherapy, patient with auto-immune disease or hypothyroidism. In any clinical setting, acute dyspnoea, chest pain, tachycardia, with haemodynamic instability and increased central venous pressure should trigger a POCUS scan.

Although a multimodality imaging approach is recommended for the diagnosis of pericardial disease [1–3], in the acute settings, echocardiography, which is widely available, rapid, repeatable, and non-invasive, is the modality of choice, and the gold-standard.

Historically, one of the first applications of echocardiography was the detection of pericardial fluid [4] and this remains one of the main targets of focused and point-of-care echocardiography [5]. Physical examination is notorious for missing a pericardial effusion (PEF) because of its non-specific presentation. Chest radiography has limited value except in the cases of a massive effusion causing cardiomegaly with clear lungs or of calcified pericardium. Echocardiography detects a pericardial effusion with an accuracy of almost 100% and allows both anatomic and haemodynamic evaluation of a PEF. POCUS rather than departmental comprehensive echocardiography allows an earlier identification of pericardial effusion and possibly shortens the time to a life-saving intervention such as pericardiocentesis [6]. Focused echocardiography in the hands of trained emergency physicians detects PEF in patients at high risk with a sensitivity of 95% and a specificity of 98% [7]. Repeatability of POCUS is an additional asset that allows serial assessment and monitoring of haemodynamics in the setting of a PEF.

Anatomy and Physiology of the Pericardium

The pericardium consists of a fibrous sac (*fibrosa*) and a serous membrane (*serosa*) that encircle the heart and the proximal part of the great vessels.

The fibrous sac attaches to the great vessels, the sternum, the vertebral column, and the diaphragm. The inner serous membrane (*visceral pericardium or epicardium*) extends to the proximal portions of the aorta, pulmonary artery, the anterior and lateral side of the vena cavae, and the anterior side of the pulmonary veins, and then reflects back along the underside of the fibrous sac. The ascending aorta and the main pulmonary artery are completely enclosed within the visceral pericardium. The *parietal pericardium* consists of the fibrosa with the serosa lining the inner side of it. The mediastinal surface

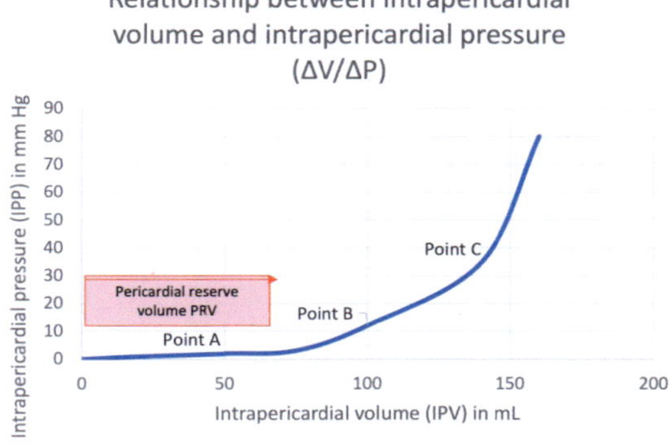

Fig. 1 Changes in intrapericardial pressure with progressive increases in intrapericardial volume. The importance of the pericardial reserve volume

of the parietal pericardium is covered by adipose tissue (*epi-pericardial fat*).

Importantly, there are two sinuses that are formed from the reflections of the visceral pericardium. These are the *oblique sinus* (posterior to the left atrium, limited by the pulmonary veins and the inferior vena cava) and the *transverse sinus* (superior to the left atrium, with borders limited by the great arteries, the superior vena cava, and the roof of the left atrium). Because of these potential spaces, the *pericardial reserve volume* allows small increases in cardiac volumes without a rise in intrapericardial pressure.

In normal situations, these two layers of the pericardium cannot be differentiated on echocardiography, and the pericardium appears as a single bright echogenic line adherent to the heart.

The *pericardial cavity* is the space between the parietal and visceral pericardium and normally contains <50 ml of serous fluid. This small quantity of pericardial fluid lubricates the surface of the heart thus decreasing friction and equalising distribution of gravitational forces [8].

The main functions of the pericardium are:

– Maintaining the heart in a stable position within the thorax
– Limiting excessive acute chamber dilation
– Preserving ventricular pressure–volume relationship
– Facilitating cardiac chamber coupling
– Forming a physical barrier that limits the spread of infection or cancer.

Intrapericardial pressure (IPP) is difficult to measure. It reflects intrathoracic pressure which in turn fluctuates around atmospheric pressure during spontaneous breathing: negative during inspiration, slightly positive during expiration [8]. The pericardial pressure volume relationship is bi-linear: at low volumes pressure increases minimally but after a critical point which is the pericardial reserve volume (PRV), it increases sharply (see Fig. 1). When IPP is less than 5 mmHg the pericardium is loose and compliant. Above this it behaves like an elastic band restraining the heart [9].

Intrapericardial pressure normally follows the intrathoracic pressure, so fluctuations of the intrathoracic pressure normally lead to equal changes in pericardial pressure [8]. This in turn causes the normal, slight respiratory variation in the left ventricular (LV) stroke volume and systemic blood pressure. During spontaneous inspiration intrathoracic pressure becomes negative and this increases venous return to the right heart. The respiratory variation, consisting in a decrease in LV volume and filling during spontaneous inspiration, is caused by the pericardium restraining further expansion of the total heart volume after the initial augmented venous return to the right heart. Because of the PRV, the normal pericardium is expansive and can accommodate this increase in right ventricular (RV) filling without significantly restricting LV filling: the normal respiratory variation in LV stroke volume and systemic blood pressure is minor (<10%).

However, when intrathoracic pressure becomes excessively negative (as in acute asthma exacerbation) increased filling of the RV during inspiration might 'overcome' the pericardial reserve volume and cause pericardial restraint.

Image Acquisition and Interpretation

A pericardial effusion can develop as a response of pericardium to any kind of insult (trauma, infection, inflammation, neoplasm, radiation, metabolic disease) or because of circulatory congestion with increased central venous pressure or obstructed lymph flow. The fluid can be blood, pus, exudate, or transudate.

Transthoracic echocardiography (TTE) is the imaging modality of choice for the detection and quantification of a PEF. Transoesophageal echocardiography (TOE) is often necessary to exclude regional localized pericardial collections, especially in post-cardiac surgery patients.

With 2D echocardiography, the normal pericardium is easy to identify as the thin (1–2 mm), highly reflective (echogenic) border of the heart. The small amount of fluid that normally exists

within the pericardial sac allows for a minimal separation of the pericardial layers best seen with M-mode and during systole. In real time 2D, the myocardium and the epicardium shorten and twist within the parietal pericardium.

A PEF will appear as an echo-free space separating the visceral from the parietal pericardium (see Figs. 2 and 3, Video 1A, B). The effusion can be global or localised. A circumferential PEF is typically seen as encircling the heart on all sides although its distribution may sometimes vary. Several views are then necessary to detect and confirm the presence of PEF. If the fluid is free and there are no adhesions, any view that includes the dependent parts of the pericardium will image it. In mechanically ventilated patients, the subcostal view is often the best one to reveal a pericardial effusion as the most posterior part of the pericardium is closest to the probe and the liver generates an acoustic window. Multiple views are necessary in order to avoid missing a loculated effusion, especially following a percutaneous cardiac procedure or cardiac surgery. Loculated effusions can be of variable shape and size and can be located close to one or two cardiac chambers.

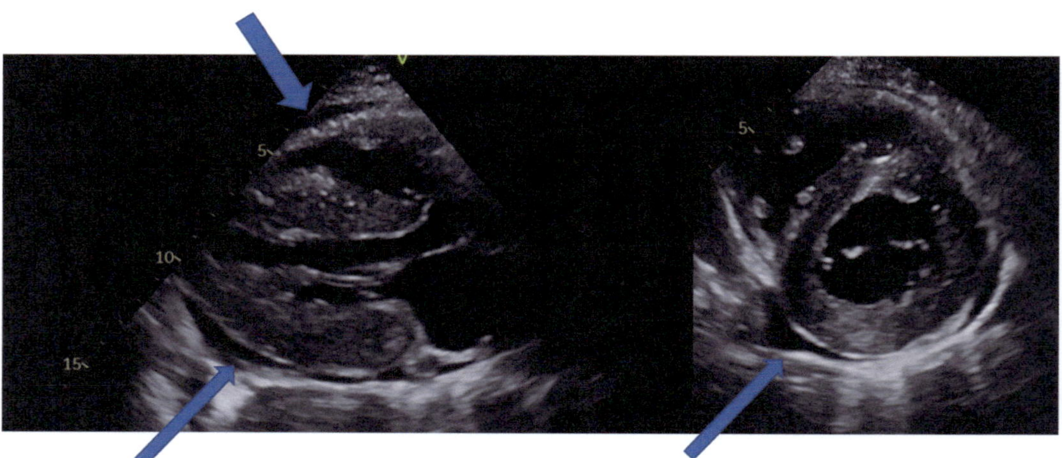

Fig. 2 TTE images corresponding to a patient with a mild pericardial collection post heart transplant. On the left, PLAX view showing mild effusion, seen anterior to the RVOT and posterior to the inferolateral wall of the LV. Measuring the depth in mm of the echo-lucent separation between the pericardium and myocardium in 2D of M mode is an accepted semi-quantitative way to assess a pericardial effusion. To the right, PSAX view of the same patient, with a mild global effusion which is more evident posteriorly. TTE: transthoracic echocardiography, PLAX: parasternal long axis view, PSAX: parasternal short axis view

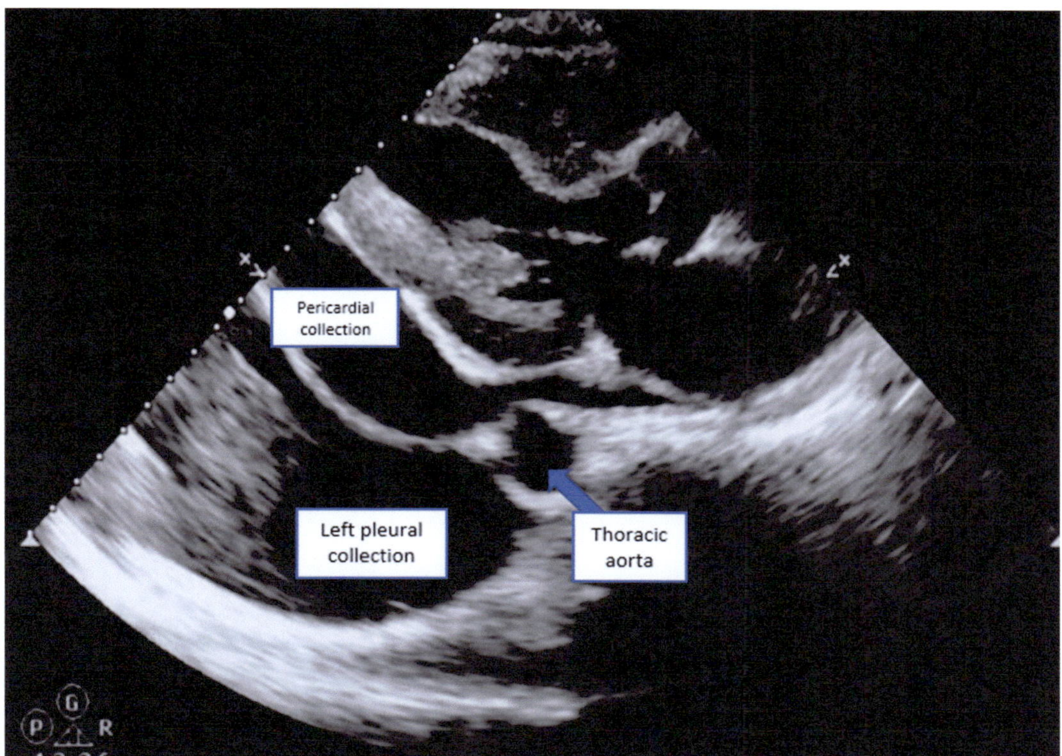

Fig. 3 PLAX view of a patient with severe (>20 mm in the inferolateral wall) pericardial collection and large left pleural collection. Note the pericardial collection sits between the heart and the descending thoracic aorta. On the contrary, the pleural collection can be seen as an echolucent space posterior to the descending aorta. PLAX: parasternal long axis view

Mostly appears anechoic, the PEF can also be of mixed echogenicity if the collection contains blood, clots, or fibrin. Complex effusions with clots can best be diagnosed with TOE (see Fig. 4, Video 1A, B). Unclotted blood in the pericardial space creates a characteristic spontaneous echo contrast in a slow twisting movement.

Primary or secondary pericardial neoplasms can appear as masses within the pericardial space usually with an effusion (see Video 2A, B).

Once the collection has been identified with 2D imaging, two crucial questions remain to be answered by the POCUS clinician: 1. How big is the pericardial effusion? 2. How is the pericardial effusion affecting haemodynamics?

Quantification of the effusion is based on the magnitude of the anechoic space between the visceral and the parietal pericardium in end-diastole: small if <10 mm, moderate if 10–20 mm, large if >20 mm, very large >25 mm [10]. If the effusion is only seen in systole, it is considered trivial and it is less than 50 millilitres. The correlation between the estimated and the actual size of the effusion is stronger for global effusions apparent from multiple views. A large effusion with no haemodynamic instability is probably a chronic one.

In order to assess the haemodynamic significance of a pericardial collection, long loops that include several cardiac cycles through inspiration and expiration should be obtained: the signs to look for are: evidence of cardiac chamber compression, venous congestion and reciprocal respirophasic changes in ventricular filling (see Table 1).

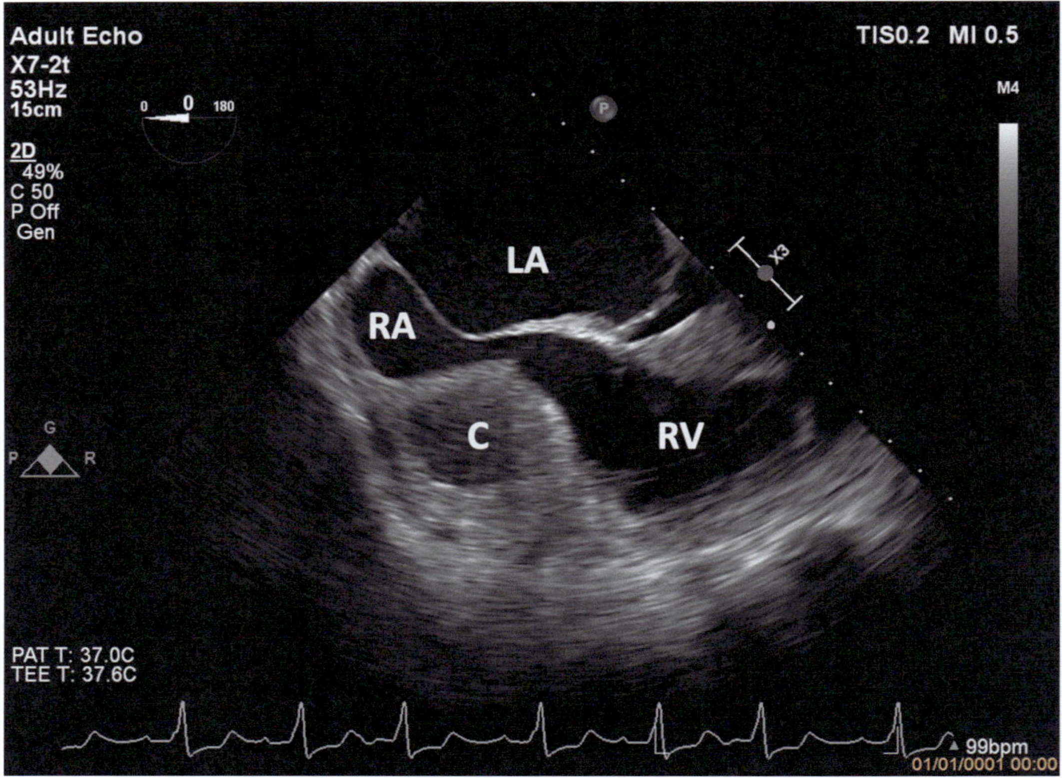

Fig. 4 Trans-oeseophageal echocardiography. Large pericardial clot (C) squeezing the right atrium (RA) in a patient post cardiac surgery. LA: left atrium, RA: right atrium, RV: right ventricle

Cardiac Tamponade

Cardiac tamponade is the clinical syndrome resulting from fluid or blood or clots or pus or rarely air accumulation in the pericardial cavity which leads to a rise in the intrapericardial pressure. Depending on the rate of fluid build-up and the mechanics of the pericardium itself, the clinical presentation of tamponade varies from acute to subacute, and from subclinical presentation with echocardiographic signs of right atrial compression to overt shock or cardiac arrest with pulseless electrical activity.

The clinical manifestations of tamponade are not specific and are a result of reduced stroke volume with compensatory increased sympathetic activity and elevated systemic filling pressures. Clinical suspicion of tamponade in the setting of undifferentiated shock should prompt immediate bedside echocardiographic examination (see Video 3A, B). However, imaging should be focused and should not delay interventional or surgical management in cases where the likelihood of tamponade is high: for example, in the case of a bleeding, hypotensive patient post cardiac surgery with a high central venous pressure.

Acute cardiac tamponade is a form of obstructive shock that is lethal if left untreated. Bleeding in the pericardial cavity as a result of trauma or myocardial rupture due to myocardial infarction is an example: the stiff pericardium cannot stretch and accommodate this abrupt rise in volume without significantly increasing the intrapericardial pressure and compressing the cardiac chambers [11]. As the pericardial reserve volume is exceeded and the pericardium stiffens,

Table 1 Summarises the echocardiographic signs of cardiac tamponadeTamponade. The most sensitive combination is probably the presence of a global PEF with inferior vena cavaInferior vena cava (IVC) plethora and a small LV cavity [3]. IVC plethora (IVC dilatation with no inspiratory collapse in self-ventilating patients) imaged from the subcostal view, will be present in >90% cardiac tamponadeTamponade cases (see Video 6). With the exception of low-pressure tamponadeTamponade, its absence makes the diagnosis of tamponadeTamponade questionable. IVC plethora can be seen in all settings associated with high RA pressures for example, pulmonary embolismPulmonary embolism, right heart failureHeart failure, positive pressure ventilation making its specificity low. Dilatation of the hepatic veins is an additional sign of systemic venous congestionVenous congestion. PEF: pericardial effusion, IVC: inferior vena cavaInferior vena cava, IPP: intrapericardial pressure, LV: left ventricle, RV: right ventricleRight ventricle, IVS: interventricular septum

Echocardiographic signs of tamponade		Mechanism
2D, M Mode	Pericardial effusion	Various causes insulting the pericardium
2D	Swinging heart	Large, global PEF allows swinging of the heart
2D, M Mode	Chamber collapse	↑IPP, ↓transmural pressure
2D, M Mode	IVC plethora. IVC ≥ 2.1 cm, inspiratory collapsibility <50%	Systemic venous congestion
2D, M Mode	LV pseudohypertrophy	Underfilled LV
2D, M Mode	Inspiratory shift of IVS to the left, reciprocal respiratory variation of RV and LV size	↑ ventricular interdependence
Doppler	Reciprocal respiratory changes in inflow velocities: >30% inspiratory reduction in peak trans-mitral velocity >60% inspiratory increase in peak trans-tricuspid velocity	↑ ventricular interdependence
Doppler	Reversed/absent diastolic antegrade hepatic vein flow	Systemic venous congestion

the cardiac chambers must compete with one another and with the pericardial content for a now fixed increased intrapericardial volume so that filling of one ventricle limits filling of the other. The respiratory variation in stroke volume which causes pulsus paradoxus (respiratory decrease in systolic blood pressure more than 10 mmHg) can be explained by the exaggerated parallel and in series interaction of the ventricles [12]. Inspiratory flow to the left heart is decreased as intrathoracic and intrapericardial pressures are now dissociated causing a decreased pressure gradient from the pulmonary veins (which are outside the pericardium) to the left atrium while flow from the systemic veins to the right atrium is maintained. The competitive ventricular filling shifts the interventricular septum to the left. Finally, there is equalisation of pericardial pressure and intracardiac diastolic pressures and cardiac filling is constrained as

transmural pressures (intracavitary minus pericardial) are diminished. This causes collapse of the cardiac cavities. The first ones to be affected are the right heart cavities because they are thin-walled with low intracavitary pressures.

In contrast, a large PEF slowly accumulating allows the pericardium to gradually increase its compliance, in this way accommodating a big intrapericardial volume without compressing the cardiac chambers. Nevertheless, when this low pressure/large volume effusion reaches the steep portion of the pressure–volume curve and the limit of pericardial stretch, tamponade ensues in a similar way (see Fig. 1).

Pearls:

- Low pressure tamponade occurs when a pericardial effusion associated with lower IPP compresses the cardiac chambers because of low filling pressure as in the case of hypovolaemia, bleeding, excessive diuresis [13]. In this case the classic signs of venous congestion may not be present.

- Mimickers of tamponade are clinical syndromes that even in the absence of pericardial effusion/pathology increase the intrathoracic pressure which is then transmitted to the pericardium, such as tension pneumothorax, positive pressure mechanical ventilation, large pleural effusions, intrabdominal hypertension/compartment syndrome.

In patients with clinical suspicion of tamponade, echocardiography is the recommended imaging modality [1]. Echocardiographic signs of tamponade depend on the increased IPP, ventricular interdependence and heart–lung interactions and the activation of compensatory mechanisms. As the haemodynamic impact of a PEF escalates, more echocardiographic signs of tamponade appear. In a subset of patients' two-dimensional echocardiography can disclose evidence of increased IPP with subtle only, if any, haemodynamic compromise [14] (see Fig. 5 and Video 4A, B). On the other hand, co-existent cardiac pathology and non- cardiac conditions may significantly alter the echocardiographic presentation of tamponade (for example an atrial septal defect, severe aortic regurgitation, pulmonary hypertension, left ventricular hypertrophy, mechanical ventilation). With all these limitations in mind, tamponade should be seen as a predominantly clinical diagnosis: any interpretation of echocardiographic findings should be done within the clinical context and any decision making will be firstly guided by the patient's clinical condition.

Cardiac chamber compression is a sensitive marker of tamponade that often precedes the clinical manifestations. *Right atrial wall collapse* occurs after atrial systole when RA volume is at its lowest is a sensitive but not specific sign of tamponade as it can appear in hypovolaemia alone. This collapse is best visualised from the apical or subcostal 4 chambers view and if it persists for more than 1/3 of cardiac cycle, specificity is improved (see Videos 5–7).

The *RV collapse happens* in early diastole after closure of the pulmonary valve when its volume is the lowest. As tamponade worsens the duration of the RV wall inversion lasts longer. The right ventricular outflow tract (RVOT) is the part of RV that is compressed first followed by the free RV wall. RVOT inversion is best seen from the left parasternal long axis view and its timing and duration can be more easily

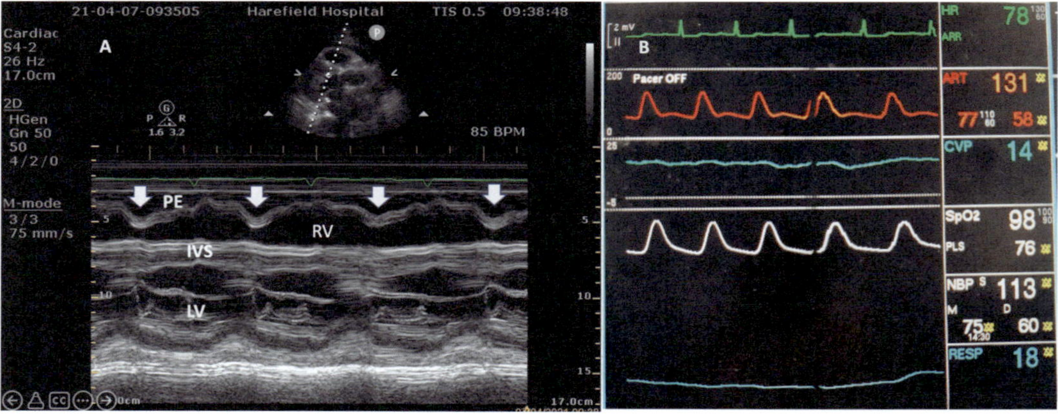

Fig. 5 A Loculated anterior pericardial effusion (PE) as seen with M-Mode from the long axis parasternal view in a patient with aortic root and valve replacement. There is early diastolic compression on the right ventricular wall (arrows). **B** Screenshot from patient's monitor at the same time as the echo scan. There was no clinical indication of haemodynamic compromise. PE: pericardial effusion, RV: right ventricle, IVS: interventricular septum, LV: left ventricle. See Video 4

understood with M-mode (see Fig. 5, Videos 4A, B). Although this is a more specific sign of tamponade, it can be absent if there is RV hypertrophy or pulmonary hypertension. In this case, the high intracavitary pressures maintain the RV transmural pressure despite the high IPP.

Compression of the left ventricle or left atrium can occur because of regional pericardial effusions or pericardial clots after cardiothoracic surgery [15]. In regional tamponade, the typical clinical and/or echocardiographic signs of tamponade maybe absent.

The exaggerated ventricular interdependence in tamponade results in reciprocal respirophasic changes in right and left ventricular dimensions with inspiratory shift of the interventricular septum to the left. Because it is typically underfilled, the LV is seen as a small cavity with thickened walls (LV pseudohypertrophy) and hyperactive due to compensatory sympathetic activation (see Video 8). Following the same pattern, Doppler echocardiography reveals changes in ventricular filling related to spontaneous breathing: mitral E wave (peak diastolic inflow to the left ventricle) decreases by more than 30% compared to expiration while tricuspid E wave (peak diastolic inflow to the right ventricle) increases by more than 60% in inspiration (see Fig. 6a, b). These reciprocal changes are best appreciated using pulsed wave Doppler with low sweep speed from the apical 4 chambers view (See Fig. 7). These signs may be masked or reversed in patients mechanically ventilated, or maybe absent if atrial septal defect or aortic regurgitation co-exist.

The hepatic vein flow can also be assessed by pulsed wave Doppler from the subcostal view or trans-hepatic mid-axillary view: antegrade flow becomes predominantly systolic, diastolic flow markedly decreases or disappears or is even reversed in expiration (see Fig. 9). Forward hepatic vein flow seen only in inspiration is an ominous sign of impending cardiac arrest [3].

Drainage

Although surgical drainage of a PEF remains the gold standard, fluoroscopy or echocardiography-guided pericardiocentesis is the procedure of choice in the emergency settings. Emergency pericardiocentesis is a life-saving procedure with no absolute contraindications in the case of life-threatening tamponade. Nevertheless, blind procedures should be avoided as they carry significant risk of laceration to the heart or other organs [1]. Traumatic pericardial effusion with tamponade is an indication for left thoracotomy rather than pericardiocentesis [16].

Echocardiography-guided pericardiocentesis starts with systematic scanning using all available windows to determine the best access approach to the point of to the largest accumulation of pericardial fluid, with the smallest skin to fluid distance, at the same time avoiding other adjacent organs. The apical and the left parasternal sites are the ones most commonly used. Real time imaging with the needle parallel to the ultrasound beam allows following of the needle trajectory. Injection of agitated saline is sometimes used to facilitate visualisation of the tip of the needle which can be difficult and to confirm positioning within the pericardial space.

Please see reference 16 for high quality video tutorial of pericardiocentesis.

Pearls and Pitfalls

- In the acute settings, ultrasound guided misdiagnoses (either overzealous or missing) can have detrimental effects on patients' outcomes [17].
- Other than pericardial effusion, hypoechoic spaces adjacent to the heart can be pleural effusions or ascites or LV pseudoaneurysms, or (rarely) pericardial cysts [18].

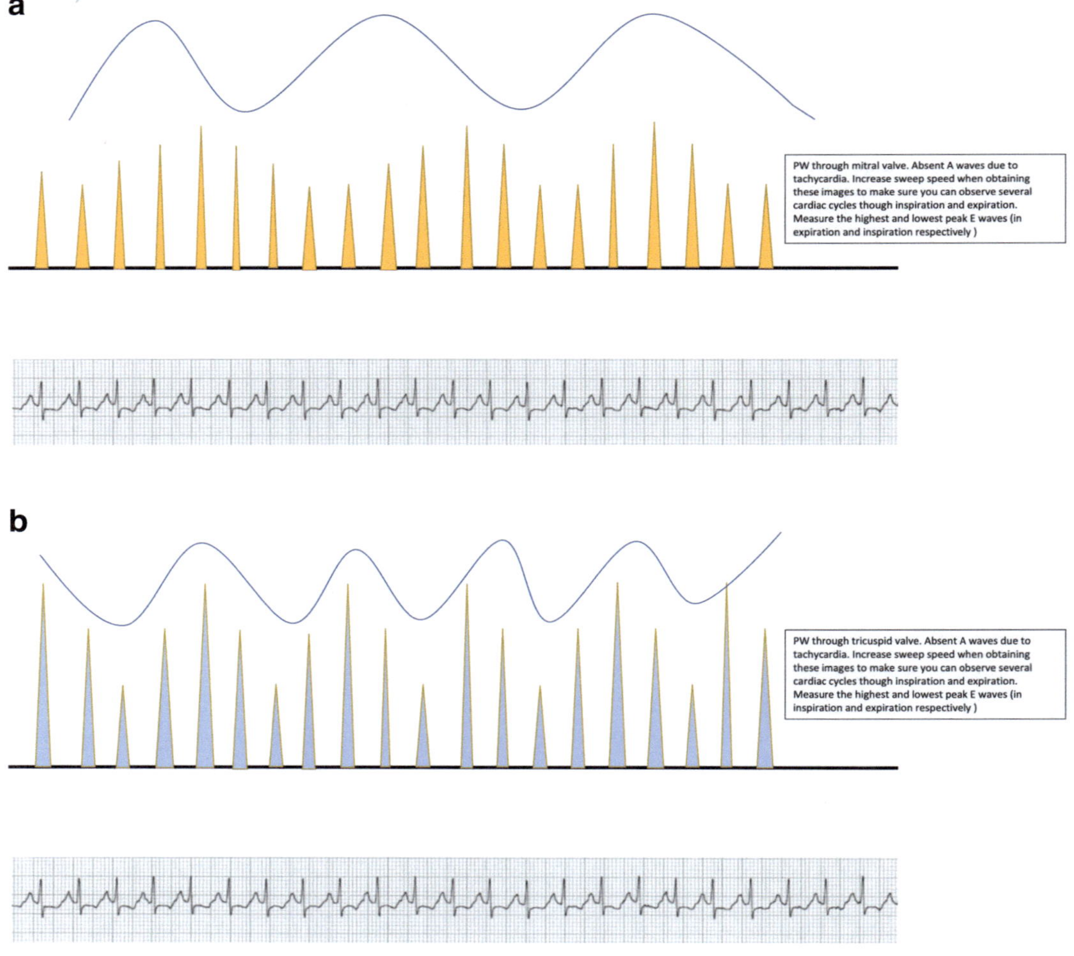

Fig. 6 a Transmitral respiratory variation of the peak E velocity in a patient with cardiac tamponade. A **drop in the peak E wave >25% during inspiration** is considered consistent with significant tamponade physiology. **b** Trans-tricuspid respiratory variation of the peak E velocity in a patient with cardiac tamponade. An increase **in the peak E wave >60% during inspiration** is considered consistent with significant tamponade physiology

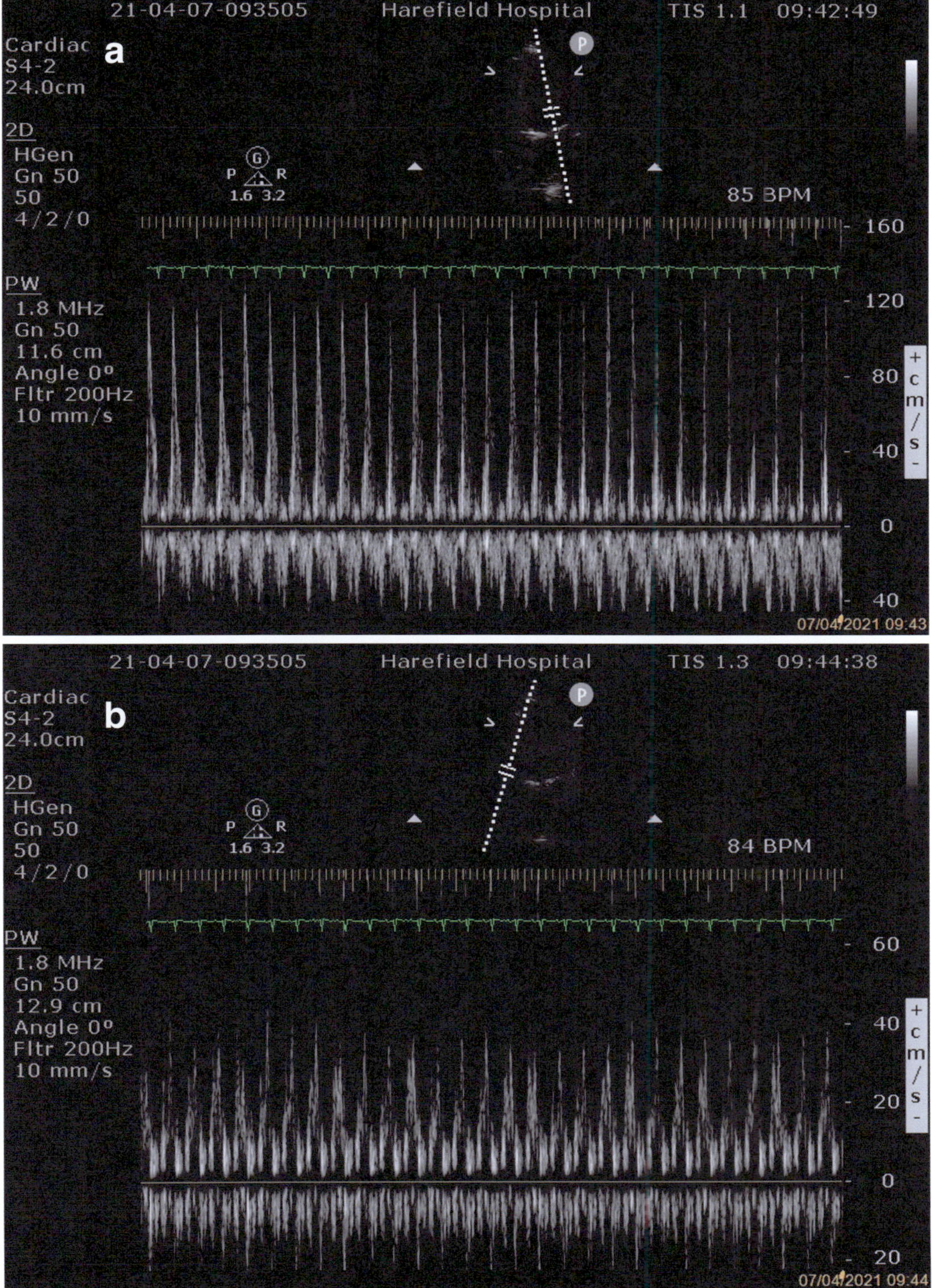

Fig. 7 Same patient as in Fig. 5 and Video 4. Pulsed wave doppler of the mitral **a** and the tricuspid inflow **b** without significant variation of the flow velocity. Slow sweep speed. Apical 4 chamber view

- Large pleural effusions can be detected from standard TTE views: a left sided pleural effusion will be posterior to the descending thoracic aorta in the left parasternal long axis view, while a right sided effusion may be seen adjacent to the right atrium from the subcostal four chamber view (see Fig. 3). Lung ultrasonography will easily localise the pleural effusion and will show the partially collapsed lung within it. (see Chap. 27 for further details).
- Large pleural effusions can cause tamponade physiology even in the absence of a pericardial effusion.
- Ascitic fluid collection can appear as an echo-free space anterior to the right heart cavities from the subcostal view. The liver and the falciform ligament can be identified within the collection [18].
- A PEF always appears around the dependent walls first: posterior, inferior, lateral.
- An anterior only, relatively hypoechoic space is likely representing epicardial fat: epicardial fat appears anteriorly only, has heterogeneous texture, and tends to move in concert with the heart while PEF is motionless.
- Presentation of PEF can be insidious. Similarly, the haemodynamics of tamponade fall in a spectrum: from subclinical normotensive phase to decompensated phase with obstructive shock. There might be discrepancies between the clinical presentation of tamponade and the echocardiographic signs which can precede overt shock.
- The association between the size of a PEF and its haemodynamic impact is often poor: large effusions that accumulate slowly can be asymptomatic; smaller effusions that build up rapidly can cause tamponade.
- Tamponade is a predominantly clinical diagnosis: any interpretation of echocardiographic findings should be within the clinical context and any decision making should be guided by the patient's clinical condition.
- The first cardiac chambers to collapse in tamponade are the right atrium and the right ventricular outflow tract (RVOT) followed by the RV free wall. In severe pulmonary hypertension, the right chambers may withstand the high IPP and may not appear collapsed.
- Be wary of a small pericardial effusion with tachycardia and small, underfilled and hypercontractile collapsing cavities: hypovolaemia may imitate diastolic collapse of the RA or the RV. In this case, a non-dilated and collapsing IVC rules out tamponade as the cause of haemodynamic instability.
- Pulsus paradoxus may appear reversed and the respirophasic flow changes in patients with tamponade who are mechanically ventilated which can be difficult to interpret (see Figs. 8a, b and 9).
- Echocardiographic signs of tamponade may be totally different in patients with mechanical circulatory support devices (see Video 9). The decision to drain pericardial collection in a patient on a peripheral veno-arterial extracorporeal mechanical oxygenator (V-A ECMO) should be based on the evidence of circuit flow or pressure compromise rather than the presence of chamber collapse. Moreover, the high risk of bleeding in these patients due to therapeutic anticoagulation should be taken into consideration.

Fig. 8 **a** Example of reverse pulsus paradoxus in a patient with tamponade while mechanically ventilated. Intrapericardial pressure rises in inspiration. Systemic arterial pressure rises, and pulmonary artery pressure decreases in inspiration (blue arrows). In expiration systemic arterial pressure decreases while pulmonary artery pressure increases (yellow arrows). **b** The same patient following pericardiocentesis. Intrapericardial pressure is now low and there is no respiratory fluctuation of systemic or pulmonary arterial pressure. This patient had long-standing pulmonary hypertension so systemic and pulmonary pressures were equal. I: inspiration, E: expiration, BP: systemic arterial pressure, PAP: pulmonary artery pressure, IPP: intrapericardial pressure

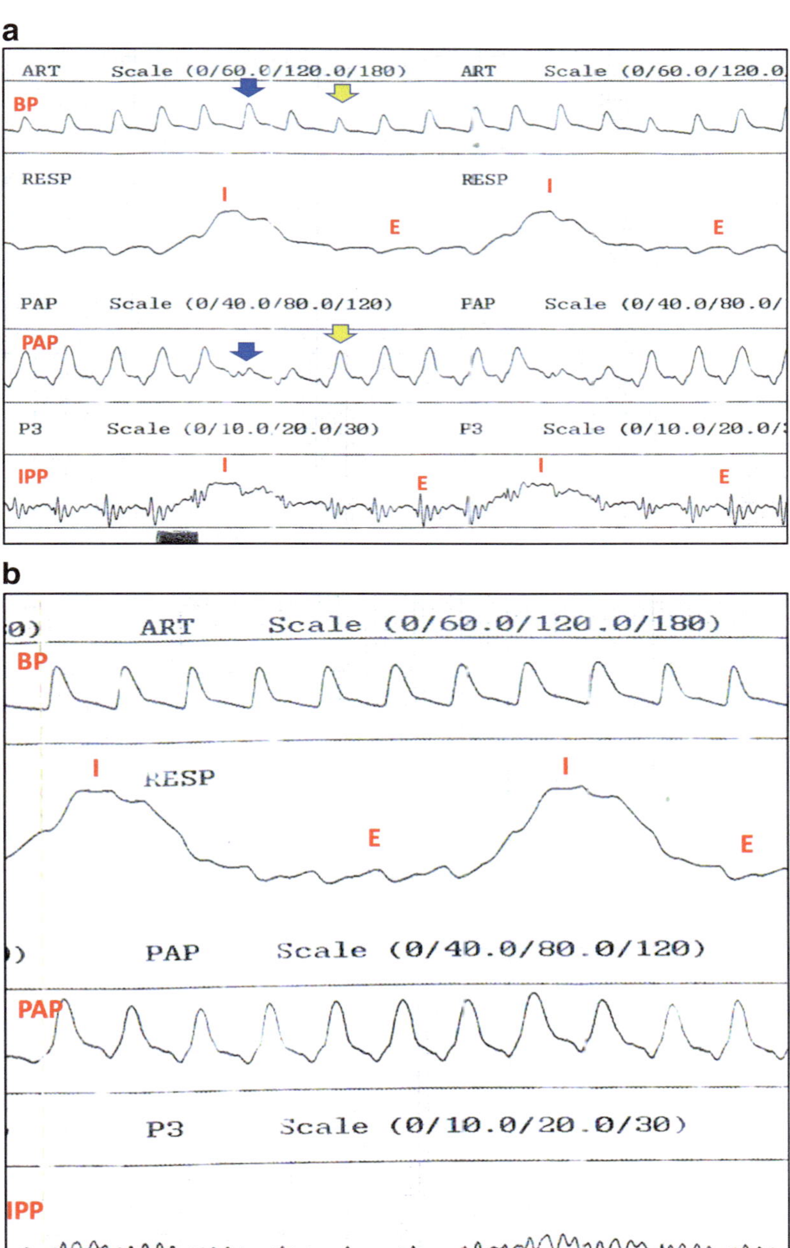

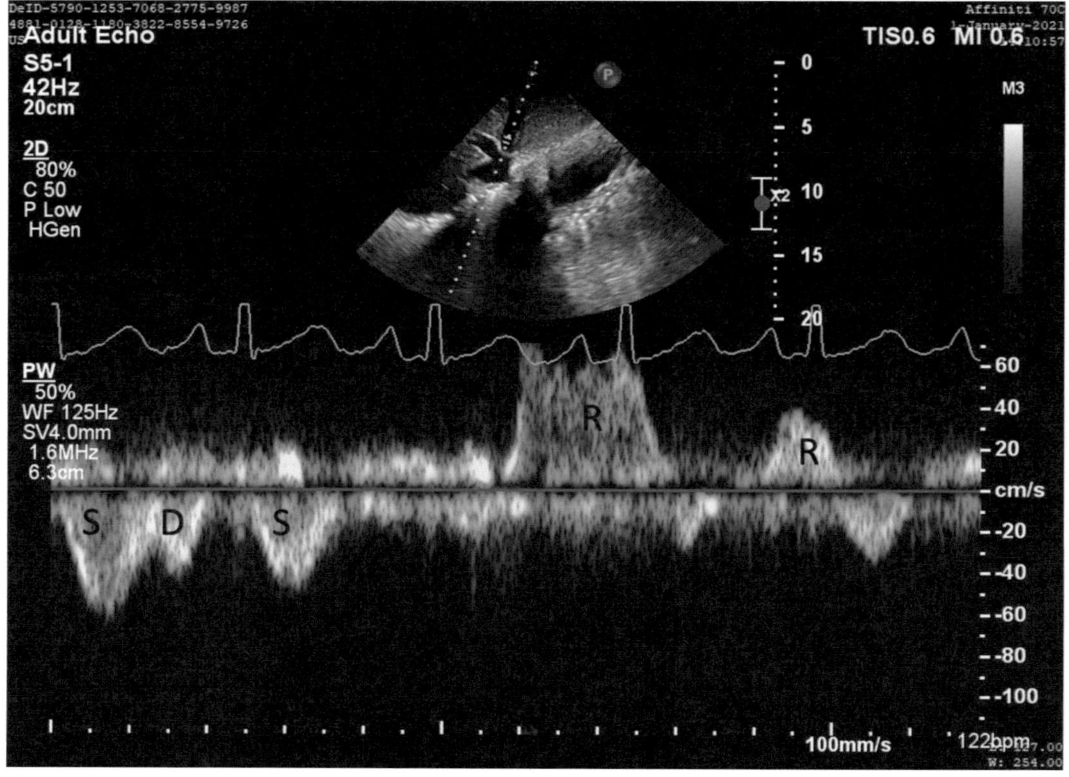

Fig. 9 Hepatic vein flow in a patient with tamponade. Forward flow is predominantly systolic (S). Diastolic forward flow is diminished (D) or reversed (R)

References

1. Cosyns B, Plein S, Nihoyanopoulos P, Smiseth O, Achenbach S, Andrade MJ, et al. European association of cardiovascular imaging (EACVI) position paper: multimodality imaging in pericardial disease. Eur Hear J-Cardiovasc Imaging. 2015;16(1):12–31.
2. Adler Y, Charron P, Imazio M, Badano L, Barón-Esquivias G, Bogaert J, et al. 2015 ESC guidelines for the diagnosis and management of pericardial diseases. Eur Heart J. 2015;36(42):2921–64.
3. Klein AL, Abbara S, Agler DA, Appleton CP, Asher CR, Hoit B, et al. American society of echocardiography clinical recommendations for multimodality cardiovascular imaging of patients with pericardial disease. J Am Soc Echocardiogr. 2013;26(9):965-1012.e15.
4. Feigenbaum H. Ultrasound diagnosis of pericardial effusion. JAMA. 1965;191(9):711.
5. Liu RB, Donroe JH, McNamara RL, Forman HP, Moore CL. The practice and implications of finding fluid during point-of-care ultrasonography: a review. JAMA Intern Med. 2017;177(12):1818.
6. Hanson MG, Chan B. The role of point-of-care ultrasound in the diagnosis of pericardial effusion: a single academic center retrospective study. Ultrasound J. 2021;13(1):2.
7. Mandavia DP, Hoffner RJ, Mahaney K, Henderson SO. Bedside echocardiography by emergency physicians. Ann Emerg Med. 2001;38(4):377–82.
8. Shabetai R, Mangiardi L, Bhargava V, Ross J, Higgins CB. The pericardium and cardiac function. Prog Cardiovasc Dis. 1979;22(2):107–34.
9. Kroeker CAG, Shrive NG, Belenkie I, Tyberg JV. Pericardium modulates left and right ventricular stroke volumes to compensate for sudden changes in atrial volume. Am J Physiol-Hear Circ Physiol. 2003;284(6):H2247–54.
10. Weitzman LB, Tinker WP, Kronzon I, Cohen ML, Glassman E, Spencer FC. The incidence and natural history of pericardial effusion after cardiac surgery–an echocardiographic study. Circulation. 1984;69(3):506–11.
11. Spodick DH. Acute Cardiac Tamponade. N Engl J Med. 2003;7.

12. Naeije R, Chemla D, Dinh-Xuan AT, Vonk Noorde-graaf A. Physiology in respiratory medicine. Eur Respir J. 2013;41(1):7.
13. Sagristà-Sauleda J, Angel J, Sambola A, Alguer-suari J, Permanyer-Miralda G, Soler-Soler J. Low-Pressure Cardiac Tamponade: Clinical and Hemody-namic Profile. Circulation. 2006;114(9):945–52
14. Levine MJ, Lorell BH, Diver DJ, Come PC. Impli-cations of echocardiographically assisted diagnosis of pericardial tamponade in contemporary medical patients: detection before hemodynamic embarrass-ment. J Am Coll Cardiol. 1991;17(1):59–65.
15. Yacoub MH, Cleland WP, Deal CW. Left atrial tamponade. Thorax. 1966;21(4):305–9.
16. Fitch MT, McGinnis HD. Emergency pericardiocen-tesis. N Engl J Med. 2012;5.
17. Blanco P, Volpicelli G. Common pitfalls in point-of-care ultrasound: a practical guide for emergency and critical care physicians. Crit Ultrasound J. 2016;8 (1):15.
18. D'Cruz IA, Kanuru N. Echocardiography of serous effusions adjacent to the heart. Echocardiography. 2001;18(5):445–56.

POCUS-Guided Assessment and Drainage of Pleural Effusion

Nora Mayer and Paras Dalal

'I had not imagined it would be necessary to give a name to such a simple device, but others thought differently. If one wants to give it a name, the most suitable would be "stethoscope."
René Laennec. French physician, and inventor of the stethoscope a (1781–1826 AD)

Abstract

Transthoracic ultrasonography as part of point of care ultrasonography (POCUS) is a well-established imaging technique which is especially useful for real-time assessment of pleural effusion. Pleural effusion is a common medical problem; with main symptom of dyspnea; and occurs on the background of various aetiologies including pleural and lung disease, systemic conditions, organ dysfunction and certain medications (1) Moreover, up to 60% of the critically ill patients present with pleural effusion (2) (3) POCUS-guided assessment and concomitant drainage of pleural effusion (thoracocentesis or chest drain insertion) provides the most cost-effective and low-risk strategy to manage pleural effusion at one time.

The following chapter on assessment and drainage of pleural effusion highlights the importance of transthoracic ultrasonography and the effectiveness of small-bore chest drains (10–14Fr) in the management of pleural effusion.

Keywords

Transthoracic ultrasonography · POCUS · Pleural effusion · Small-bore chest drains · Thoracocentesis

Abbreviations

ap	Anteroposterior
BTS	British Thoracic Society
CT	Computed tomography
Fr	French
INR	International normalized ratio
LDH	Lactate dehydrogenase

N. Mayer
Department of Thoracic Surgery, Royal Brompton and Harefield Hospitals, Guy's and St. Thomas NHS Foundation Trust, London, England

P. Dalal (✉)
Department of Radiology, Royal Brompton and Harefield Hospitals, Guy's and St. Thomas NHS Foundation Trust, London, England
e-mail: p.dalal@rbht.nhs.uk

"""

pa	Posteroanterior
POCUS	Point of care ultrasound
tPA	Tissue plasminogen activator
2-D	2-Dimensonal

Key message

Pleural effusion is a frequent medical problem which often presents with dyspnoea. Transthoracic ultrasound has emerged as a useful diagnostic tool. It can also help with safe placement of aspiration needles and drains.

Assessment of Pleural Effusion

Characteristics and impact of pleural effusion

Pleural effusion is a common medical problem; its most common symptom is dyspnoea [4, 5]. In critically ill patients, pleural effusion can lead to significant reduction in gas exchange and respiratory compliance. Multiple causes for pleural effusion have been described with congestive heart failure, malignancy, pulmonary infection and pulmonary embolism accounting for more than 90% [6, 7]. The patient's medical history and clinical examination in combination with thoracic ultrasound can effectively narrow the range of possible differential diagnoses.

Imaging modalities for pleural effusion

Chest radiography remains the primary imaging modality of choice in daily practice. However, while a pleural effusion can efficiently be diagnosed on erect chest x-rays, it is commonly underestimated on supine studies (due to posterior fluid distribution) [8, 9]. Ultrasound, however, is more sensitive than chest radiography in detection of pleural effusions, especially in identifying and quantifying small effusions [10, 11]. In comparison to chest computed tomography (CT), thoracic ultrasound provides equal sensitivity in detection of pleural effusion while offering several advantages such as dynamic imaging, portability, absence of radiation exposure and no adverse effects on kidney function [12]. In addition, for complex effusions, ultrasound even yielded a significantly higher sensitivity in detecting septate effusions when compared to CT [13, 14]. Therefore, thoracic ultrasound has been well established and described for the assessment of pleural effusion [6, 15] (Fig. 1).

Ultrasonographic features of pleural effusion

Different ultrasonographic presentations of effusion (e.g. echogenic, anechoic and septated) can help to distinguish between the different types of effusion. In this way, a simple effusion (homogenously anechoic) can be morphologically

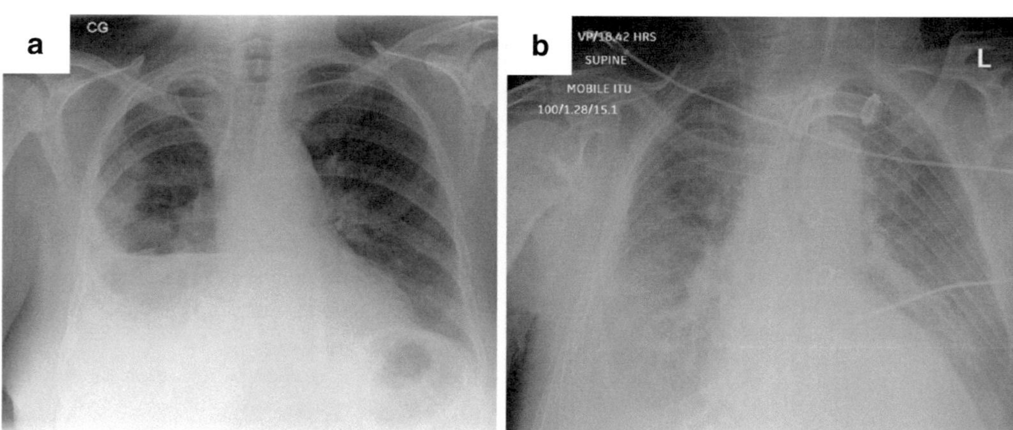

Fig. 1 Similar volume of right pleural effusion in posteroanterior (PA) chest x-ray (**a**) and supine antero-posterior (AP) chest x-ray (**b**)

differentiated from a complex effusion/empyema (echogenic, septated) as further specified and visualised in Table 1. The "haematocrit sign" (a surface layer of anechoic fluid sitting on top of a settled sediment) is highly suggestive for a haemothorax.

Table 1 Typical ultrasonographic features of different types of pleural effusion

Type of pleural effusion	Ultrasonographic features	Ultrasonographic 2D images
Simple effusion	Homogeneously anechoic	
Complex effusion/empyema	Echogenic "plankton sign": hyperechoic floating foci septations with multiple loculations	

(continued)

Table 1 (continued)

Type of pleural effusion	Ultrasonographic features	Ultrasonographic 2D images
Haemothorax	Echogenic septations "haematocrit sign": surface layer of anechoic fluid sitting on top of a settled sediment/different layer	
Chylothorax	Homogeneously anechoic septations	

Drainage of Pleural Effusion

Indications

National and international guidelines are well established for aspiration and drainage of pleural effusion [1, 16, 17]. In general, drainage of pleural effusion is either indicated for diagnostic or therapeutic reasons. Conservative therapeutic measures (e.g. increasing heart failure and diuretic medications) are usually considered prior to proceeding with invasive interventions (especially in bilateral, most likely transudative, effusions without suspicion for malignancy).

The major criteria for proceeding to aspiration or drainage are: symptomatic with respiratory compromise, suspicion of infected effusion/empyema or requirement of a precise differential diagnostic categorization [18, 19].

In spontaneously breathing patients, relief of dyspnoea symptoms and increase in lung function testing after thoracocentesis has been proven [20]. In the critically ill patients, drainage of especially large pleural effusion has been shown to be associated with improved oxygenation (improved PaO_2: FiO_2 ratio) and respiratory mechanics [21]. The size of effusion, however, is not an absolute indication for drainage. Drainage of even small effusions may be clinically important and has been shown to improve oxygenation significantly in patients with acute respiratory failure [22].

Patients with pleural effusion >10 mm in depth in association with a pneumonia, sepsis, recent chest trauma or surgery may benefit from diagnostic pleural fluid sampling. Drained pus is diagnostic for empyema and is a usual indication for chest drain insertion and antibiotic treatment (and surgical considerations). In non-purulent effusions, where infection is suspected, pleural fluid pH < 7.2 has been shown to be the single most powerful indicator predicting the need for chest drainage [23, 24].

In cases with diagnostic uncertainty, especially in suspected malignant pleural effusion, diagnostic sampling is mandatory to define diagnosis; malignant effusion can be diagnosed by fluid cytology in around 60–90% of the cases [25–27].

Fluid characteristics of pleural effusions have shown to be the most accurate test to guide further therapy [28]. Light's criteria are applied to aspirated fluid to distinguish between transudate and exudate and narrow the range of differential diagnoses [1] (Box 1). The most common causes of transudative pleural effusion are left ventricular failure, liver cirrhosis and hypalbuminemia whereas exudates most commonly appear in malignancies, parapneumonic effusions and pulmonary embolism [29].

> **Box 1.** Light's criteria: a pleural effusion is an exudate if at least one of the criteria [1–3] is met.
>
> A pleural effusion is an exudate if at least one of the criteria [1–3] is met.
>
> (1) Protein concentration in effusion divided by serum protein concentration >0.5
> (2) Lactate dehydrogenase (LDH) concentration in effusion >200 IU
> (3) LDH concentration in effusion divided by serum LDH concentration >0.6.

Preassessment and Requirements

Written consent

Informed consent is an essential and important step prior to any invasive procedure.

The commonest complications from pleural aspiration/drainage are pneumothorax, procedure failure and haemorrhage, and a most serious complication is visceral injury. These complications must be discussed with the patient to achieve formal informed consent. In the critical care setting however, informed consent is rarely possible and so decision making may require a multidisciplinary approach.

Clotting disorders and anticoagulation

In anticoagulated patients or patients at risk of coagulopathy (e.g. thrombocytopenia or hepatic/renal failure), the risk of bleeding should be assessed prior to any invasive procedures. Existing guidelines of the British Thoracic Society (BTS) suggest, non-urgent aspiration/chest drain insertion should be postponed in patients with International Normalized Ratio (INR) >1.5 and Platelets count <50 × 10^9/l [31]. Urgent procedures (especially in patients who do fulfil these criteria) may be carried out after seeking specialist hematology advice.

> **Box 2.** Requirements for chest drain insertion.
>
> Written consent
> Resolving of clotting disorders and discontinuation of anticoagulation.
> Cardiovascular monitoring.
> Ultrasound and drain insertion kit and competent operator available.
> Staff familiar with drain management.

Chest drains and equipment

A sterile technique with full aseptic barrier precautions (including cleaning solution (chlorhexidine, alcohol based)), draping of the sterile drain insertion area and surgical gown, surgical cap, face mask and sterile gloves are recommended to avoid infections of both drain insertion site and chest cavity. Fully equipped pre-prepared chest drain insertion kits are available in many hospitals (Box 3).

> **Box 3.** Equipment required for chest drain insertion.
>
> 2 × 10 ml skin antiseptic solution (Chlorhexidine in Alcohol or Iodine).
> Sterile drapes.
> Sterile gloves, gown,
> Surgical cap and face mask.
> Gauze swabs.

Local anaesthetic (e.g. Lidocaine 1% (dose dependent on weight but normally at least 10 ml).

Scalpel and blade.

A selection of syringes (10 ml, 20 ml) and needles (21–25 gauge).

Stiff guide wire and dilators for Seldinger technique.

Chest tube.

Closed drainage system (including connection tubing and water).

Suture (e.g. 0 or 1–0 silk).

Dressing.

Small bore chest drains (10–14 Fr) inserted via Seldinger technique have shown to be as effective as large bore drains (>14 Fr) while being reported as less painful and are considered first-line treatment of pleural effusion and empyema [16, 32, 33]. In most studies, small bore chest drains <14 Fr were found to be effective in draining the effusion and even reduced the frequency of surgical referral and length of hospital stay after application of intrapleural fibrinolytic agents [34]. Even though small bore catheters have been reported to be more susceptible to blockage and kinking, these complications can be avoided with regular and careful review of the drains to avoid kinking and flushing the drain in case of blockage [32, 33, 35]. Large bore (20–32 Fr) surgical drains may be considered if small bore drains fail.

Thoracocentesis and chest drain insertion

POCUS-guided bedside pleural effusion drainage performed by experienced physicians has shown to be a safe option to ensure effective drainage and prevent complications, independent of the size of the pleural effusion [35–38]. Depending on the indication, either thoracocentesis or drain insertion can be undertaken. In order to prevent repeat thoracocentesis, insertion of a drain (Fig. 2) is recommended if recurrence of effusion is expected. Thoracocentesis in malignant effusion is associated with high recurrence rate and is

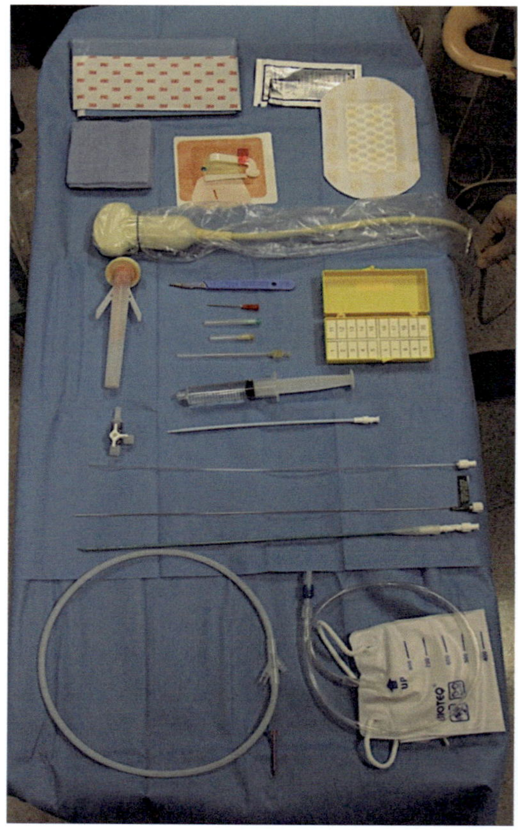

Fig. 2 Pigtail chest drain insertion kit (Seldinger technique). The ultrasound probe is added to the sterile field

not recommended if life expectancy is >1 month [16].

As chest drain insertion has reported to be a painful procedure (with 50% of patients describing pain), a combined systemic and local analgesia regimen is recommended [39]. Small-bore drains have also been shown to have significantly lower analgesia requirements than large-bore drains (when they have been inserted for the same indication) [40]. As a result, small-bore drains have become the first choice for effusion drainage. Local anaesthetic (e.g. lidocaine) (up to 3 mg/kg) is usually infiltrated subcutaneously into the intended puncture site. POCUS-guidance can allow visualisation of the needle and accurate deployment of the anaesthetic. In sedated patients, temporary increase of the established pain regimen, deepening of sedation and occasional paralysis to reduce movement during the procedure may be considered.

The patient's position is dependent on the operator preference and the site of the pathology. The patient may sit upright leaning forward, or lying supine or on their side with the respective arm underneath their head, exposing the area of the "triangle of safety" [41]. Potential immobility of the critically ill patients may restrict possible drain insertion areas; leaving the supine position as the most frequently used. Ultrasound guidance is the most helpful tool to localize a safe puncture site [35]. An anecdotal 'rule of thumb' is to avoid positioning a posterior drain closer than a hands-breath to the spine, considering that the neurovascular bundle is usually more exposed in posterior position [42]. A fluid depth of at least 10 mm at the site of puncture is recommended [35]. Important intrathoracic anatomical structures including the diaphragm, the lung and heart as well as intraabdominal structures like spleen and liver should be clearly identified when selecting the puncture site.

'Step by step'

Ideally local anaesthesia is performed using a series of needles, progressing gradually deeper in to the chest wall and finally to the parietal pleura (Fig. 3).

Under ultrasound guidance, a needle (connected to a syringe) is introduced into the pleural space under constant aspiration. The trajectory of the needle can be seen and should be along the upper border of the respective rib; it should be advanced slowly until aspirating pleural fluid to confirm the needle position in the pleural space (Fig. 4).

A guidewire is then inserted through the needle into the pleural space and its position checked using ultrasound. The needle is then removed (while keeping the guidewire secure) (Fig. 5).

A small skin incision next to the guidewire entry point is then made. Using sequential dilator sizes, dilatation of the incision is performed by advancing the dilators deeper in a twisting motion over the fixed guidewire. Once the track around the guidewire has been dilated, the drain is inserted over the guide wire until the last drainage hole is positioned well inside the pleural space. The drain is then held in a fixed position and the guidewire is removed. The drain is then connected to the prepared drainage system. All drains other than pigtail systems should be secured with skin sutures to prevent accidental removal (Fig. 6) [35].

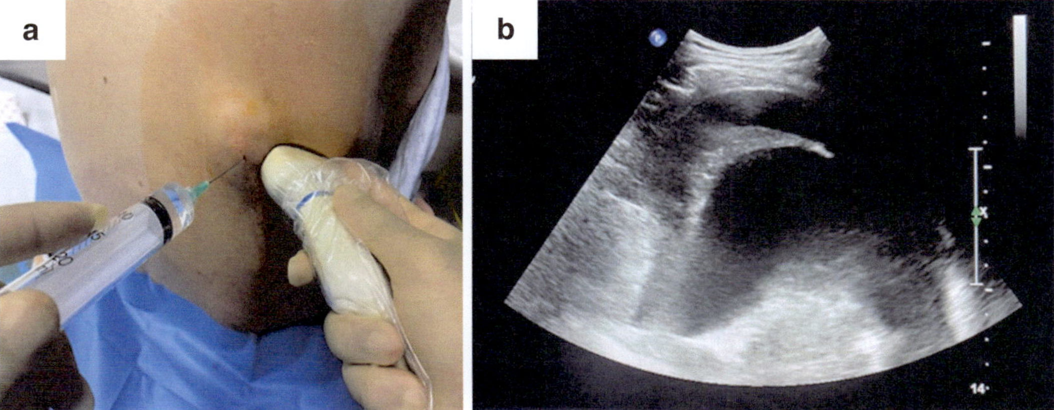

Fig. 3 Local anaesthesia is applied to the skin and following chest wall levels (**a**). Pleural effusion is confirmed with ultrasound (**b**)

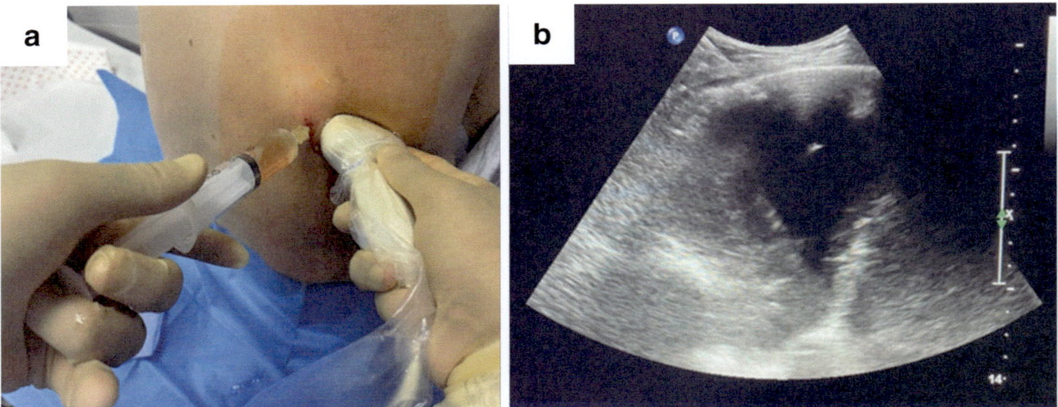

Fig. 4 A needle, connected to a syringe, is introduced into the pleural space and pleural fluid is aspirated (**a**) Sonographic verification of the intrapleural needle position (**b**)

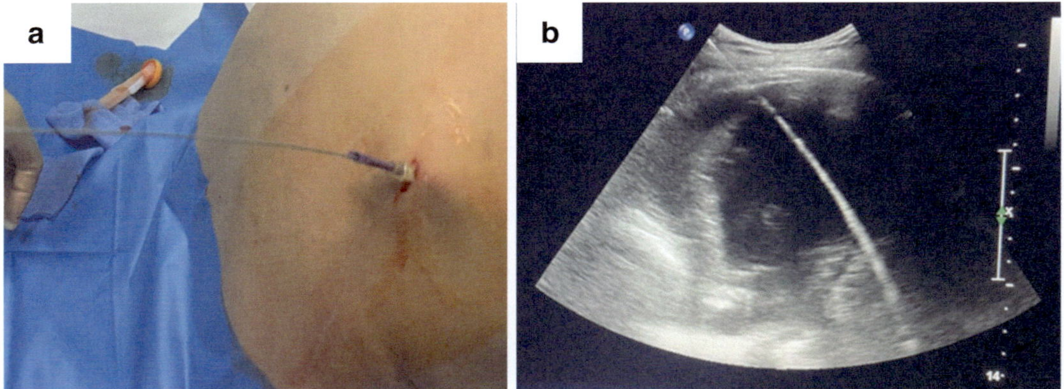

Fig. 5 Guidewire insertion under ultrasound-guidance with position of guide wire in patient (**a**) and in the pleural space (**b**)

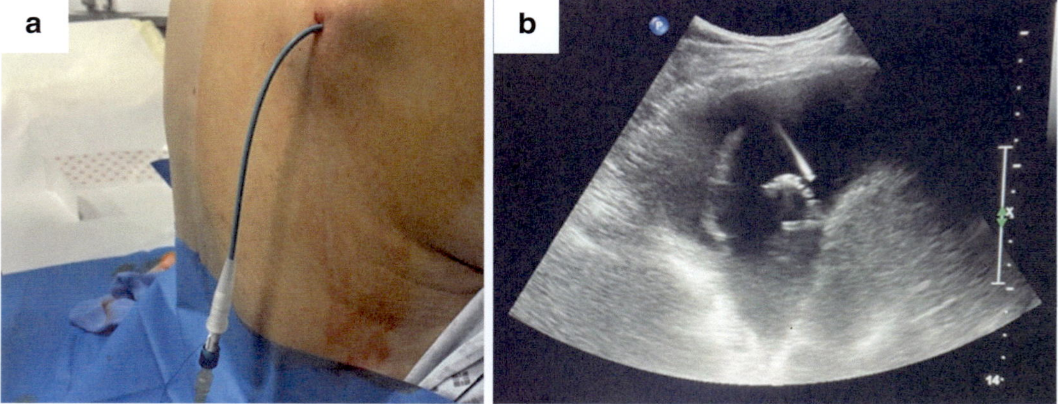

Fig. 6 Inserted small bore pigtail chest drain (**a**) and ultrasound confirmation of pigtail drain inside the pleural cavity (**b**)

Fibrinolytic agents and pleurodesis

As mentioned above, small-bore catheters (10–14 Fr) have shown to be effective for drainage of empyema [34]. On occasion, multiloculated, drainage-resistant effusion may only be effectively drained with the intrapleural application of the combination of DNase and tissue plasminogen activator (tPA); this has been shown to work with good effect [34, 43, 44], with referral rates for surgical treatment and hospital stay significantly reduced without increase in advert events [45]. However, current literature still remains controversial and guidelines do not support the routine use of intrapleural fibrinolytic agents.

If pleurodesis is indicated (e.g. in malignant effusion), a bedside Talc slurry pleurodesis can be performed through a small-bore (10–14 Fr) chest drain. This method has been shown to be as effective as thoracoscopic Talc pleurodesis in preventing recurrence of effusion in patients who were not fit for surgery or able to have thoracoscopy [16, 46–48].

Complications and chest drain management

In general, complications following thoracocentesis and small-bore chest drain insertion under ultrasound guidance are rare. The most important are pneumothorax, injury to spleen and liver, failed procedure, infection and bleeding [16, 36]. Awareness of potential complications, operator experience and POCUS guidance improve outcome and safety [35, 49–51]. Of note, the use of a trocar has shown to be associated with the highest complication rate and is now considered obsolete [52].

Ultrasound precisely demonstrates needle position and any underlying abnormalities such as cardiac enlargement, raised hemidiaphragm or adherent lung, minimizing the risk of thoracic or abdominal organ injuries, which represent the most severe complication. Use of POCUS-guided thoracocentesis has significantly reduced the rate of post-interventional pneumothorax to around 1–4% [51, 53]. A post-procedural chest x-ray is no longer mandated in asymptomatic patients, as an ultrasound can confirm sliding lung in the absence of pneumothorax [54]. Infectious complications following chest drain insertion like empyema can occur in up to 25% but can be reduced to a minimum using the previously described strictly aseptic technique [35, 55].

The volume of pleural effusion drainage within the first hour should not exceed 1.5 L to prevent the physiological complication of re-expansion pulmonary oedema [56, 57]. Assessment of the chest drain at regular intervals, supervised by a team experienced with drain management, is recommended to ensure patency. If blocked, the drain can be flushed with 20–30 ml of normal saline, however, regular flushing to ensure patency is not recommended.

Pitfalls

See Table 2.

Table 2 Pitfalls in POCUS-guided small-bore chest drain insertion

Pitfall	Solution
Incorrect sizing of effusion in ultrasound single plane view	Always show two planes (longitudinal and transverse)
Changing patient position in between marking of optimal drainage site and procedure (The "x marks the spot" method)	Live bedside POCUS-guided drainage
Differentiating pleural effusion from pleural thickening	Use of color Doppler in addition to grey-scale ultrasound [15], less likely with increased operator experience [58, 59]

Conclusion

Pleural effusion is a common medical problem and can be precisely diagnosed with the help of point of care thoracic ultrasound in addition to patient's medical history and clinical assessment. Beyond its excellent diagnostic sensitivity, POCUS guidance allows safe aspiration and drainage of pleural effusion (for symptomatic treatment or further diagnostic analyses), minimizing complications like pneumothorax in experienced hands. Small-bore catheters (10–14 Fr), inserted using a Seldinger technique, should be considered first-line treatment in effusions and empyema, and provide an option to enhance patient outcome with administration of fibrinolytic agents and Talc pleurodesis treatment if required.

References

1. Hooper C, Lee YCG, Maskell N. Investigation of a unilateral pleural effusion in adults: British thoracic society pleural disease guideline 2010. Thorax. 2010;65(Suppl 2):ii4–17.
2. Mattison LE, Coppage L, Alderman DF, Herlong JO, Sahn SA. Pleural effusions in the medical ICU: prevalence, causes, and clinical implications. Chest. 1997;111(4):1018–23.
3. Fysh ETH, Smallbone P, Mattock N, McCloskey C, Litton E, Wibrow B, et al. Clinically significant pleural effusion in intensive care: a prospective multicenter cohort study. Crit Care Explor. 2020;2(1): e0070.
4. Jany B, Welte T. Pleural effusion in adults—etiology, diagnosis, and treatment. Dtsch Ärztebl Int. 2019;116(21):377–86.
5. Thomas R, Jenkins S, Eastwood PR, Lee YCG, Singh B. Physiology of breathlessness associated with pleural effusions. Curr Opin Pulm Med. 2015;21(4):338–45.
6. Brogi E, Gargani L, Bignami E, Barbariol F, Marra A, Forfori F, et al. Thoracic ultrasound for pleural effusion in the intensive care unit: a narrative review from diagnosis to treatment. Crit Care. 2017;21(1):325.
7. Marel M, Zrůstová M, Stasný B, Light RW. The incidence of pleural effusion in a well-defined region. Epidemiologic study in central bohemia. Chest. 1993;104(5):1486–9.
8. Henschke CI, Yankelevitz DF, Wand A, Davis SD, Shiau M. Accuracy and efficacy of chest radiography in the intensive care unit. Radiol Clin North Am. 1996;34(1):21–31.
9. Ruskin JA, Gurney JW, Thorsen MK, Goodman LR. Detection of pleural effusions on supine chest radiographs. AJR Am J Roentgenol. 1987;148(4):681–3.
10. Eibenberger KL, Dock WI, Ammann ME, Dorffner R, Hörmann MF, Grabenwöger F. Quantification of pleural effusions: sonography versus radiography. Radiology. 1994;191(3):681–4.
11. Kocijančič I, Vidmar K, Ivanovi-Herceg Z. Chest sonography versus lateral decubitus radiography in the diagnosis of small pleural effusions. J Clin Ultrasound. 2003;31(2):69–74.
12. Volpicelli G, Elbarbary M, Blaivas M, Lichtenstein DA, Mathis G, Kirkpatrick AW, et al. International evidence-based recommendations for point-of-care lung ultrasound. Intensive Care Med. 2012;38(4):577–91.
13. Kearney SE, Davies CW, Davies RJ, Gleeson FV. Computed tomography and ultrasound in parapneumonic effusions and empyema. Clin Radiol. 2000;55(7):542–7.
14. Doelken P, Strange C. Chest ultrasound for "Dummies." Chest. 2003;123(2):332–3.
15. Lipscomb DJ, Flower CD, Hadfield JW. Ultrasound of the pleura: an assessment of its clinical value. Clin Radiol. 1981;32(3):289–90.
16. Roberts ME, Neville E, Berrisford RG, Antunes G, Ali NJ, BTS pleural disease guideline group. Management of a malignant pleural effusion: British thoracic society pleural disease guideline 2010. Thorax. 2010;65(Suppl 2):ii32–40.
17. Bibby AC, Dorn P, Psallidas I, Porcel JM, Janssen J, Froudarakis M, et al. ERS/EACTS statement on the management of malignant pleural effusions. Eur Respir J. 2018;52(1).
18. Karkhanis VS, Joshi JM. Pleural effusion: diagnosis, treatment, and management. Open Access Emerg Med OAEM. 2012;22(4):31–52.
19. Fartoukh M, Azoulay E, Galliot R, Le Gall J-R, Baud F, Chevret S, et al. Clinically documented pleural effusions in medical ICU patients: how useful is routine thoracentesis? Chest. 2002;121(1):178–84.
20. Wang L-M, Cherng J-M, Wang J-S. Improved lung function after thoracocentesis in patients with paradoxical movement of a hemidiaphragm secondary to a large pleural effusion. Respirol Carlton Vic. 2007;12(5):719–23.
21. Razazi K, Thille AW, Carteaux G, Beji O, Brun-Buisson C, Brochard L, et al. Effects of pleural effusion drainage on oxygenation, respiratory mechanics, and hemodynamics in mechanically ventilated patients. Ann Am Thorac Soc. 2014;11(7):1018–24.
22. Miller KS, Sahn SA. Chest tubes. Indications, technique, management and complications. Chest. 1987;91(2):258–64.
23. Heffner JE, Brown LK, Barbieri C, DeLeo JM. Pleural fluid chemical analysis in parapneumonic

effusions. A meta-analysis. Am J Respir Crit Care Med. 1995;151(6):1700–8.

24. Davies HE, Davies RJO, Davies CWH. Management of pleural infection in adults: British thoracic society pleural disease guideline 2010. Thorax. 2010;65 (Suppl 2):ii41–53.

25. Salyer WR, Eggleston JC, Erozan YS. Efficacy of pleural needle biopsy and pleural fluid cytopathology in the diagnosis of malignant neoplasm involving the pleura. Chest. 1975;67(5):536–9.

26. Garcia LW, Ducatman BS, Wang HH. The value of multiple fluid specimens in the cytological diagnosis of malignancy. Mod Pathol Off J U S Can Acad Pathol Inc. 1994 Aug;7(6):665–8.

27. Hsu C. Cytologic detection of malignancy in pleural effusion: a review of 5,255 samples from 3,811 patients. Diagn Cytopathol. 1987;3(1):8–12.

28. Potts DE, Levin DC, Sahn SA. Pleural fluid pH in parapneumonic effusions. Chest. 1976;70 (03):328–31.

29. Pneumatikos I, Bouros D. Pleural effusions in critically ill patients. Respiration. 2008;76(3):241–8.

30. Light RW, Macgregor MI, Luchsinger PC, Ball WC. Pleural effusions: the diagnostic separation of transudates and exudates. Ann Intern Med. 1972;77 (4):507–13.

31. McVay PA, Toy PT. Lack of increased bleeding after paracentesis and thoracentesis in patients with mild coagulation abnormalities. Transfusion (Paris). 1991;31(2):164–71.

32. Horsley A, Jones L, White J, Henry M. Efficacy and complications of small-bore, wire-guided chest drains. Chest. 2006;130(6):1857–63.

33. Keeling AN, Leong S, Logan PM, Lee MJ. Empyema and effusion: outcome of image-guided small-bore catheter drainage. Cardiovasc Intervent Radiol. 2008;31(1):135–41.

34. Rahman NM, Maskell NA, West A, Teoh R, Arnold A, Mackinlay C, et al. Intrapleural use of tissue plasminogen activator and dnase in pleural infection. N Engl J Med. 2011;365(6):518–26.

35. Havelock T, Teoh R, Laws D, Gleeson F. Pleural procedures and thoracic ultrasound: British Thoracic Society pleural disease guideline 2010. Thorax. 2010;65(Suppl 2):i61–76

36. Vetrugno L, Guadagnin GM, Orso D, Boero E, Bignami E, Bove T. An easier and safe affair, pleural drainage with ultrasound in critical patient: a technical note. Crit Ultrasound J. 2018;10(1):18.

37. Liang S-J, Tu C-Y, Chen H-J, Chen C-H, Chen W, Shih C-M, et al. Application of ultrasound-guided pigtail catheter for drainage of pleural effusions in the ICU. Intensive Care Med. 2008;35(2):350.

38. Lichtenstein D, Hulot JS, Rabiller A, Tostivint I, Mezière G. Feasibility and safety of ultrasound-aided thoracentesis in mechanically ventilated patients. Intensive Care Med. 1999;25(9):955–8.

39. Luketich JD, Kiss M, Hershey J, Urso GK, Wilson J, Bookbinder M, et al. Chest tube insertion: a

prospective evaluation of pain management. Clin J Pain. 1998;14(2):152–4.

40. Clementsen P, Evald T, Grode G, Hansen M, Krag Jacobsen G, Faurschou P. Treatment of malignant pleural effusion: pleurodesis using a small percutaneous catheter. A prospective randomized study. Respir Med. 1998;92(3):593–6

41. Laws D, Neville E, Duffy J. BTS guidelines for the insertion of a chest drain. Thorax. 2003;58(Suppl 2): ii53–9.

42. DeBiasi EM, Puchalski J. Thoracentesis: state-of-the-art in procedural safety, patient outcomes, and physiologic impact. PLEURA. 2016;3:237399 7516646554.

43. Laisaar T, Püttsepp E, Laisaar V. Early administration of intrapleural streptokinase in the treatment of multiloculated pleural effusions and pleural empyemas. Thorac Cardiovasc Surg. 1996;44(5):252–6.

44. Bouros D, Schiza S, Panagou P, Drositis J, Siafakas N. Role of streptokinase in the treatment of acute loculated parapneumonic pleural effusions and empyema. Thorax. 1994;49(9):852–5.

45. Corcoran JP, Rahman NM. Point: should fibrinolytics be routinely administered intrapleurally for management of a complicated parapneumonic effusion? Yes CHEST. 2014;145(1):14–7.

46. Dresler CM, Olak J, Herndon JE, Richards WG, Scalzetti E, Fleishman SB, et al. Phase III intergroup study of talc poudrage vs talc slurry sclerosis for malignant pleural effusion. Chest. 2005;127(3):909–15.

47. Clive AO, Jones HE, Bhatnagar R, Preston NJ, Maskell N. Interventions for the management of malignant pleural effusions: a network meta-analysis. Cochrane Database Syst Rev. 2016;(5):CD010529.

48. Reddy CB, DeCamp MM, Diekemper RL, Gould MK, Henry T, Iyer NP, et al. Summary for clinicians: clinical practice guideline for management of malignant pleural effusions. Ann Am Thorac Soc. 2018;16(1):17–21.

49. Collins TR, Sahn SA. Thoracocentesis. Clinical value, complications, technical problems, and patient experience. Chest. 1987;91(6):817–22.

50. Gordon CE, Feller-Kopman D, Balk EM, Smetana GW. Pneumothorax following thoracentesis: a systematic review and meta-analysis. Arch Intern Med. 2010;170(4):332–9.

51. Mayo PH, Goltz HR, Tafresh M, Doelken P. Safety of ultrasound-guided thoracentesis in patients receiving mechanical ventilation. Chest. 2004;125 (3):1059–62.

52. Remérand F, Luce V, Badachi Y, Lu Q, Bouhemad B, Rouby J-J. Incidence of chest tube malposition in the critically ill: a prospective computed tomography study. Anesthesiology. 2007;106(6):1112–9.

53. Cavanna L, Mordenti P, Bertè R, Palladino MA, Biasini C, Anselmi E, et al. Ultrasound guidance reduces pneumothorax rate and improves safety of thoracentesis in malignant pleural effusion: report on

445 consecutive patients with advanced cancer. World J Surg Oncol. 2014;2(12):139.

54. Dancel R, Schnobrich D, Puri N, Franco-Sadud R, Cho J, Grikis L, et al. Recommendations on the use of ultrasound guidance for adult thoracentesis: a position statement of the society of hospital medicine. J Hosp Med. 2018;13(2):126–35.

55. Kwiatt M, Tarbox A, Seamon MJ, Swaroop M, Cipolla J, Allen C, et al. Thoracostomy tubes: a comprehensive review of complications and related topics. Int J Crit Illn Inj Sci. 2014;4(2):143–55.

56. Mohammed HM. Chest tube care in critically ill patient: a comprehensive review. Egypt J Chest Dis Tuberc. 2015;64(4):849–55.

57. Echevarria C, Twomey D, Dunning J, Chanda B. Does re-expansion pulmonary oedema exist? Interact Cardiovasc Thorac Surg. 2008;7(3):485–9.

58. Wu RG, Yuan A, Liaw YS, Chang DB, Yu CJ, Wu HD, et al. Image comparison of real-time gray-scale ultrasound and color Doppler ultrasound for use in diagnosis of minimal pleural effusion. Am J Respir Crit Care Med. 1994;150(2):510–4.

59. Kalokairinou-Motogna M, Maratou K, Paianid I, Soldatos T, Antipa E, Tsikkini A, et al. Application of color Doppler ultrasound in the study of small pleural effusion. Med Ultrason. 2010;12(1):12–6.

Teaching and Accreditation in Cardiopulmonary POCUS

Serena Rovida, Giampaolo Martinelli, and Nick Fletcher

Tell me and I forget. Teach me and I remember. Involve me and I learn

Benjamin Franklin—American scientist and polymath (1705–1790 AD)

Abstract

Over the last 20 years, the demand for cardiopulmonary ultrasound training has led to the 'ground up' development of courses and educational resources. Relevant specialist societies have followed with formal curricula and accreditations. E-learning and simulation with metrics have expanded the possibilities and accelerated the potential for acquiring knowledge and technical skills. A global competency framework has developed initially from a small number of enthusiasts and these fields are now established as key competencies across critical care and emergency medicine in addition to the traditional disciplines of radiology and cardiology. Knowledge and skills can be divided into basic and advanced levels of competency and this has been reflected in the accreditations that have developed. Echocardiography goes from a focused 2D protocol up to a comprehensive examination with all Doppler modalities directed at critically ill patients including TOE. Lung ultrasound has also become ubiquitous during COVID-19. The availability of skilled and dedicated mentors and supervisors is key to the further roll out of these disciplines. The future direction is to incorporate them in the formal training programmes of the bodies responsible for training in the various global healthcare systems.

Keywords

Lung ultrasound · Cardiac ultrasound · Echocardiography · Training · Accreditation

S. Rovida (✉) · N. Fletcher
Department of Cardiothoracic Anaesthesia,
St George's University Hospital, London, UK
e-mail: sererovida@gmail.com

G. Martinelli
Department of Cardiothoracic Anaesthesia,
Barts Health NHS Trust, London, UK
e-mail: giampaolo.martinelli@nhs.net;
snick@doctors.org.uk

© The Author(s), under exclusive license to Springer Nature Switzerland AG 2023
H. Soliman-Aboumarie et al. (eds.), *Cardiopulmonary Point of Care Ultrasound*,
https://doi.org/10.1007/978-3-031-29472-3_28

355

Key Messages

- Basic and Advanced POCUS accreditations for cardiac and pulmonary pathologies are now well established in the emergency medicine and critical care settings
- Experienced and skilled mentor and supervisor availability are key to further roll out of competency in these fields
- Simulation with accompanying metrics can aid the development and acceleration of technical competency
- Incorporation in the formal training programs for emergency and critical care medicine is the next big step in making these disciplines available to improve the management of patients in these areas.

Introduction

Physician use of cardiopulmonary ultrasound in intensive care, anaesthesiology, acute and emergency medicine is now clearly established and is recognized to be one of the key development areas for the current generation of clinicians. In addition to point of care diagnosis, this can guide interventions and is complementary to many of the existing forms of monitoring. More affordable portable ultrasound machines with good quality linear,, curvilinear, phase array and transoesophageal (TOE) probes are now available. Many of the technological barriers to adoption have therefore been removed. The issue of physician training has sparked the interest of educators. Cardiopulmonary ultrasound training requires both a technical apprenticeship and a significant knowledge curriculum. For an individual to gain competence even in basic POCUS, it will take a minimum of 6 months. Those with the ambition to educate trainees to gain this competence are trying to determine how to achieve this within a limited time and constantly expanding medical curriculum. The manpower, expenses and time required for supervision and training is considerable. This chapter will look at how this has been achieved thus far and will discuss some of the concepts involved [1].

The Educational Challenges

It is important here to consider how cardiopulmonary ultrasound has developed from a point where it was practised and delivered almost solely by cardiologists or echocardiography technicians 20 years ago, to the point where it is ubiquitous and delivered predominantly in many units by critical care and emergency physicians. The challenges and solutions can be summarised here:

1. *Rapid expansion despite a limited number of educators:* A few enthusiasts started to push for critical care echocardiography skills initially in cardiac units. A network of trainers and courses developed who used the new accreditations to develop new mentors and trainers. Everyone who trained became an educator and resulted in an almost viral spread of competency.
2. *Resistance:* There has been resistance to a new group of specialists entering this space. This may be due to payments for service, territorial anxiety or concerns regarding governance and quality. This has varied between healthcare systems and has been mitigated by various strategies including engagement, development of an evidence base and demand for service provision. The support of specialist societies and development of education and accreditation programmes with attention to the quality agenda has been pivotal in this regard.
3. *Curriculum development and training time:* Again, the engagement of specialist societies in this regard has been essential to support the development of training networks. This has been very much a bootstrapping phenomenon, driven by enthusiasts and doctors in training who appreciated the value of POCUS for their patients. As this is a training intensive process, creation of service posts with a dedicated ultrasound training element has been a positive and engaging route to competency attracting a generation of interested trainees into critical care.
4. *Digital media development:* This has accompanied roll out of ultrasound and acted as both a driver and a recipient. Digital images

captured from ultrasound lend themselves to dissemination via media platforms such as teaching sites and increasingly social media. The current generation have an increasing visual literacy in ultrasound images and they often act as signposts into training material and an appetite for further material. Whereas there are privacy concerns, medical regulators have strict positions on any patient identifiable material.

5. *Integration of ultrasound information with patient clinical and other monitoring information:* This interface is the most difficult and crucial educational step and takes the most time to master. High quality mentoring and supervision is required for this process and will take varying lengths of time for each learner depending on their ability and experience.

Key Education Concepts

Clearly defined areas can be identified for training; there is a knowledge-base required for ultrasound practice, there are the technical aspects and there is reporting which integrates the two into a defined outcome that should be standardised and recorded.

Knowledge Base

This is the theoretical basis, including physics of ultrasound, probe selection, cardiopulmonary anatomy, sonoanatomy, cardiopulmonary function and pathological findings. For basic level POCUS, the curricula are similar and limited. This can be taught through lectures, self-directed e-learning and tutorials. The development of e-learning packages has allowed broader roll out and can be directly linked with an accreditation.

Technical Skills

Technical skills involve both motor skills and spatial awareness and can only be taught at the bedside with a skilled mentor. This is the more time-intensive aspect which requires time and availability of mentors. There is always much discussion about the number of cases needed to develop competence and indeed it will vary between trainees. We are used to the concept of competency-based learning. There is evidence that the learning curve seems to level out above 30 cases and 50 cases is commonly taken as the required logbook number for basic competence to ensure all have attained the required level. For more advanced levels, logbook numbers are higher with a wider spread—and generally assume the basic level has been previously attained. The use of simulators and metrics has proved important in embedding and accelerating technical competence.

Simulation

Simulation has been recognised to aid and accelerate the development of echocardiography competence in particular. Studies conducted on cohorts of learners randomised to groups with or without simulation have shown that it is beneficial to the learning process, both in terms of technical and anatomical progress. Sophisticated high-fidelity simulators for TTE and lung US are useful adjuncts to actual scanning, but it is for TOE where the biggest potential gains exist. There is potential harm associated with TOE probe movements and this can be an impediment to the early-stage learner. A particularly helpful feature of simulators is a 3D model of the heart with a haptic interface, allowing visualisation of the ultrasound plane position in relation to cardiac anatomy as the dummy probe is manipulated [2].

Reporting

Reporting is a quality issue which can be standardised and measured as an indicator of progress. It demonstrates the integration of the two other educational tracks and the interpretation for patient management is the final common pathway into improving patient outcomes and the most important goal of training and practice.

Mentoring/Supervision

This is the most important element of the whole educational project. Access to a dedicated and supportive mentor who is able to provide time and teaching opportunities is highly likely to produce the most successful learning outcome. A mentor may not be trained in the learner's own speciality and may not necessarily be a doctor. The mentor may be an effective tutor for technical skills without the associated relevant clinical content. This is where a supervisor is needed to work with the mentor and provide quality assurance for the learner and ensure that all objectives have been met and to sign off that competence has been achieved. A supervisor's role is also to educate the mentor and possibly to provide a local network with an educational framework, whereby competent learners become mentors once competence is achieved. Group teaching sessions whereby learners can interact with others is also very useful and this is increasingly happening in the virtual space, particularly following COVID-19.

Cardiac ultrasound training and accreditation in anaesthesia and intensive care:

Pocus in Anaesthesia and Intensive Care:

Echocardiography has been utilized for a long time as a diagnostic modality in cardiac anaesthesia, critical care and emergency medicine, however, it was mainly performed by cardiologists and trained echocardiography technicians. More recently, the focus has been on echocardiography practice by clinicians themselves. Training has been broadly defined as either basic or advanced in line with the complexity of the information sought. Basic competence encompasses mostly a limited set of 2D transthoracic imaging planes to diagnose severe and potentially life-threatening pathology, otherwise referred to as focused echocardiography with additional imaging for diagnosis of pneumothorax and pleural effusion. Advanced practice utilizes a full range of anatomical and Doppler imaging via TTE or TOE to diagnose pathologies and monitor hemodynamic interventions. Advanced pulmonary ultrasound has extended to the diagnosis of a number of lung conditions. We will first consider educational concepts related to cardiac ultrasound followed by lung ultrasound. Whereas they are often taught together and are in many ways integrated; the origins, techniques, evidence and knowledge base are distinct.

Development of Basic Cardiac Ultrasound Teaching Protocols

Basic cardiac ultrasound is essentially based on the focussed assessed transthoracic echocardiography (FATE) developed by Sloth and colleagues. The imaging used the long and short parasternal axis views, together with the apical four chamber and the subcostal long axis view. This is common to all of the basic training views with the addition of a pleural view. Training assumes the clinician has no prior competence in ultrasound of the heart and no knowledge of sonoanatomy. The trainee is likely to have some basic knowledge of ultrasound-guided vascular access which is now ubiquitous in critical care.

Cardiology led the way with training and education in echocardiography. An early example was for cardiac physiologists in the UK with the TTE accreditation from the British Society of Echocardiography. Professor Eric Sloth and the Aarhus group first developed the concept of a focussed scan and education programme for non-cardiologists in anaesthesia and critical care in the late 1980s. These focused applications of echocardiography used a 4-plane cardiac scan with the addition of a pleural view. The package was delivered in a standardised one-day course and certification which did not include a logbook for sign off. Teaching was limited by the number of non-cardiology experts in POCUS for this group of patients. It was limited to a small number of mainly tertiary centres and postgraduate practical courses by major societies such as the European Society of Intensive Care Medicine (ESICM). A big step in the UK was the establishment of two accreditations resulting from a collaboration of the Intensive Care Society and the British Society of Echocardiography (FICE) and the Resuscitation Council (FEEL). FICE (Focused Intensive Care Echocardiography) currently named FUSIC (Focused Ultrasound in Intensive Care) had a structured course, a system of mentors and supervisors, a logbook and a final assessment.

Advanced Echocardiography

Cardiac anaesthetists were the first non-cardiology specialty to adopt echocardiography in a structured way. Competency in intraoperative TOE for diagnosis and monitoring of the cardiac surgical patient has now become essential for all specialist practitioners and teaching programmes embedded in training schemes and accreditations are well established. Professional societies in different regions of the world have evolved systems of accreditation and training to develop the required level of competency, these programmes have much in common even though the caseload requirements may differ significantly. Critical care clinicians have developed their own systems of accreditation adapted to the specialized needs of their patients. These training and accreditation programmes necessarily contain much more in the way of knowledge content and include a formal examination and a significant training logbook and require a much higher level of technical competence embedded into a framework for translation into clinical management. Most of the advanced accreditations are separated into the mode of echocardiography, whether TTE or TOE. It can be argued that the knowledge base for more advanced forms is similar, whether in both, it is the technical skills that diverge. The exception is the ESICM

European Diploma in Advanced Critical Care Echocardiography (EDEC) which incorporates both modalities within the accreditation package.

Intermediate and Modular Accreditations

It was anticipated that there was a gap between basic POCUS and advanced status that would fuel demand for progression for those who wanted more quantitative cardiac US but without the resources to pursue the commitment to an advanced accreditation. There are a number of iterations of this, probably the first attempt to provide a wide roll out being FATE+. More recently in the UK FUSIC HD [3] and the BSE Level 1 Ultrasound are noted attempts. Increasingly training and accreditation will be seen as a series of accumulative modular blocks which can be gained at a rate and stage determined by the trainee according to their need, interest and stage of training. At each stage, the trainee becomes the trainer for the previous stage thus sustaining and consolidating the progressive uplift of the competency pyramid. Matching modular educational online resources and course configurations can be developed in parallel to the sophistication of the accreditation.

Lung Ultrasound Training and Accreditation

Over the last two decades, the use of Lung Ultrasound (LUS) has increased substantially in several settings such as Emergency Department as well as surgical and medical units. Together with its diagnostic accuracy. LUS is a reliable monitoring tool for the most common causes of acute respiratory failure including pneumothorax, pulmonary edema, consolidations and pleural effusion. Rapid, reproducible and radiation-free, LUS is nowadays integrated in the bedside assessment and increasing evidence is supporting its role and applications among acute and chronic pulmonary conditions. Medical specialists other than radiologists are undertaking ultrasound examinations on patients referred to them for their clinical opinion as a direct extension of their clinical examination. Several international societies have developed their own guidelines for LUS accreditation, however a unique standardized rotation route in education and competency assessment is not available yet. In this section we summarize the current state of development of LUS accreditation options from different national and international societies including their training programs and certifications.

Development of Lung Ultrasound Teaching Protocols

Several LUS scanning protocols have been developed by local teaching faculties and most of them are modified version of the initial Bedside Lung Ultrasound in Emergency (BLUE)-protocol proposed by Lichtenstein back in the nineties. The BLUE protocol algorithm allows the immediate diagnosis of acute respiratory failure by a quick scanning technique which aims to assess the main anterior chest area and lung bases. Overall, 10 signs have been described which are able to guide the physician through the diagnosis and definition of lung profiles for main pathologies including pneumonia, congestive heart failure, COPD, asthma, pulmonary embolism, pneumothorax with an accuracy up to 90% [4]. Later on Volpicelli et al. proposed a lung scanning approach for the assessment of acute interstitial syndrome based on 8 scanning zones, 4 for each hemithorax covering the anterior and the lateral lung zone further divided in superior and inferior quadrants [5]. More extensive protocols providing full chest assessment including the posterior chest zones have been introduced as well as a LUS scoring system (LUSS) has been adopted by intensivists for estimation of the aeration score and follow up during patients stay in ITU [6]. Despite being complete and appropriate, these protocols are usually quite challenging since the majority of the patients are bedbound, lying semi recumbent or usually in respiratory distress which significantly limits patient cooperation and mobility.

According to ATLS algorithm, the standard Focused Assessment with Sonography in Trauma (FAST) has been recently implemented with lung ultrasound anterior chest views and now known as extended FAST (e-FAST) for quick identification of pneumothorax [7].

During resuscitation the fluid administration limited by lung sonography (FALLS) protocol has been also proposed for the management of acute circulatory failure and expedite the diagnosis of distributive (usually septic) shock.

Intermediate and Modular Accreditations

Similar to other ultrasound modalities, including bedside echocardiography and abdominal ultrasound, the LUS accreditation process is comprehensive and consists of three steps. The first one generally consists of modules of lectures and theoretical knowledge covering the basic principles of LUS and ultrasound-guided procedures. Due to the current COVID-19 pandemic and the technological advances of internet-based virtual platforms, the majority of the courses are currently being held online, allowing participants to complete their e-learning modules remotely at their own pace. Once the participants have successfully completed their first part demonstrating their knowledge throughout a theory assessment test, they can join the second step. A one or two-day practical course featuring clinical observation, hands-on training with volunteers and simulation training will provide the skills to the candidates to create their own portfolio made of an established number of examinations with a minimal logbook of pathological scanning reports. Following successful completion of the theoretical and hands-on course, the LUS candidate will have a mentor who will guide them with the initial scanning. After the initial supervised scanning, the candidate will submit a portfolio of a predefined number of reported scans followed by a triggered assessment usually run by the program director or by a POCUS supervisor.

These three steps are mandatory for LUS accreditation; however, they can slightly differ from a society or a country to another due the number of required supervised scans, the courses modality and the medical specialties the participants belong to.

In 2012, a group of international experts wrote the first consensus recommendations for LUS with the intent to summarize the available evidences and elaborate a unified approach as well as common language for LU clinical applications [8]. Nowadays several societies provide detailed guidelines including description of logbook, number of supervised examinations and basic knowledge required prior to become an independent sonographer. Advantages of having established roles from official institutions ensure quality of theoretical and practical skills, however a unique route is not available yet and a substantial variability between different accreditation pathways and trainees' portfolio exists. According to a systematic review of published literature in clinical LU training, the educational programs proposed are heterogenous and this discrepancy is primarily due to different LU application among specialties [9].

Some effort has been initiated to incorporate LUS into specialty curricula, however the majority of training programs proposed by the accreditation bodies currently remains extra-curricular for trainees. The American College of Emergency Physicians (ACEP) developed in 2008 the first guidelines for the ultrasound portfolio for residency training and it recently implemented the program by introducing dedicated fellowship aiming to develop a deeper comprehension of ultrasound in acute settings. In UK, the Royal College of Emergency Medicine introduced in 2009 two levels of ultrasound practice: the first one, which is encompassing the core elements for basic chest ultrasound, is mandatory while the second level remains optional for specialty trainees. Publications by the Royal College of Radiologists and a joint document by the Association of Anaesthetists of UK and Ireland, Intensive Care Society and Royal College of Anaesthetists also provide guidance for LUS training program. The Intensive Care Society launched an accreditation pathway known as Core Ultrasound in Intensive Care (CUSIC) in which includes all the key aspects of bedside LUS. The CUSIC has been subsequently substituted by FUSIC which includes cardiac, lung, abdominal and vascular ultrasound modules.

As the integration of POCUS along with the standard assessment moves forward, attempts to integrate LUS teaching into undergraduate medical education have been initiated. As an example, in 2020 the statement from Canadian ultrasound Consensus for the undergraduate medical education elaborated a focused ultrasound curriculum for medical students including LU basic knobology [10]. Several small pilot studies demonstrated that, among the medical students without ultrasound experience, limited LUS education could successfully improve their knowledge, image acquisition, and interpretation ability [11–13].

Future Perspectives

LU is a relatively quick technique to grasp with a steep learning curve. The advent of hand-held devices, the development of artificial intelligence (AI) and the increase of demand of lung ultrasound training programs makes the accreditation essential for the medical community. Ideally a common pathway should facilitate evidence collection and standardize the educational goals, however there is a consistent variation between specialties as well as national healthcare systems. Specialist societies have led the way with cardiopulmonary POCUS training and accreditations are becoming more established with increasing uptake. The next step is for educational bodies to formalize the network of supervisors and mentors and incorporate existing educational structures into the formal training curricula of relevant specialties including emergency medicine, general medicine, anaesthesia and critical care.

References

1. Vieillard-Baron A, Millington SJ, Sanfilippo F, Chew M, Diaz-Gomez J, McLean A, et al. A decade of progress in critical care echocardiography: a narrative review. Intensive Care Med. 2019;45(6):770–88.
2. Clau-Terre F, Sharma V, Cholley B, Gonzalez-Alujas T, Galinanes M, Evangelista A, et al. Can simulation help to answer the demand for echocardiography education? Anesthesiology. 2014;120(1):32–41.
3. Miller A, Peck M, Clark T, Conway H, Olusanya S, Fletcher N, et al. FUSIC HD. Comprehensive haemodynamic assessment with ultrasound. J Intensive Care Soc. 2021.
4. BLUE-protocol and FALLS-protocol: two applications of lung ultrasound in the critically ill. Daniel A Lichtenstein).
5. Volpicelli G, Mussaa A, Garofalob G, Cardinaleb L, Casolia G, Perottob F, Favab C, Frascisco M. Bedside lung ultrasound in the assessment of alveolar-interstitial syndrome.
6. Mongodi S, Bouhemad B, Orlando A, Stella A, Tavazzi G, Via G, Iotti GA, Braschi A, Mojoli F, Modified lung ultrasound score for assessing and monitoring pulmonary aeration.
7. Bloom BA, Gibbons RC. Focused assessment with sonography for trauma
8. International evidence-based recommendations for point-of-care lung ultrasound. Intensive Care Med. 2012;38:577–91.
9. Pietersen PI, Madsen KR, Graumann O, et al. Lung ultrasound training: a systematic review of published literature in clinical lung ultrasound training. Crit Ultrasound J. 2018;10:23. https://doi.org/10.1186/s13089-018-0103-6.
10. Ma IWY, Steinmetz P, Weerdenburg K, Woo MY, Olszynski P, Heslop CL, Miller S, Sheppard G, Daniels V, Desy J, Valois M, Devine L, Curtis H, Romano MJ, Martel P, Jelic T, Topping C, Thompson D, Power B, Profetto J, Tonseth P. The Canadian medical student ultrasound curriculum. J Ultrasound Med. 2020;39:1279–87. https://doi.org/10.1002/jum.15218.
11. Lim JS, Lee S, Do HH, Oh KH. Can limited education of lung ultrasound be conducted to medical students properly? A pilot study. BioMed Res Int 2017;2017:6. Article ID 8147075. https://doi.org/10.1155/2017/8147075
12. Steinmetz P, Oleskevich S, Dyachenko A, McCusker J, Lewis J. Accuracy of medical students in detecting pleural effusion using lung ultrasound as an adjunct to the physical examination. J Ultrasound Med. 2018;37:2545–52. https://doi.org/10.1002/jum.14612.
13. Paganini M, Bondì M, Rubini A. Evaluation of chest ultrasound integrated teaching of respiratory system physiology to medical students. Adv Physiol Educ. 2017;41(4):514–7.

Safety and Governance in Cardiopulmonary Ultrasound

Thor Edvardsen and Lars Gunnar Klaeboe

The very first requirement in a hospital is that it should do the sick no harm

Florence Nightingale—English social reformer and the founder of modern nursing (1820–1910 AD).

Abstract

Point-of-Care Ultrasound (POCUS) is a focused ultrasound examination that allows clinical staff to answer specific questions related to diagnosis and patient management in a bedside setting. Portable, easy-to-use scanners that can provide high quality imaging at low-cost have made POCUS widely available. The expanded application of POCUS, however, raises important questions regarding requirements for safe and cost-effective use. These questions do not only involve certification and training requirements described in previous chapters. This chapter aims to put focus on safety aspects related to clinical implementation of POCUS.

Keywords

Point-of-Care ultrasound · POCUS · Safety · Governance

T. Edvardsen (✉) · L. G. Klaeboe
Department of Cardiology, Rikshospitalet, Oslo University Hospital, Oslo, Norway
e-mail: thor.edvardsen@medisin.uio.no

Key messages

- POCUS is an important diagnostic tool that can improve patient safety through enhanced bedside diagnostics.
- Implementing POCUS in clinical practice would benefit from quality-controlled programs organizing education, infrastructure and scope of practice.

Introduction

Point-of-care ultrasound (POCUS) is a focused ultrasound examination performed at the bedside, aiming to solve specific clinical questions. POCUS has been shown to be a powerful extension of the physical examination that may improve bedside diagnostics [1–3] even when performed by relatively inexperienced operators [4–9]. Traditionally, the use of POCUS has been regarded as risk-free, considering its non-invasive nature and lack of harmful ionizing radiation. However, improper use of this diagnostic technology raises the possibility of misdiagnosis, unnecessary treatment and increased patient risk. This may not only be related to errors in imaging acquisition and interpretation, but also to how application of this imaging technology is organized, supervised and quality controlled.

Availability, A Safety Concern?

Small, portable and low-cost ultrasound devices have made POCUS widely available and an integral part of clinical practice for a wide range of health care professionals. POCUS is a complex exercise that requires integration of practical skills and theoretical knowledge together with clinical experience and awareness of limitations related to the imaging technology. Education and training described in previous chapters are regarded as essential for safe application of POCUS [9]. Understandably, there might be concerns related to POCUS being performed by non-imaging experts. However, as POCUS is already a well-established clinical tool in everyday practice, it is inevitable that a large proportion of users will not hold certification when first introduced to bedside ultrasound. This lack of formal imaging competency along with fear of wrong decision-making have been reported as barriers for performing focused ultrasound among anesthesiologists [10]. However, the fact that malpractice lawsuits have been linked to POCUS not being performed when indicated rather than to POCUS-related misdiagnosis and interpretation [11] should be encouraging for expanded use.

The availability of POCUS is likely to increase the frequency of incidental findings. Once identified, these findings might require further diagnostic resources to clarify their significance. Also, exposure to side effects of examinations and treatment that otherwise would not have been initiated might be a concern. Although the use of POCUS is emerging, there is still a large evidence gap regarding its impact on economic and clinical variables. POCUS has been shown to be useful in increasing diagnostic precision and shortening the time to diagnosis [3]. Even though POCUS is likely to be beneficial for patients, evidence is still evolving regarding whether POCUS implantation translates into improved outcomes or false positive findings and subsequent overtreatment. Randomized controlled trials evaluating the use of focused ultrasound on factors like length of hospital stay, morbidity and mortality are needed and are expected to provide more understanding of consequences related to POCUS implementation [12].

Structure and Organization of POCUS

Implementation of POCUS will require quality assurance to manage patient safety and increase competency. For better organization of POCUS, it has been suggested to focus on the five following areas or pillars: governance, infrastructure, administration, education and quality [13].

To ensure clinical competency, hospital executive operational endorsement and necessary resources, a mixed board of clinical and key hospital personnel could facilitate incorporation of POCUS in clinical practice [14] that is in accordance with recommendations and societal guidelines[15].

A POCUS program will require infrastructure for image acquisition and analysis. Ultrasound scanners have become more affordable and thus more available. Nevertheless, diagnostic performance, service agreements and compatibility with existing systems are factors of consideration during procurement processes to maintain quality.

Images and cine loops recorded during POCUS should be archived according to relevant general data protection regulations (GDPR), and ideally in a picture archiving and communication system (PACS) [16]. The increased use of smaller, wireless devices may open up for cloud-based storage solutions. Storage of image loops for later re-evaluation is important not only for safety, but also for supervision, and allows remote expert re-evaluation for educational purposes and quality control. Artificial intelligence (AI) tools are increasingly becoming available in traditional ultrasound systems and are expected to improve efficiency and accuracy. AI has perhaps even greater potential in POCUS, where the variation in user ultrasound experience is higher. By providing guidance during acquisition, AI tools can improve study quality [17], and even help novice ultrasound users capture diagnostic images [18, 19]. By automating or assisting measurements and aiding diagnosis [20], AI is expected to reduce variability, and may somewhat alleviate the need for manual POCUS review.

When implementing POCUS as accessible, reliable and verifiable diagnostic service, dedicated department responsibility will be important. A multidisciplinary POCUS committee that defines scope of practice in accordance with professional recommendations and that ensures that necessary technology and competence is available when needed, has been suggested to provide governance of clinical application of POCUS [13].

Reporting POCUS

Repeated POCUS examinations may be necessary to monitor the patient's treatment. Information obtained during POCUS will form the basis for further decisions and treatment. These data would be essential to compare clinical status over time, document clinical decision-making and provide important information for further referral when an expert opinion is needed. Accordingly, these data should be formally reported in electronic medical records and made available to relevant personnel involved in care of the patient [21]. Reporting POCUS using a standard form stating the indication for examination, summary of findings and an interpretation is one of the few quality improvement projects that has been published lately to promote governance and safety in POCUS [22].

Conclusion

POCUS is an important diagnostic tool that can improve patient safety through enhanced bedside diagnostics. Implementing POCUS in clinical practice would benefit from quality-controlled programs organizing education, infrastructure and scope of practice. AI tools assisting the POCUS user may become an important driver of adoption.

References

1. Moore CL, Copel JA. Point-of-care ultrasonography. N Engl J Med. 2011;364:749–57. https://doi.org/10.1056/NEJMra0909487.
2. Morrow D, Cupp J, Schrift D, Nathanson R, Soni NJ. Point-of-care ultrasound in established settings. South Med J. 2018;111:373–81. https://doi.org/10.14423/smj.0000000000000838.
3. Smallwood N, Dachsel M. Point-of-care ultrasound (POCUS): unnecessary gadgetry or evidence-based medicine? Clin Med (Lond). 2018;18:219–24. https://doi.org/10.7861/clinmedicine.18-3-219.
4. Jacoby J, Cesta M, Axelband J, Melanson S, Heller M, Reed J. Can emergency medicine residents detect acute deep venous thrombosis with a limited, two-site ultrasound examination? J Emerg Med. 2007;32:197–200. https://doi.org/10.1016/j.jemermed.2006.06.008.
5. Bonnafy T, Lacroix P, Desormais I, Labrunie A, Marin B, Leclerc A, et al. Reliability of the measurement of the abdominal aortic diameter by novice operators using a pocket-sized ultrasound system. Arch Cardiovasc Dis. 2013;106:644–50. https://doi.org/10.1016/j.acvd.2013.08.004.
6. Kobal SL, Trento L, Baharami S, Tolstrup K, Naqvi TZ, Cercek B, et al. Comparison of effectiveness of hand-carried ultrasound to bedside cardiovascular physical examination. Am J Cardiol. 2005;96:1002–6 https://doi.org/10.1016/j.amjcard.2005.05.060.
7. Andersen GN, Graven T, Skjetne K, Mjølstad OC, Kleinau JO, Olsen Ø, et al. Diagnostic influence of routine point-of-care pocket-size ultrasound examinations performed by medical residents. J Ultrasound Med. 2015;34:627–36. https://doi.org/10.7863/ultra.34.4.627.
8. Maw A, Jalali C, Jannat-Khah D, Gudi K, Logio L, Evans A, et al. Faculty development in point of care

ultrasound for internists. Med Educ Online. 2016; 21:33287. https://doi.org/10.3402/meo.v21.33287.

9. Watson K, Lam A, Arishenkoff S, Halman S, Gibson NE, Yu J, et al. Point of care ultrasound training for internal medicine: a Canadian multicentre learner needs assessment study. BMC Med Educ. 2018;18:217. https://doi.org/10.1186/s12909-018-1326-8.

10. Conlin F, Connelly NR, Eaton MP, Broderick PJ, Friderici J, Adler AC. Perioperative use of focused transthoracic cardiac ultrasound: a survey of current practice and opinion. Anesth Analg. 2017;125:1878–82. https://doi.org/10.1213/ane.0000000000002089.

11. Reaume M, Farishta M, Costello JA, Gibb T, Melgar TA. Analysis of lawsuits related to diagnostic errors from point-of-care ultrasound in internal medicine, paediatrics, family medicine and critical care in the USA. Postgrad Med J. 2021;97:55–8. https://doi.org/10.1136/postgradmedj-2020-137832.

12. Cid X, Canty D, Royse A, Maier AB, Johnson D, El-Ansary D, et al. Impact of point-of-care ultrasound on the hospital length of stay for internal medicine inpatients with cardiopulmonary diagnosis at admission: study protocol of a randomized controlled trial—the IMFCU-1 (Internal Medicine Focused Clinical Ultrasound) study. Trials. 2020;21:53. https://doi.org/10.1186/s13063-019-4003-2.

13. Cormack CJ, Wald AM, Coombs PR, Kallos L, Blecher GE. Time to establish pillars in point-of-care ultrasound. Australasian J Ultrasound Med. 2019;22:12–4. https://doi.org/10.1002/ajum.12126.

14. Strony R, Marin JR, Bailitz J, Dean AJ, Blaivas M, Tayal V, et al. Systemwide clinical ultrasound program development: an expert consensus model. West J Emerg Med. 2018;19:649–53. https://doi.org/10.5811/westjem.2018.4.37152.

15. Guidelines U. Emergency, point-of-care and clinical ultrasound guidelines in medicine. Ann Emerg Med. 2017;69:e27–54. https://doi.org/10.1016/j.annemerg med.2016.08.457.

16. Mani N. Implementing a quality framework for storing emergency department point-of-care ultrasound examinations on a picture archiving and communication system. Ultrasound. https://doi.org/10.1177/1742271x21990069.

17. Chen X, Owen CA, Huang EC, Maggard BD, Latif RK, Clifford SP, et al. Artificial intelligence in echocardiography for anesthesiologists. J Cardiothorac Vasc Anesth. 2021;35:251–61. https://doi.org/10.1053/j.jvca.2020.08.048.

18. Narang A, Bae R, Hong H, Thomas Y, Surette S, Cadieu C, et al. Utility of a deep-learning algorithm to guide novices to acquire echocardiograms for limited diagnostic use. JAMA Cardiol. 2021. https://doi.org/10.1001/jamacardio.2021.0185.

19. Cheema BS, Walter J, Narang A, Thomas JD. Artificial intelligence–enabled POCUS in the COVID-19 ICU: a new spin on cardiac ultrasound. JACC: Case Reports. 2021;3:258–263. https://doi.org/10.1016/j.jaccas.2020.12.013.

20. Akkus Z, Aly YH, Attia IZ, Lopez-Jimenez F, Arruda-Olson AM, Pellikka PA, et al. Artificial Intelligence (AI)-Empowered echocardiography interpretation: a state-of-the-art review. J Clin Med. 2021;10. https://doi.org/10.3390/jcm10071391.

21. Clevert D-A, Nyhsen C, Ricci P, Sidhu PS, Tziakouri C, Radziņa M, et al. Position statement and best practice recommendations on the imaging use of ultrasound from the European Society of Radiology ultrasound subcommittee. Insights Imaging. 2020;11:115. https://doi.org/10.1186/s13244-020-00919-x.

22. Aziz S, Bottomley J, Mohandas V, Ahmad A, Morelli G, Thenabadu S. Improving the documentation quality of point-of-care ultrasound scans in the emergency department. BMJ Open Q. 2020;9: e000636. https://doi.org/10.1136/bmjoq-2019-000636.

Future Applications of Handheld POCUS

Craig Fryman and Paul H. Mayo

We believe this 'ultrasound stethoscope' is very useful for the differential diagnosis ... it allows quick screening of ill patients with doubtful physical symptoms and signs since visualization of intra-abdominal organs or processes is readily available. The instrument can therefore be considered as an "extended palpation" ... Immediate and on-the-spot assessment of patients is now possible with this miniaturized, self-contained and battery powered ultrasound device ... It is expected that this miniaturized and automated instrument will have an important impact on the diagnostic use of ultrasound and the further development of ultrasonic equipment.

Professor Jos Roelandt, Dutch Cardiologist & POCUS Pioneer (1938–2014 AD)

Abstract

Handheld POCUS devices are a disruptive technology that will have major impact on the future of POCUS. Similarly, advances in the field of artificial intelligence are likely to have multiple applications for ultrasonography in critical care practice. This chapter will review the utility of handheld devices and artificial intelligence with emphasis on POCUS.

Keywords

Hand-held ultrasonography device · Point of care ultrasonography · Artificial intelligence · Machine learning · Deep learning

Handheld Ultrasonography Devices

Hand-held ultrasonography devices (HUD) are a disruptive technology that will have major impact on the future of point of care ultrasonography (POCUS) in the intensive care unit (ICU). The ultrasonography (US) machine manufacturers, recognizing that there might be a market niche for the HUD, brought out the first reasonable quality HUD in 2012. Since that time, there has been major improvement in HUD capability and reduction in acquisition cost [1].

While the details of machine design vary, the typical HUD is comprised of a probe that is connected to a standard smartphone or tablet.

C. Fryman (✉) · P. H. Mayo
Division of Pulmonary, Critical Care, and Sleep Medicine, LIJ/NSUH Medical Center, New Hyde Park, NY, US
e-mail: cfryman@northwell.edu

Donald and Barbara Zucker School of Medicine at Hofstra/Northwell, Hempstead, NY, US

© The Author(s), under exclusive license to Springer Nature Switzerland AG 2023
H. Soliman-Aboumarie et al. (eds.), *Cardiopulmonary Point of Care Ultrasound*,
https://doi.org/10.1007/978-3-031-29472-3_30

With few exceptions, the screen component is purchased separately from the proprietary probe and may be used as a multifunction device when not connected to the probe. The typical HUD probe is designed to be pocket sized. Most models connect to the screen with a proprietary cord, but some models have wireless connection. Most systems have connectivity to the Internet. This allows for image storage, remote image review, remote training and testing, peer to peer interaction, and telemedicine. Some models allow for real-time transmission of the US image to a larger screen for group review at the bedside in the ICU.

One HUD that is in widespread use has a unique probe design that replaces the standard piezoelectrical crystal with a microprocessor array. This allows use of a single probe for vascular, cardiac, and abdominal scanning thereby obviating the need for multiple probes of different frequencies with consequent reduction in cost of the device. The cost of a capable HUD has fallen in recent years within the range of $2000 to 10,000 USD depending on probe selection and Internet connectivity subscription. Highly capable lower cost models are within the budget range of the individual POCUS clinician. Due to the low cost of the HUD, we envision that the interested clinician may acquire one as a routine part of their personal clinical equipment.

In our own use of a variety of devices, we have observed some of their limitations. Compared to the typical US probe, the HUD probe is larger, heavier, and has a bigger probe face area. Few HUD platforms currently has pulsed wave Doppler while continuous wave Doppler remains a technical challenge due to the space constraints related to probe size and the requirement for two transducers within the probe.

The ergonomics of machine operation may be problematic. As a practical issue, the operator is tasked with probe manipulation while holding the screen with the other hand. This makes it difficult to alter machine settings unless the screen is placed on a stable surface. This is challenging with the critically ill patient. There are a variety of aftermarket solutions that allow connection of the screen component of the HUD to fixed elements of the patient bed. Some manufacturers are developing probes that have the machine controls (e.g., gain, depth, zoom) embedded in the probe. This may ultimately be combined with a heads-up display worn by the operator. The operator would then use the free hand, now unencumbered by the need to touch the screen, to guide real-time needle insertion.

Image quality of the available HUD varies between machines. While image quality is somewhat inferior to higher quality cart mounted machines, our experience with HUD is that they are often adequate for most applications of POCUS in the ICU. One study compared routine echocardiography with a HUD against a high-end machine in 349 patients demonstrating that no clinically relevant findings were missed when the study was performed by expert echocardiographers [2]. HUD may also be used to reliably quantify pleural or pericardial effusion [3] and for identification of B-lines in patients with heart failure [4]. Evidence is limited regarding acquisition of skills and competency using HUD [5]. Their low cost and functionality are two elements that are a strength of the HUD, but this presents a risk in the hands of intensivists who are not competent in their use. Widespread acquisition of these devices by clinicians who are not well trained to use them will potentially bring harm to patients and discredit to the field.

We predict that the increasing availability of HUD will have a major impact on the future of POCUS. Their portability, clinical utility, ease of use, and excellent Internet connectivity are obvious to the clinician who is competent in POCUS. Their affordability will lead to the democratization of POCUS, as the critical care clinician will no longer need to rely on hospital administrative entities to purchase ICU based machines. We envision that many clinicians will acquire a HUD to extend the use of POCUS in their practice beyond that which is feasible with a cart mounted machine. With foreseeable improvements in machine design and Internet connectivity, the HUD is expected to have far-reaching clinical applications including telemedicine, distance learning, peer to peer consultation, and provision of POCUS capability in remote enviroments such as the battlefield [6] and outer space [7].

Artificial Intelligence and POCUS

Artificial intelligence (AI) is a component of computer science that focuses on the development of programs capable of performing tasks that generally require human cognition [8]. As innovation within the field continues to advance, the integration of AI with clinical medicine is becoming a reality. AI systems have multiple potential applications, including image analysis, pattern recognition, data interpretation, and prognostication [9]. While the development of AI algorithms has shown promise in a variety of subspecialties [10], much of its development has focused on automated image interpretation within the field of radiology [10, 11]. Clinical applications of machine learning (ML), a form of AI, using various imaging modalities including computed tomography (CT), magnetic resonance imaging (MRI), positron emission tomography, and US have been described [8].

Deep learning (DL) programs, a subset of ML, are designed to self-learn and extract unique features from an image [12]. This involves the use of artificial neural networks to process raw input images and is commonly used in medical image analysis [12], notably within the field of US [13]. The application of AI technology for analysis of US images has the potential to improve identification of pathological findings, to extract quantitative data from images that would otherwise be difficult to perform based on visual inspection alone, to enhance workflow, and to reduce variability between examiners [13]. The latter is of interest given the operator-dependent nature of US.

AI algorithms have been developed that focus on ultrasonographic detection of abnormalities within a variety of organ systems [14–17]. These also include the use of US and AI to characterize musculoskeletal disorders [18], identify fetal abnormalities [19], quantify carotid plaque [20], and improve competency-based training protocols [21]. To date, there are 11 US-based AI algorithms approved by the Food and Drug Administration [22]. With the widespread use of POCUS in critical care and emergency medicine, AI algorithms that improve the efficiency and diagnostic capabilities of echocardiography and thoracic US evaluation have been a focus of research which may be useful in critical care medicine.

Artificial Intelligence and Echocardiography

Incorporation of AI programs into bedside echocardiographic evaluation has the potential to improve image acquisition, to classify pathological patterns, and to automate quantification of clinically relevant parameters such as cardiac output, myocardial velocities, and wall motion abnormalities [23]. A study demonstrated an overall accuracy of 97.8% using a DL algorithm trained to identify 15 common echocardiographic views [24]. On single low-resolution images, accuracy was greater than 91.4% compared to an average of 79.4% to 84% accuracy by board-certified echocardiographers [24]. An AI program allowed automatic calculation of the left ventricular outflow tract velocity time integral (VTI) in order to derive stroke volume and cardiac output; measurements using an experimental animal model more closely correlated with cardiac output measured by thermodilution compared to those obtained manually [25]. Automated VTI calculation may confer advantages over manual assessment, including more accurate contour tracing and the ability to simultaneously average multiple VTI measurements. AI algorithms have been used to calculate ejection fraction (EF) from apical 4 and 2 chamber views for 2D biplane calculations. When compared to manually made calculations by expert cardiologists, automated calculation using an AI algorithm was accurate with better reproducibility [26]. Another study demonstrating the utility of automated EF analysis established reproducibility as well as rapid assessment of EF, end-diastolic volume, end-systolic volume, and longitudinal strain. The average time for obtaining automatically-derived EF was eight seconds per patient [27].

Advanced echocardiographic imaging modalities, such as speckle tracking and 3D echocardiography, are not utilized in POCUS due to their lack of feasibility at the beside. The use of AI may facilitate their use, permitting rapid and accurate assessment of volumetric chamber measurements as well as intrinsic mechanical properties of the myocardium [28]. This may be useful in assessment of the right ventricle given its complex shape and motion relative to the left ventricle [28].

Artificial Intelligence and Lung Ultrasonography

The qualitative and often binary nature of LUS is particularly well suited for AI. Correa et al. developed an AI algorithm using LUS to detect pneumonia based on the presence of alveolar consolidation with a sensitivity and specificity exceeding 90% [29]. Another algorithm was able to distinguish between the presence and absence of B-lines although with only moderate ability to score severity of B-line number [30]. We anticipate the development of AI programs that will be able to identify lung sliding, A-lines, B-lines, consolidation, and pleural effusion with potential integration into an algorithm that develops a differential diagnosis of the cause for respiratory failure [31].

As an adjunct to qualitative assessment, the quantification of LUS findings has clinical utility. To date there are no integrated AI systems in clinical practice that accomplish this task. As computational power continues to improve and larger data sets with which to develop and train algorithms become available, quantitative LUS will likely be incorporated into standard POCUS assessment. This is expected to improve accuracy, decrease impact of user variability, and improve workflow by cutting down the time required for each exam when performing quantitative scoring of LUS.

A unique feature of DL-based image interpretation is the capacity to detect patterns that are not readily obvious to the human eye [32, 33]. While there are subtle differences in B-line distribution and pleural line morphology that may help differentiate cardiogenic pulmonary edema from other etiologies, the ability to reliably detect these differences is limited by human analysis alone [33]. The development of algorithms that can recognize subtle changes between US images may overcome this limitation. For example, the existence of US markers that suggest the presence of viral pneumonia caused by severe acute respiratory syndrome Coronavirus 2 (SARS-CoV-2) are currently under investigation [33–35]. Arntfield et al. developed a model that outperformed the ability of physicians trained in POCUS to distinguish B-line patterns in patients with hydrostatic pulmonary edema, pneumonia due to SARS-CoV-2, and non-SARS-CoV-2-related acute respiratory distress syndrome [33].

Telemedicine and the use of remote monitoring are increasingly being utilized [36]. There are a few platforms commercially available that facilitate tele-US and permit healthcare professionals and patients to interact remotely. In one scenario, a US technologist or novice clinician could scan a patient in a remote location while a distant expert views the images in real-time. The expert could guide the user to improve image quality. AI-assisted image acquisiton might prove helpful in the event a human is not available or able to effectively guide the probe. The algorithm could instruct a user to adjust the probe until an optimal image is detected [37]. This type of technology has the potential to improve diagnostic capabilities and standardize image acquisiton amongst clinicians and trainees with varying degrees of expertise. Such standardization is a key component for effective use of AI algorithms.

Limitations of Combining AI and POCUS

ML programs are trained to recognize patterns, so their performance is based upon the training set that is utilized to develop the pattern recognition system. The resulting program can have poor performance outside the scope of the data used to train it. This presents a problem in combining AI with POCUS. Differences in probe design and processing of the US image differs between machines, so any training set must be developed to account for cross machine differences. This problem is compounded by the operator effect. Operator capability is less problematic with CT or MRI compared to POCUS, where the quality of the image is very dependent on the skill of the operator at image acquisition. This is further amplified by the difficult scanning conditions that are often encountered at the bedside in the ICU. It is not appropriate to assume that the operating characteristics of an AI program that has been developed by a team of expert scanners using one type of US machine in a controlled unpressured clinical environment will necessarily have utility in real world ICU scanning. This challenge must be met before AI systems can be applied in field conditions in the emergency settings and ICU. A key aspect in resolving this problem is to focus on training acute care clinicians and intensivists to a high skill level in image acquisition and developing training sets that are representative of the ICU environment to which they will be applied.

Blaivas et al. developed an AI algorithm using open-source software and images publicly available on the Internet [38]. The algorithm was designed to classify images into specific categories that would enable its distribution to specific faculty and ultimately facilitate more comprehensive review and quality assurance of image sets. While the algorithm accurately classified 98% of new images related to its training set, performance diminished considerably when the algorithm was applied to unrelated images obtained from different US equipment [38]. This limited generalizability is often described as overfitting [13]. Overfitting is one of several biases related to AI [39].

There are ethical concerns to address on data ownership, patient anonymity, and transparency with regard to the complex processes that result in AI-derived decision and prediction [39, 40]. These issues take on heightened significance in light of increased accessibility and utilization of US machines throughout the healthcare system, particularly with use of HUD.

Conclusion

The use of the HUD will become widespread in the ICU. Their low cost, ease of use, clinical utility, and Internet connectivity will greatly increase the use of POCUS. We can expect further improvement in their design. A major challenge to the widespread adoption of HUD is the need to assure competence in their use.

It is inevitable that AI will be used to augment the utility of POCUS. The clinician approaches the use of AI by being cognizant of the pitfalls of ML. These include the need to assure the use of an appropriate training set that addresses the variability of machine design, the variable skill of the operator, and the challenging frontline scanning conditions in the acute care and emergency settings.

References

1. Rykkje A, Carlsen JF, Nielsen MB. Hand-held ultrasound devices compared with high-end ultrasound systems: a systematic review. Diagnostics (Basel). 2019;9(2). https://doi.org/10.3390/diagnostics9020061.
2. Prinz C, Voigt JU. Diagnostic accuracy of a hand-held ultrasound scanner in routine patients referred for echocardiography. J Am Soc Echocardiogr. 2011;24(2):111–6. https://doi.org/10.1016/j.echo.2010.10.017.
3. Graven T, Wahba A, Hammer AM, Sagen O, Olsen Ø, Skjetne K, et al. Focused ultrasound of the pleural cavities and the pericardium by nurses after cardiac surgery. Scand Cardiovasc J. 2015;49(1):56–63. https://doi.org/10.3109/14017431.2015.1009383.

4. Platz E, Pivetta E, Merz AA, Peck J, Rivero J, Cheng S. Impact of device selection and clip duration on lung ultrasound assessment in patients with heart failure. Am J Emerg Med. 2015;33(11):1552–6. https://doi.org/10.1016/j.ajem.2015.06.002.

5. Nielsen MB, Cantisani V, Sidhu PS, Badea R, Batko T, Carlsen J, et al. The use of handheld ultrasound devices—an EFSUMB position paper. Ultraschall Med. 2019;40(1): e1. https://doi.org/10.1055/a-0881-5251.

6. Nations JA, Browning RF. Battlefield applications for handheld ultrasound. Ultrasound Q. 2011;27 (3):171–6. https://doi.org/10.1097/RUQ.0b013e31822b7c14.

7. Hamilton DR, Sargsyan AE, Martin DS, Garcia KM, Melton SL, Feiveson A, et al. On-orbit prospective echocardiography on international space station crew. Echocardiography. 2011;28(5):491–501. https://doi.org/10.1111/j.1540-8175.2011.01385.x.

8. Hosny A, Parmar C, Quackenbush J, Schwartz LH, Aerts HJWL. Artificial intelligence in radiology. Nat Rev Cancer. 2018;18(8):500–10. https://doi.org/10.1038/s41568-018-0016-5.

9. Ramesh AN, Kambhampati C, Monson JR, Drew PJ. Artificial intelligence in medicine. Ann R Coll Surg Engl. 2004;86(5):334–8. https://doi.org/10.1308/147870804290.

10. Topol EJ. High-performance medicine: the convergence of human and artificial intelligence. Nat Med. 2019;25(1):44–56. https://doi.org/10.1038/s41591-018-0300-7.

11. Syed AB, Zoga AC. Artificial intelligence in radiology: current technology and future directions. Semin Musculoskelet Radiol. 2018;22(5):540–5. https://doi.org/10.1055/s-0038-1673383.

12. Akkus Z, Cai J, Boonrod A, Zeinoddini A, Weston AD, Philbrick KA, et al. A survey of deep-learning applications in ultrasound: artificial intelligence-powered ultrasound for improving clinical workflow. J Am Coll Radiol. 2019;16(9 Pt B):1318–28. https://doi.org/10.1016/j.jacr.2019.06.004.

13. Park SH. Artificial intelligence for ultrasonography: unique opportunities and challenges. Ultrasonography. 2021;40(1):3–6. https://doi.org/10.14366/usg.20078.

14. Schmauch B, Herent P, Jehanno P, Dehaene O, Saillard C, Aubé C, et al. Diagnosis of focal liver lesions from ultrasound using deep learning. Diagn Interv Imaging. 2019;100(4):227–33. https://doi.org/10.1016/j.diii.2019.02.009.

15. Minoda Y, Ihara E, Komori K, Ogino H, Otsuka Y, Chinen T, et al. Efficacy of endoscopic ultrasound with artificial intelligence for the diagnosis of gastrointestinal stromal tumors. J Gastroenterol. 2020;55(12):1119–26. https://doi.org/10.1007/s00535-020-01725-4.

16. Choi YJ, Baek JH, Park HS, Shim WH, Kim TY, Shong YK, et al. A computer-aided diagnosis system using artificial intelligence for the diagnosis and characterization of thyroid nodules on ultrasound: initial clinical assessment. Thyroid. 2017;27(4):546–52. https://doi.org/10.1089/thy.2016.0372.

17. Mango VL, Sun M, Wynn RT, Ha R. Should we ignore, follow, or biopsy? Impact of artificial intelligence decision support on breast ultrasound lesion assessment. AJR Am J Roentgenol. 2020;214 (6):1445–52. https://doi.org/10.2214/AJR.19.21872.

18. Shin Y, Yang J, Lee YH, Kim S. Artificial intelligence in musculoskeletal ultrasound imaging. Ultrasonography. 2021;40(1):30–44. https://doi.org/10.14366/usg.20080.

19. Drukker L, Noble JA, Papageorghiou AT. Introduction to artificial intelligence in ultrasound imaging in obstetrics and gynecology. Ultrasound Obstet Gynecol. 2020;56(4):498–505. https://doi.org/10.1002/uog.22122.

20. Biswas M, Saba L, Chakrabartty S, Khanna NN, Song H, Suri HS, et al. Two-stage artificial intelligence model for jointly measurement of atherosclerotic wall thickness and plaque burden in carotid ultrasound: a screening tool for cardiovascular/stroke risk assessment. Comput Biol Med. 2020;123: 103847. https://doi.org/10.1016/j.compbiomed.2020.103847.

21. Bowness J, El-Boghdadly K, Burckett-St Laurent D. Artificial intelligence for image interpretation in ultrasound-guided regional anaesthesia. Anaesthesia. 2020.https://doi.org/10.1111/anae.15212.

22. FDA Cleared AI Algorithms. https://models.acrdsi.org. Accessed February 14 2021.

23. Alsharqi M, Woodward WJ, Mumith JA, Markham DC, Upton R, Leeson P. Artificial intelligence and echocardiography. Echo Res Pract. 2018;5(4):R115–25. https://doi.org/10.1530/ERP-18-0056.

24. Madani A, Arnaout R, Mofrad M. Fast and accurate view classification of echocardiograms using deep learning. NPJ Digit Med. 2018;1. https://doi.org/10.1038/s41746-017-0013-1.

25. Bobbia X, Muller L, Claret PG, Vigouroux L, Perez-Martin A, de La Coussaye JE, et al. A new echocardiographic tool for cardiac output evaluation: an experimental study. Shock. 2019;52(4):449–55. https://doi.org/10.1097/SHK.0000000000001273.

26. Asch FM, Abraham T, Jankowski M, Cleve J, Adams M, Romano N, et al. Accuracy and reproducibility of a novel artificial intelligence deep learning-based algorithm for automated calculation of ejection fraction in echocardiography. J Am Coll Cardiol. 2019;73(9_Supplement_1):1447. https://doi.org/10.1016/S0735-1097(19)32053-4.

27. Knackstedt C, Bekkers SC, Schummers G, Schreckenberg M, Muraru D, Badano LP, et al. Fully automated versus standard tracking of left ventricular ejection fraction and longitudinal strain: the FAST-EFs multicenter study. J Am Coll Cardiol. 2015;66 (13):1456–66. https://doi.org/10.1016/j.jacc.2015.07.052.

28. Chen X, Owen CA, Huang EC, Maggard BD, Latif RK, Clifford SP, et al. Artificial intelligence in echocardiography for anesthesiologists. J Cardiothorac Vasc Anesth. 2021;35(1):251–61. https://doi.org/10.1053/j.jvca.2020.08.048.

29. Correa M, Zimic M, Barrientos F, Barrientos R, Román-Gonzalez A, Pajuelo MJ, et al. Automatic classification of pediatric pneumonia based on lung ultrasound pattern recognition. PLoS ONE. 2018;13 (12): e0206410. https://doi.org/10.1371/journal.pone.0206410.

30. Baloescu C, Toporek G, Kim S, McNamara K, Liu R, Shaw MM, et al. Automated lung ultrasound b-line assessment using a deep learning algorithm. IEEE Trans Ultrason Ferroelectr Freq Control. 2020;67(11):2312–20. https://doi.org/10.1109/TUFFC.2020.3002249.

31. Lichtenstein DA, Mezière GA. Relevance of lung ultrasound in the diagnosis of acute respiratory failure: the BLUE protocol. Chest. 2008;134 (1):117–25. https://doi.org/10.1378/chest.07-2800.

32. Poplin R, Varadarajan AV, Blumer K, Liu Y, McConnell MV, Corrado GS, et al. Prediction of cardiovascular risk factors from retinal fundus photographs via deep learning. Nat Biomed Eng. 2018;2(3):158–64. https://doi.org/10.1038/s41551-018-0195-0.

33. Arntfield R, VanBerlo B, Alaifan T, Phelps N, White M, Chaudhary R, et al. Development of a deep learning classifier to accurately distinguish COVID-19 from look-a-like pathology on lung ultrasound. medRxiv. 2020:2020. https://doi.org/10.1101/2020.10.13.20212258.

34. Roy S, Menapace W, Oei S, Luijten B, Fini E, Saltori C, et al. Deep learning for classification and localization of covid-19 markers in point-of-care lung ultrasound. IEEE Trans Med Imaging. 2020;39 (8):2676–87. https://doi.org/10.1109/TMI.2020.2994459.

35. Born J, Brändle G, Cossio M, Disdier M, Goulet J, Roulin Jee, et al. POCOVID-net: automatic detection of COVID-19 from a new lung ultrasound imaging dataset (POCUS). ArXiv. 2020;abs/2004.12084.

36. Pourmand A, Ghassemi M, Sumon K, Amini SB, Hood C, Sikka N. Lack of telemedicine training in academic medicine: are we preparing the next generation? Telemed J E Health. 2021;27(1):62–7. https://doi.org/10 1089/tmj.2019.0287.

37. Muse ED, Topol EJ. Guiding ultrasound image capture with artificial intelligence. Lancet. 2020;396 (10253):749. https://doi.org/10.1016/S0140-6736 (20)31875-4.

38. Blaivas M, Arntfield R, White M. DIY AI, deep learning network development for automated image classification in a point-of-care ultrasound quality assurance program. J Am Coll Emerg Physicians Open. 2020;1(2):124–31. https://doi.org/10.1002/emp2.12018.

39. Brady AP, Neri E. Artificial intelligence in radiology-ethical considerations. Diagnostics (Basel). 2020;10 (4). https://doi.org/10.3390/diagnostics10040231.

40. Wang F, Kaushal R, Khullar D. Should health care demand interpretable artificial intelligence or accept "Black Box" medicine? Ann Intern Med. 2020;172 (1):59–60. https://doi.org/10.7326/M19-2548.

Index

A

Accreditation, 274, 276, 353–359
Acute heart failure, 79, 80, 114, 147, 273–275
Acute kidney injury, 197
Acute respiratory distress syndrome (ARDS), 70, 113, 120, 137, 147, 148, 153, 155, 159, 160, 163–166, 170–173, 178, 182, 211, 235, 244, 306, 309–312, 368
Aliasing, 16, 24–26, 45–47, 255, 263, 269
Aortic valve, 16, 26, 33–38, 48, 49, 54–58, 86, 104, 105, 210, 222, 224, 252–258, 270, 278, 292, 293
Artefacts, 7, 9–11, 15, 16, 19–21, 23, 24, 26, 27, 68, 107, 153, 253, 254, 264, 274, 304, 310, 311
Artifacts, 2, 19–24, 26, 27, 59, 63–65, 67, 69–71, 87, 123, 125, 138, 161, 162, 164, 171, 197, 309
Artificial intelligence, 174, 359, 362, 365, 367, 368
Attenuation, 7, 10, 11, 14, 15, 20, 21, 107, 125

B

B-lines, 79, 82, 87–90, 106, 123, 125, 130, 135, 138–140, 142, 144, 153–155, 159–163, 165, 170–173, 302, 304, 309–311, 366, 368

C

Cardiac arrest, 4, 38, 112, 115, 139, 140, 275, 286, 289, 290, 297, 306, 315–323, 325, 326, 332, 335
Cardiac output, 87, 105, 177–180, 184, 186, 187, 191, 209, 215–219, 226, 244, 269, 273, 276, 278, 280, 281, 284, 285, 290, 367
Cardiac surgery, 55, 75, 76, 94, 104, 226, 273, 275, 276, 278, 281–284, 328, 330, 332, 338
Cardiac ultrasound, 29, 79, 80, 99, 202, 276, 356
Cardiogenic shock, 106, 148, 215, 216, 218, 235, 274, 275, 284, 289–291
Chest ultrasound, 359
Clinical ultrasound, 174
Community acquired pneumonia, 118, 129
Compression ultrasound, 114
Computer Aided Diagnosis (CAD), 118
Consolidation, 63, 65, 70, 71, 112, 117–123, 125, 126, 128–130, 138, 139, 159, 161–163, 165, 170–173, 304, 306, 307, 310–313, 357, 368
Cor pulmonale, 84, 85, 113, 298

COVID-19, 76, 77, 89, 117–120, 122, 169–175, 353, 356, 358

D

Decongestion, 147, 154, 205
Deep learning, 174, 367
Diaphragm and lung, 75
Diastolic function, 81, 86, 98, 201–212, 240, 243, 277, 279, 280, 283, 285
Doppler, 7, 11, 15–17, 20, 24, 26, 30, 38, 43–49, 56, 58, 59, 81, 86, 87, 97, 98, 114, 122, 125, 153, 180, 181, 191–197, 203–205, 207, 209, 215–217, 220, 222, 223, 235, 240–243, 245–247, 252, 255–270, 277, 279, 280, 283, 284, 293, 333, 335, 337, 349, 353, 366
Doppler imaging, 7, 16, 17, 24, 26, 47, 49, 80, 86, 201, 203–205, 207, 209, 216, 223, 240, 282, 356

E

Echocardiography, 3, 9, 13, 21, 23, 29, 30, 51, 53, 59, 60, 63, 80–82, 85, 86, 90, 93–96, 98, 101, 103, 107, 148, 177, 178, 180, 183–188, 194, 202, 207, 215–219, 222, 223, 231, 232, 235, 236, 240, 242–245, 247, 251, 252, 256, 259, 260, 262, 265–270, 273–278, 280, 284–286, 289–291, 294–298, 316, 327–330, 332, 334, 335, 353–358, 366–368
End-expiratory occlusion, 178, 179, 184–186
Extracorporeal membrane oxygenation (ECMO), 274, 280, 281, 290–295, 311, 338

F

Filling pressures, 81, 86, 87, 89, 98, 201–212, 256, 278, 292, 332, 333
Fluid balance, 192
Fluid challenge, 177, 184, 186, 188, 285
Fluids, 1, 21, 64, 65, 70, 84, 112, 122, 123, 144, 148, 153, 154, 159–161, 170, 173, 177–186, 188, 192, 197, 201, 202, 211, 219, 274, 276, 280, 285, 286, 302–305, 310, 317, 327–330, 332, 335, 338, 342–345, 347, 348, 358

Focused cardiac ultrasound (FoCUS), 30, 79–82, 85–87, 90, 113, 115, 116, 202, 232, 234, 276, 289–292, 294, 295, 343

G
Governance, 354, 362, 363

H
Hand-held ultrasonography device, 365, 366, 369
Heart failure, 79, 80, 87, 98, 106, 112, 125, 147, 148, 153–155, 170, 201, 202, 211, 223, 235, 276, 278, 290, 342, 344, 358, 366

I
Inferior vena cava, 40–42, 72, 77, 80, 82, 85–87, 89, 114, 147, 154, 164, 177, 178, 183, 194–196, 203, 209, 267, 275, 277, 285, 319, 329
Ischaemia, 93–96, 98, 99, 101, 104–108, 224, 226, 278, 280, 318
Ischaemic cascade, 95, 96, 99

L
Lung aeration, 123, 125, 129, 160–162, 164, 173, 309–313
Lung aeration score, 310–313
Lung contusion, 304–307
Lung point, 70, 135, 139–144, 302, 306, 319
Lung ultrasound, 10, 21, 63, 64, 79–81, 87, 106, 112, 117–119, 121, 125, 135–144, 147, 153, 162, 166, 169, 170, 173, 211, 212, 274, 309, 310, 353, 356–359
Lung ultrasound score, 160, 164, 311

M
Machine learning, 367
Mechanical circulatory support, 273, 274, 280, 289, 290, 338
Mitral valve, 33–37, 40, 43, 44, 49, 56–58, 81, 85–87, 97, 99, 203–205, 209, 210, 212, 240, 255, 256, 259–261, 263–266, 274, 275, 277, 284, 293
Multiorgan ultrasound, 111
Myocardial contractility, 215, 216, 218, 219, 226, 278
Myocardial infarction, 85, 87, 94, 105, 106, 216, 259, 261, 262, 293, 318, 328, 332

N
Non cardiogenic pulmonary oedema, 163

P
Passive leg raising, 177–179, 184, 186–188, 285
Pleural effusion, 34, 63–65, 69–71, 79, 82, 84, 89, 90, 112, 114, 122, 126–129, 144, 153, 154, 161, 163–165, 171, 173, 302, 305, 334, 335, 338, 341–347, 349, 350, 356, 357, 368
Pleural sliding, 65, 69, 135, 302
Pneumothorax, 63–65, 68–70, 88, 112, 114, 135–144, 275, 299, 300, 302, 306, 307, 316, 319, 334, 345, 349, 350, 356–358
Point of care ultrasonography, 341, 365
Point of care ultrasound (POCUS), 1–5, 7, 17, 27, 30, 50, 51, 60, 70, 71, 76, 79–82, 85, 86, 88, 93–96, 104–106, 108, 111–115, 117, 118, 120, 122, 128–130, 141, 142, 147, 148, 153–155, 159, 160, 163, 165, 166, 170, 178, 179, 181, 188, 191, 201–203, 206, 207, 210, 212, 215, 216, 223, 224, 226, 227, 231, 232, 235–237, 241, 243, 247, 251, 263, 270, 275–278, 281, 284–286, 299, 302, 304–307, 310, 315–317, 319–328, 331, 341, 346, 349, 350, 354, 355–359, 361–363, 365–369
Pulmonary artery pressures, 89, 231, 232, 243–246, 284, 339
Pulmonary embolism, 111, 113, 153, 160, 244, 246, 275, 280, 284, 316, 317, 342, 345, 358
Pulmonary hypertension, 104, 113, 153, 155, 231, 232, 235, 236, 241, 243, 244, 246, 247, 266, 269, 270, 275, 283, 284, 334, 335, 338, 339
Pulmonary oedema, 64, 70, 88, 89, 106, 121, 147, 148, 153, 155, 159, 160, 162–164, 175, 179, 186, 211, 278, 291, 304, 310, 313, 349

R
Regional Systolic Function, 215, 224
Regional wall motion abnormalities, 41, 50, 81, 83, 94, 95, 99, 153, 205, 215, 224, 275, 278, 318
Resolution, 7–9, 11–15, 46, 58, 65, 67, 99, 101, 122, 141, 154, 202, 219, 261, 313, 367
Resuscitation, 38, 80, 179, 191, 197, 286, 290, 297, 315, 316, 319–326, 357, 358
Reverberation, 7, 10, 20, 21, 64, 65, 68, 87, 136, 253, 254, 304
Right ventricle, 21, 36, 37, 39, 40, 42, 53, 56, 58, 79, 104, 106, 112, 182, 192, 193, 226, 231–239, 242, 278, 290, 305, 317, 319, 332, 334, 335, 368

S
Safety, 30, 51, 52, 59, 170, 274, 306, 307, 347, 349, 361–363
SARS CoV2, 169, 170
17-segment model, 83, 99, 106, 224, 225, 278

Shock, 4, 84, 112–115, 177, 179, 186, 211, 216, 217, 219, 220, 227, 275, 284, 285, 324, 327, 328, 332, 338, 358
Small-bore chest drains, 341, 346, 349
Spectral Doppler, 15, 16, 47, 58, 284

T
Tamponade, 82, 84, 113, 114, 153, 273, 275–277, 289, 305, 316, 317, 327, 328, 332–336, 338–340
TEE, 274
Thoracocentesis, 341, 344, 346, 349
Training, 3–5, 30, 59, 60, 81, 96, 97, 153, 166, 274, 276, 278, 289, 291, 297, 315, 316, 320–322, 353–359, 361, 362, 366, 367, 369
Transesophageal echocardiography (TOE), 20, 23, 26, 51–53, 55, 56, 59, 60, 164, 217, 239–241, 255, 261–263, 273, 274, 276, 278, 281, 282, 284, 285, 289–297, 330, 331, 353–357
Transthoracic ultrasonography, 341
Trauma, 3, 4, 136, 137, 140, 142–144, 266, 299, 300, 302, 304–307, 316, 328, 330, 332, 344, 358
Tricuspid annular plane systolic excursion, 113, 232, 235, 239, 240
Tricuspid valve and pulmonary valve, 36, 42, 242

U
Ultrasound, 1–5, 7–12, 14–17, 19–24, 26, 27, 30, 35, 52, 53, 56–58, 63–65, 71, 72, 75–77, 89, 90, 95, 101, 108, 119, 129, 135–139, 141, 142, 144, 148, 153, 154, 159, 160, 162, 171, 174, 181, 184, 191, 192, 231, 232, 241, 247, 257, 300, 302, 304, 305, 307, 315, 316, 321–323, 335, 342, 345–350, 353–359, 361–363, 365
Ultrasound technology, 2

V
Valvular heart disease, 81, 85, 216, 271, 284
Venous congestion, 191–197, 211, 235, 278, 331, 333, 334
Venous excess ultrasonography (VExUS), 5, 191–193, 195–197, 235
Ventilator-associated pneumonia, 118, 120, 128, 310, 312, 313
Volume expansion, 178–180, 184, 188

W
Wavelength, 8, 10–12, 15